Tips and Tricks in Orthopedic Surgery

Tips and Tricks in Orthopedic Surgery

Ajit N Damle MS(Ortho) MS(GS) D Ortho
Consultant
Ratna Hospital and Joshi Hospital
(Maharashtra Medical Foundation)
Pune, Maharashtra, India

Foreword
Anand S Kelkar

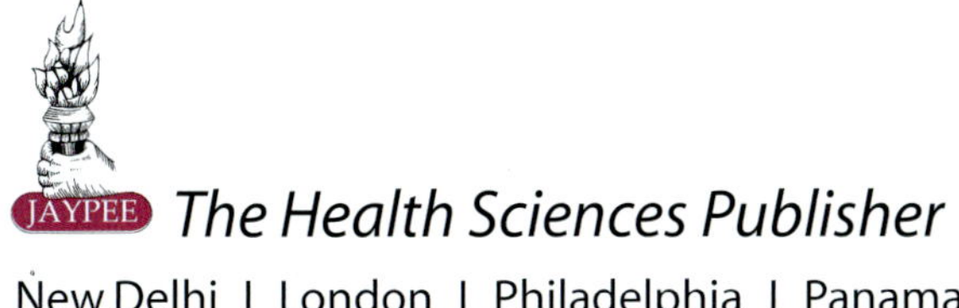

The Health Sciences Publisher
New Delhi I London I Philadelphia I Panama

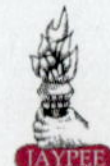

Jaypee Brothers Medical Publishers (P) Ltd.

Headquarters
Jaypee Brothers Medical Publishers (P) Ltd.
4838/24, Ansari Road, Daryaganj
New Delhi 110 002, India
Phone: +91-11-43574357
Fax: +91-11-43574314
E-mail: jaypee@jaypeebrothers.com

Overseas Offices

J.P. Medical Ltd.
83, Victoria Street, London
SW1H 0HW (UK)
Phone: +44-20 3170 8910
Fax: +44(0)20 3008 6180
E-mail: info@jpmedpub.com

Jaypee-Highlights Medical Publishers Inc.
City of Knowledge, Bld. 237, Clayton
Panama City, Panama
Phone: +1 507-301-0496
Fax: +1 507-301-0499
E-mail: cservice@jphmedical.com

Jaypee Medical Inc.
The Bourse
111, South Independence Mall East
Suite 835, Philadelphia, PA 19106, USA
Phone: +1 267-519-9789
E-mail: jpmed.us@gmail.com

Jaypee Brothers Medical Publishers (P) Ltd.
17/1-B, Babar Road, Block-B, Shaymali
Mohammadpur, Dhaka-1207
Bangladesh
Mobile: +08801912003485
E-mail: jaypeedhaka@gmail.com

Jaypee Brothers Medical Publishers (P) Ltd.
Bhotahity, Kathmandu, Nepal
Phone: +977-9741283608
E-mail: kathmandu@jaypeebrothers.com

Website: www.jaypeebrothers.com
Website: www.jaypeedigital.com

Tips and Tricks in Orthopedic Surgery

First Edition: **2015**

ISBN: 978-93-5152-484-7

Printed at : Samrat Offset Pvt. Ltd.

Dedicated to

My wife, Dr Nalini
—An anesthesiologist and a perfect homemaker

Foreword

I have been associated with Dr Ajit N Damle for over the past fifty years, as a colleague and friend.

One starts the clinical practice after having a formal training and education. In early days of practice, one relies on textbooks to guide us in managing both common and unusual situations. Quite a few cases are rarely a textbook features and what one needs is hidden in between the lines of a textbook. This book will help us read in between the lines.

Dr Damle has been meticulous person since his training days. He has built up a large collection of clinical material, which includes clinical and operative notes, clinical and radiography photographs. This book is a compilation of this enormous resource in a systematic and useful format.

The author has taken immense task to have clarity in presentation and the well-taken photographs are self-explanatory. This book exemplifies the spirit of a senior surgeon, passing the baton to the colleagues of the next generation.

Clinical work and practice is a continuous learning process: we have problems, may make some errors, and develop technique to address them and overcome such a situation. These techniques, which are very useful, are often unreported, thus denying benefit to many others facing a similar situation. Making the same error again and correcting it is like reinventing the wheel!

This book will help many surgeons in learning from his experience of over the four decades and also help a patient receive a better care. Acquisition of this book is highly recommended to improve surgical techniques.

Anand S Kelkar
MS(Ortho) MS(GS) D Ortho
Consultant
KEM Hospital
Pune, Maharashtra, India

Preface

From my training days, I have been taking down notes of whatever I learn—both in clinical non-operative and operative methods of patient management. Hobby of photography has helped me to document many things as well. Having seen the collection, my teachers, seniors and colleagues, especially, Dr Anand S Kelkar, insisted that I must write my experiences, which would benefit many clinicians and surgeons in making.

I have discussed my thought process in some cases, when the patient consulted me. Hence, at places, I have presented them as my thought process. A procedure , therefore, is so described, that the reader can visualize it well. Precise management needs a tender patient care, well-planned procedure, including availability of various implants and instrumentation. This is possible only with intense desire, dedication and discipline.

The practical features of management will enhance the understanding of the principles and rational therapy. Many textbooks mention a few methods of managing a given type of injury and then mention what the author prefers. I have mentioned, the one, which I find useful in my hands.

The methods described are not necessarily my creations, but gathered from my teachers, be revered masters; or from young colleagues. Going through this book, prior to a procedure, would help the surgeon. It would also serve as a source of revision and mental stimulation. Experienced surgeons too would enjoy reading this, would spot some omissions, and suggest some corrections or additions.

Emergency room care is written in a manner that is easy-to-recall, in a pictorial manner, while studying away from bedside. A few readers may learn something new: many, I hope, will be assisted in their revision of knowledge already acquired; and, perhaps, some will be stimulated to look deeper into the methods mentioned.

I thank Dr Rahul A Damle, for sharing his suggestions, especially, mechanical aspects in operative methods. Many tricks I have learnt from him, who has been very meticulous in arranging the patient positioning personally before he proceeds for any case. I have always enjoyed working with and learning from him, and it has been a wonderful period in my life.

It is a great pleasure to present this work to the interested ones, who desire to treat the injured ones in a safe manner and in the pursuit of excellence.

Ajit N Damle

Acknowledgments

I would like to thank all the members of my team—emergency care givers, colleagues, medical and nursing staff, technicians from radiology department, operation room, laboratory and splint makers. Colleagues from internal medicine have been always of great help in patient care. All of them have been of great help in both non-operative and operative methods of treatment.

I appreciate the patience and understanding of patients, who accepted, with a broad mind, things which came their way. This is more so for those, who had to undergo a secondary procedure.

I am indebted to my colleague, Dr Anand S Kelkar, with whom I worked since my residency days. Dr Kelkar has been after me to write this and willingly went through the manuscript.

My son, Dr Rahul A Damle, has been contributing to my understanding of mechanical principles every day, because of whom, I am still progressing. My daughter Mrs Swati, a computer engineer, extended all the technical support to prepare this book.

My wife, Dr Nalini, an anesthesiologist, has very graciously tolerated my being in front of the computer to prepare the work and photography for long hours. Our family still continues to be well-knit.

Contents

Section I Upper Extremity

Section II Lower Extremity and Pelvis

Introduction

Aim of fracture management is to treat every injury, in the best manner as one can. Good clinical examination, assessment, efficient and necessary splint application on arrival and arranging necessary X-ray examination form the basis of treatment and its planning. Every orthopedic trainee must know a few things regarding X-ray positioning and avoid pitfalls in the technique.

One should attempt to reduce the patient discomfort and keep any chance of complication to a minimum. Such a care would help to restore the function, close to the pre-injury status.

Having organized and planned steps in any procedure, one should continue to carry out a procedure in the same order. This improves the speed and efficiency of the entire team. Thus, in an operation room, placement of gadgets should be exactly at the same place with respect to the patient position.

In a case, after induction of anesthesia, once I observed that the 'C' arm did not start! Lesson learnt is, prior to induction of anesthesia, one should check that all gadgets are in order and working. It must be confirmed that they are functioning properly, prior to induction of anesthesia and it is a safe and necessary step. This is very much needed in a small and mid-size organizations, where the infrastructure is just adequate and spare equipment may not be available. Pneumatic tourniquet, electro-cautery and 'C' arm unit are important gadgets and if, unfortunately, one of them does not function well, one knows what one is likely to face during a procedure!

The operation instruments and implants, including power tools, video equipment, etc. be sterile and ready. Every OT should have all the instruments packed and arranged, as per the system and be sterile all the time. This is because, one may need few additional instruments during a surgical procedure, unexpectedly.

In spite of advances in technology, instrumentation, implants and availability of gadgets such as 'C' arm unit along with basic surgical skills, pre-operative planning and thinking of likely alternative steps, continue to have their place.

It is necessary to know what the purpose of an implant is, such as an interlocking nail or an LCP. One should know, how much stability a plate will confer and in what mode it is used, i.e. tension band or a neutralization mode. If this is not understood and one expects too much from an implant, it is likely to fail.

In the last few years, it is seen that immediate internal fixation being done in a fracture case, soon after arrival. Quite a few unfortunate results are noted in such cases. I feel this could have been avoided, if immediate closed reduction and appropriate external immobilization or skeletal traction was administered as a stage I of the procedure. This improves venous drainage and keeps the tissue reaction leading to hematoma and edema formation to a minimum. If an injury is left without a formal reduction and immobilization, blister formation around the ankle is a common phenomenon. If the planned procedure is delayed judiciously, and is done at the right time, the outcome would be far superior and a secondary procedure could be avoided. This is especially observed in fractures in subtrochanteric area, lower end of femur, upper end of tibia and ankle fractures. Unfortunate result is often seen in such an injury that was the only injury in the person. In such a case, immediate fracture stabilization, to make the patient stable, is not always essential. The time interval between the initial reduction and definitive fixation offers the body, time to recover from the initial injury and the surgeon has some time to plan and think every option and keep necessary equipment ready.

Radiographic examination should be done with correct patient positioning, to give the necessary information. Certain intra- and juxta-articular injuries need further CT scan with a 3D reconstruction, to have a correct definition of the injury and avoid surprises on the table.

In nearly all bone and joint injuries, I would prefer to carry out first a closed reduction and immobilize in a plaster support. Certain hip and knee injuries are better immobilized with a Thomas' splint. One should take a pride to have a good splint room, next to the emergency room. If a CT scan is felt necessary, then instead of a Thomas' splint for the knee, one can apply a padded plaster slab support. The patient comfort increases while a CT scan is done.

This observation period stabilizes both the young and the elderly patients, for different reasons. In the young, the tissue reaction is quite some, for which, one needs to wait. The teaching is to keep femur and pelvic fractures in skeletal traction. In quite a few cases, it does help a lot. Pre-operative planning and arranging the necessary equipment usually needs some time. In the elderly, often the blood sugar needs to be controlled, fresh 2D echo study needs to be done and anti-platelet drugs need to be stopped. Many of them are not well-hydrated and anemic too. Waiting judiciously for a few hours or days is thus well-utilized and well-rewarded.

If one decides to operate a case of multiple fractures admitted, outside working hours, many considerations are required: More number of trained OT staff, more number of sterile instrumentation sets for different limbs, assured sterilization and a few other supporting things are needed. I wonder, how many operation theater units have a dedicated area, separate sets of instruments and team, in general, for emergency procedures, different from that for a planned surgery. If such a separate facility is available, it also protects the principal operation area complex. Besides this, the principal surgeon should not be 'a tired surgeon' at the end of a given day and has to stabilize a few challenging fractures, one after the other.

One needs to remember a few aphorisms:

- There are no errors. These are only experiences to learn from.
- Pathway to success is paved with failures and experience means remembering one's failures and manage the future cases accordingly.
- Success is not a key to happiness. Happiness is the key to success. If one loves what one is doing, one would be successful.
- Do not read success stories. All you will get is a message. Read failure stories and surely you will get ideas to make a success story!
- To me fascinating statistics are not important. Any given procedure when being done, should be well-indicated, have its utility and be a safe one. One should do what is safe in one's hand.
- Perhaps one cannot make all the mistakes in one's life and hence, it is better to learn from each other's as well. Intelligent ones learn from their own mistakes, while the genius ones learn from others' mistakes as well.

Rapid growth of knowledge and newer implants are available. However, the place of earlier implants still continues, e.g. in a Barton injury of the wrist, each case does not need a locking plate and some cases can still be well managed by a buttress plate, which we have been using for the last many years. Often a decision is difficult and the treating clinician may be torn between the ideal method available today and financial constraint of the patient.

When a case comes to me for a second or a third opinion, I carefully take the history, do a clinical examination and try to know the purpose of his visit to me. I look at the day 1 X-ray films and think, as to what I would do in such a situation. Then I see the films, to know, what was done in the given case. This improves my learning and thinking process, so I can make an honest plan of action. For such a situation quoted in this book, I have given analysis of my thoughts, which would be useful to the reader.

I would always prefer a neat and precisely carried out procedure with good judgment and safety in a reasonable operative time, rather than a fast surgery. The speed always comes when specified steps and protocol are followed for each procedure.

A balanced approach to manage a case is important. This led me to the idea of publishing a compact book in orthopedic surgery. It is hoped that the reader will welcome this concise format, practical tips and steps in patient management.

The aim has been to promote a careful and safe technique, with regards to soft tissue respect.

Thus, this book *Tips and Tricks in Orthopedic Surgery* is a collection of ideas put together. I am sure, the reader will find them useful and interesting. Some ideas, I have learnt from my students and colleagues and I have acknowledged them. Whatever I am today, is because of my teachers—may be directly or indirectly. Teachers have been torch-bearer for me and I am indebted to them forever.

The entire photography is done by myself. While digitizing a photo from an analogue slide, I am aware, some loss of quality is inevitable.

When a case comes to me for a second or a third opinion, I carefully take the history, do a clinical examination and try to know the purpose of his visit to me. I look at the day 1 X-ray films and think as to what I would do in such a situation. Then I see the films to know what was done in the given case. This improves my learning and thinking process, so I can make an honest plan of action. For such a situation quoted in this book I have given analysis of my thoughts, which would be useful to the reader.

I would always prefer a neat and precisely carried out procedure with good judgment and safety in a reasonable operative time, rather than a fast surgery. The speed always comes when planned steps and protocol are followed for each procedure.

A balanced approach to manage a case is important. This led me to the idea of publishing a compact book in orthopedic surgery. It is hoped that the reader will welcome the concise format, practical tips and steps in patient management.

The aim has been to promote a careful and safe technique with regards to soft tissue respect.

Thus, this book *Tips and Tricks in Orthopedic Surgery* is a collection of ideas put together. I am sure the reader will find them useful and interesting. Some ideas, I have learnt from my patients and colleagues, and I have acknowledged them. Whatever I am today, is because of my teachers, may be directly or indirectly. I am blessed to have had the best teachers for me and I am indebted to them for ever.

The entire photographs are taken by myself. While digitizing a photo from an analogue slide, some loss of quality is inevitable.

Section I

Upper Extremity

CHAPTER

1

Clavicle Fracture

OBSERVATIONS

The time-honored treatment for a fracture of clavicle has been non-operative. With the advent of procedures such as, external fixation, intramedullary closed wire fixation under `C` arm control, precontoured locking plate, etc. fracture stabilization is possible by operative method. Currently, with high energy road traffic accidents, more than one fracture in a limb are observed. Thus if in addition to a clavicle fracture, if there is presence of another fracture in upper limb, clavicle stabilization has become necessary. Due to increase in patient's expectations, spreading knowledge and availability of alternative procedures, one needs to be aware of scope of each technique, its advantages, disadvantages and limitations.

INTRODUCTION

A closed fracture clavicle with 2 fragments or with a displaced 3rd fragment usually unites with nonoperative method, using a figure of 8 bandage technique. Today, a readymade clavicle brace is available. My preference is for a figure of 8 bandage to a brace. This method is satisfactory, when a fracture of clavicle is the only injury in a patient.

Figure of 8 Bandage: Technique and Principle

- The crepe bandage width should be 8 or 10 cm. First a cotton roll or a gamjee roll is applied in a figure of 8 method and then the crepe bandage is added on it (Details of application technique are not described here). The figure of 8 bandage needs to be changed every 5 to 7 days. After 2 weeks, when the fracture becomes sticky, the patient can remove it at home, have a bath and come for reapplication. Due to the wide cushion under the bandage in the axilla, the elbow remains away from the chest wall and hence it is uncomfortable to use a conventional sling and the person can walk with, the injured side wrist supported by other hand. This leads to a mechanism like a rope over a pulley, keeping the fracture reduced, reducing any overlap of the fracture ends.
- Duration of the figure of 8 bandage is 4 weeks initially. Thereafter it is continued, as per the pain and the discomfort without bandage/morphology of the fracture/X-ray appearance, etc. It is preferable to have it on for 5 weeks at least, when the fracture is consolidating. Usually a patient prefers to have the bandage on, as it offers more comfort and sense of security.

- Resuming normal activities: Light work as in an office may be started at the end of three weeks. However, one should avoid load on the injured limb, such as taking a hand support while rising/riding a bicycle, etc. till the abnormal mobility disappears, the clavicle has become pain free and the fracture has clinically united.

Available Clavicle Fracture Brace

- The strap is narrow and hence uniform support all along the entire width of the lateral fragment is not achieved.
- The belt is narrow in the axilla and rope over pulley effect of a figure of 8 bandage is not observed.

TREATMENT METHODS AVAILABLE

- *Non-operative* method is usually successful in obtaining bony union, in majority of cases, with a low energy injury. This is especially true in young adults below the age of 35 years, when healing potential is good. However, when
  - The initial displacement is wide, the soft tissue attachment to the fracture ends is stripped off.
  - Presence of many fragments
  - Presence of a segmental fracture.

Then clavicle fracture fixation be considered on day 1. One prefers a Titanium Elastic Nail, which can be passed usually by a closed method under 'C' arm control. I prefer to have a complementary figure of 8 bandage on, for at least 4 weeks. This supports the shoulder girdle and reduces the girdle load on the implant at the fracture site.

While the non-operative treatment is on:

If at an expected duration of 4 to 5 weeks, a clinical union is not achieved with abnormal mobility, one should assess, if there is local pain. If the pain is progressively reducing, one may continue the bandage for further 3 weeks, as in a slow union. Surgery is necessary in the presence of a painful fibrous union or non-union. However, the treatment of an ununited fracture of clavicle is rather demanding, due to its subcutaneous position, presence of neurovascular structures nearby and the bone contour itself.

- If the fracture morphology demands internal fixation on day 1, my preference is for closed IM wire fixation, with all the advantages of a closed procedure.
- At times in 3 or 4 part fractures, at the end of six weeks, fracture has not consolidated, one may recommend internal fixation and bone grafting. Due to soft callus formation and closure of the medullary cavity, at this stage of fracture healing, a closed IM wire fixation is not possible and a surface fixation is needed.

Radiological Union

With non-operative method, usually at the end of five weeks, the fracture pain, local tenderness and abnormal mobility reduce. It is an observation, that most persons prefer to have the figure of eight bandage on, for further a week or two, as they find it more secure. However, on an X-ray film, the fracture line continues to be visible. It is usually at the end of four months, that either external callus bridge is visible or the fracture line disappears (Fig. 1.1).

Delayed Union

At the end of six weeks of non-operative method, if surgery is advised, at times, a patient opts for alternative method of therapy. Information tells, they have taken some oral medication from alternative therapy and at the end of a year, one observes radiological union. Hence I respect his/her choice. Of course, some cases do continue to have a fibrous or a non-union (Figs 1.2 to 1.4).

In an undisplaced fracture being treated nonoperatively, the position is noted to be well-maintained for the initial 2 to 3 weeks. Later on, at times, one observes fragment displacement and/or angulation at the end of 6 to 7 weeks. I have no explanation why this happens. Therefore, if all fractures should be recommended a closed IM wire method, remains to be answered (Fig. 1.5).

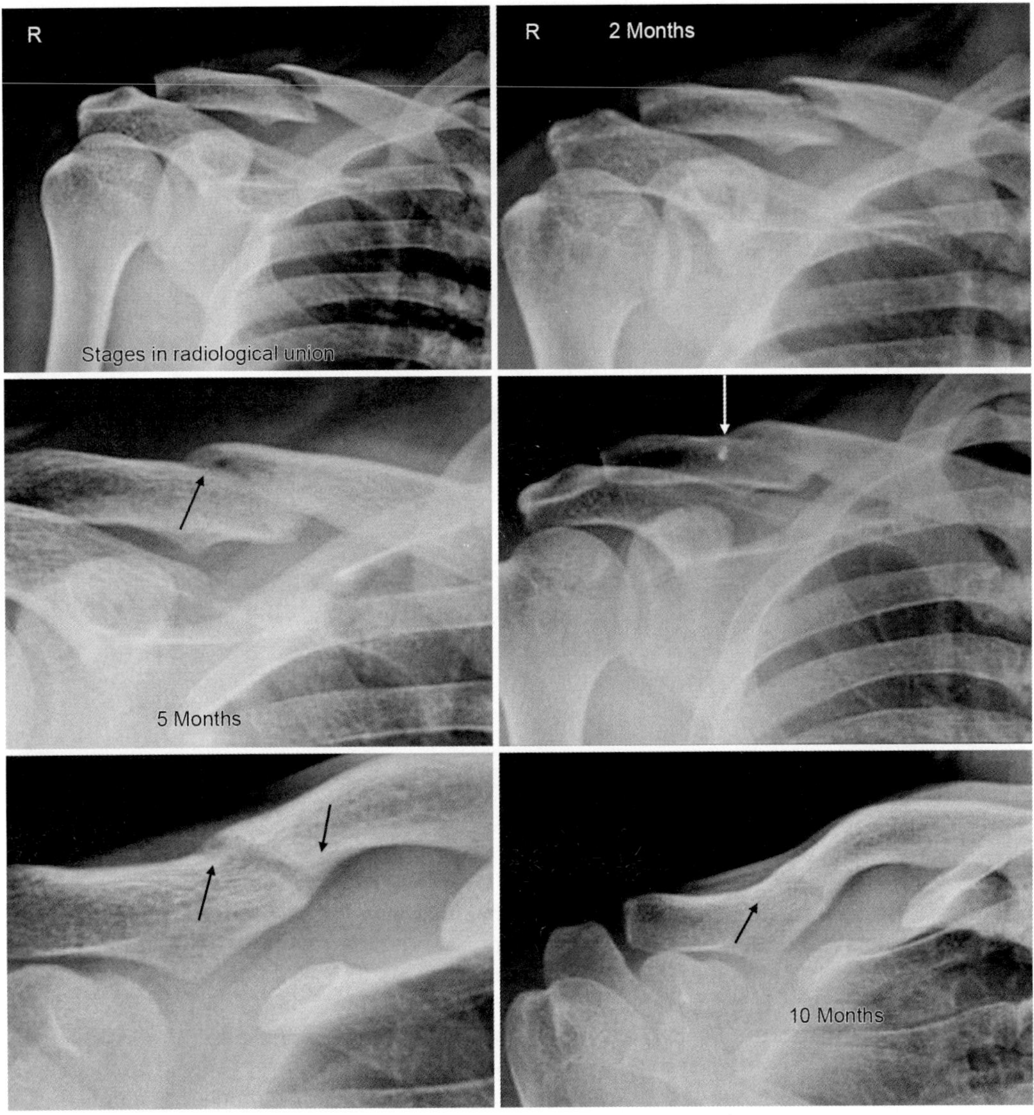

Figure 1.1 Radiological union stages

Few surgeons prefer external fixation for almost all fractures of the clavicle as a method of choice. I have no experience in different morphological types of fractures of clavicle and the outcome. I believe, this method be reserved for an open fracture with a bone loss, as a primary method (Theoretically, an external fixator is not so rigid to ensue a primary bone union, nor elastic enough to promote a secondary union).

- *ORIF with a plate*: A precontoured locking compression plate (LCP) is coming in vogue and time will tell us its utility. The muscle attachments and hence the blood supply to the clavicle is as it is less, which may further be jeopardized. However, the stability obtained by the well-contoured plate will overcome the above drawback. It is certainly useful in a case with multiple fractures in one limb. Its stabilization reduces local pain

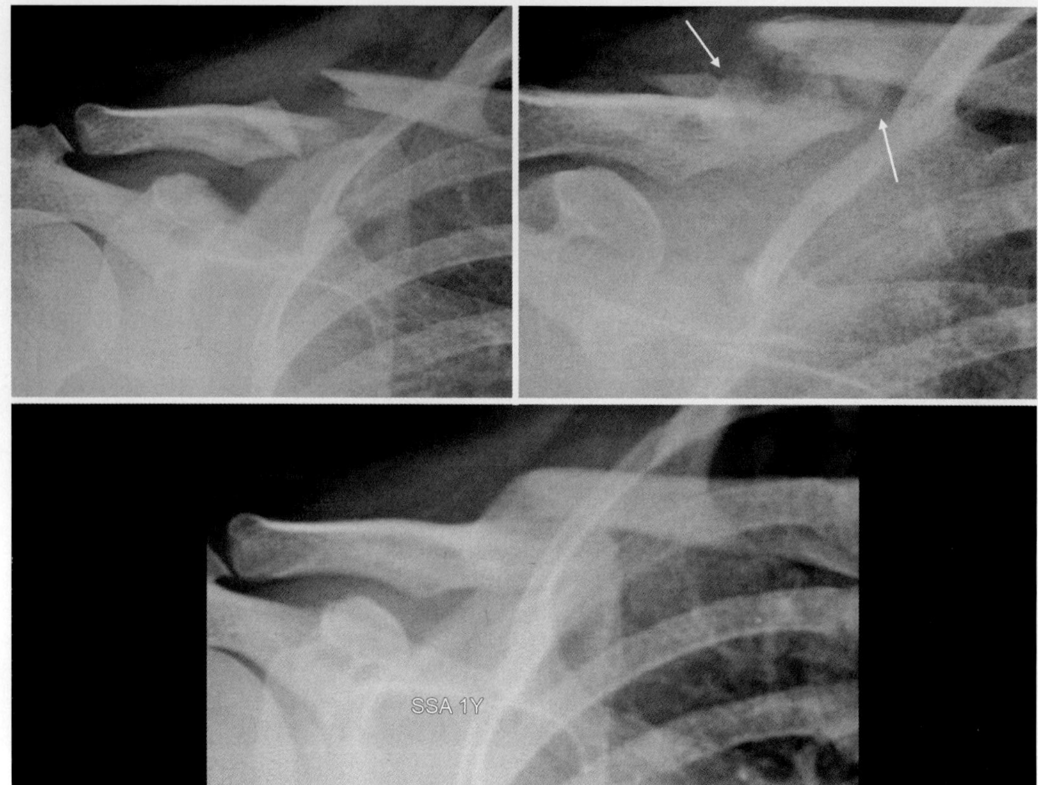

Figure 1.2 Slow union

and allows comfortable movements of the shoulder joint (Fig. 1.6).

The plate needs to have adequate strength and meant for a clavicle. Use of another design may fail, due to less strength (Fig. 1.7).

A transverse fracture with overlapping ends or a segmental fracture with overlap, usually leads to shortening. Especially in young and active persons, this may lead to:

- Cosmetic problem, as that side of the girdle appears narrower
- May come in the way of physical fitness in armed forces services or elsewhere.

Hence, it is a good idea to consider a closed reduction under anesthesia and assess. Choice is between a closed IM wire or external fixation (Figs 1.8 and 1.9).

In a long oblique fracture, the fracture plane is usually horizontal, with more chances of soft tissue interposition. If treated nonoperatively, soft tissue interposition is more likely to occur. This may lead to a slow and perhaps non-union also. If a closed IM wiring is attempted, at least the bone length would be restored and the soft tissue sleeve around the fracture would stretch out. Thus a chance of delayed union, due to the soft tissue interposition would reduce. A successful closed IM fixation or with minimal exposure, is a procedure of less magnitude with assured result.

Closed IM Method

Technique

The IM wire reduces local abnormal mobility. It keeps the medullary canal patent and helps

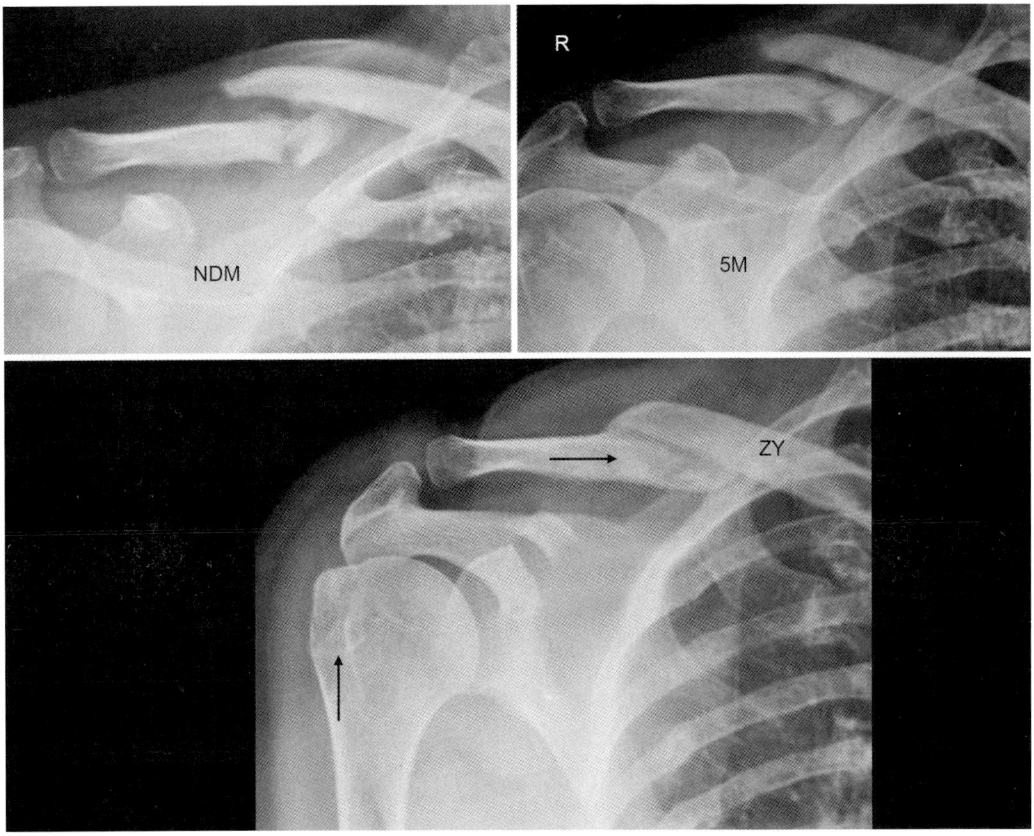

Figure 1.3 Slow union

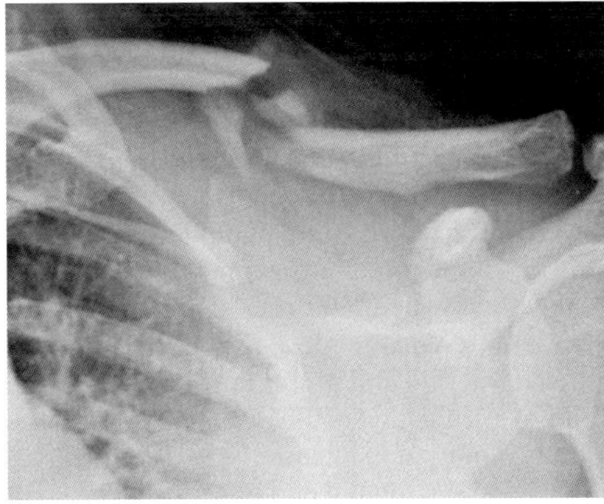

Figure 1.4 Non-union

bone bridge formation all around and thus helps union. The stability which the IM wire offers, reduces the abnormal mobility in the fragments and thus a bony union is expected. A successful closed IM fixation is cosmetically well accepted by the patient.

However, if in spite of the advice of operative method, if the patient opts for non-operative method, one treats it accordingly (If after a week or so, patient demands operative method, during this period, soft callus forms around the fracture ends, the medullary cavity is filled with granulation tissue and hence, a closed elastic nailing may not be successful and one may need an open reduction).

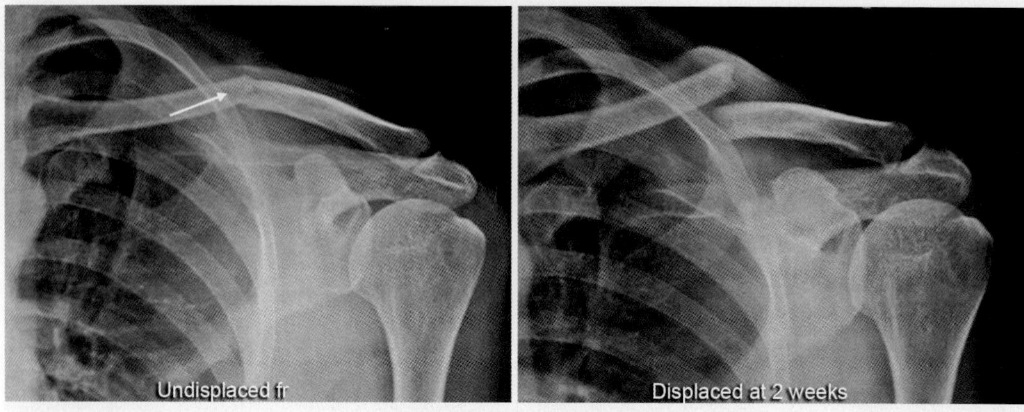

Figure 1.5 Late displacement

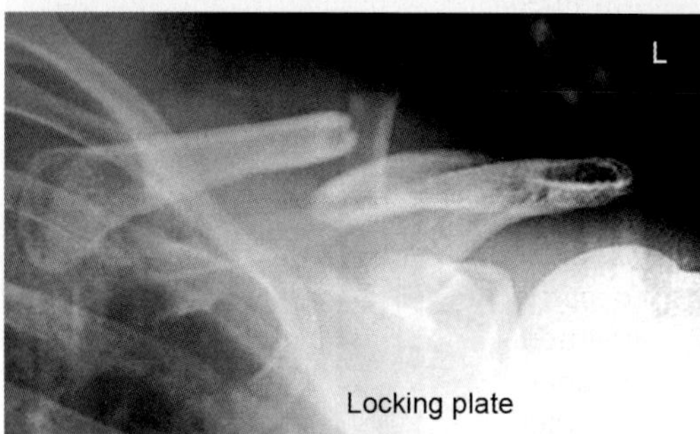

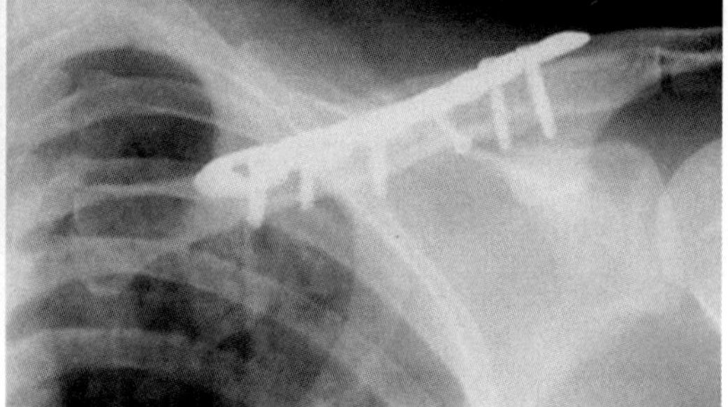

Figure 1.6 Locking plate

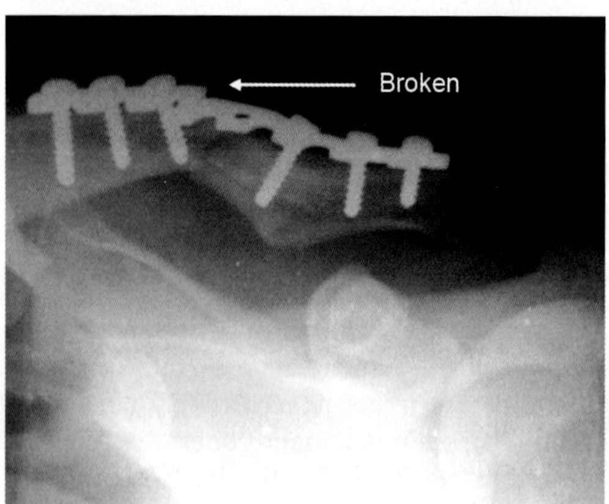

Figure 1.7 Failed RECO plate

Position of the patient, arrangements around the operation table should be as in surgery for fracture of lateral/4 of clavicle or acromio-clavicular dislocation. A transverse horizontal incision on medial end clavicle. Erase periosteum. Make a drill hole with 3.5 mm bit. Only 10 mm of drill bit has to be kept outside the chuck, so accidentally it cannot over pierce the medial end clavicle. The track is made oblique and slightly wider, with a cobbler awl.

A titanium wire 1.8 mm diameter is prepared. One end is cut and made rounded with a file. It is also slightly bent, like that of an olive wire in an interlock nail, to slide along bone cavity. This wire countering and preparation is better done prior to sterilization of the instrumentation. The wire is mounted in a cannulated T handle and inserted in the medial end of the clavicle along its long axis. It is further advanced towards the lateral end with a slight rotary motion. The fracture is manipulated and once the wire

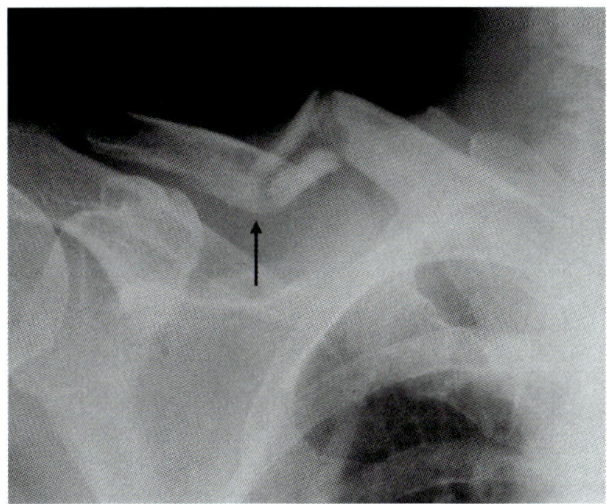

Figure 1.8 Segmental fracture

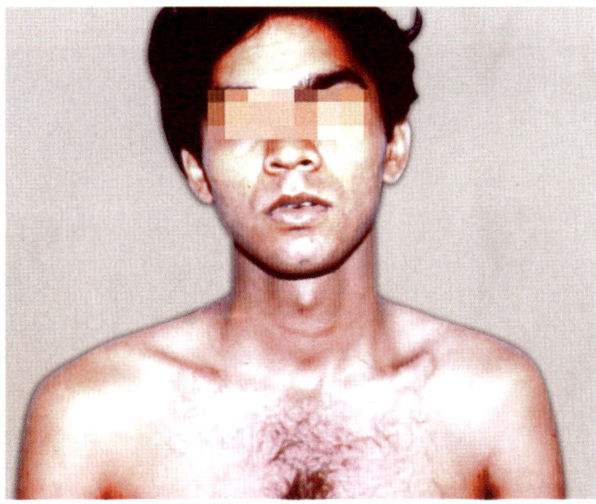

Figure 1.9 Clavicle shortening

tip enters the lateral fragment, it is advanced further.

A K-wire is more stiff than a titanium wire. The later tends to take shape of the curved bone easily. The clavicle cavity being narrow, needs some rotary force to be applied. The choice of the wire diameter is as per the cavity seen on an X-ray film. While the final seating of a wire is done, both the shoulders should be compressed together. It prevents fracture distraction, while the wire tip is entering the narrow and hard lateral fragment. If this care is not taken, the distraction may persist or the wire may back out, while the fracture settles and fracture ends come closer.

The wire end is slightly bent at 3 mm outside the entry hole and cut off with a side wire cutter.

Problems Faced during the Procedure

- In a fracture at the mid/3 area, while the wire is traversing the lateral fragment, one notices some distraction at the fracture site. *Answer*: Withdraw the wire to some extent and give lateral to medial compression and then while rotating through 90 deg, advance the wire. Often this technique is successful and the wire negotiates the lateral fragment well. Still, one may have to be satisfied by passing the wire, may be only 2 cm beyond the fracture site. The reduction and intramedullary presence of the implant is checked under C arm in two views, at least at an angle of 70 deg to each other, to overcome any illusion.
- There could be few small fragments in the fracture area which may have impaled in the cavity. In such a situation, one may have to carry out open reduction, retrieve the fragments and then advance the wire.
- Preoperative radiological assessment of the fracture may suggest a reasonably wide medullary cavity. However, on table one finds it difficult to pass even a 1.6 mm wire. In such a situation, one may have to stabilize the fracture with preferably a locking plate, which needs to be ready.
- The lateral part of the clavicle is flat, with nearly no cavity and the wire will not advance adequately to have a good fixation (Figs 1.10 and 1.11).

Message

In a fracture at lateral/3 area, this procedure of closed IM nailing is more likely to fail. One often has to open the fracture to prepare a canal in the lateral fragment and the purpose of closed nailing may fail.

Postoperatively, usually an elbow pouch usually suffices. In the elderly patient, especially with diabetes, one must start the external rotation exercises early, to prevent a stiff shoulder. A neutral position shoulder splint to

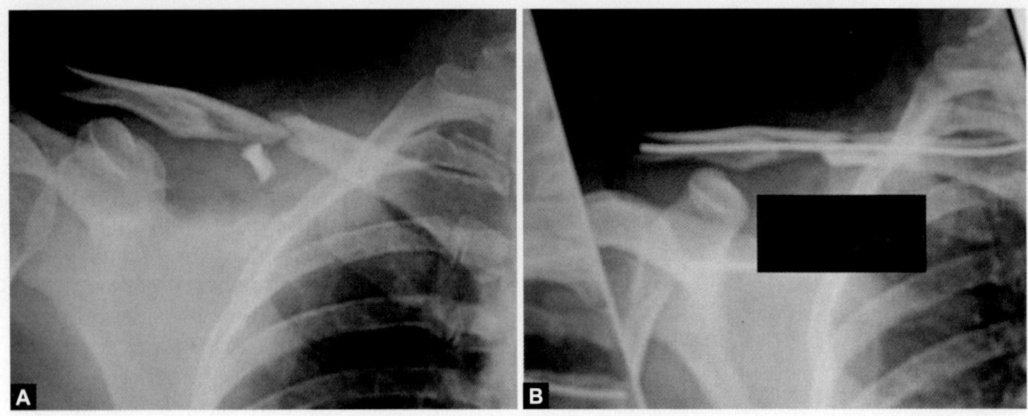

Figures 1.10A and B IM K-wire

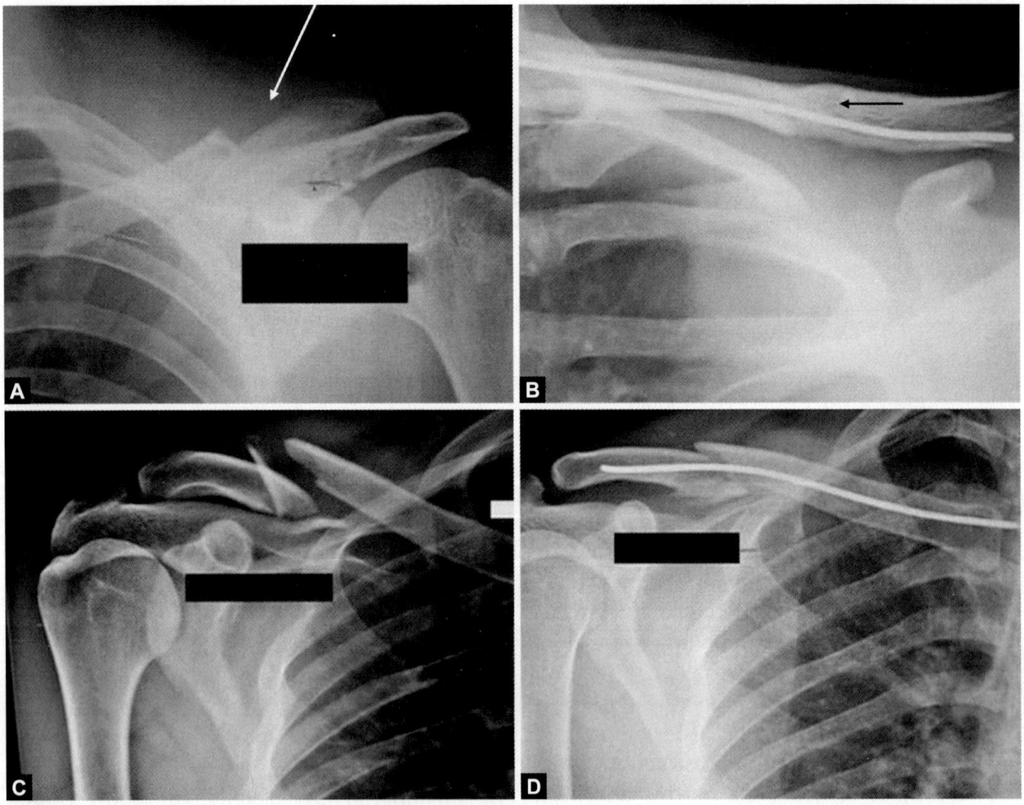

Figures 1.11A to D IM K-wire

keep the shoulder in neutral position for initial 10 days at least, would prevent a chance of stiff shoulder (see fracture neck Humerus).

External Fixation: Tips

- *Antero-posterior drilling*: Be careful of nerves posterior to the clavicle.
- *Supero-inferior drilling*: Be careful of the vessels inferior to the clavicle.
- The drill bit may have a depth guard or, if not, the length of the bit outside the chuck be just 2 mm more than the expected thickness of the bone. This trick and care taken during the use of the drill will make the procedure safe.
- In a tibia, the bone being a straight one, all four Schanz's pins can be linked to a single tube. The clavicle being a curved bone, one needs to use 2 Schanz`s pins in each fragment. The medial 2 pins are attached to a short bar and lateral 2 pins to another one. The two assembly bars are linked by a 3rd bar, after the fracture is reduced and stabilized.
- As a principle of external fixation, the assembly is too rigid to allow contact opposition and controlled collapse. At appropriate time, when a clinical union is observed, it should be removed and may be a figure of 8 bandage/a clavicle brace or a shoulder pouch be given, so good co-ption and consolidation occurs.

Place of Bone Grafting

While treating an ununited fracture clavicle, in addition to some form of fixation, cancellous bone grafting is necessary. The undisturbed soft tissue cover, with good blood supply is present more on the posterior surface of the bone. The grafts are first laid posterior to the fracture area, prior to fracture reduction, alignment and fixation. Once fracture is reduced and stabilized, it is not possible to harvest grafts, posterior to the fracture area and make a bed for the bone ends. This applies more so, when a plate is used. The available bone surface for bone grafts is posterior and it is here that a bone union will take place. Besides, the skin closure is easy, when the grafts are laid deep to the bone.

CHAPTER 2

Fracture of Lateral End of Clavicle

Some persons have congenital prominent lateral ends of the clavicle and are bilaterally symmetrical (Fig. 2.1).

CLINICAL DIAGNOSIS

Presence of an abrasion posterior to the acromion is a hall-mark of injury at lateral end of the clavicle or acromio-clavicular joint injury (Fig. 2.2).

The stability of the lateral end of the clavicle is maintained by the conoid and the trapezoid parts of the coraco-clavicular ligaments. If they are intact/partially injured, then the displacement is less and the end result of a treatment is superior. A transverse or oblique fracture with fracture direction from below upwards and laterally is relatively more unstable. Due to the fracture geometry, the medial fragment gets displaced superiorly, due to unopposed action of trapezius muscle.

A reverse oblique fracture is more stable and result of non-operative method is better than in the other types.

CLINICAL ASSESSMENT OF REDUCIBILITY

The patient is made to sit on a stool and clinician standing behind him. The clinician keeps the

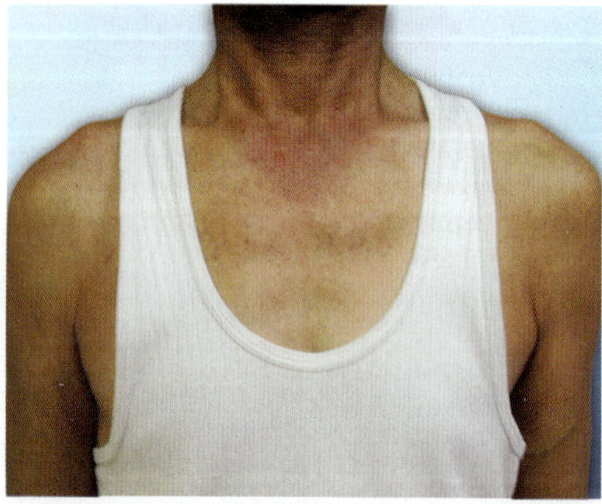

Figure 2.1 Bilateral prominent lateral end clavicles

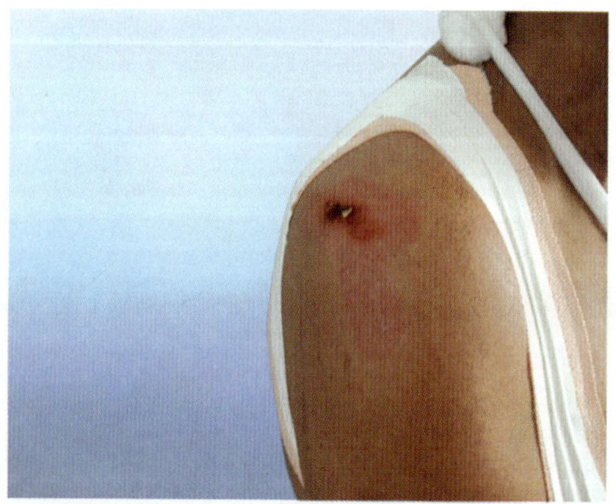

Figure 2.2 Abrasion posterior to clavicle is a hallmark

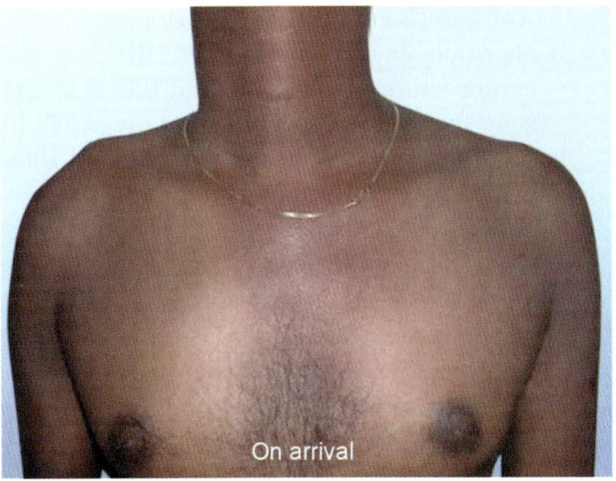

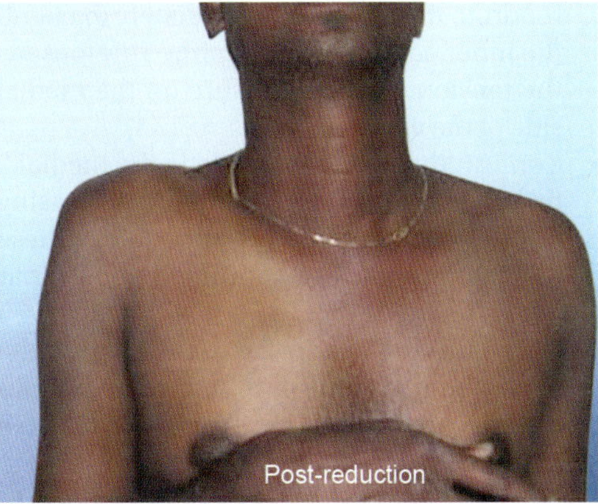

Figure 2.3 Clinical assessment

mid-portion of clavicle depressed down and with the other hand presses the point of a flexed elbow upwards. In a reducible fracture, the deformity reduces easily and to a good extent (Fig. 2.3).

Radiological Examination

Standing X-rays of both the shoulders are taken, with weights hanging from the wrist. Comparative study of both the shoulders is more useful and easy to demonstrate, document and for better understanding for the patient. (*Please note, the weights are to be suspended from the wrist and not to be held by the patient under examination.*)

TREATMENT: NON-OPERATIVE

In a reducible fracture with a displacement up to 8 to 10 mm, non-operative method of treatment is possible. Robert Jone's strapping is applied.

Steps of Strapping

- Patient sitting on a stool and clinician standing behind him. The assistant stands in front of patient
- Care of arm pit
- Elbow flexed to 120 deg and a pad kept on the medial humeral epicondyle to protect the ulnar nerve.
- 6 cm adhesive elastic strapping is started from the midtrapezial area and goes over the scapula. It thus starts medial to the fracture site on the clavicle and body of the scapula and then after stretching is taken around the elbow, 3 fingers width distal to the point of elbow and handed over to a trained assistant. The surgeon applies differential pressure—downwards pressure on the clavicle medial to the fracture area, to reduce it, while the point of elbow is pressed upwards, to bring the lateral fragment towards the medial fragment. The assistant takes the strap from behind to the front of the upper forearm, vertically upwards and medial to the fracture site. This strapping band overlaps the starting end. It, thus, does not cover the lateral fragment, which is lifted up by the upward pressure on the elbow by the clinician.

  Over this elastic adhesive strapping, a cloth adhesive strapping of 5 cm is added. Elastic adhesive does not bite in the skin, is more comfortable, while the cloth adhesive strapping is non-yielding and maintains the reduction well.
- A sling is given maintaining the hand across the chest. The elbow continues to be in 120 deg of flexion.

Instructions for Patient

- Instruct the patient to observe, if he gets tingling on the medial two fingers. If so, report to the clinician immediately to cut off the inner edge of the strapping. This loosens the tension and the pressure on the medial side of the elbow.

- Confirm that the tingling along the medial 2 fingers is reduced and fanning and closing of stretched fingers is possible. These movement indicates continued good ulnar nerve function.
- Grip and static arm exercises within the strapping is carried out. Both the exercises are extremely important ! This maintains the arm muscle tone well (Figs 2.4 and 2.5).

Further Course

- The strapping is elastic and with gravity and weight of the limb it stretches. The next strapping is added on the previous one every alternate day. It is necessary to keep the earlier strapping in place and the next one is added on the previous one only. After 10 days, the muscle spasm reduces and then twice a week strapping is adequate.

The previous strapping is maintained as such, so at least some reduction is maintained and the skin soreness is avoided by daily removal and reapplication. In fact, daily removal is not necessary as well. The hold of the first strapping on the skin continues and usually after 4 to 5 applications of strapping, the entire mass falls out. At this point, usually 12 to 14 days are over. When this happens at home, patient can remove the entire of it, have a bath and then attend the clinic for further strapping.

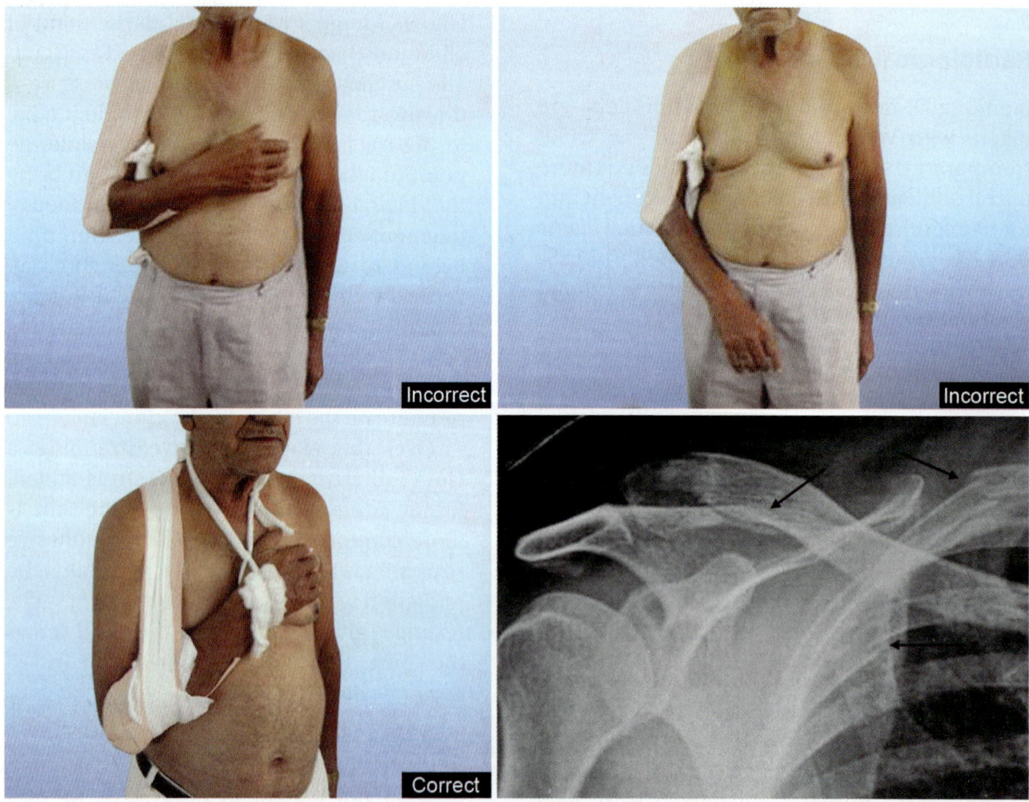

Figure 2.4 Method of strapping

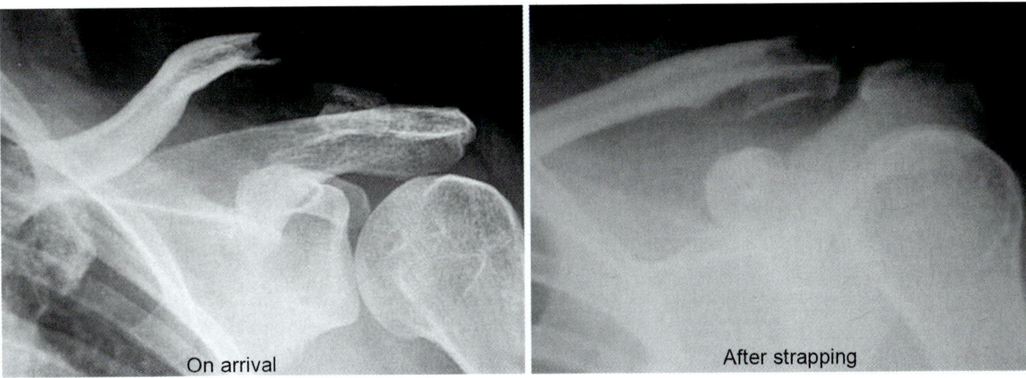

Figure 2.5 Post-strapping reduction

- Persons over 40 years of age and those having diabetes, need to carry out the shoulder external rotation exercises, twice a day. This can be done with the strapping in place. If this is not practised, troublesome shoulder stiffness ensues.

  During the course of the therapy, the shoulder joint is maintained in internal rotation and the post-immobilization stiffness can be troublesome. So much so that one may consider internal fixation and early mobilization of the shoulder as a definitive method of treatment.
- Gravity tends to displace the fracture and hence the strapping needs to be applied often and thus maintained for 5 weeks at least. Weekly X-ray examination of the shoulder is done in standing posture to confirm that the reduction is maintained well.

INDICATIONS FOR INTERNAL FIXATION

- Irreducible displacement, which may have soft tissue interposition
- Skin problem or soft tissue injuries in the area, which would not permit strapping.
- Associated injuries, due to which outdoor ambulatory care is not practical or with associated ipsilateral upper limb injuries.
- Patient's preference to the method of treatment (Fig. 2.6).

Surgical Technique of Internal Fixation

Position and draping for operations on the fracture of clavicle and AC joint:

- *Propped up position*: Upper part of the body is flexed to about 30 degrees. Slight upward tilt in the lower segment of table, to bend the hips and the knees and prevent patient sliding down. A pillow below the knee maintains the knee flexion and prevents sciatic nerve stretching.
- *A Thin pillow below the ipsilateral scapula*: With the conventional table, the metal accessories at the head end of the table, especially the side bars for the clamps, come in the way of 'C' arm beam. Hence I prefer to turn around the table—the foot end of the table is kept towards the head end. The anesthesia machine and thus the patient's head is rested on the foot end of the table. After induction of anesthesia, a test exposure with a 'C' arm is taken to confirm that one gets a clear picture on the screen, without any metal parts of the table coming in the way of X-ray beam. True AP view and with 30 degree tilt on either side is confirmed.

The head is rested over a head ring and turned towards the opposite side and an adhesive strapping is added over the forehead of patient to stabilize it. A protective eye ointment is usually applied by the anesthesiologist and the upper eye

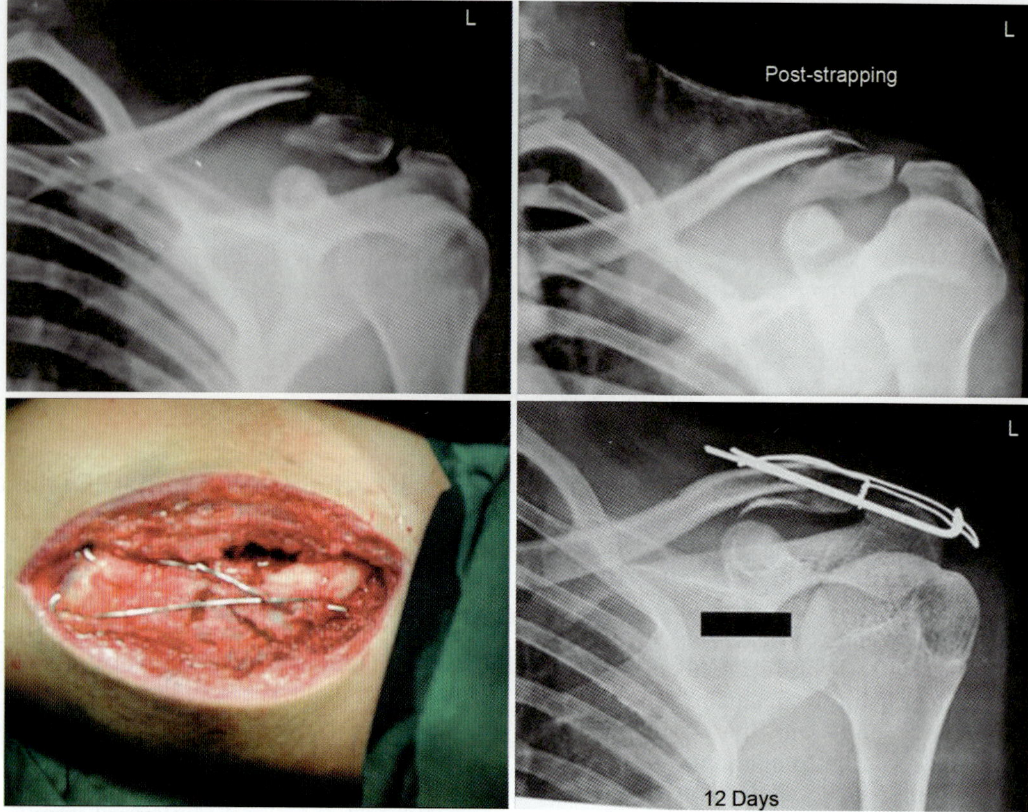

Figure 2.6 Locked fragments

lid closed down, to protect the eye, especialy the cornea, by a small adhesive strip.

- `C` arm is brought from the head end of the table, so surgeon can stand on the side to be operated. The X-ray tube is given a tilt to be at right angle to the clavicle.
- The anesthesia team and the machine are on the opposite side. The `C` arm monitor is placed on the opposite side at the calf level and the power and monitor cables are taken beyond the anesthesia machine. The surgical cautery unit and the vacuum suction unit are at the foot end of the table.
- The shoulder to be operated is brought at the edge of the table, and the elbow is supported by a short and wide wooden plank, tucked under the shoulder, under the mattress. Prior to painting and draping, C arm image must be checked, to avoid intraoperative difficulty. One needs to have a clear and unobstructed view of the operative area in the X-ray monitor. The shoulder position may need some adjustment, to confirm that metal parts of the operation table do not come in the way of the X-ray beam.
- On the first occasion, this position is better rehearsed a day prior to the surgery, so no time is wasted on the day of surgery.
- Limb to be operated is draped separately.

INCISION

A gentle curved incision is preferred. After marking the incision, lignocaine and adrenaline infiltration is done. Thick skin flaps are raised. Fracture is located and one extends the incision from the lateral part of the acromion, medially approx 3 cm medial to the fracture area. It is necessary to confirm that the exposure is till the extreme outermost part of the angle of the acromion.

Soft tissue interposition, if any is removed and fracture reduced by gentle upwards pressure on the elbow, while the medial clavicle is depressed with a broad and blunt tool like a periosteum elevator or a punch.

A cordless power drill is a great asset. A 1.8 mm K-wire is kept like a template on the superior surface and the direction in which it is to be inserted is judged. Usually the entry is slightly anterior on the acromion, so the tip exits posteriorly, approximately 2.5 cm medial to the fracture site. This is a point where the clavicle curvature changes. A 4 mm elevator is pressed against the posterior surface of the clavicle, so it protects the soft tissues as well. Accordingly, two 1.8 mm K wires are drilled across the fracture area separated by a distance of 4 mm in ant-posterior plane. Approximately, 5 mm of each wire is kept protruding beyond the posterior surface of the clavicle. A 1 mm soft bone wire (cold drawn) is put as a figure of 8 loop, round the medial and lateral ends of two K wires. The figure of 8 wire is loaded gently with a tractor bow. Laterally, the loop is taken just deep to the K wires and not deep to the deltoid muscle, as it may crush the fleshy deltoid origin.

One observes that while the tractor bow loads the circlage, the K wires slightly bend, indicating they are loaded well. If the local situation permits, the medial tip of the K wires may be slightly bent in appropriate direction, to prevent circlage wire slipping out. This is better done, prior to passing the circlage around. The lateral end of each K-wire is bent and cut. They are slightly rotated if needed and buried well and gently tapped home.

The circlage crossing and the knot if possible is done at postero-superior to the clavicle, where adequate soft tissue cover is available.

Assess the lengths of the medial ends of the K wires protruding from posterior surface of the clavicle. If an end is rather long, it is carefully held in a small narrow pliers and cut with a small, pointed and flat wire cutter. These tools are very important in this situation and are a must! This makes the wire end blunt and should it migrate medially, is less likely to penetrate an important structure.

Appropriate closure of deeper layers is done and skin closure is done with subcutaneous monocryl. Steri-strips may be used. This makes a straight scar without cross hatchings.

Postoperative Care

- A pillow is kept under the elbow.
- Shoulder pouch during ambulation.
- Static arm and grip exercises are mandatory.

At times, the strength and stability of the TBW assembly may not be adequate enough to counteract the gravity and the weight of the limb, in a well-built, muscular or obese person. In such a situation, one may add Robert Jone strapping for 3 weeks at least. This is important to counteract the effect of gravity. During the postoperative period, with or without the strapping, external rotation exercises for the shoulder are important, to prevent shoulder stiffness.

In place of a Robert Jone's strapping, one may use a rib belt and a sling as per the convenience and need of the patient. The belt is taken around the operated limb and across the chest. This restrains unnecessary use of the affected limb.

In a patient with diabetes and elderly person, I would prefer a neutral shoulder splint (as used after internal fixation of fracture neck humerus). It may appear inconvenient, but in the long run, the return of shoulder range of motion is indeed satisfactory and avoids periarthritis of shoulder joint.

Warning and Implant Removal

Mechanically, it is difficult to pass K wires from the lateral end of the clavicle, as it participates in formation of acromio-clavicular joint. Hence it needs to be driven in from the lateral end of the acromion.

During the shoulder girdle motion, some gliding movement occurs at the AC joint, which may lead to breakage of the K wires and/or the circlage. The medial part of the broken K-wire migrates medially. Hence, they need to be removed usually at the end of six months or so, as per the radiological union. Hence, regular follow up and X-ray examination every six to eight weeks is necessary. If this is not strictly followed, the wire may break and migrate towards the root of the neck and its retrieval is difficult (Fig. 2.7).

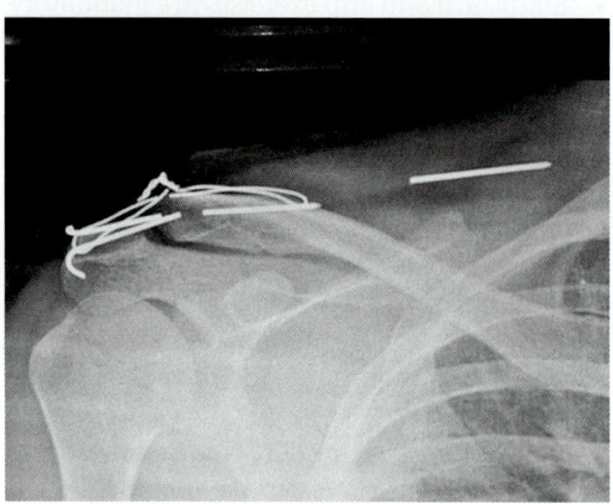

Figure 2.7 Wire migration

With availability of a hook plate, inserting a K-wire or a screw across the AC joint could be avoided. However, the hook plate is said to have its own problems also.

Recovery Period

- Office work can be begun approx 7 to 10 days after the surgery. However driving a car is usually safe after 6 weeks from surgery, as per the ROM achieved, local pain and clinical status.
- Driving a scooter/bike usually would take at least 2 months, depending on above factors and X-ray appearance, etc. This is important for student population.

Complications/Sequela

If the K wire tip at the lateral end is not properly turned/bent and buried, it may cause a sinus and may be associated with pain. If the K-wire is thicker than 1.8 mm, usually this problem of bending and cutting of the wire comes up. Removal of the K-wire settles the sinus problem (Fig. 2.8).

ASSOCIATED INJURIES

When an X-ray for the shoulder injury is taken, it is safe to include the adjacent portion of the

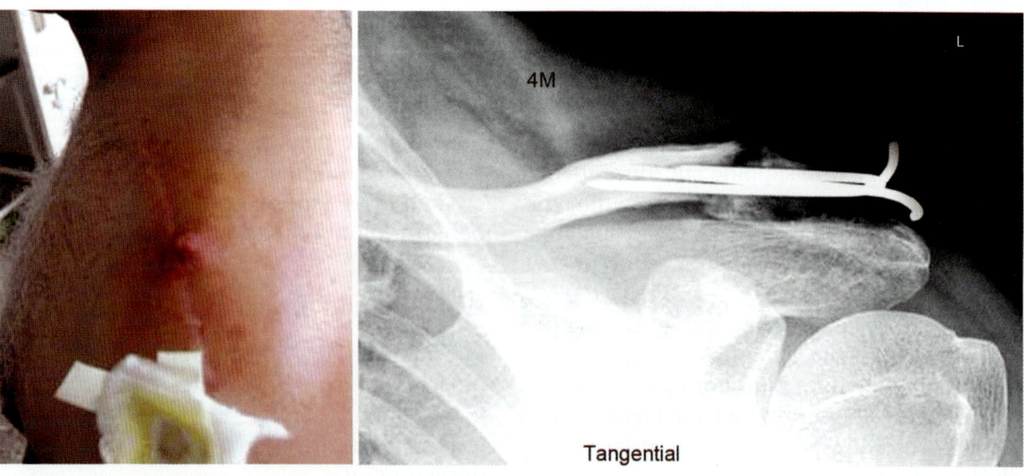

Figure 2.8 Sinus

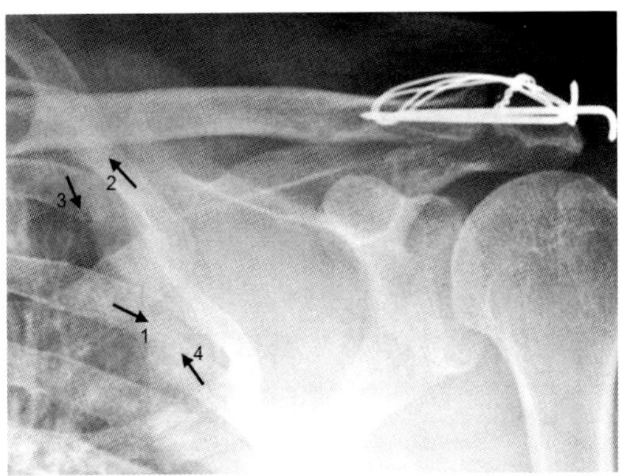

Figure 2.9 Associated rib fractures

rib cage. Associated fractures of upper ribs is known to occur. Clinically, it may be difficult to assess the cause and origin of pain (from the rib fractures) and hence the day 1, X-ray taken in two views settles the diagnosis.

After a fracture of the clavicle is noted, still one should carefully look for a rib fracture, if any, and MARK that rib fracture on the X-ray film. The first occasion of clinical and X-ray film study is the best time to detect any bone injury, if any. During follow up, when one sees the X-ray film, the arrow marks catch one's attention and every time one may need not examine the film in great details (Fig. 2.9).

CHAPTER

3

Acromioclavicular Dislocation

X-ray with weights suspended from the wrist reveals grade of an injury. If, patient holds a weight in a hand, the muscles tend to be tight and the skiagram may not reveal exact nature and degree of the AC joint injury.

Prior to innovation of a good method of internal stabilization of the acromioclavicular joint, one would treat such an injury by a Robert Jone strapping method with a satisfactory outcome (Fig. 3.1).

Today, especially in cases with multiple fractures in one limb, stabilization of this joint permits early mobilization of adjacent joints.

For internal fixation, following technique is useful (Fig. 3.2):

PATIENT POSITION AND SURGICAL TECHNIQUE

The steps in patient positioning and surgical exposure are the same as in surgery for fracture of lateral/4 clavicle.

Gelpi retractor is a useful instrument for good exposure. A transverse incision is taken on the lateral/3 clavicle, such that the medial end of the incision is slightly posterior to the clavicle,

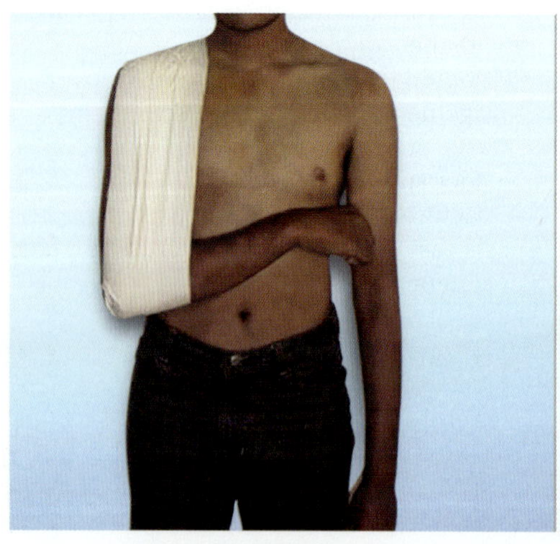

Incorrect method

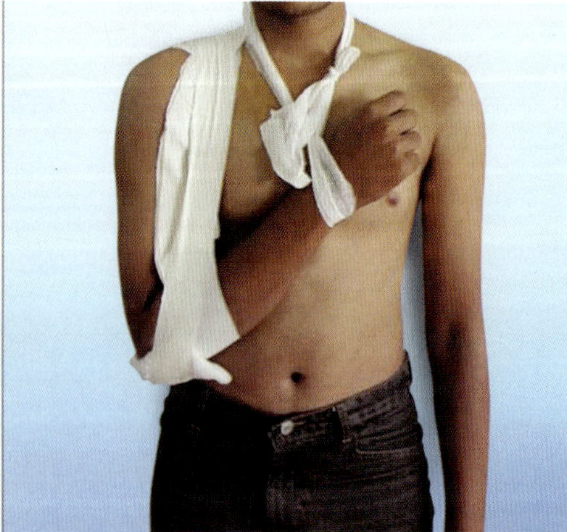

Correct method

Figure 3.1 Strapping

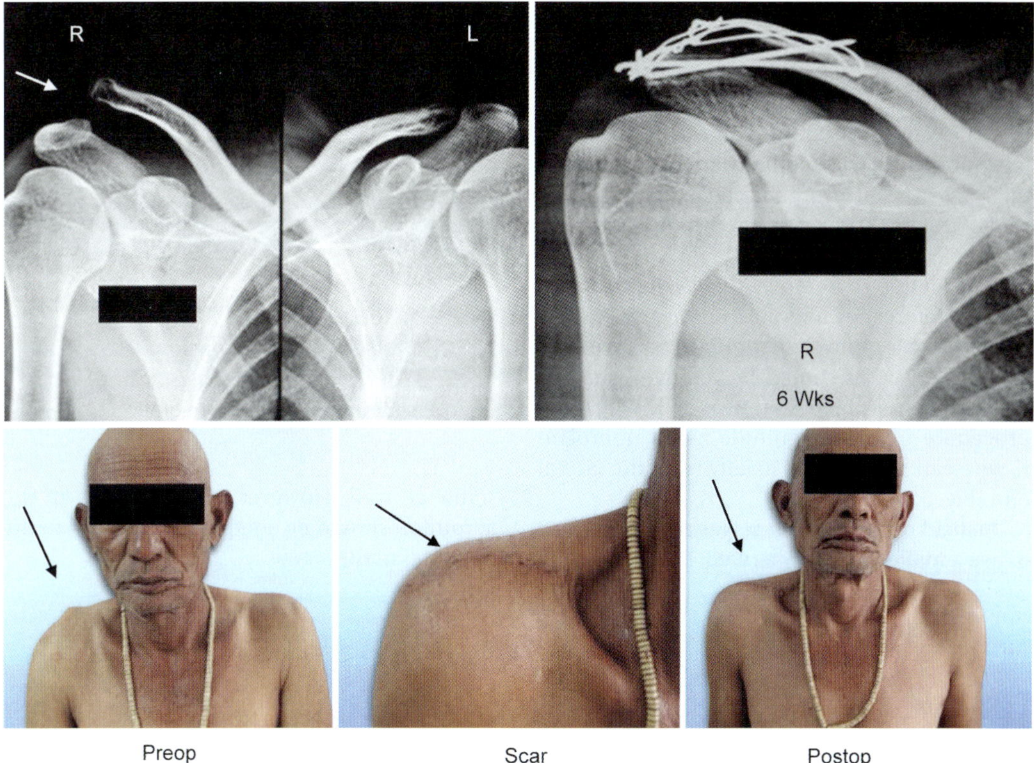

Figure 3.2 X-ray and operative technique

where the K-wire exits from the clavicle. Both the clavicle and the acromion are exposed well and provisional reduction done by pushing the elbow proximally and upwards.

Coraco-clavicular ligaments are studied and possibility of their suturing/reconstruction is assessed.

After passing each K-wire, one should confirm in exact AP and both tangential projections in a 'C' arm and that the K wire is intra-osseous. This is important, as though clinically, the wire may appear to be in the center of the acromion, it could be close to the inferior plate of acromion.

In the recovery room, and later on, while the patient lying on the back, a pillow support under the elbow makes the patient comfortable.

During the follow up, one should encourage active external rotation movement of the shoulder to prevent a stiff shoulder. This is especially important in the elderly and patients with diabetes, in whom, post-immobilization stiff shoulder is common. As in postoperative management of a case of fracture lateral/4 clavicle, it is important to use a neutral shoulder splint. This prevents internal rotation contracture, keeps the patient pain-free and assists easy restoration of the external rotation movement.

FOLLOW UP AND IMPLANT REMOVAL

At the end of 6 weeks, usually the shoulder range is restored well. However, one must follow up the case every month, for first three months, and then, every 2 months. At the end of five to six months, the implants are to be removed and this MUST be emphasized to the patient or else an X-ray taken after six to twelve months shows a broken and migrated K-wire! This instruction should be given on the discharge card as well.

It is observed that often a K-wire breaks at the AC joint level due to some motion in the joint and then the medial part of the K-wire migrates medially from the clavicle towards the root of the neck, towards important nerves and vessels.

It is better to remove the implant at the earliest before they migrate quite away from the clavicle and is quite challenging to remove it. At least, the K wires should be removed, leaving the circlage in place. Removal of K wires is a procedure of less magnitude as an unbroken K-wire can be removed axially from the lateral end (Fig. 3.3).

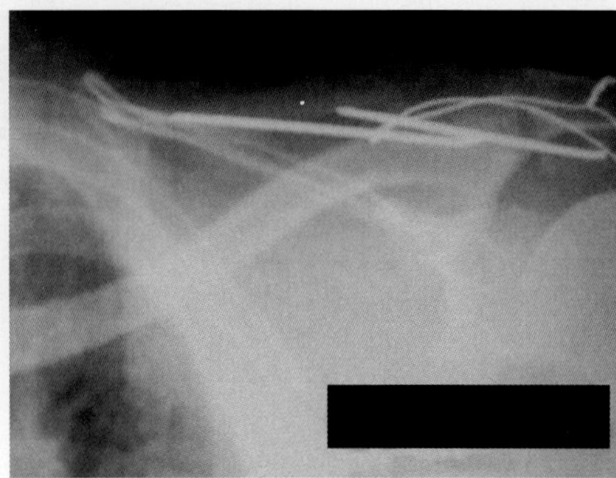

Figure 3.3 K-wire migration

Instead of the K wires, it was recommended to use a malleolar screw as well. I have used the screw as well. However, the thickness of the acromion should be adequate compared to the diameter of the screw.

CHAPTER

4

Posterior Dislocation of the Shoulder

- A posterior dislocation of shoulder is less common than the anterior dislocation.
- The casualty clinician and the X-ray technician, both are likely to miss the injury, both clinically and radiologically. Hence, there is a possibility that the patient might be sent home as a shoulder sprain. (As in a case of an uncertain fracture of carpal scaphoid/ an impacted fracture neck femur or fracture of a pubic ramus or a compression fracture spine.)
- Orthopedic surgeon on call must see and examine such a case personally and be aware of pitfalls. It is necessary to take axillary X-ray view personally if needed, to avoid any missed injury. The `cost` and efforts required to carry out this exercise of diagnosis of posterior dislocation of shoulder is much less than that of a missed injury.

CASE STUDY

Following is a case story, which is self-explanatory and an eye opener for everybody concerned in establishing a diagnosis of a not so common an injury.

After an injury, a patient attended a casualty department with shoulder pain at midnight. I received a call from the CMO 'here is a case with severe pain in the shoulder, but X-ray appeared normal' 'I thought of a possibility of an uncommon situation, like a posterior dislocation and attended immediately. My observations:

- The contour of the shoulder was altered, though is not as much angular as seen in an anterior dislocation.
- All active movements were associated with severe pain and muscle spasm.
- Dugas test positive (Could not touch the opposite shoulder tip with the injured hand (Fig. 4.1).

In a Normal Ap View of a Shoulder

There is some overlap of head humerus on the glenoid. The so called joint line is not visible.

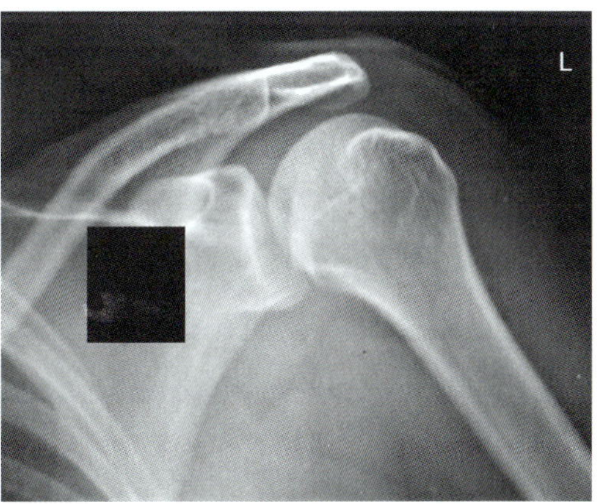

Figure 4.1 Arrival AP of shoulder

Posterior Dislocation

The shape of the head of the humerus is not as usual. Has a pear shape or an electric bulb like appearance.

Though, the diagnosis of a posterior dislocation of the shoulder is clear in an AP view, it is important and safe for documentation (and confirmation beyond doubt) to have an axillary view.

Parental analgesic was given and then gently and with perseverance, patient was made to lie on an X-ray table and an axillary view was personally taken. (In fact to make the patient lie on a table is in itself a challenging procedure, because of the pain, that he has!) (Fig. 4.2).

The glenohumeral congruity was absent and a diagnosis of posterior dislocation confirmed. Immediate closed reduction under anesthesia was done and was successful. AP and axillary check X-ray examination done and films taken. A shoulder immobilizer was given.

The patient was discharged the next day, with a request to keep shoulder immobilized and grip and static arm exercises to be done. Follow up at appropriate time was advised. A better method of immobilization is to give a shoulder splint with a waist belt and an attached device to keep the shoulder in neutral position, with hand pointing forward and avoiding any internal rotation movement. (If the shoulder is immobilized with hand across the chest with a sling, there is a possibility of re-dislocation of head humerus. This is more so, when there is an associated impacted fracture in the anterior segment in the head humerus. The overall shape of the head humerus becomes flat and easily slides, to slip over the posterior lip of the glenoid cavity). This splint keeps the shoulder in neutral rotation and prevents any possibility of posterior dislocation occurring again (Figs 4.3 and 4.4).

Patient reported only after 3 weeks, for completion of insurance papers.

The patient made a good recovery in a reasonable time. As per my habit, I thought of

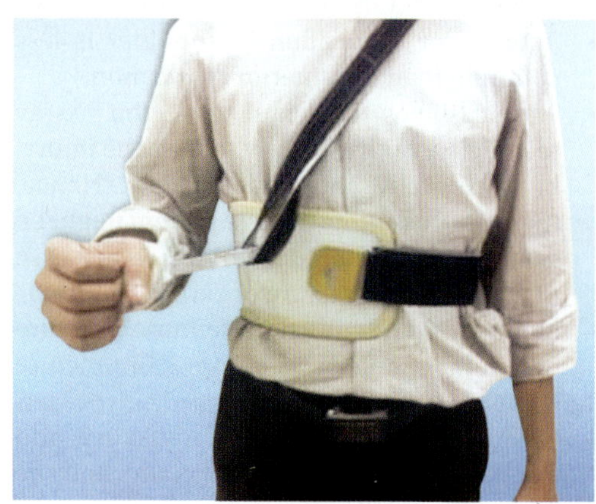

Figure 4.3 Shoulder splint I

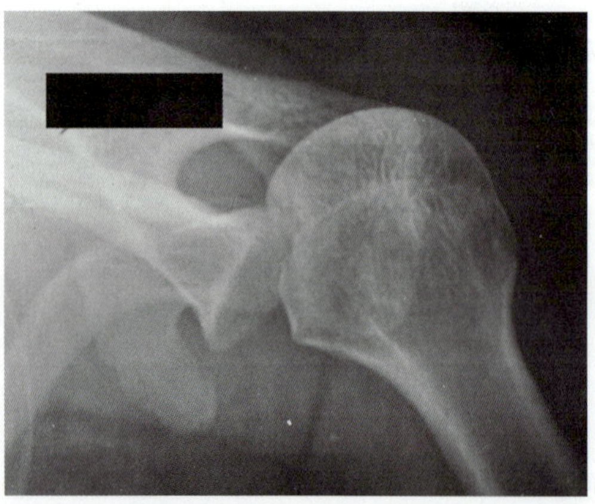

Figure 4.2 Arrival axillary view

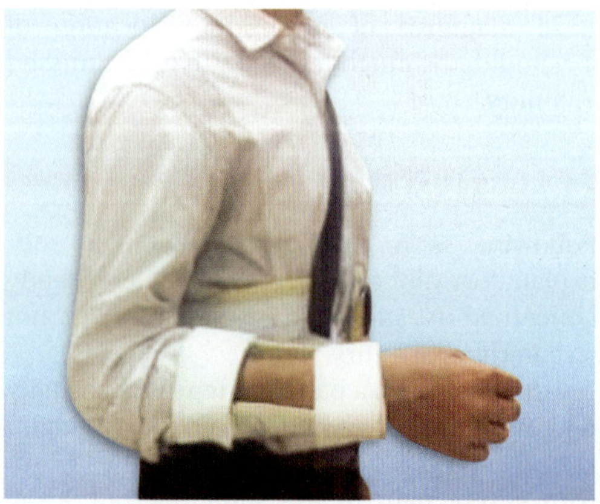

Figure 4.4 Shoulder splint II

reviewing all the films. I took out the first X-ray film from the envelope, I happened to see the radiologist report on both AP and axillary views. To my surprise, it was reported as normal X-ray without a bone or joint injury by the radiologist!

To avoid any administrative problem, I went to the radiologist to discuss and ratify the result. To my surprise, even after seeing AP and axillary views, both on arrival and post-reduction films, the radiologist refused to accept it as a case of a posterior dislocation of the shoulder! (Figs 4.5 and 4.6).

Here Arise Few Questions

1. Was there indeed a posterior dislocation ?
2. When on X-ray examination of both the AP and the lateral views, the posterior dislocation is clear, is it necessary to arrange a CT scan with a 3D reconstruction to prove the point.
3. Is the CT worthwhile, spending half an hour more, and keep the patient in painful state in the CT gantry, rather than carrying out immediate closed reduction? If necessary, the scan be always done at a later stage, to know any associated injury, especially in the anterior part of the head of humerus, but then the initial dislocation would not be seen.

If I had allowed to continue to carry the X-ray report as 'no bone/joint injury', the insurance company or any one may have raised a point, that the entire surgical procedure of a closed reduction was not needed, because, the report says, there is no bone and/or joint injury! Of course, I would have contested and won the discussion. But it puts everybody to inconvenience and the community would have a ground to doubt regarding the diagnosis and scientific basis for the procedure. This would have arose in spite of a so efficiently and correctly diagnosing a rare condition and immediately carrying out a procedure under anesthesia, in the middle of a night.

In yester years, often the midnight analogue film processing would be less than satisfactory and the last stage of 'Fixing' process in chemical development may not be done adequately to have a good quality film. Today, with a digital technology, the images can be stored and even if one film is spoilt or lost, we do have access to the data of a study done at the time of arrival.

Fortunately, for everyone, reluctantly though, the radiologist changed the report!

Lessons Learnt

1. When a discharge is planned, read X-ray report of all the films. Confirm that the patient's name, the side of body part examined is correctly mentioned on the film. At the end, go through the laboratory and

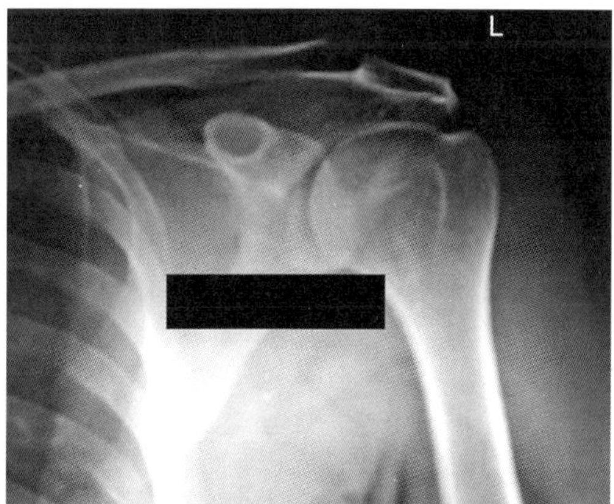

Figure 4.5 Post-reduction AP view

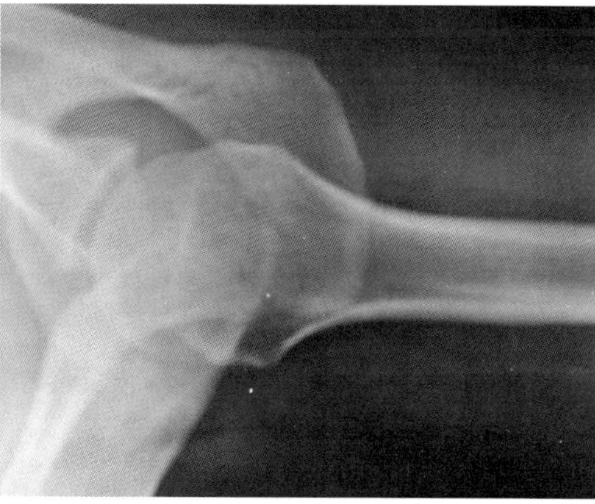

Figure 4.6 Post-reduction axillary view

imaging report. The bone and joint injury is preferably marked by a marker pen, so every time one sees the film, it is immediately eye catching.

2. The X-ray report may not be delivered at the time of discharge, as it may be half-a-day stay, especially on a holiday. During follow up, one needs to spend time and energy to see all the paper work. This would avoid unnecessary (and avoidable) situations.
3. I have also come across situations, where a clinician, including myself, has missed an associated injury in an X-ray film and one noticed it later on after going through the radiologist's report. Thus, we need to work in harmony, for a better patient care.
4. It is safer to see all the X-ray and imaging reports, and if in doubt, have an open discussion with the colleague. Everyone learns with time.

CHAPTER

5

Fracture Dislocation of the Shoulder

A fracture dislocation of shoulder joint is a major injury, due to severe violence. It is commonly seen after an episode of convulsions or electric shock, which leads to severe jerks to the shoulder area and spine.

After an attack of convulsion, one should check thoracolumbar spine as well, to exclude any associated compression fracture of a vertebra.

Following observations are based on clinical findings and data available.

In the two shoulder cases shown, the injuries and their mechanism are similar ones.

CASES 1 AND 2

Injuries

- On the (R) side
  - Displaced fracture of greater tuberosity
  - Displaced vertical fracture of neck humerus
  - Anterior dislocation of head humerus
- On the (L) side
  - Displaced fracture of greater tuberosity
  - Anterior dislocation of head humerus.

Treatment

- *On arrival*: (L) shoulder could be reduced at bedside with Kochar method soon after arrival. Slow sustained external rotation at the shoulder and taking the elbow medially across the chest usually leads to a successful reduction and Dugas test turns negative. The relocation is confirmed by X-ray examination, done in neutral position of the shoulder—palm facing forward position. Then under anesthesia, closed reduction on the right side was attempted.
- (R) *shoulder*: Due to break in continuity (due to the vertical fracture neck humerus) the reduction is usually unsuccessful. In spite of local pressure on the head of humerus to reduce it back in the glenoid cavity the reduction was unsuccessful as expected.
- This fracture with a large fragment of the head with a medial vertical break, almost always needs open reduction and internal fixation. This should be carried out as early as possible. If one tries to reduce it under anesthesia, as an emergency measure or prior to the definitive internal fixation, the fragment displacement increases, with loss of medial soft tissue continuity. At the time of open reduction, this continuity does help in relocating the displaced head of humerus back in the glenoid. The required efforts are less and maintaining the medial contact opposition, the blood supply is also preserved well. Hence, I suggest, with this fracture morphology, one should straightway proceed to an immediate open reduction and internal fixation at the earliest.

Definitive Treatment and Surgery

An open reduction of the right fracture dislocation of the shoulder was carried out. The upper end of right humerus was fixed by a locking plate. During this procedure, the greater tuberosity was reduced and placed under the plate and stabilized.

Further Therapy

- Immediate finger/elbow and static arm exercises were started.
- The left shoulder was already treated by a closed reduction and the immobilization by an arm to chest band was continued. It was actively mobilized after 3 days. It is an observation that whenever there is associated fracture of the greater tuberosity of humerus in a dislocation of shoulder, recurrent dislocation is uncommon. Hence, one may not rigidly immobilize such an injury, which makes restoration of movements rather difficult.

The greater tuberosity fragment was not internally fixed and one needs to take care during mobilization.

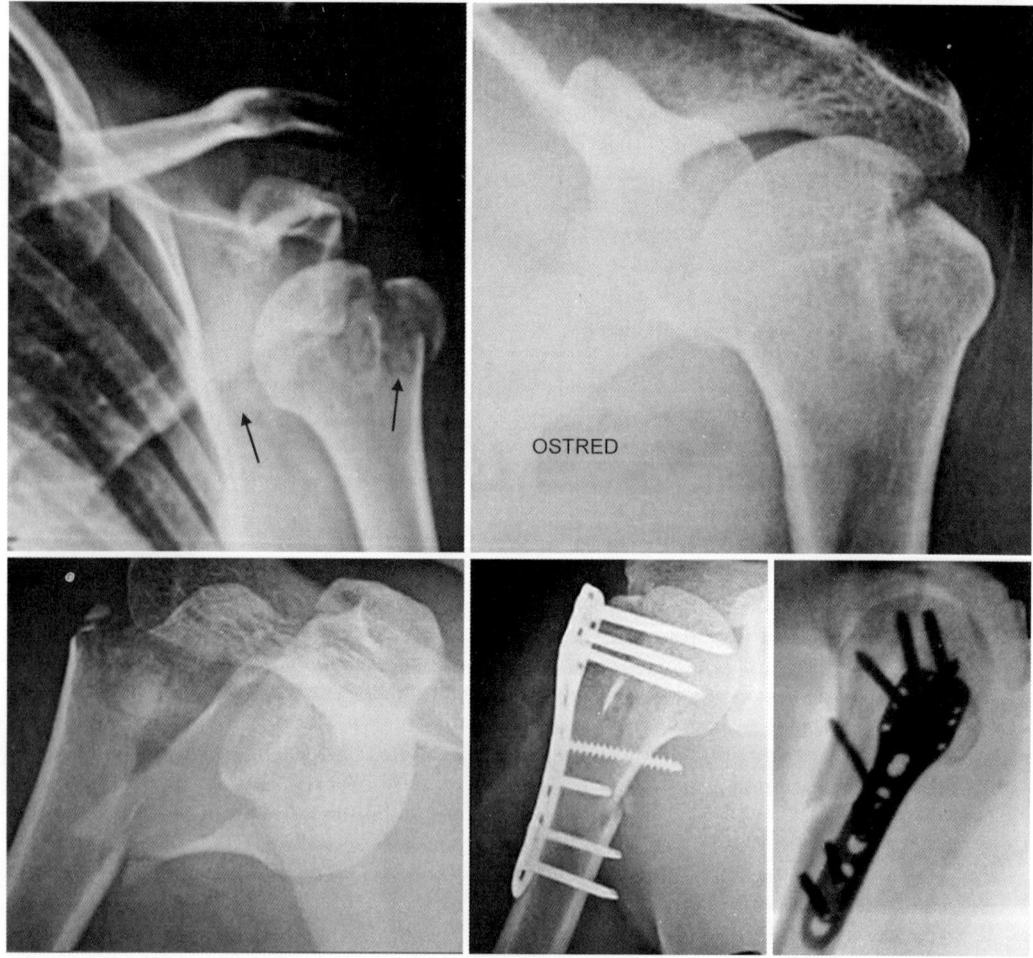

Figure 5.1 Post-convulsion bilateral fracture dislocation

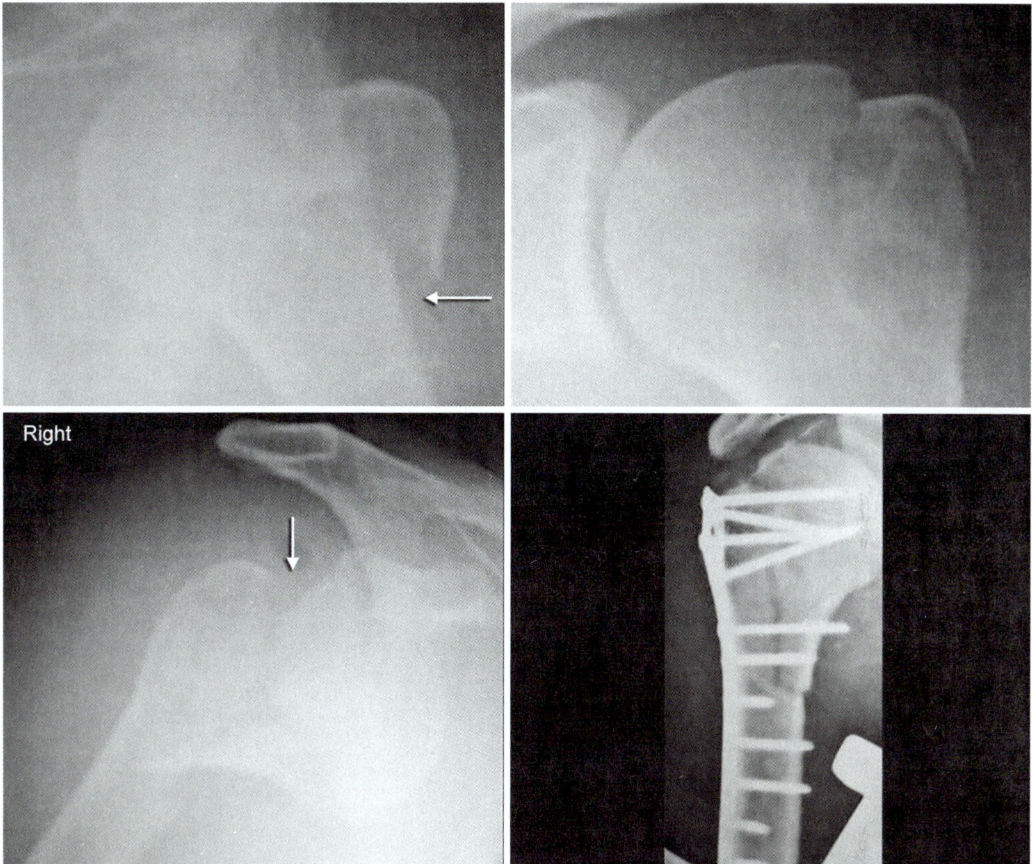

Figure 5.2 Postconvulsion bilateral fracture dislocation II

Initially active external rotation of shoulder is emphasized, especially after anterior approach. Assisted glenohumeral abduction is delayed, as the tuberosity fragment was not fixed.

- The right shoulder after ORIF with a locking plate was immobilized in a neutral shoulder splint, to keep the shoulder in neutral position: Fingers pointing straight forward. From a day after the surgery, first flexion and extension and then assisted external rotation and abduction exercises are encouraged. The surgeon should personally supervise the active and assisted mobilization of the shoulder and the elbow joint. This is important to prevent any additional injury during mobilization. It is easier to mobilize the shoulder joint, at this stage, than attempting it after 10 days. (Remember 90-90 elevation of the knee after ORIF of injury around the knee, which helps early and pain free good restoration of the knee range of motion).
- Follow up X-ray every 10 days on two occasions is carried out. Thus at the end of three weeks from surgery, further X-ray examination can be decided (Figs 5.1 and 5.2).

FEW OBSERVATIONS

Recurrent anterior dislocation shoulder is observed, following dislocation alone, but

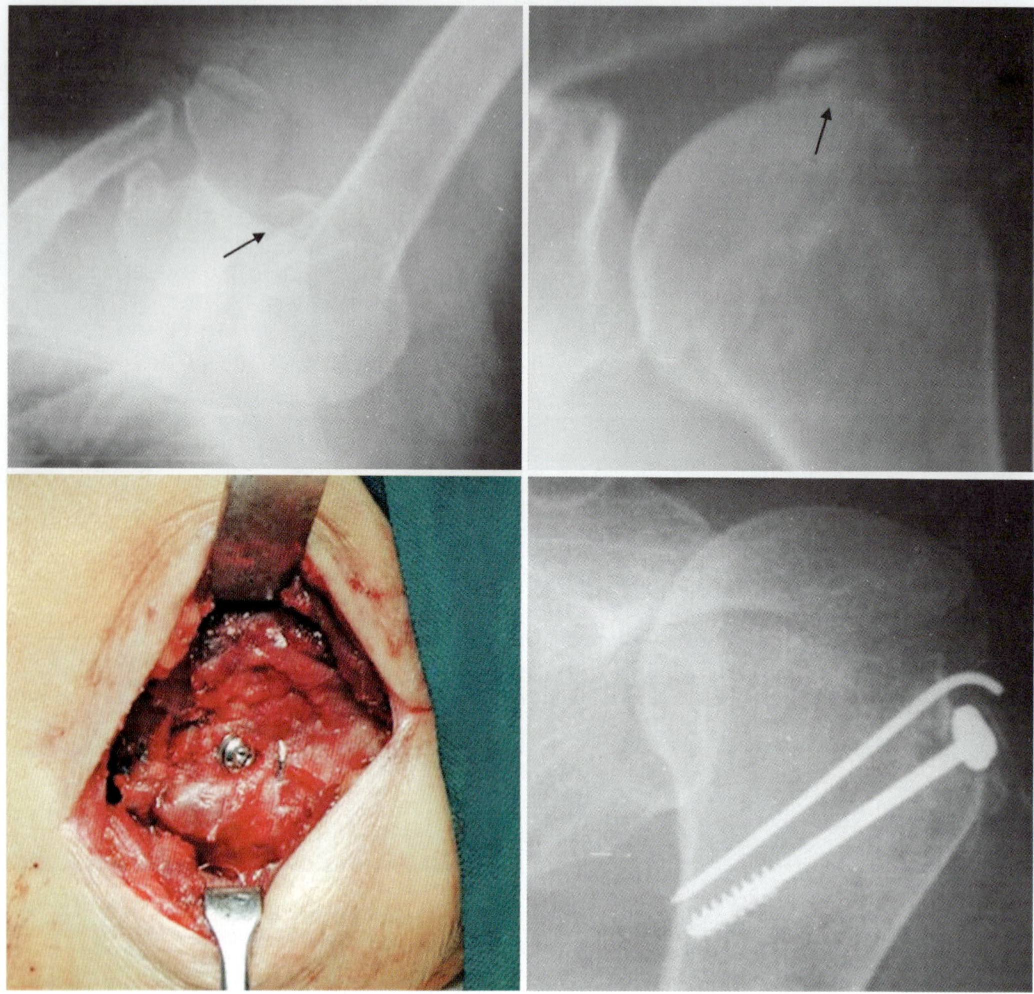

Figure 5.3 Luxatio erecta

not after a fracture dislocation. The displaced fracture of greater tuberosity, as a part of anterior fracture dislocation of the shoulder, falls back into position, after a closed reduction. To date, non-operative method for the associated fracture of greater tuberosity was carried out. Today, with availability of 'C' arm and 4 mm shaft screw, small 7 mm washer, it is possible to fix this fragment. This internal fixation can be done through a direct deltoid splitting approach, reaching the greater tuberosity. This keeps the fragment well reduced and prevents sub-acromial impingement during glenohumeral abduction.

The radiological union takes about 10 to 12 weeks.

The nature of injuries and treatment given were exactly as above.

Case 3

A patient more than 80 yrs of age, slipped and had a fall. Presented with abduction deformity in the (L) shoulder and attended the hospital with the left arm raised fully upwards. Clinically, diagnosis of Luxatio erecta type dislocation of the left shoulder was made and X-ray examination confirmed it. A fracture of the greater tuberosity was noted.

The dislocation could be reduced at bedside. Check X-ray showed a displaced fracture of the greater tuberosity, under the arch of acromion. This required open reduction and was done through a direct vertical incision, locating the level and planning the incision. Distal limit of the incision is carefully planned due to presence of the circumflex nerve (Fig. 5.3).

Case 4

A lady past 50 years of age, sustained a fall and pain and limitation of motion in the right shoulder while on a tour. She attended a local clinic, who arranged for an X-ray and shoulder immobilizer. On returning back home 2 days later, a repeat X-ray done, which indicated more than 4-part anterior fracture dislocation of the shoulder. A CT scan with a 3D reconstruction made the picture clear.

For a pain free shoulder, hemiarthroplasty of the shoulder was planned and executed (Figs 5.4 and 5.5).

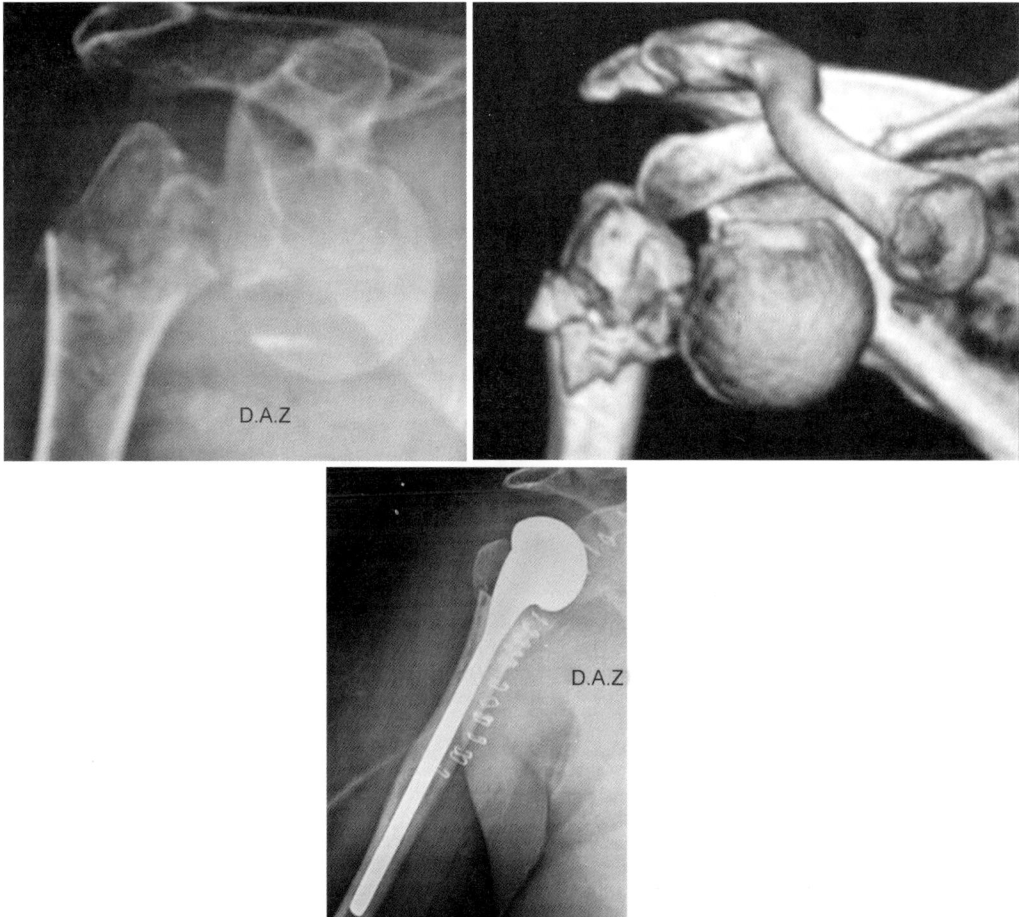

Figure 5.4 Partial shoulder replacement

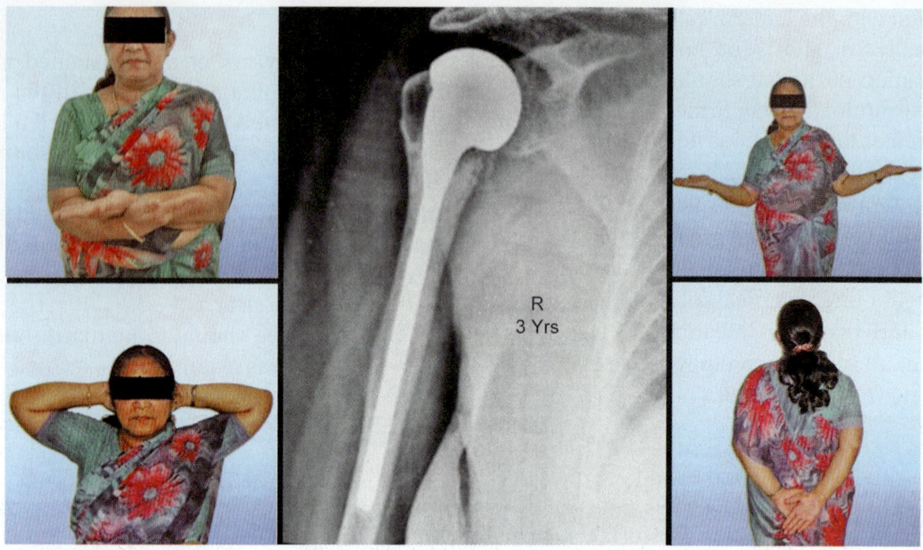

Figure 5.5 Partial shoulder replacement clinical result

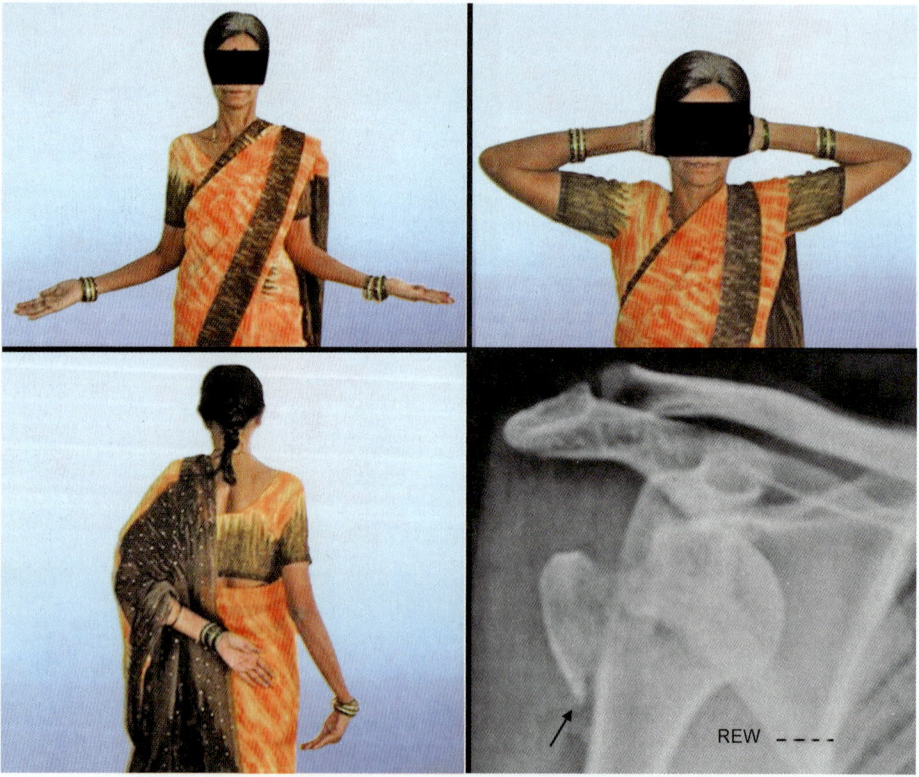

Figure 5.6 Missed anterior fracture dislocation of shoulder

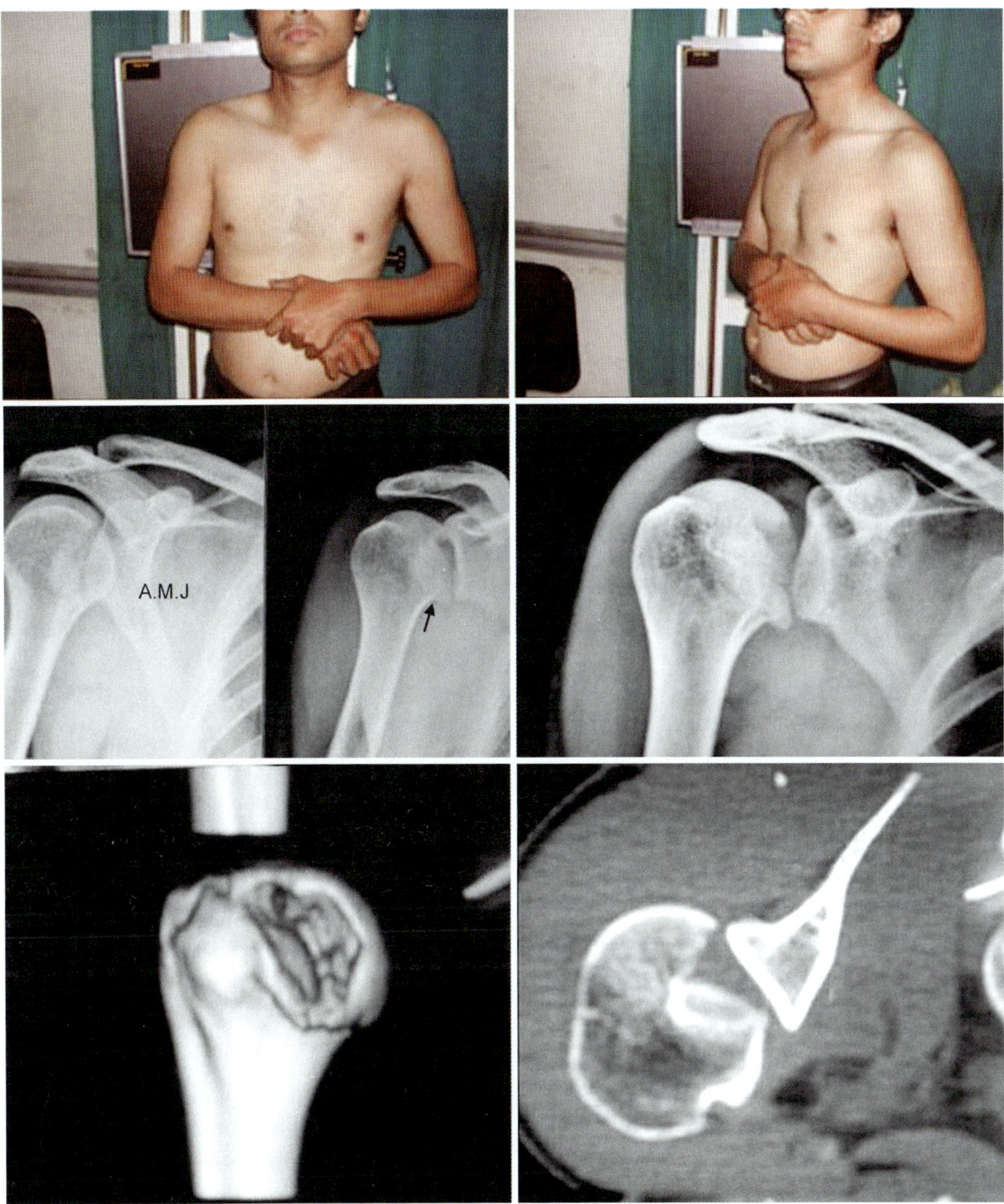

Figure 5.7 Posterior fracture dislocation of shoulder. Impaction in anterior head humerus

A lady presented to the clinic with restriction of motion of (R) shoulder for two months.

Following an electric shock to the right hand, there was forceful jerk to the right limb. As per the history given by the patient, she had attended a clinic of a family physician, who thought it to be a sprain of the shoulder. It was two months later that she consulted me for pain and some restriction of motion in the affected shoulder.

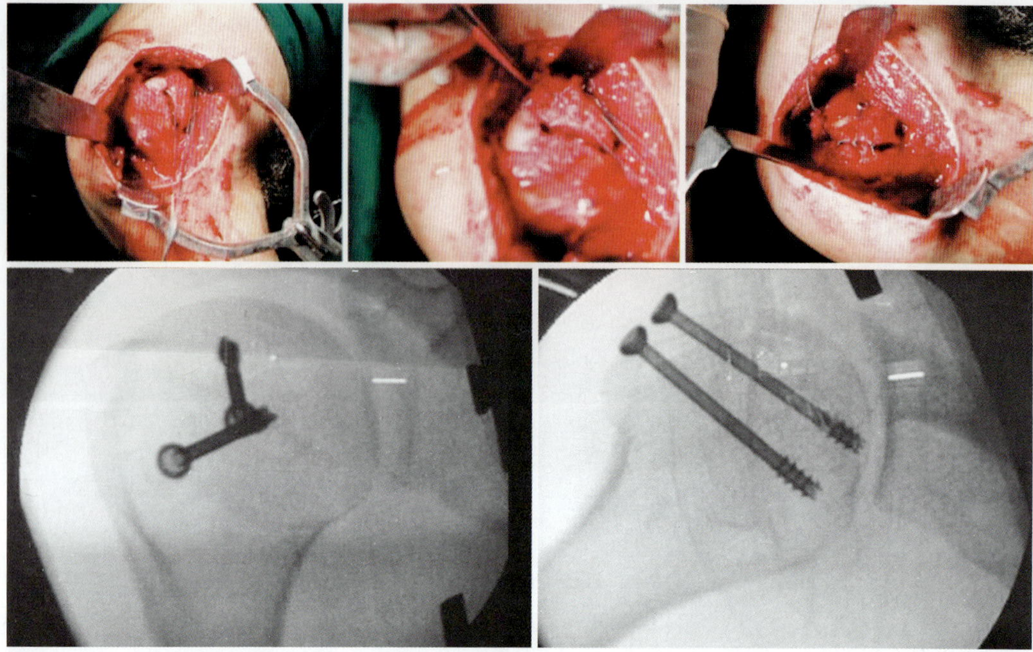

Figure 5.8 Cicac osteotomy

Clinically

- Loss of shoulder roundness
- No palpable head humerus under the deltoid
- Palpable head antero-medial to the upper end of the arm
- *Dugas test*: Positive
- Range of motion, as in illustration
- Due to the anterior dislocation of the head, internal rotation was restricted.

X-ray examination revealed anterior dislocation of head humerus with a displaced fracture of the greater tuberosity.

The patient was not keen for further tests like a CT scan and desired to accept the shoulder state as of then. Since she has nearly 70 to 80% range of motion and very little shoulder pain.

Message: After an electric shock injury, besides clinical examination, a proper radiological examination is very much necessary and essential. It is possible to achieve a successful closed reduction, which would help one to restore a good range of motion (Fig. 5.6).

A young man of 30 years sustained a jerk to the right hand, may be due to an electric shock, which he was not sure. Had severe pain and spasm in the right shoulder. The shoulder contor was less rounded than the opposite side and had associated severe spasm.

Immediately X-ray films in two positions taken personally, as shown. It showed a pear or electric bulb shape head humerus, indicating a posteriorly dislocated head humerus, with an impacted segment in the anterior part of the head of the humerus. During the position for axillary view, it was found to be unstable and extremely painful and hence any attempt to reduce it again, after the X-ray examination, was abandoned.

Soon an examination under anesthesia was done. However, any degree of internal rotation from the neutral, would redislocate it. Arm to chest brace was given and a CT examination done. As expected after the first X-ray, the scan revealed a depressed segment in the head humerus. Unless, the depression is elevated, the posterior dislocation would recur.

The impaction is on the anterior segment, which was approached by the anterior approach. The depression was identified and tagged by no 5 Ethibond sutures and was elevated.

From the lateral part of the head humerus, two canulated cancellous screws were inserted. This elevated the impacted segment. Postoperative, a neutral shoulder splint was given to prevent any internal rotation position and prevent posterior dislocation (Figs 5.7 and 5.8).

MESSAGE

- Fracture dislocation of the shoulder is a painful injury.
- As a result of convulsions, usually a bilateral injury is observed.
- A jerk to the upper limb, following an electric shock, may lead to a similar injury.
- Initial clinical assessment for stability and good radiological examination is necessary.

CHAPTER 6

Humerus Neck Fracture

After a fall in an elderly person presenting with a painful limitation of motion in the shoulder, a fracture of neck of humerus is taken, till proved otherwise.

FEW COMMON OBSERVATIONS

- After fracture of neck of humerus, almost always, a bruise appears on anteromedial arm, after 2 to 3 days. Often a person reports, because of the bruise, rather than pain and restricted range of motion. The bruise takes at least 3 weeks to disappear and any form of local cream does not hasten its resolution (Fig. 6.1).
- Fallacies in X-ray of shoulder after an injury: After a shoulder injury, when the person comes walking, a good practice is to do X-ray examination with patient standing, whenever possible.

  Even when the shoulder injury is the only injury, almost always an X-ray is taken in lying down position or standing position, with palm across the chest (i.e. internal rotation at the shoulder). This gives appearance of the shoulder as in (Fig. 6.2):

Correct radiological positioning, if possible:

The palm must face forwards, so shoulder is in neutral position and a neck of the humerus injury is less likely to be missed.

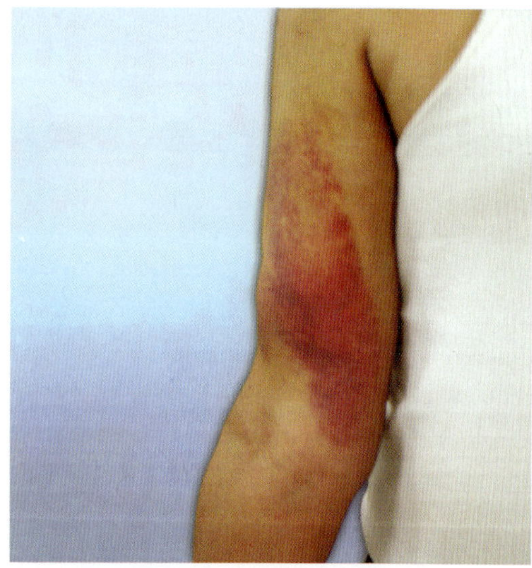

Figure 6.1 Bruise of neck of humerus

If shoulder cannot be brought to a neutral position, the patient is made to stand with the uninjured shoulder towards the X-ray tube.

Thus, the X-ray beam is so directed, that one gets a true AP view of the shoulder.

This demonstrates a fracture of greater tuberosity, missed in the other view (Fig. 6.3).

- Following any method of treatment for a fracture neck of humerus or after any injury around shoulder area, static arm exercises to

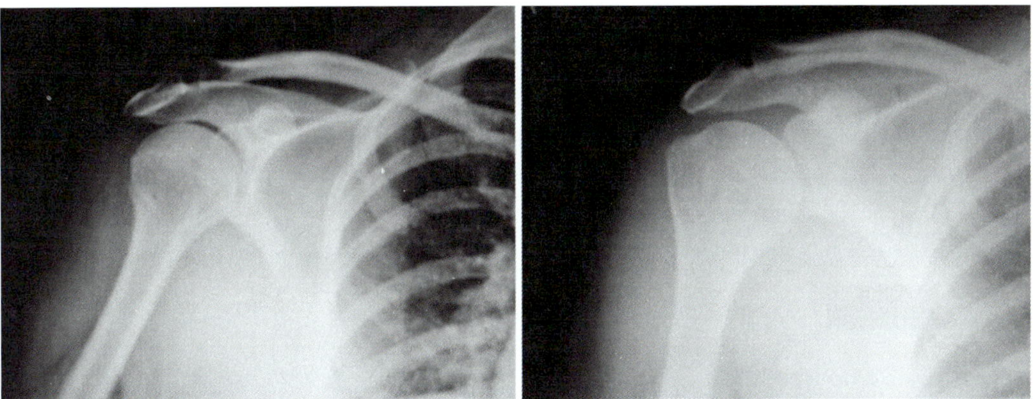

Figure 6.2 Shoulder position

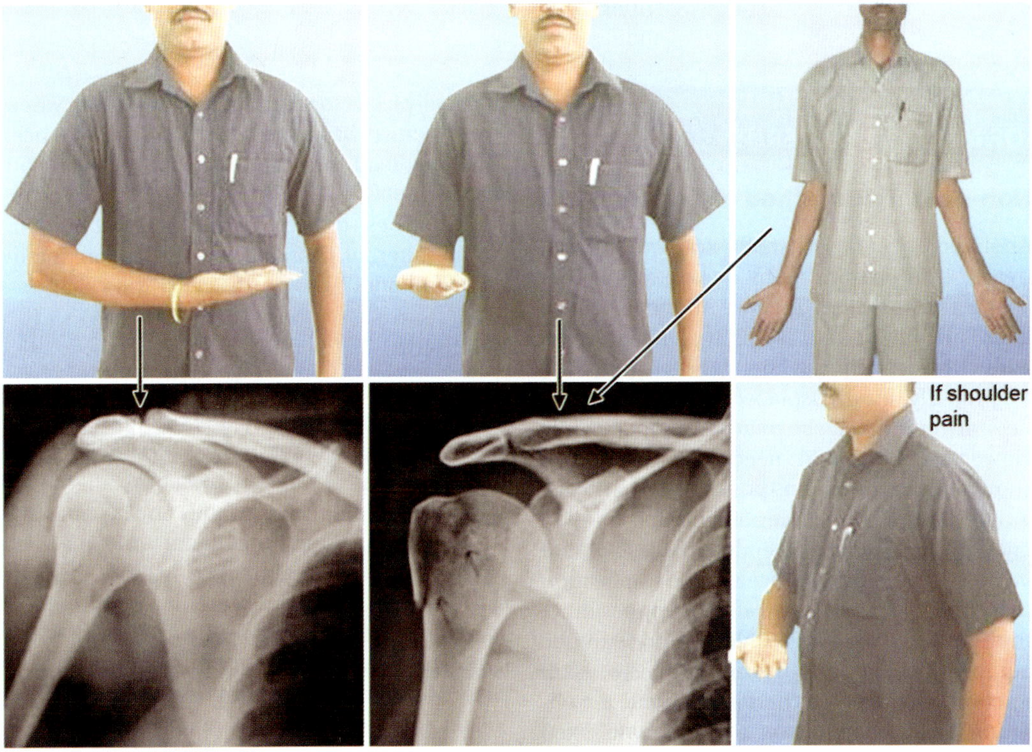

Figure 6.3 Shoulder position for X-ray

tighten the biceps and triceps are necessary. If this is not carried out, because of gravity and reduced tone in the arm muscles, the humerus sags down and X-ray of shoulder in standing gives an appearance of subluxated shoulder joint.

After static arm exercises, tone is restored well (Fig. 6.4).

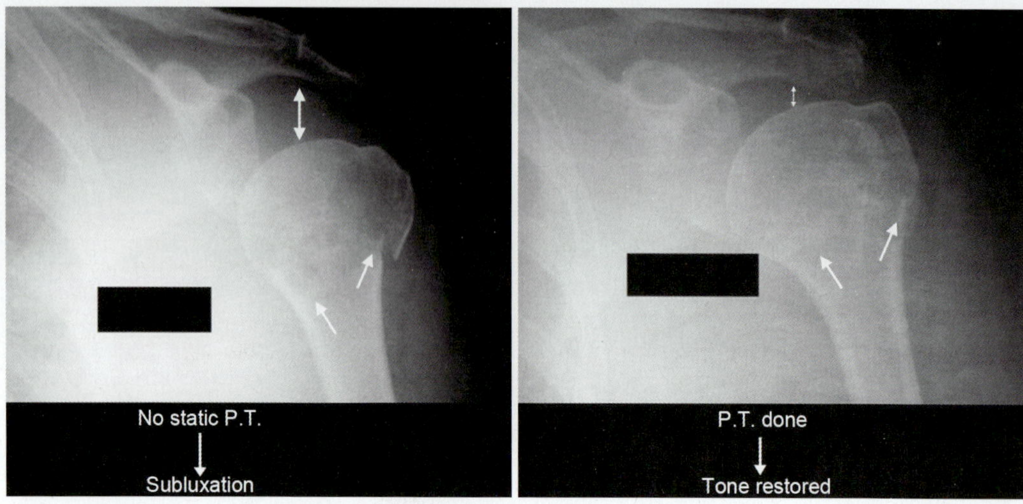

Figure 6.4 Fallacy

TWO-PART FRACTURE OF NECK OF HUMERUS

Non-operative Method of Treatment

An inter-trochanteric stable fracture can be treated non-operatively by a skeletal traction, keeping the hip in abduction. Abduction offers good alignment and stability and prevents adduction deformity at end of the treatment.

Similarly, an undisplaced 2 part fracture of neck of humerus can be treated nonoperatively. However, this would need maintenance of shoulder in abduction position for at least 3 weeks and would certainly offer a good anatomical outcome. The ideal method would be indoor care for three weeks and application of a Thomas splint for the affected upper limb. In the past, this was possible and done by the author, with good outcome. Adhesive skin traction is applied to the forearm and a well-fitting splint is put over it. Adequate fixed traction is applied. The shoulder is maintained at approx 30 deg flexion and abduction in neutral rotation. Thereby the axial compressive forces keep the fracture stable, being at right angle to the fracture line.

If a shoulder immobilizer or a shoulder sling pouch is given, with arm by the side of the chest, it usually leads to an adduction deformity when the fracture has united. In clinical practice, this may lead to some restriction of overhead movement (Fig. 6.5).

If one desires to have a full range of motion, stable internal fixation is needed to maintain the alignment.

Decision

If either the clinician or the patient or both feel that the fracture be treated nonoperatively, there has to be an understanding between the two, that should the fracture alignment change (which occurs usually in the first two to 3 weeks), then immediately the plan be changed to a surgical method without delay. If further delay is done for internal fixation, then restoration of alignment is not easy. If non-operative treatment is continued, some fibrosis may occur on the fracture surface area and may lead to delayed or fibrous union also.

THREE OR MORE PARTS IMPACTED/ MINIMALLY DISPLACED FRACTURES

Non-operative Method

After a domestic fall, such injuries are observed more in women, perhaps due to osteoporosis.

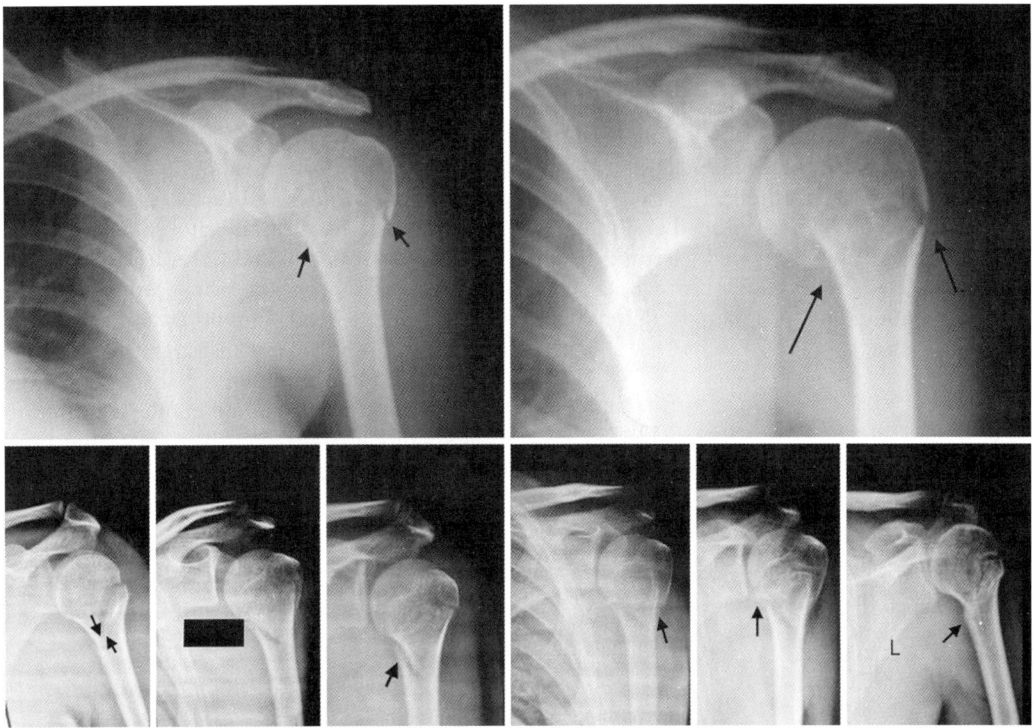

Figure 6.5 Non-operative method leads to varus

The head neck and shaft angle of the humerus: The angle with respect to the shaft and the relationship with the glenoid cavity is maintained well. The greater tuberosity, though displaced in some cases, may not cause impingement, because, usually, the greater tuberosity is tilted backwards and does not impinge the acromion. Clinically, the pain is less in comparison to the multiple part fracture. The patient is also able to some active movements of the shoulder joint. This indicates a possibility of impaction at the fracture site. In such a situation, if one is considering a non-operative treatment, the fracture should not be reduced, or otherwise, it will get disimpacted and lose the stability.

A CT scan with 3D reconstruction for further study and evaluation is advised, but often the patient refused the scan and opted for non-operative method of treatment and was prepared to accept, whatever may be the outcome.

Management

- Can be managed by an arm to chest belt and a sling.
- Immediate exercises for grip and static arm exercises are started. Isometric exercises for the biceps and triceps help to maintain the fracture alignment. It also helps to maintain the head of humerus in the glenoid cavity well. If this is not followed, the head of humerus tends to subluxate inferiorly. Once this happens, due to loss of muscle tone, more efforts are needed to restore it back.
- The arm to chest belt can be removed for sponge bath and reapplied.
- Appropriate dress, going over the shoulder and arm is needed, putting the arm through any dress sleeve is avoided to help maintain the limb position, close to the chest. Care of the axilla is taught to prevent skin chafing.
- Follow-up X-ray is done every week to confirm that position is maintained well.

- At the end of two weeks, belt is removed for bath and in the evenings. On these occasions, gradual, gentle and assisted mobilization of the shoulder is started. The external rotation exercises are begun. This is initially done under observation of the clinician. No forced mobilization is permitted.
- *Further*: When pain is reduced and fracture position is maintained well, circumduction is started.
- The rehabilitation program is tailored for each person.

Discussion

In the young, the healing potential is good.

In the elderly, primary osteoporosis exists. The head fragment is small and even a locking plate may not have adequate hold on the head fragment, which is like an egg shell. Besides, with this non-operative method, the blood supply to small fragments is left undisturbed which contributes towards good healing within time. If one had chosen and carried out anatomical reduction and a locking plate fixation, one wonders what would be the viability of the head of humerus and how much hold the screw ends wound have in the bone. Bone grafting would fill the voids and help the healing. However, the hold of the screw tips on the small egg shell-like fragment of the head humerus cannot be altered (Figs 6.6A to C).

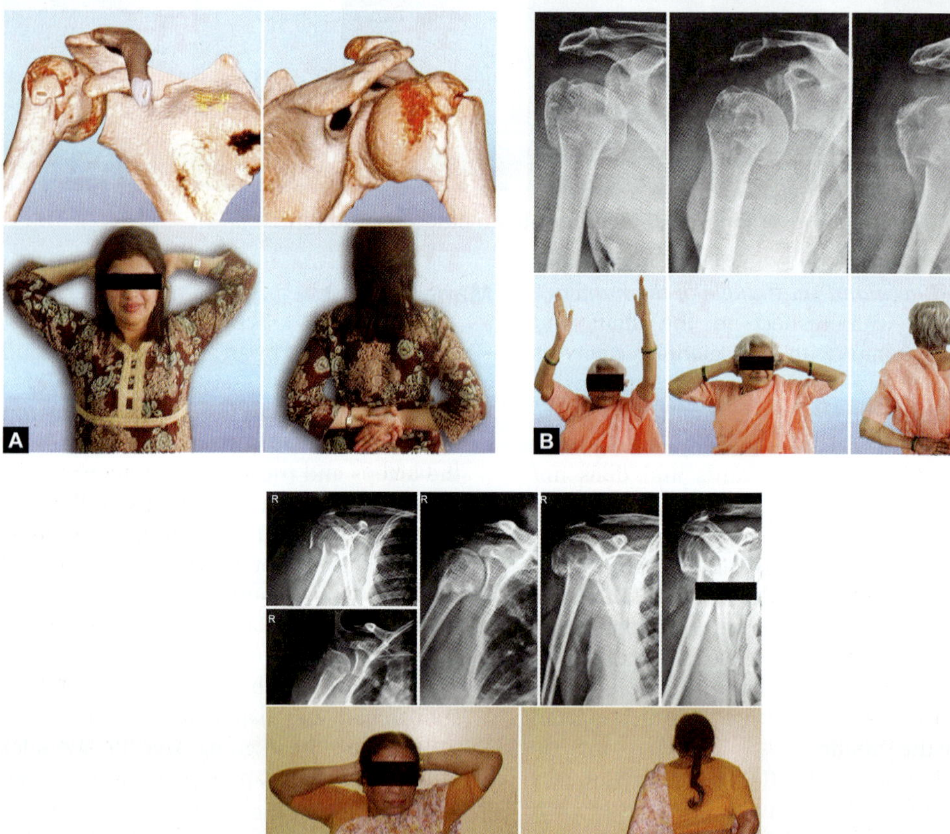

Figures 6.6A to C Non-operative method

Having seen the fracture pattern in above cases, one wonders:

In above cases:

1. How much more stability would LCP have offered?
2. How early mobilization could be started compared to the non-operative method?
3. How much more range would have achieved with internal fixation?
4. In osteoporotic bones, there is always a likelihood of screw pullout.
5. How much more benefit would partial shoulder replacement would have offered?

A locking screw has no deep buttress threads (like 4 mm cancellous screw) and the hold on the bone is mainly due to the obliquely set screws at 50 deg, which prevent its pullout.

Operative Methods and Rationale

On arrival, if the fracture is angulated more than 30 deg, then a definitive surgical treatment is advised and explained.

In Pre-locking Plate Era

Implants available in the recent past:

- 1/3 tubular plate was not strong enough, while 12 mm plate was rather too thick. In the later, only the end screw hole accepted a 6.5 mm screw.
- In a 1/3 tubular plate, it is possible to insert 4 mm cancellous screws in the head. However, due to the non-locking mechanics, some toggling was possible. This is because there was no mechanical anchor and angular stability between the screw head and the plate (Fig. 6.7).
- Some form of internal fixation was necessary. In presence of osteoporosis, screw pullout is known to occur. \`C\` arm was available. During such an era, when \`C\` arm was available, but locking plates were yet to be invented, percutaneous K-wire fixation gave a fairly good outcome.

LOCKING PLATE

It is a good addition of a long needed implant for proximal humerus. Perhaps proximal humerus locking plate is the most used implant of all the locking plates.

- Anatomical and pre-contoured plate.
- Plate thickness is less, so impingement under the acromial arch is less likely.
- The wide proximal end of the plate is a square and is adequate to accept 4 to 5 screws.
- The proximal locking holes are set at 50 deg angle, so once inserted in the head humerus and locked, in the plate, screw pullout is less likely, due to the angular stability achieved.
- Presence of holes for stabilizing K wires is an excellent addition. This helps to maintain formal reduction and stability. The fracture fragments are reduced and are appropriately assembled and a plate is laid over it. Provisional stability is achieved by inserting few K wires through the holes provided at the border of the plate. The position and direction of the holes is such that the K wires do not come in the way of screws to be inserted later.

Technique suggested for the 3.5 mm locking screw insertion:

- For the 3.5 mm locking screws, drill bit of 2.8 mm diameter is recommended. It should be used to make a track for only the outer ¼ th part of the expected length of a screw. The drill bit is removed and a 2 mm K-wire is used to make rest of the track. Thus the distant track is narrower in the depth of the head of humerus. Now, when a self-tapping and locking 3.5 mm screw is inserted, it enters the track well and the screw shaft gets a better purchase in the head of humerus.
- I feel the 3.5 mm locking screw needs to be modified. It should have a screw with buttress thread design like 4 mm shaft screw. I predict, this difference between the core and thread diameter would come in the near future. In addition, the buttress threads would offer a better hold in the bone.

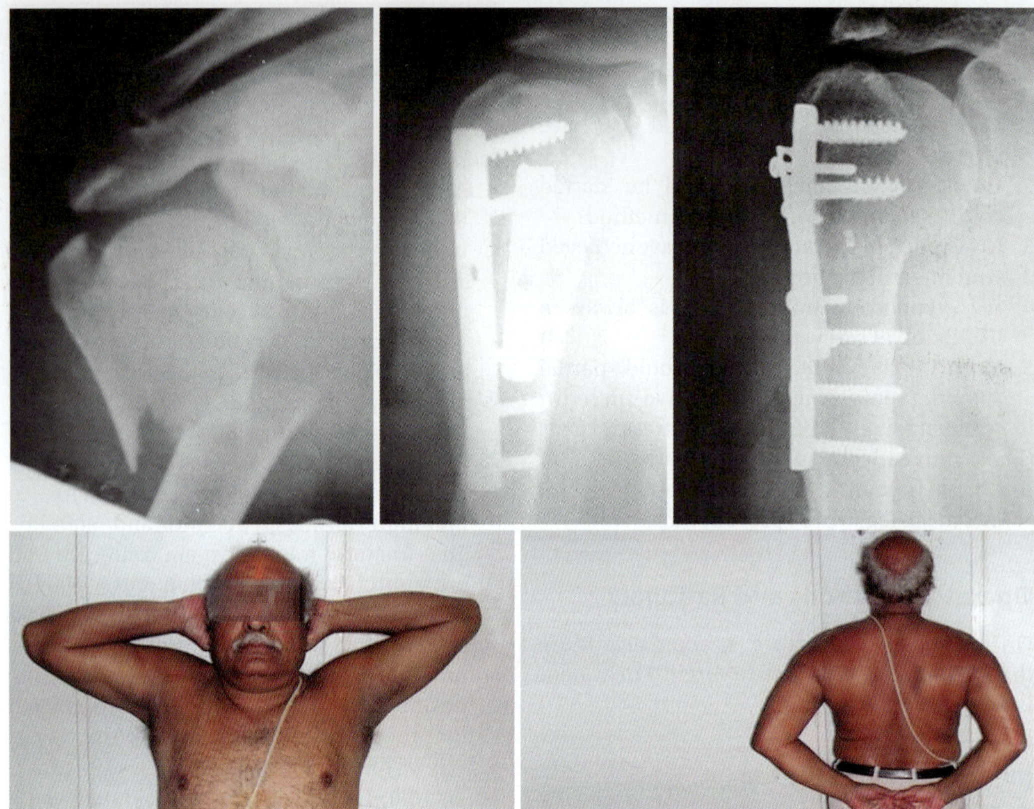

Figure 6.7 ORIF with 1/3 tubular and 12 mm plates

Such a design for the shaft and a locking head would have a benefit of both a good hold in a soft bone and angular stability (Figs 6.8A and B).

Final clinical result:

- 90% range should be taken as an excellent result.
- Some degree of loss of terminal external rotation and external rotation with abduction, is a common observation.

THREE OR MORE PARTS FRACTURE OF NECK OF HUMERUS: DISPLACED

Internal Fixation

Displaced fractures do need internal fixation to achieve stability, early mobilization, union in expected duration and good final range of motion.

When

- Displacement is severe, with chances of soft tissue intervention,
- There is a likelihood of acromial impingement, open reduction and stable internal fixation is necessary.
- Care needs to be taken to have correct rotational alignment during reduction and provisional fixation prior to final internal fixation. Often there is cominution in the anterior part of the fracture area and the fracture tends to settle in an internal rotation position. If this is accepted, there would be limitation of external rotation and thus abduction as well, as an end result.

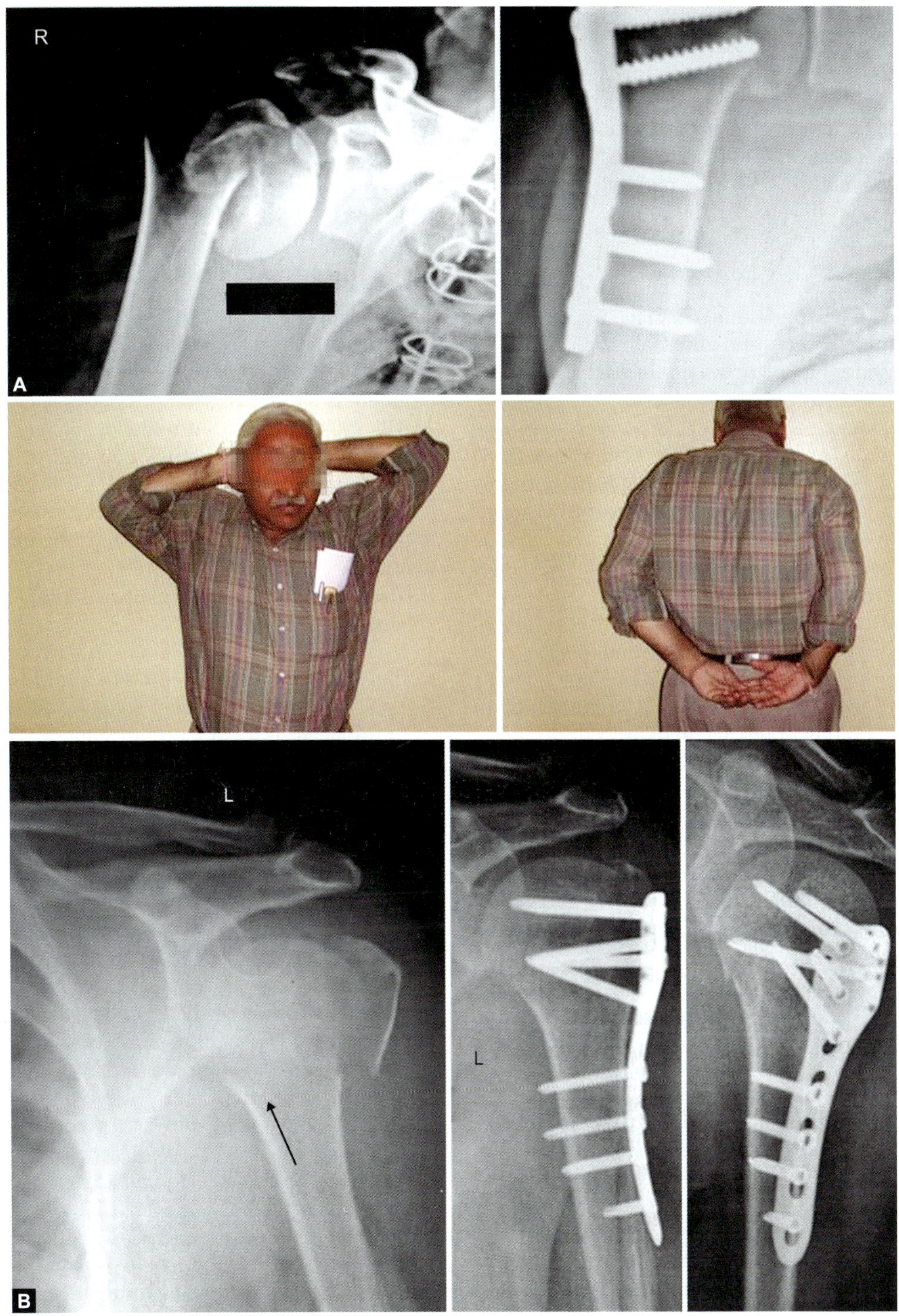

Figures 6.8A and B Locking plate

- Following a displaced fracture, local tissue reaction and swelling is likely to be severe. If the case presents with huge swelling, it is preferable to wait for a few days. In elderly patients who are on oral anti-diabetic and anti-platelet drugs, one needs some time to stabilize BSL with parental insulin and reduce the effect of the later.

Decision

If it is planned and agreed to carry out, open reduction and internal fixation, still, a consent must be obtained for partial shoulder replacement.

Should patient agree for surgery and one attempts to do ORIF, then as the fracture is reduced, the small fragment of head humerus may get separated and chances of avascular necrosis increase. This may need change of decision to carry out a partial shoulder replacement.

(However, as seen by the clinical results of non-operative method, the end results of a non-operative method are at par or perhaps better compared to the final range of motion with a shoulder replacement procedure).

Under anesthesia the position of the shoulder with respect to the operation table, has to be different as per the procedure to be done.

With gentle traction, the shoulder is examined under a "C" arm and a decision made as to whether ORIF or replacement is to be carried out.

Position of the Patient on the Operation Table

For either internal fixation or hemi-shoulder replacement, position of the table and equipment arrangement should be as in surgery for fracture of lateral/4 clavicle (Described elsewhere).

If internal fixation is planned, then the patient is slightly moved towards the midline of the table, so the 'C' arm image can be clear and the side metal bars of the table do not come in the way of X-ray beam. A short 8 wide wooden plank is tucked under the shoulder and coming out obliquely, to support the elbow, is a useful aid.

If replacement of the head humerus is planned, the patient is moved slightly lateral, till the edge of the table. This helps to extend the shoulder, so the elbow can be taken below the table top, for insertion of the prosthesis.

Mechanics and Reduction Technique

The proximal fragment in a fracture of neck humerus is a short lever arm with osteoporosis and hence the hold of screws on the proximal fragment is rather poor.

Till 2004 (prior to introduction of locking plate for proximal humerus), one had to use available implants. If the bone stock was good, it worked well. Often one had to take recourse to tension band wire to stabilize few fragments together.

- The normal retroversion of head of humerus needs to be maintained.
- In extrusion fracture of the tuberosities, they are reduced back into place and held by K wires. Then the shaft is finally aligned to the head. If the fracture is reduced, with the shaft humerus in internal rotation, in the end result, the external rotation is restricted and is an important setback to final range of motion. It is observed that in spite of good anatomical reduction visually and radiologically, still the external rotation remains restricted, as seen at the final outcome and hence the precaution needs to be exercised.
- The greater tuberosity is often displaced posteriorly. This is difficult to visualize on table. It may not be appreciated in a `C` arm image, but becomes more visible on follow up X-ray. However, if one has a preoperative CT scan with a 3D reconstruction, the fragment is clearly seen on the scan and one should look for it on table.
- How to bring the posteriorly displaced greater tuberosity fragment in its place ?

An Ethibond suture with a needle is used to take two independent sutures through the greater tuberosity. These two sutures are held and with traction and gentle manipulation, the fragment is brought anteriorly (Dr Rahul Damle).

Having pulled the posterior fragment forwards, a K-wire is inserted from posterior side, through the intact skin, about 4 to 5 cm posterior to the incision, through the reduced greater tuberosity fragment and then in the head of humerus. This helps to stabilize the head fragments, on which an LCP can be fixed (Dr Hemant Shirali). Having thus reconstructed the head of humerus, the shaft alignment is confirmed and one can proceed to fix the plate. The K wires inserted for provisional fixation, through the skin are later removed.

A few clinical examples:

There was comminution of a large 3rd fragment. To fill the voids and have good contact opposition, bone grafts were placed medially, intramedullary and on the surface of the bone. The large fragment was stabilized by interfragmentary screw fixation. This was followed by locking plate fixation.

Uneventful recovery. The lateral X-ray view depicts how the upper screws cross at 50 deg, adding to stability of fixation and prevention of pullout (Fig. 6.9).

A decade ago, the available indigenous implant screws had more diameter. Now the 3.5 mm screws are available (Fig. 6.10).

COMMENT ON BONE GRAFTING

With absolute stability after a locking plate, there is no micromotion in the fragments, to stimulate callus formation. The bone union is at bone contact points only. Hence to create good contact opposition, one needs to add bone grafts. Bone grafting helps to fill the voids, good bridging across the fracture area and fracture union in an expected duration.

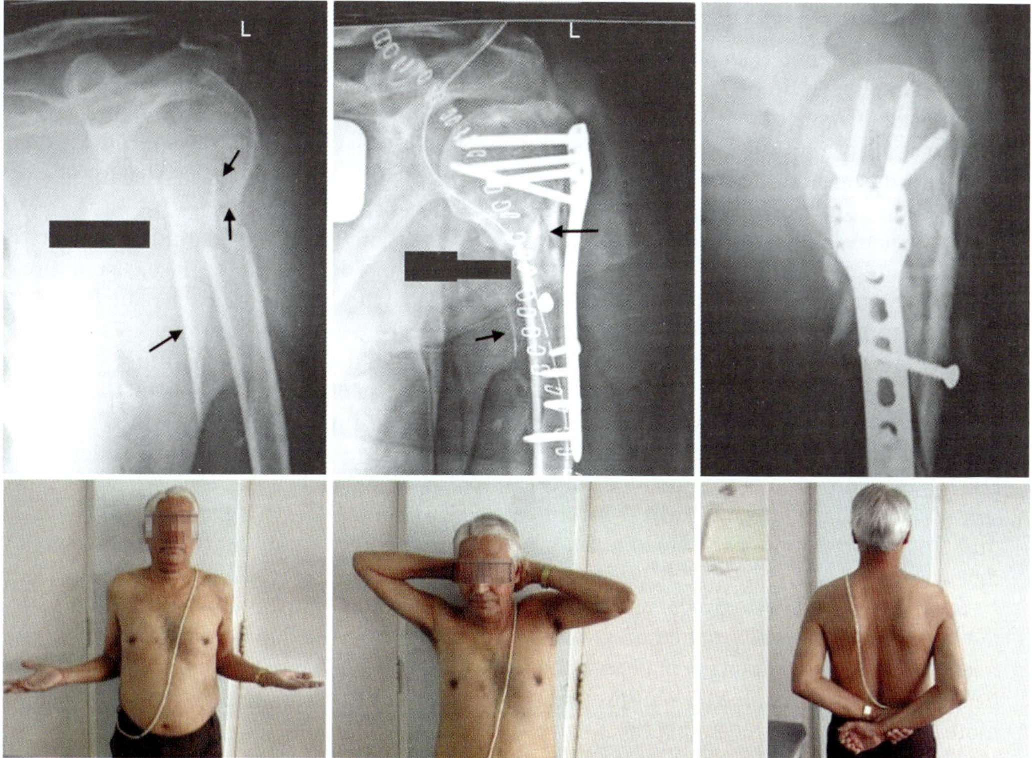

Figure 6.9 LCP and bone grafts

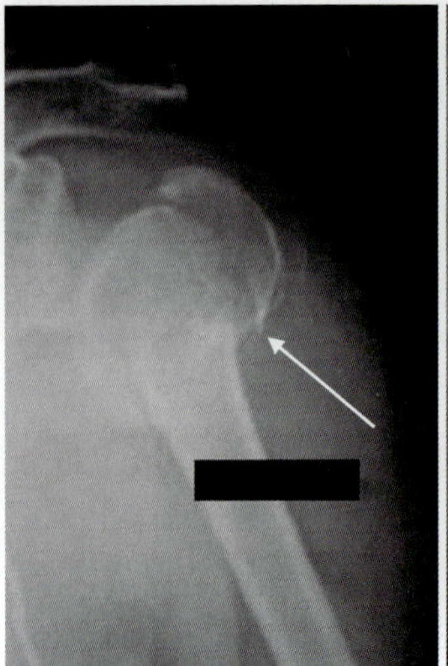
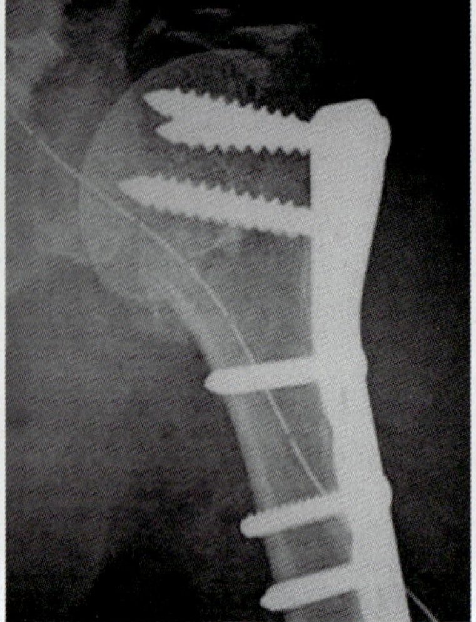
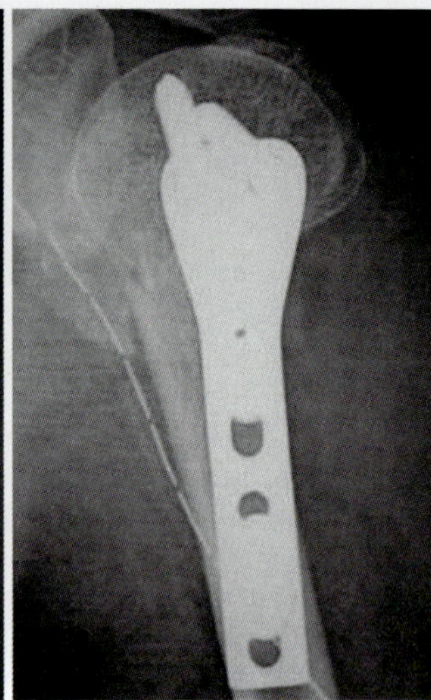

Figure 6.10 Indigenous implant

STEPS OF BONE GRAFTING AND PLATE FIXATION

When in doubt, draping is so planned that the donor site iliac crest is draped and ready.

- A provisional reduction is done to assess the steps of fixation. Iliac crest cancellous grafts are taken and laid in the medullary cavity at the comminuted area and possibly intramedullary and on the endosteal surface of humerus.
- Once the fragments are opposed, then locking plate is laid over the bone ends and held by few stabilizing K wires in the head and neck area. The lower part of the plate is held opposed to the bone by an assistant's fingers or a medium self-centering forceps. Use of this forceps may demand erasing soft tissue at that place, medially from the humerus, to be able to insert tip of a jaw of the forceps.

  Having thus stabilized the assembly, the humerus is internally rotated, to see the relation of the upper part of the plate with the head. At times, one may need to slide the plate more posteriorly (after changing the K-wire placement and loosening the self-centering forceps). This step allows the posterior screw to be placed more posteriorly on the head of the humerus. This screw passes from posterior to anterior obliquely, to hold the anterior part of the subchondral head. This step facilitates ease of insertion of the sleeve in the posterior most hole on the plate and subsequent steps. While placing the proximal end of the plate, one confirms that the greater tuberosity is brought under it.
- The assembly is checked under `C` arm. If one finds that at some place, usually just distal to the fracture area, the plate is slightly away from the bone, then a 3.5 mm non-locking screw is fixed first at this level. This hole is usually the upper hole on the shaft of the plate. The screw, while finally tightened, brings the plate and the bone together. It also helps to achieve a good anatomical alignment. Though, it is said that LCP is an internal fixator and there is no necessity to have plate in contact with the bone, I am comfortable with the above technique. I feel, though the titanium implants can tolerate stresses, why not attempt to reduce the stress on the screw shaft by achieving good plate to bone contact?
- *The locking screws in the head of humerus*: It is often difficult to have a screw of precise

length as per the depth gauge reading. The screws are in 5 mm increments. It is safer to take 3 mm shorter than indicated by a depth gauge. The screw holes are at angle and confer good angular stability. After passing each screw, better to check under `C` arm. And after passing of 2 screws, rotate the shoulder to confirm, there is no grating palpable, indicating, the screw tip has not penetrated the head cartilage. If unfortunately a screw penetrates the head humerus and is detected in post-operative period, to remove exactly that irritating screw only, is a job by itself.

On a few occasions: One finds on table 'C' arm and X-ray image, that the screw tips are quite away from the articular surface of the head of humerus. However, during follow up, one finds that few screw tips are beyond the articular surface. I feel, this 'Medialization' phenomenon does occur. It is due to fracture morphology at the lateral part of the head, local crushing, so that the shaft with the plate moves medially, till a stable contact is found by the fracture fragments. (I would compare this with auto-medialization seen in an intertrochanteric fracture after an anatomical reduction and fixation with a DHS). Hence, it is preferable to keep the screw length in the proximal fragment rather shorter than indicated by the depth gauge.

I have seen this happening, in spite of the angular geometry of the plate hole design. Intra-operative and some postoperative even 3 views did not reveal this and it was only after a few months that some X-ray view demonstrated this. It is important to prevent this, because should a screw tip irritate the glenoid, to identify exactly, which screw is responsible, is quite difficult on an X-ray film. Even if one can localize it, one wonders if just that screw can be removed percutaneously using a 'C' arm. It may be safer to reopen the proximal humerus again, rather than removing another screw.

- On the shaft of humerus, 3 or even 2 bicortical and 2 unicortical locking screws do offer adequate stability. The rest holes may be left as such. This depends on fracture morphology, built of the patient, associated injuries and load on the fracture site, etc.

POSTOPERATIVE CARE

- Local dressing and I prefer to have an arm to chest elastic belt. This helps to reduce the movements in the shoulder and reduce pain.
- A pillow support below the elbow helps to keep the elbow elevated and add to the comfort.

After the patient has recovered from anesthesia, a shoulder splint (a metal or a plastic padded belt) round the waist, with a support for the elbow, to keep the shoulder in neutral position, is added. This device needs to be kept ready pre-operatively and explained to the patient well, so its acceptance in the recovery period is easy.

- The drain is removed at 24 to 48 hrs, as per the volume drained.
- The shoulder splint keeps the shoulder joint in a neutral position. From here onwards, it is easy to regain further external rotation movement.
- Active exercises for grip/static exercises for the arm and gentle mobilization at the earliest, would help to restore a good range of movement.
- Delay in active mobilization of the shoulder, leads to adhesions and stiffness around the shoulder. The therapist needs to be trained, regarding how much assistance to be given and passive force to be applied. In the illustrated case, which came for X-ray opinion after a complication, one noticed that in this patient with diabetes, the mobilization was started three weeks after the surgery and during assisted mobilization, developed a fracture through the distal hole! This example is an eye opener to use the shoulder splint and practice early mobilization and that no excess force is to be used (Fig. 6.11).

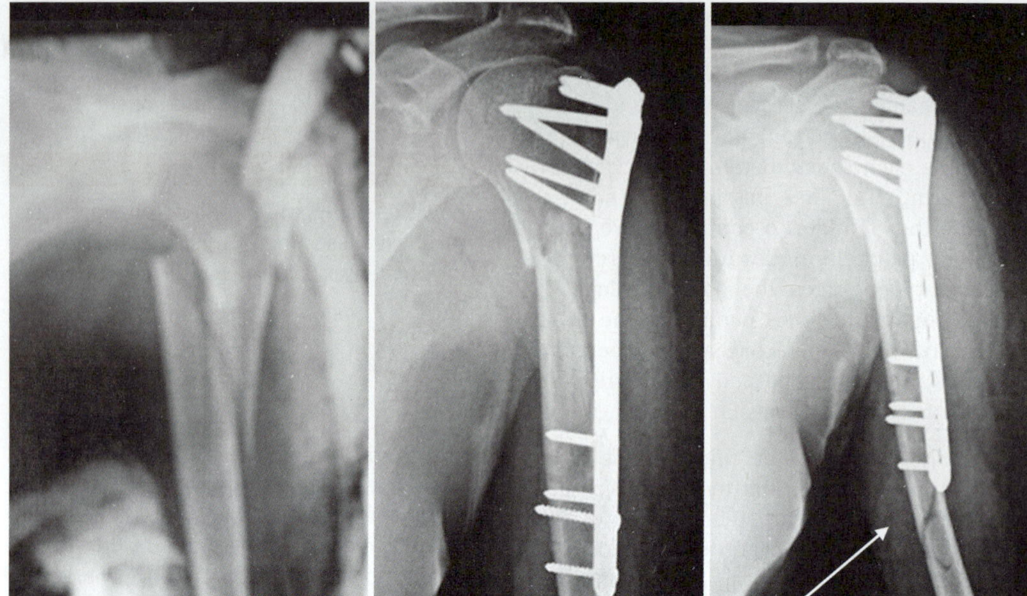

Figure 6.11 Fracture during mobilization

NON-UNION OF FRACTURE OF NECK OF HUMERUS

Problem in Juxta-articular Non-Union

The proximal fragment is a small fragment: In a case of un-united fracture of neck of humerus, there is a likelihood that the head fragment may not be mobile within the glenoid cavity and glenohumeral joint might have become stiff. One should do an examination under a 'C' arm to know the mobility of the head humerus within the glenoid cavity. If the head is found to be mobile in the glenoid, then it is safe to carry out above procedure, without a fear of screw cut out, when the arm is mobilized. If the head is not mobile within the glenoid, one should review the case again, whether internal fixation is possible and worthwhile.

A case report: An elderly person sustained a fracture of neck of a humerus and was treated by an arm to chest strapping by a surgeon, perhaps not trained in the field of orthopedics and traumatology. At the end of about 4 weeks, the fracture continued to be un-united and reported to me with only AP view of the shoulder. I, therefore, advised another view, which showed a displaced fracture, without bone to bone contact. By this time, the bones had become osteoporotic and I did not have an assured method of internal fixation, which will hold the bones well and lead to union (Pre-locking plate era).

In the meanwhile, unfortunately patient had a fracture of the tibia and was managed successfully. Thereafter he reported and requested to do something for the non-union in the neck of humerus, which by then had made the bone ends atrophic and rounded. Just then the proximal humerus locking plate was introduced. Osteosynthesis using this implant and bone grafting was done. The fracture united.

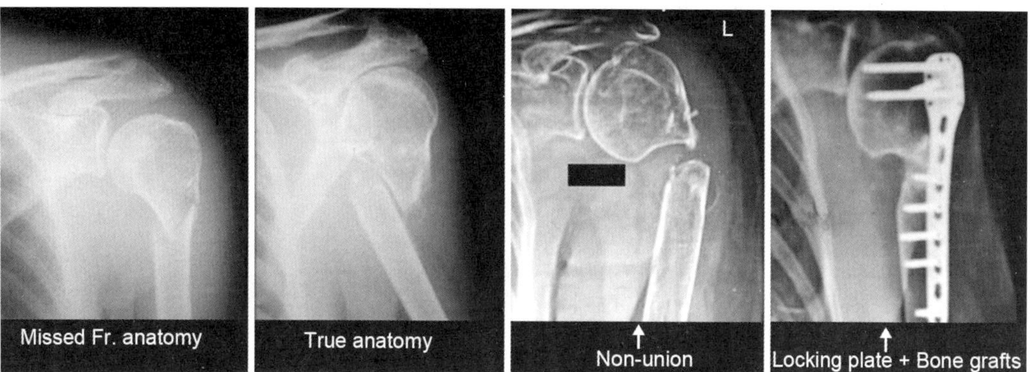

Figure 6.12 Nonunion fracture of neck of humerus

If one observes the fracture geometry, the later version of the plate, the proximal humerus internal locking system (PHILOS) would have been ideal, as it has an oblique, so called 'Calcar' screw, which offers more angular stability (Fig. 6.12).

CHAPTER

7

Humerus Shaft Interlock Nailing

INTERLOCKING NAILING IN HUMERUS

In any long bone, intramedullary nail and extra-medullary plate as a fixation devices, have their advantage and disadvantages. One needs to consider fracture morphology, energy level of injury, associated diseases, patient expectations and what is expected from the treatment.

CASE 1: PALLIATIVE SURGERY TO ALLEVIATE PAIN

In an elderly patient with malignancy and metastases, leading to pathological fractures, aim is to offer stability to the fracture and thus relief from the fracture pain. The necessary treatment for the primary malignancy was already given and we are expected only to offer some relief in pain (Fig. 7.1).

CASE 2: LONG OBLIQUE FRACTURE OF UPPER/3 AREA

In long oblique fractures, a procedure of closed nailing may not offer good contact opposition, which a plate fixation can offer.

If such a fracture is treated by a locking nail by a closed method, anatomical reduction is not always achieved and perhaps a delayed or a non-union may occur.

Hence, in a long oblique fracture, if one observes that good contact opposition is not obtained after passing a nail, the nail needs to be removed and an open nailing is done. A successful closed nailing is usually achieved in a transverse or a spiral fracture with good contact opposition, than an oblique fracture. If a successful closed nailing is achieved, but good contact opposition is not obtained, one needs to carry out an open reduction. Fracture is exposed and reduction is achieved by holding the fracture ends together with a reduction forceps and then the nail is advanced further. If open reduction is also not able to offer a good contact opposition, one may change the method of internal fixation from a nail to a plate in the same sitting. Such a situation can come across any surgeon, especially when the medullary cavity is quite wide and the fracture site is away from the mid/3 level. Therefore, necessary instrumentation and implants for plate fixation must be available in every case, when IM nailing is planned.

A closed interlocking nailing was done elsewhere. However, reduction was not anatomical and there was no adequate bone to bone contact. Bone grafting and de-rotation plate fixation lead to union (Fig. 7.2).

CASE 3: SEGMENTAL LONG OBLIQUE FRACTURE

In a segmental fracture, a successful closed nailing is a better choice, because it preserves the

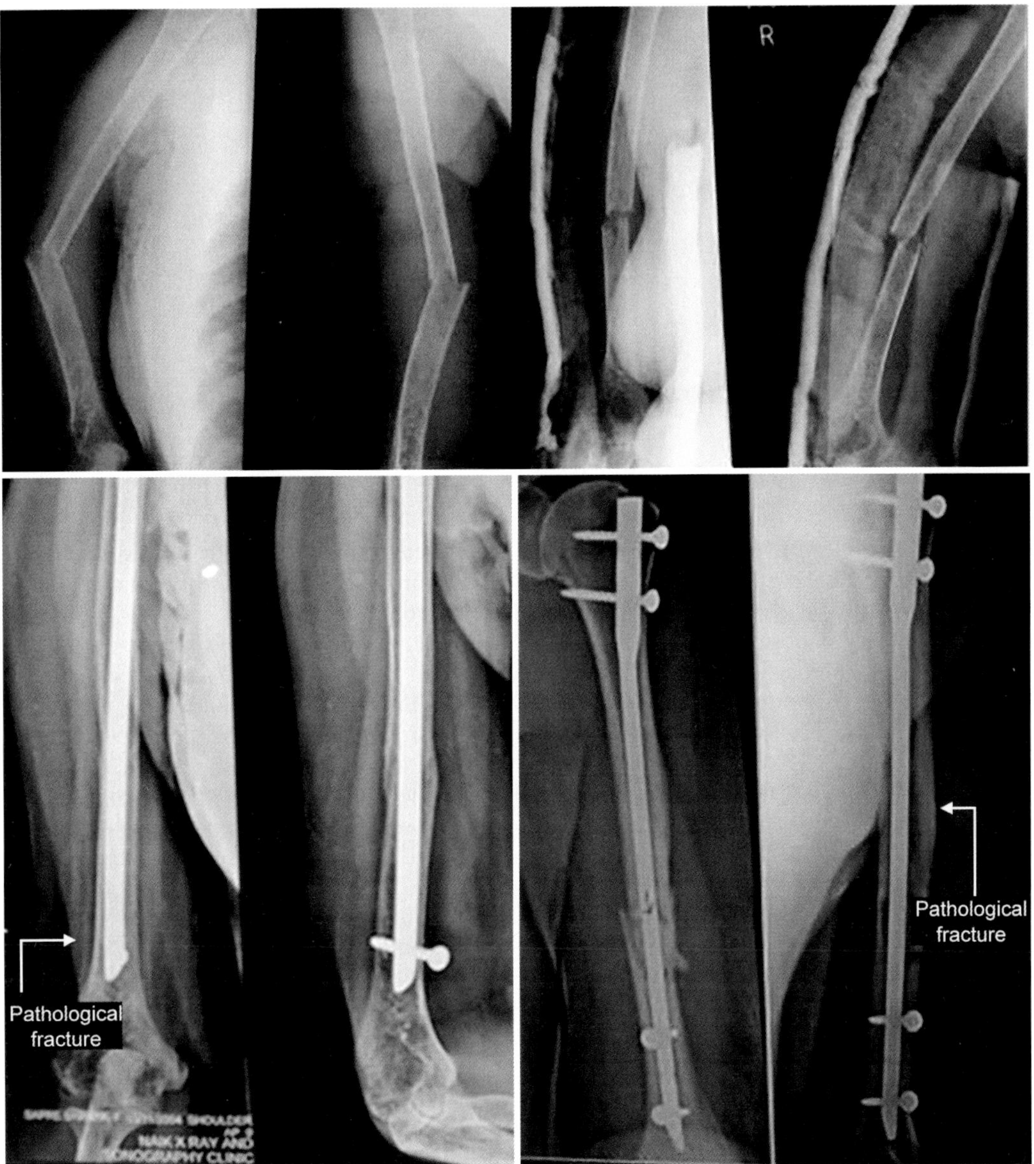

Figure 7.1 Pathological fracture

soft tissues, especially to the middle fragment. Of the two fractures, the transverse or short oblique fracture has a better chance of good contact opposition, leading to good healing. However, a long oblique fracture usually does not achieve a good contact opposition. The undisplaced upper fracture united, while the lower oblique fracture, which was not well-opposed by the closed method, did not unite. Decortication, bone grafting and addition of a

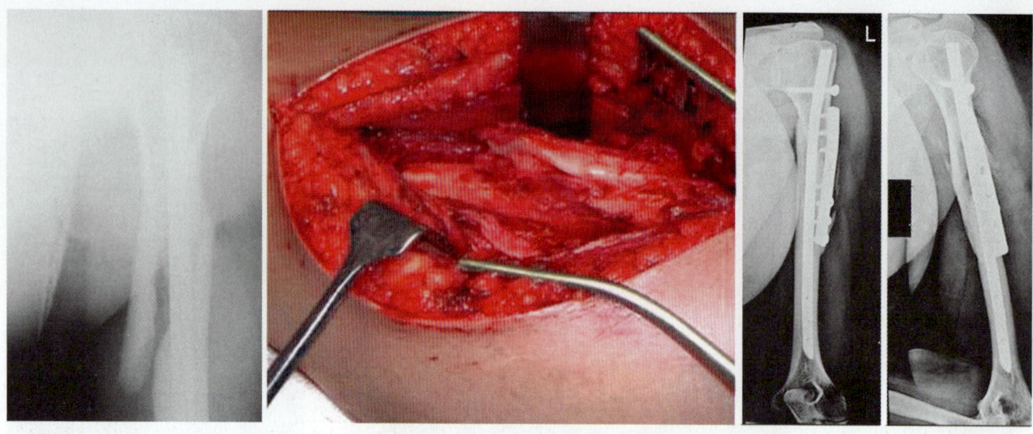

Figure 7.2 Oblique fracture

de-rotation plate lead to a good consolidation (This was prior to locking plate era).

With this experience to credit, in a next such a case, one would choose to do a plate fixation by an open technique, which permits IFS as well (Fig. 7.3).

The medullary cavity of humerus is not quite wide at the lower end, to accept a nail of adequate diameter in relation with the length of the bone.

- Besides, reaming in the distal segment is tricky. The distal humeral cortex being quite hard and strong, one is concerned about possible splintering. Besides, the medullary cavity in most humeri is narrow, considering its length and cortical thickness.
- In a humerus with a cavity having a narrow diameter, a nail of small diameter has to be passed. In a nail with a 7 or 8 mm. diameter, the distal locking screw is of a smaller diameter. With such a narrow distal locking screw, the interlock nail construct cannot adequately resist torsional stresses, to achieve a stable fixation.
- In a fracture at lower third level, with a narrow medullary cavity, the nail segment length beyond the fracture site is short and the nail tip may not reach the distal most end of the bone. In such a situation, two locking screws cannot be inserted distal to the fracture. This leads to inadequate purchase on the distal fragment, leading to suboptimal stability and resistance to the torsional forces.
- The nail length has to be precise.
  - In the presence of some distraction at the fracture site, thumping the elbow proximally is needed.
  - If the thumping technique is successful, the nail tip will be more prominent at the proximal end and cause soft tissue irritation near the shoulder area, leading to loss of good range of motion (In a gluteal area, if a femur nail is slightly more protruding proximally, the soft tissues would accommodate it).
  - If the distraction continues, it may lead to a delayed and perhaps non-union.
  - In such a morphology, a plate would be a better option, with assured union.

CASE 4: REPEAT SURGERIES

Interlocking nail in a nonunion after plate fixation: Around 2000 AD for a fracture of lower/3 humerus in a young lady anterior 12 mm plate fixation was done by a colleague. The plate avulsed and she consulted me for further treatment.

I advised her a revision surgery, a posterior plate fixation and bone grafting. She chose to go to her surgeon friend in her home town.

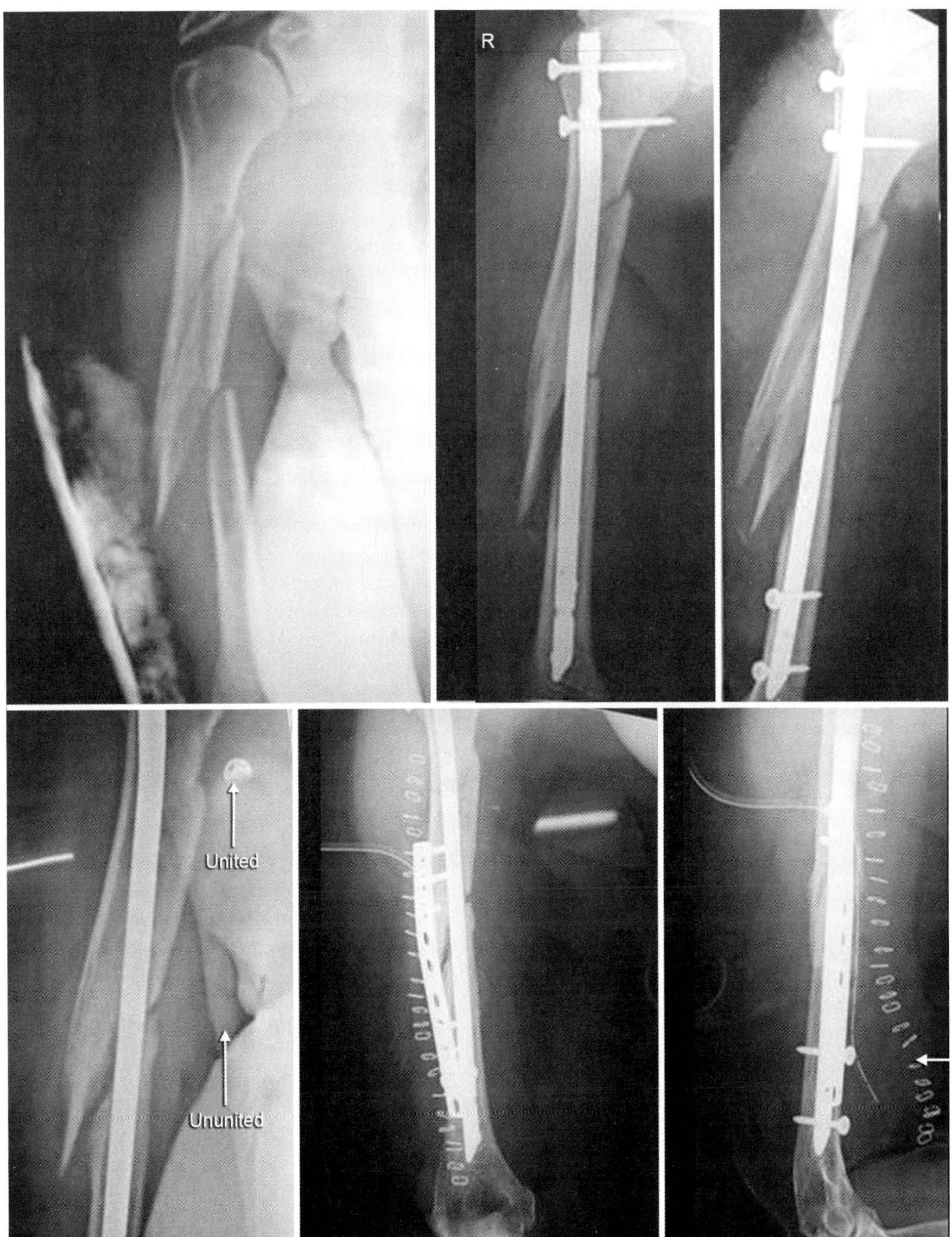

Figure 7.3 Segmental fracture

My Plan

The steps would be: In supine position, by anterior approach, remove the plate and anteriorly gently decorticate the bone, just to make it raw. If one decorticates it more, the screw hold in the revised plate will be poor. Close the anterior wound and turn the patient on a side or make prone and by posterior approach, fix a 16 mm wide and well-contoured plate (Prebent) and add bone grafts (Pre-locking plate era).

Tips in a plate fixation technique:

- Iliac crest bone grafts need to be laid on the side opposite on which the plate would be fixed. Laying down of grafts has to be done prior to fracture reduction and plate fixation.
- Plate must be prebent, so that the opposite bone cortex would come under compression.
- As per the fracture line direction, the plate to be fixed on the distal fragment first, so the apex of the distal end of proximal fragment will be wedged between the distal fragment and the plate adequately under load.
- The angular and rotary alignment needs to be confirmed, prior to the plate fixation.
- *Order of screw fixation*: In a transverse fracture: The holes close to the fracture site are left unused initially. The plate is so positioned, that new screw holes do not match with the old ones.
- The distal screw second from the fracture area, is passed first and fully tightened and the elbow is firmly pressed axially proximally towards the shoulder, to achieve contact opposition and avoid any void at the fracture site. While this is so held, second screw proximal to the fracture is passed in the DCP with a load guide. Because of manual axial compression, possible void at the fracture site is nearly absent. Then the additional load, exerted by the DCP stabilizes the fracture further. Then both the screws are alternately tightened.
- If it is possible to extend the surgical exposure adequately on either side of the fracture, I would prefer to load the fracture with an articulated tension device, also called an outboard device. I feel, the load of 60 to 80 kp is better generated by this device than the gliding hole principle in an oval hole of the DCP.

What the patient chose and what was the outcome in the given case?

The colleague operated her. Removed the anterior plate and carried out an interlocking nail fixation with bone grafting. After getting operated in other city, patient arrived back and came to see me and showed the X-ray after this procedure:

I requested her to carry out controlled exercises and to come for follow up and X-ray examination every six weeks.

X-ray at the end of six months from the revision surgery of interlocking nail, did not show bony union and hence I was not sure, if the fracture would consolidate, if left as such. The patient was advised to come for X-ray examination every month, till the fracture unites well. However, the patient came only after approx four years for ache in the arm. X-ray taken now, showed ununited fracture with the interlocking nail *in situ*.

This Required Again a Revision Surgery

She went back to the previous surgeon, who had done the interlocking nailing. As per the latest information, removal of the nail and a locking plate fixation on the posterior surface was done. The fracture united in due course (Fig. 7.4).

CASE 5: FRACTURE OF LOWER/4 AREA

20 years ago, for a fracture of humerus in lower/4 area with a 3rd fragment, IM nailing was done elsewhere and the fracture did not unite at the end of a year. There was no halo around the nail, indicating stability was good.

I had two options:

1. Decorticate and bone grafting.
2. Change the nail to a plate and graft.

I chose the second option and the fracture united (Fig. 7.5).

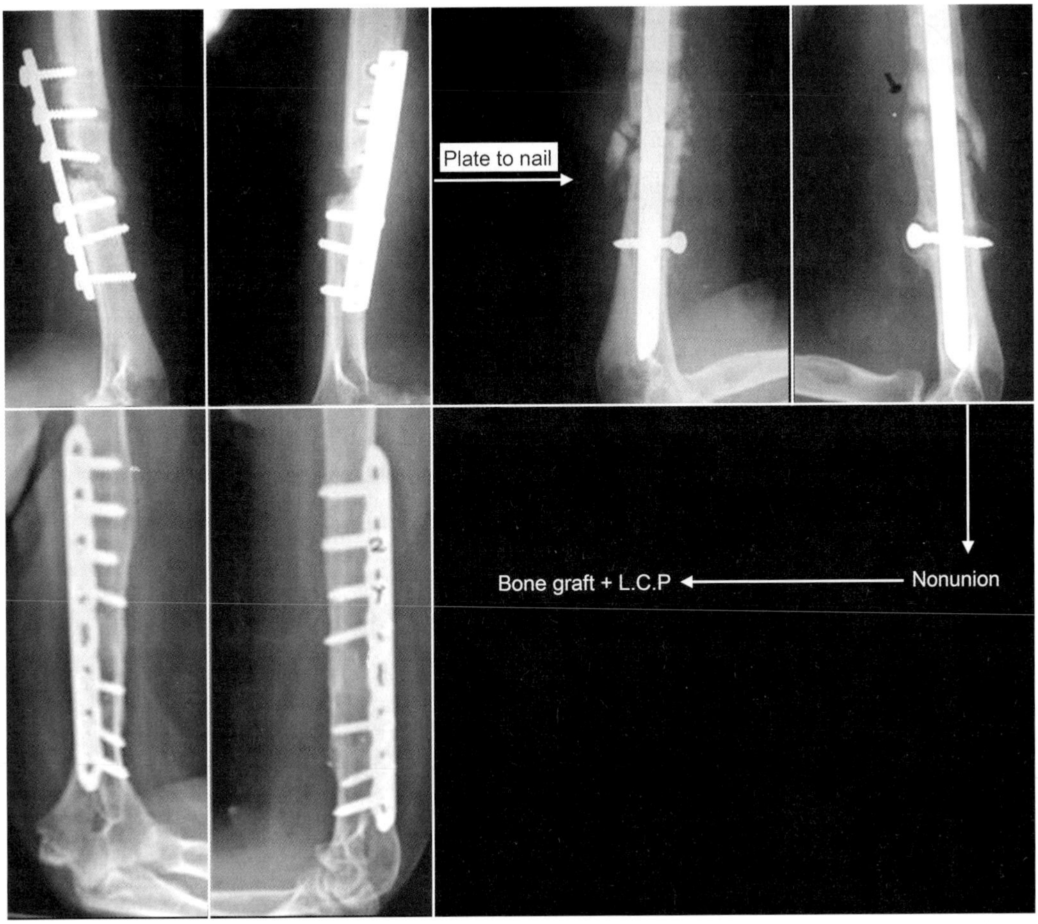

Plate to nail

Nonunion

Bone graft + L.C.P

Figure 7.4 Plate to nail to plate

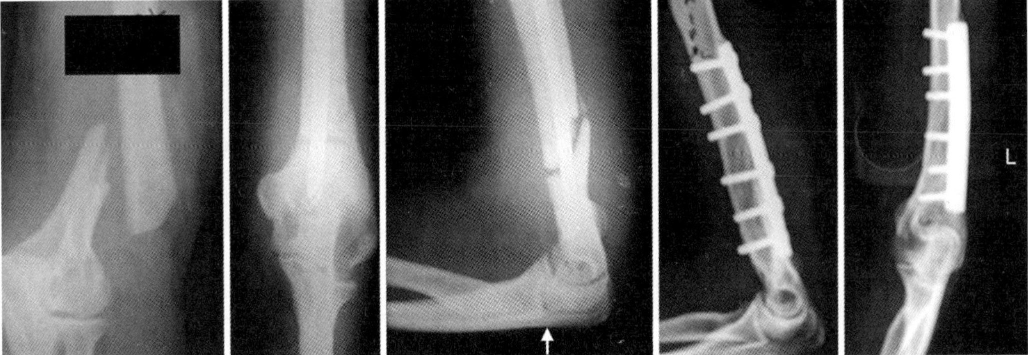

Figure 7.5 Nail to plate

CASE 6: FRACTURE OF LOWER/3 AREA NAIL TO PLATE

For this 3-part long oblique fracture of humerus, someone did a nail fixation and added synthetic bone substitute. The nail was quite narrow, with respect to the medullary cavity. The fracture limb was immobilized, yet did not unite. The nail was removed, may be because it backed out. At the end of 15 months, the fracture did not unite and at this stage the patient consulted me. The fracture required to be stabilized with a plate and addition of bone grafting. I did it by anterior approach. The fracture was exposed and soft tissues were cleared from the fracture ends and the bone grafts were laid on the opposite side of the fracture, prior to the plate fixation.

The distal end of the proximal fragment was a thin beak. It was stabilized by an interfragmentary screw through the plate. The narrow fragment required use of a 3.5 mm cortical screw for the IFS and was done so, passing the screw through a plate hole. The head of screw being small, a 7 mm washer was used, so the screw head has a purchase on the plate hole (Fig. 7.6).

CASE 7: FRACTURE OF LOWER/4 AREA

This patient was treated elsewhere and reported for further treatment. Pre- and immediate post-operative X-ray films were not available. Possibly, had a fracture in the lower third of humerus. An interlocking nail fixation was done. As seen in the follow-up X-ray (Fig. 7.7).

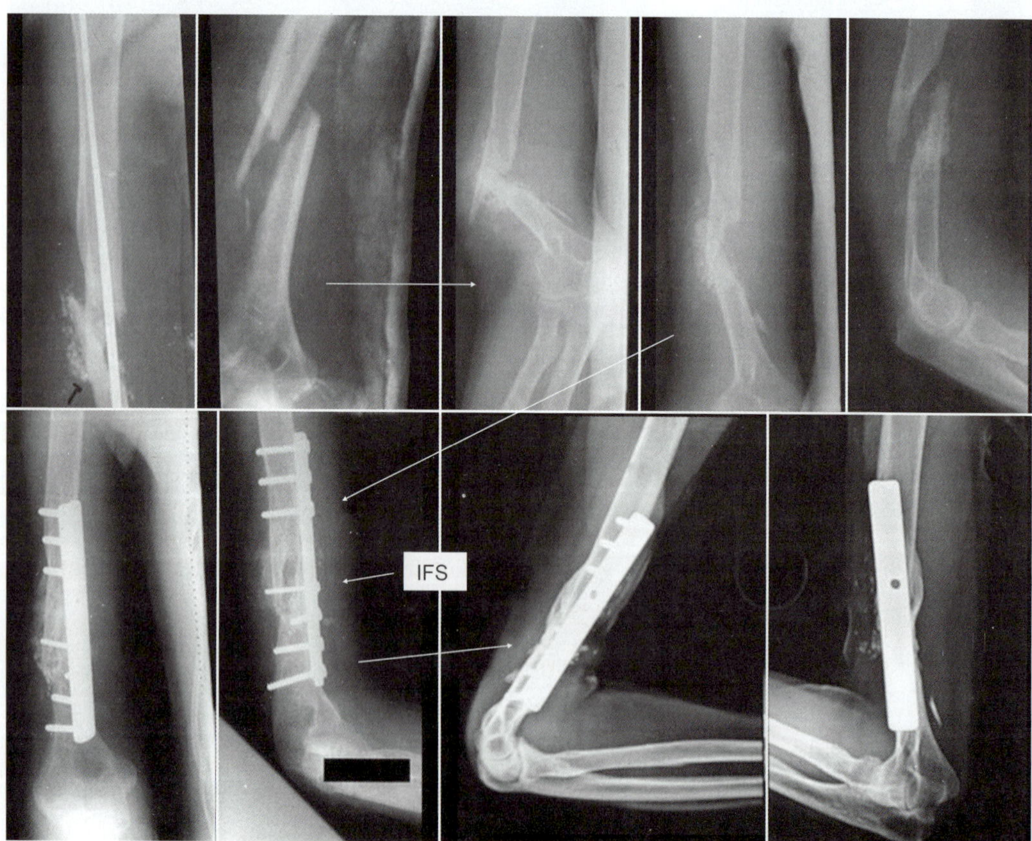

Figure 7.6 Lower/3 fracture–Nail to plate

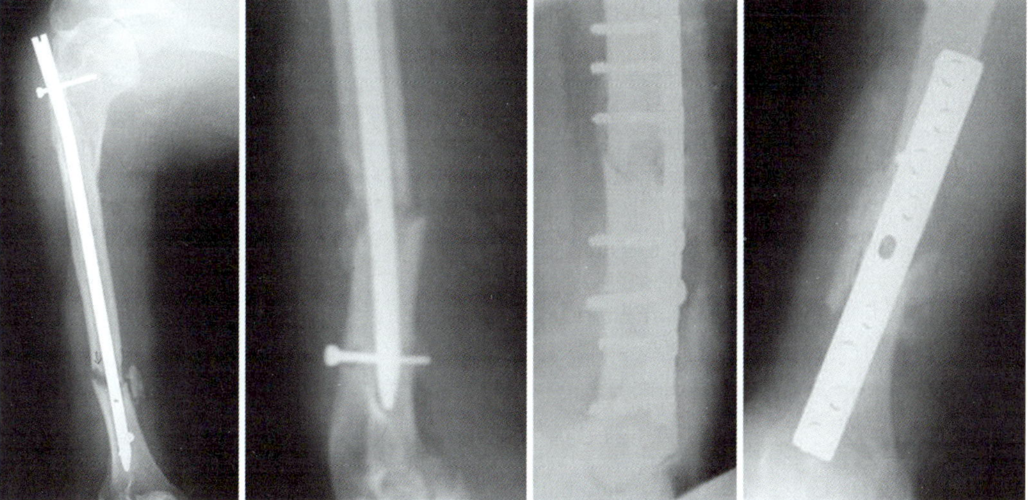

Figure 7.7 Fracture in lower/4–Nail to plate

Observations on X-ray taken now:

- The nail entry is much lower.
- Possibly during the nail entry, a fracture occurred (may be the first X-ray was a small film and this upper fracture may have been missed then).
- The second hole from below was close to the fracture area and hence was not used. Thus only one screw in the distal fragment did not confer stability. The result: was a non-union of the fracture.

The un-united fracture was treated by internal fixation by a plate and bone grafting by a posterior approach. Note the prebending of the plate, which brings the opposite surface under compression.

I have made custom-made plates, where the central span is increased to 40 mm, so the plate strength is maintained well over the fracture site.

As is necessary, a 16 mm broad plate was used with articulated tension device on the proximal fragment.

CASE 8: 3-PART FRACTURE OF MID/3

In some cases, a 3rd fragment is seen at the fracture area and is attachment to one of the major fragments. The fracture geometry was such that an IFS through or outside was not possible. In such a situation, I use a custom-made 16 mm wide plate. The central span of standard 26 mm is increased to 45 mm, as per the need. This makes the central bridge area of the plate strong, as there is no unused screw hole. This makes mechanical plate failure less likely (Fig. 7.8).

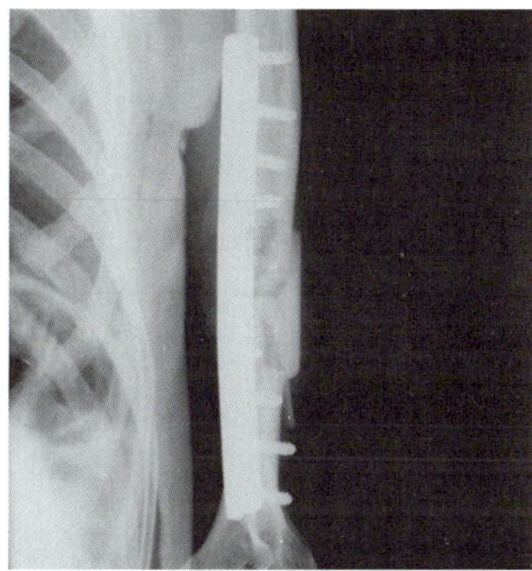

Figure 7.8 3-part fracture of mid/3–Span plate

As seen in a few cases shown, often there is a local comminution or a 3rd fragment, so few holes in the central area of the plate need to be left unused. This area tends to be a potentially a weak spot in the construct. Hence few plates are manufactured with central span in between two central holes. The standard span of 26 mm is increased to 40 or 45 or may be 50 mm also.

I have preferred to use round hole plates. Once a screw is well inserted, it is less likely to toggle in the round hole. In a situation, where the screw needs to be inserted in a tilted way, the oval hole geometry of a DCP is very beneficial (Fig. 7.9).

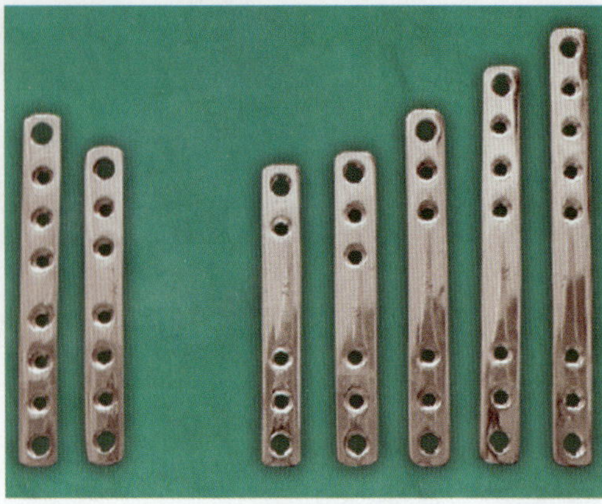

Figure 7.9 Implants–Span plate

CONCLUSIONS FROM THE ABOVE CASES

- For a long oblique fracture, a closed nailing may not obtain anatomical reduction. If anatomical reduction/cooption is not obtained, it is better to open the fracture on the first occasion and do an open reduction. I do not find a good result after a circlage wire and is biologically inferior.
- If a long oblique fracture continues to be unreduced, plan early bone grafting to achieve bone union in expected time. Success rate of interlock nail in humerus is less than that in femur, tibia, radius and ulna.
- If the primary fracture treatment does not lead to union, the secondary procedure be so planned that it should assuredly give a good result. Help from a competent colleague is worthwhile in decision making/ pre-operative planning and in the surgery as well.
- In interlock nailing, the nail entry site be precise. May take help of `C` arm to locate it. Or else, a fracture may occur at the entry site.
- Synthetic bone substitute is no substitute for good reduction, stable fixation and good bone to bone contact.
- For both, a primary or asecondary procedure (revision surgery for a non-union), autologous bone grafts are far superior to bone substitutes.

CHAPTER

8

Humerus Holstein and Lower Shaft Fracture

HOLSTEIN FRACTURE AND FRACTURES IN LOWER/4 HUMERUS

Holstein fracture is a spiral fracture at the lower/3 shaft humerus. At this level, the radial nerve is closely winding around the bone, penetrating the lateral intermuscular septum, to come in the anterior compartment. It is, thus, not freely mobile in this area. During the mechanical displacement of the fracture, sharp bone edge is very likely to damage the nerve at the time of injury. The fracture geometry is such that, this two-part fracture is less amenable to non-operative method of treatment and hence needs internal fixation. Often, there is a 3rd fragment, attached to the distal fragment and we should carefully look for it. During surgery, every care is necessary to prevent this fragment getting displaced.

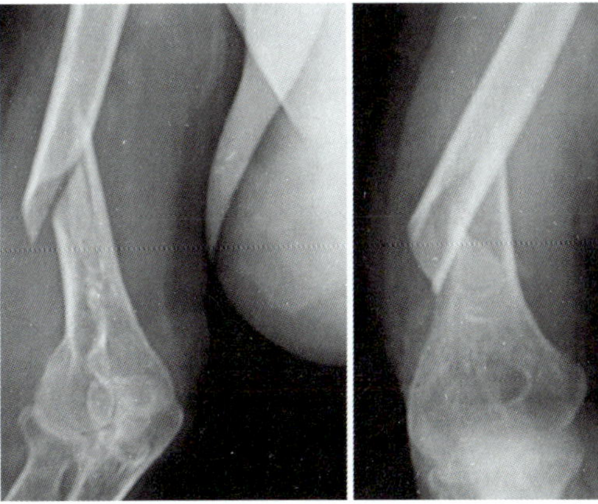

Figure 8.1 Arrival

The illustrated case had rheumatoid disease, with restricted motion in the ipsilateral shoulder and elbow joint. Associated osteoporosis was expected. The radial nerve was not injured at the time of the accident (Fig. 8.1).

Management

Immediately on arrival, padded axilla to mid forearm POP slab was given in sitting position. In a sitting position, due to the gravity, the fragments remain aligned and parallel to each other. If one does this plaster immobilization in supine position, the fracture tends to sag down. Besides, in spite of every care taken, the sagging may cause stretching of the radial nerve.

Operative Technique

The case was managed in the pre-locking plate era.

- *Lateral position*: The shoulder flexed to 90 deg and the arm was rested on a bolster kept on the front of the patient. Padding was needed on the bolster, so that the surface on which the arm (humerus) would rest, will have a stable and flat support under it. Iliac crest was also draped. Surgeon stands in front of the patient, with assistant next to him. At times, the assistant needs to stand on the dorsal side of the patient, at some stage of the procedure. The vacuum suction and electro-cautery are better located at the foot-end of the table.

- Posterior triceps splitting approach was taken. On the medial side ulnar nerve was kept in the mind.
- The radial nerve with accompanying vessels were located and the soft tissue envelope around it was maintained. An osteotome or a periosteum elevator was used close to the distal end of the proximal fragment to clear the tissues near the fracture edge. Assistant held the forearm to reduce the fracture, so the surgeon could remove the soft tissue interposition. Both the fragment ends of the bones were sharp and pointed apical ends were nibbled out. This step helped good contact opposition and reduction of the fracture. A provisional trial reduction was done and a suitable plate was selected.
- Bone grafts were taken from the iliac crest and were laid on the anterior surface of the fracture and a few small cancellous slivers were inserted in the medullary cavity of both the fragments. This step is important. (It is this fracture area, through which later an interfragmentary screw would be passed and where the fracture union is expected to occur). Once the fracture was reduced and a posterior plate was applied, the soft tissues are stretched and they fall back in their place. At this stage of procedure, it is difficult to lay down the grafts anteriorly, where they should exactly lie. Hence, it is necessary to lay them, prior to fracture reduction is done. From this deep muscular layer, the grafts receive the blood supply and have a good soft tissue bed as well.
- The teaching has been to use a 16 mm broad plate in the proximal limb segment, i.e. femur and humerus.

For a fracture of shaft humerus, a 16 mm plate is necessary. In this fracture morphology, compression across the plate is not needed and a round hole plate is acceptable. When a screw is placed in a round hole, it sits close to the plate and does not toggle compared to that in a DCP. Additional advantage of a DCP oval hole is that it permits tilting of the screw in either plane, as per the need, according to the fracture geometry.

The lady had a small frame. If a 16 mm broad plate is put on the bone, then it is difficult to centralize it and to know if the screw will be exactly in the center of the bone, holding both the cortices. If the plate is slightly misaligned along the long axis of humerus, then, as one goes towards the end of the plate, the end screws may not have adequate hold on the bone. However, if a 12 mm plate is used, this difficulty is avoided.

The plate used in this case was 12 mm broad and was a custom made. It had a central span of 30 mm (as against standard 26 mm) in between the central two screw holes. If a conventional plate is used, often a screw hole over the fracture area is seen to lie on the fracture line and has to be left void. It is through this hole that a mechanical failure of the plate occurs in a delayed union of a fracture. Thus a plate with extended central span enhances the strength of the plate over the fracture site and reduces a chance of mechanical failure of the plate. In any fracture, the fracture healing must occur in expected time or else a mechanical failure is likely. Primary bone grafts do assist bone union in expected duration, especially in a case with osteoporosis and immuno-compromised disease like a rheumatoid arthritis.

Steps in Plate Fixation

- The selected plate was matched to the length of fracture fragments.
- The distal fragment permitted 3 screws till the olecranon fossa. However, if one tilts the plate slightly, and move more distally on the lateral column, one can insert 4 screws, which is more important for better hold and stability. Thus if the distal part of the plate is placed on the lateral column, then the proximal part of the plate goes more medially, resulting in mild varus angulation

at the fracture site. This is preferred to having a less number of screws in the distal osteoporotic fragment, which is under more stress during postoperative mobilization. In an upper limb, to have few degrees of varus is preferable than to have less hold in an osteoporotic fragment.

- Often one is tempted to use bone levers, for easy and good exposure of the fracture area. In this anatomical situation, without one's knowledge, the bone lever may cause undue pressure on the radial nerve. Langenbeck retractors rather than bone levers are safer in this place.
- At this stage if there are two assistants, procedure becomes easy. One retracts to expose the proximal fragment and the other controls the distal fragment, holding the forearm.
- It may be possible to use a self-centering forceps to hold the proximal fragment with the plate and another pointed reduction forceps to hold the reduction across the fracture area. (The bone grafts are already laid in.) Now the second hole from the distal-most end of the plate is used to insert a 4.5 mm positional screw and is not fully tightened.
- Use of the second last screw allows some change of plate alignment in relation to bone easily. If one fixes the far-most screw in the plate first, this is not possible.
- At this stage, assistant manually gives some axial pressure to achieve a good contact opposition and alignment. Then proximal to the fracture line, second screw from the fracture line is inserted. The two screws thus inserted are alternately tightened. This results in good provisional stability. Then alternately, one screw on either side is inserted.
- One finds a suitable position to insert one interfragmentary screw outside the plate. The screw has to be at right angle to the fracture line. A 4 mm shaft screw was planned. This needs use of a 2.5 mm drill bit with a drill sleeve. In osteoporotic bone it works well. (In a normal bone, a 2.5 mm drill bit on a humerus may break, as the torque required to drill the bone is more.) Screw length was measured with a depth gauge: A cancellous 3.5.mm tap was used for just few turns and a 4 mm shaft screw of necessary length with a 7 mm washer was inserted.
- While the plate was placed on the bone, it was seen that a hole on the fracture could be used for an IFS through the plate. This hole was used for a 3.5 mm cortical screw as an IFS. The direction of the screw was decided by the direction of the underlying fracture line. Standard technique: Near hole 3.5 mm drill → Insert sleeve → 2.5 mm drill → depth gauge → Tap far cortex with 3.5 mm and screw with a 7 mm washer is inserted. This completes the fixation. (In a large plate the holes are meant 4.5 mm screw and we are using a 3.5 mm screw. This permits tilting the screw, but needs use of a 7 mm washer, so the screw head is held well over the hole edge.) In the illustrated case, the oblique screw through the plate is a 3.5 mm cortical screw inserted over a 7 mm washer. If one is not versed with these steps and the implants, it is necessary to study it on a bone model, study the implants prior to the surgery, before the instruments are sterilized. The above step nos 7, 8 and 9 are important to confer more stability to the fixation.
- The fixation was completed by inserting alternately the rest of the screws. The remaining bone grafts were laid around the fracture area. Drain was placed and wound closed.
- One would observe that once the bone is aligned and stabilized, the tension on the adjacent tissues, especially the radial nerve, remarkably reduces and it lies in its bed (Fig. 8.2).

The lady with rheumatoid arthritis had a stiff shoulder and one expected that she may exert more load on the fracture area in the initial post-operative period. Hence, a short above elbow POP slab was applied, over a padded crepe bandage. This support protected the fracture and exercise for the shoulder is also possible.

In the AP view, one notices that the lower end of the plate is on the lateral column of the humerus, to have one additional screw in the plate. This necessitates to direct the upper end of plate medially. As depicted in Fig. 8.5, the lower humeral plate has overcome this anatomical difficulty) (Fig. 8.3).

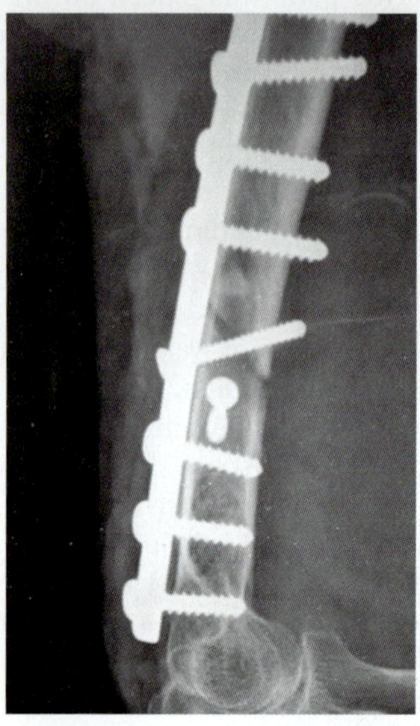

Figure 8.2 Post-op lateral view

End result: The radial nerve function was well preserved. It took about 10 to 12 weeks, as expected, to show evidence of bone union.

Exercises for the shoulder/elbow/static arm and the grip are important and were religiously carried out by her.

DECADES AGO

Fracture in the lower 3rd and lower 4th of shaft of humerus, plate fixation by a posterior approach was an accepted method of treatment. The distal fragment must have a hold by at lest 3 bicortical screws for the necessary stability. To achieve this, it was necessary to apply the plate on the lateral column on the posterior surface, so that it could be adequately cover an area, which will accommodate 3 screws. This directs the plate towards the medial humeral cortex. In this situation, to keep the plate well-aligned on the proximal fragment, an alignment of the plate in varus was necessary. The fracture union was of more importance than some varus and hence one had to accept it (Fig. 8.4).

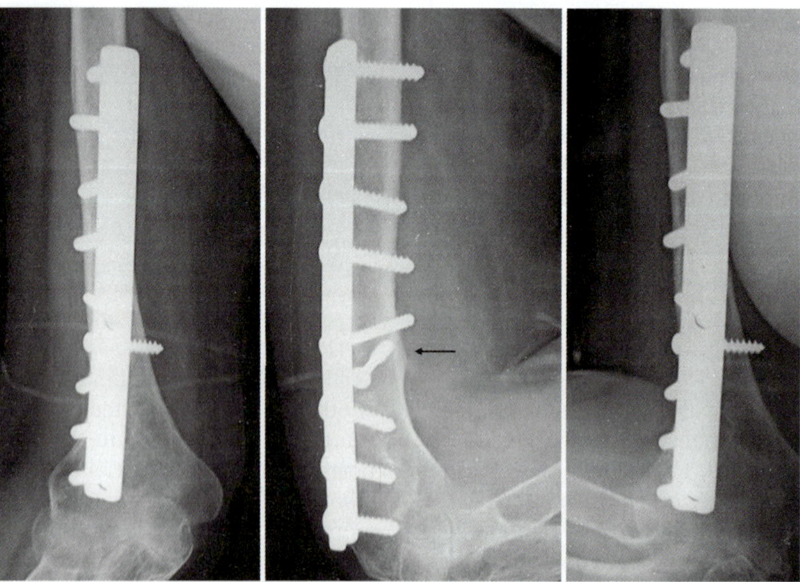

Figure 8.3 18 months post-op

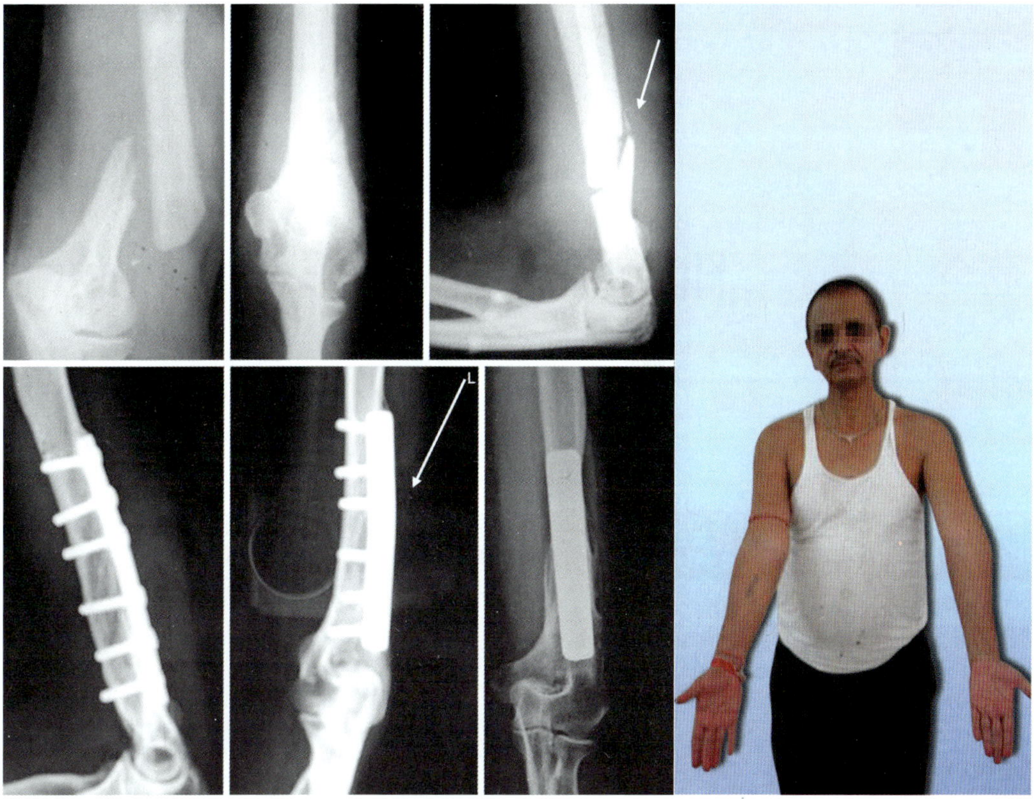

Figure 8.4 Varus unavoidable

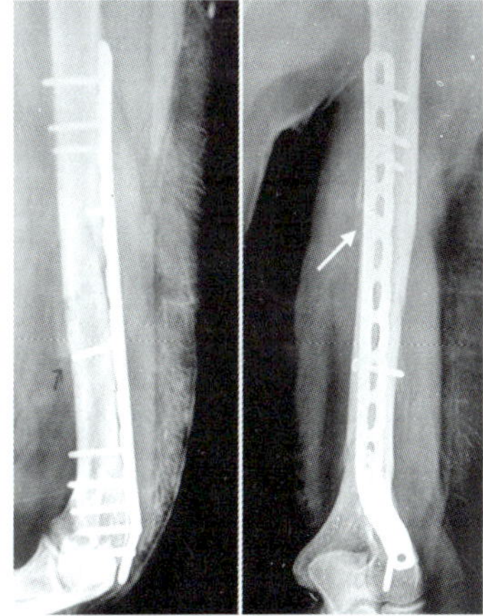

Figure 8.5 Lower humeral locking plate

FUTURE

Today a locking plate is available. As a further development, we have side specific lower humeral plate. The lower end is anatomically contoured to lie on the lateral column on the posterior surface. This has made it possible to have the proximal part of the plate well-aligned on the proximal fragment, unlike what is described above. This has made the fracture reduction and plate placement easier. Still the operative skill to preserve the soft tissue attachment to bone ends, and therefore, to preserve the blood supply to the bone ends, remains the important feature of the procedure (Fig. 8.5).

CHAPTER

9

Humerus Lower-End Exposure

POSTERIOR EXPOSURE FOR FRACTURE OF LOWER/4 HUMERUS

Fracture morphology in the given case: Supracondylar fracture with extension upwards and laterally, like a step fracture. There was no intra-articular extension (Fig. 9.1).

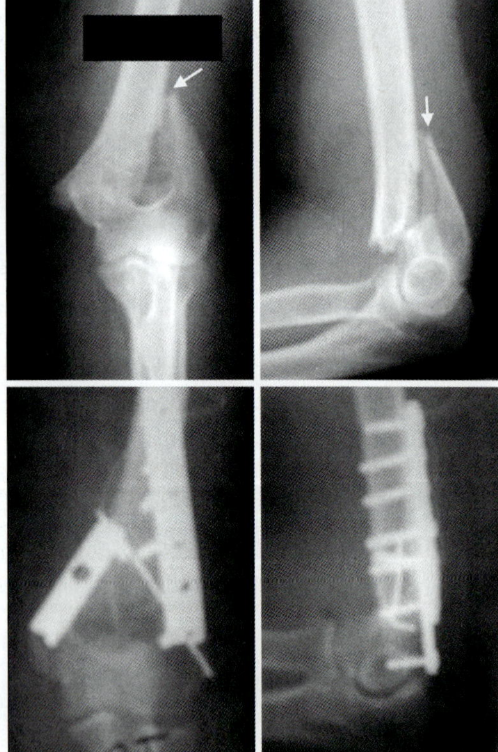

Figure 9.1 Lower humerus fracture

Options in Exposure

- *Bringing down a tongue of triceps*: One must know the area, where one is likely to encounter the radial nerve. Active mobilization of the elbow has to be slow, as the muscle repair needs time to heal well.
- *Olecranon osteotomy*: It is needed, when an intra-articular fracture extension is present. In this case, there was no intra-articular fracture and hence the osteotomy was not needed.

Position: Lateral with arm on a bolster, with ability to flex the elbow to 100 deg. If possible, a pneumatic tourniquet should be used because of its advantages.

Midline posterior approach, extending little beyond the olecranon. Thick subcutaneous flaps are raised. Either sides of the triceps are palpated and exposed.

Medially the ulnar nerve is identified and the triceps is lifted and shifted laterally. Carefully, the dissection is done till the tip of the medial epicondyle, so that medial plate can be fixed as low as possible.

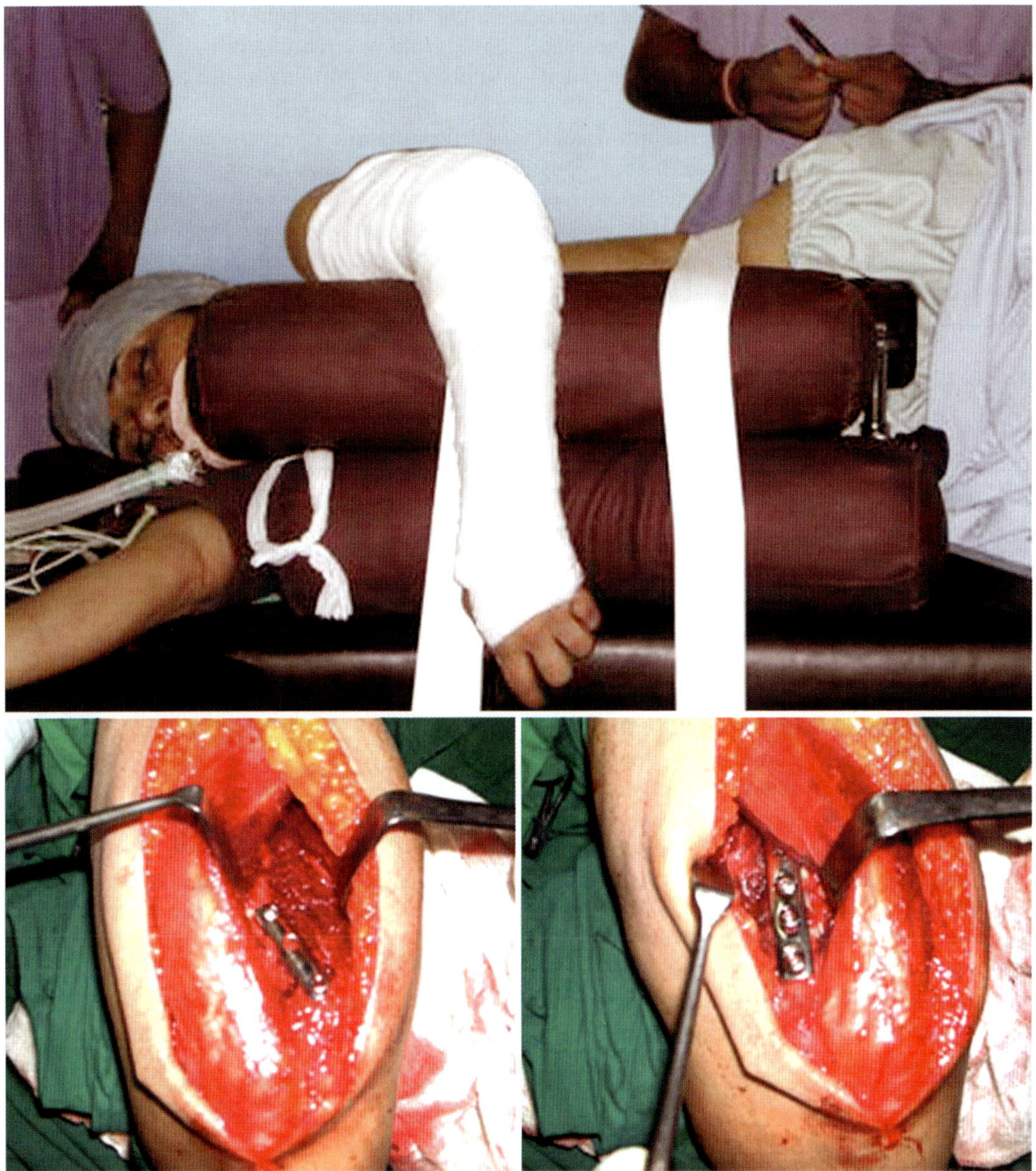

Figure 9.2 Operative position and exposure

Caution: Here quite a few vas nervosa come across. If seen, catch with a hemostat and keep it so, till the end of procedure. Use of an electrocautery generates local current, which may affect the ulnar nerve, unless a bipolar handpiece is used.

Laterally, the lateral triceps head is moved medially by a finger dissection, till the fracture is well visualized. The radial nerve penetrates the lateral intermuscular septum at the junction of upper 2/3 and lower 1/3 of a line joining insertion of deltoid to the lateral condyle.

Distal to this point, it comes anterior to the septum. It is surrounded by profunda vessels, which is a guide to the presence of the radial nerve.

For exposure of the fracture, the soft tissues are retracted by Langenbeck retractors. It is tempting to use a bone lever on either side of the humerus for ease of exposure. This should be avoided, as it can easily press the nerve under it. The surgeon needs to watch this all the time and guide assistants (Fig. 9.2).

Reduction Technique

The fracture surface is cleared by manipulating the upper forearm the fracture reduction is achieved and held by pointed reduction forceps/towel clips.

It is necessary to lift and pull the lateral skin edge towards the midline and stretch the skin flaps and palpate the lateral condyle. Then a 1.8 mm K-wire is inserted through the skin into the condyle. This is important to avoid skin puckering after closure, around the K-wire. It is necessary to know the direction of the wire, by visual judgment. To have an AP image with `C` arm is difficult in this position, before the fracture is stabilized.

A 1.8 mm K-wire is inserted from the tip of the lateral condyle till is seen in the fracture site. Then from lateral humeral condyle, the K-wire is advanced further across the fracture till it engages the medial supracondylar ridge. This provisional fixation is very necessary, helpful and makes plate application easy.

For the lateral column, a 3.5 mm system DCP plate of adequate length from SFS set is selected. It is prebent, as per the bone contour and applied in DCP mode. Initially the two screws, one on either side of the fracture line, are used to stabilize and load the fracture. Then on the medial pillar posteriorly a 1/3 tubular plate is contoured and fixed. One needs to see the lower end carefully, its relation with ulnar nerve, etc. to prevent pressure on the nerve. If necessary, the plate corners are bent. I prefer 1/3 tubular to a reconstruction plate here. The lateral plate fixation is completed. Mechanically, it is a good idea to have the medial plate contoured to sit on the medial supracondylar ridge. However, it needs to nibble the ridge to make it flat, to accommodate the drill bit, and prevent the drill bit from slipping over the bone ridge.

The provisional K-wire is bent, cut and tapped to bury the tip under the skin. It certainly confers additional axial stability to the fixation. I prefer to keep it as such.

If applied, the tourniquet is released and wound closed over a drain.

Message: On one column at least, preferably the lateral one, a DCP of 3 mm thickness is used. The other plate could be 1/3 tubular on the medial side. This combination makes the assembly quite strong. Today with titanium locking plates, fixation has taken a different turn. However, the exposure would remain the same. The triceps muscle is intact and hence early mobilization can be safely undertaken.

CHAPTER

10

Elbow Fracture Dislocation

ELBOW LATERAL DISLOCATION WITH SECTORAL FRACTURE OF HEAD OF RADIUS

Following a fall from a bike, a patient sustained lateral dislocation elbow with a sectorial fracture of head of radius.

- Immediate closed reduction was done and a padded crepe and AE POP slab was applied. This immediate closed reduction is necessary to have the following advantages:
  - Pain is reduced immediately.
  - After restoration of the anatomy and with added padded crepe bandage support, edema and blister formation is less likely.
- A CT scan with 3D reconstruction was done.
- *Operation*: 2 days later, the displaced sector fracture comprising 35% of the head radius was excised. The elbow was stable. Checked under `C` arm, with elbow at 100 deg. of flexion. The padded crepe needs to be given, while elbow is held at 100 deg flexion to keep it stable. Above elbow, POP slab is added on it and kept for 2 weeks.
- After completion of the plaster support, the elbow is checked again under 'C' arm to confirm that it continues to be well- located. For documentation, an X-ray is taken through the plaster support on table.
- (Due to the dislocation of the elbow, the ligaments are torn and hence, after excision of head radius, there is more likelihood of a dislocation). Re-dislocation is a known complication, especially after total excision of head radius, in a case of fracture dislocation of the elbow. This often happens, while the dressing and crepe application is done. Often, the assistant fails to hold the elbow continuously at 100 degree of flexion and hence, the elbow gets dislocated.
- After 10 days, sutures are removed while the crepe support and the back slab are continued. Gradually active intermittent mobilization is done. Improving the grip strength is the key to a good outcome. The plaster slab is removed twice a day and only active exercises and mobilization is carried out and the back slab is reapplied. At the end of four weeks, the back plaster slab is discarded, while the crepe support is continued.
- *Care*: Only active mobilization is carried out. No passive stretching/massage is permitted, as it is known to lead to myositis ossificans. Exercises must be done under supervision initially. Active mobilization after cast removal may take six to eight weeks to regain a pre-operative range.

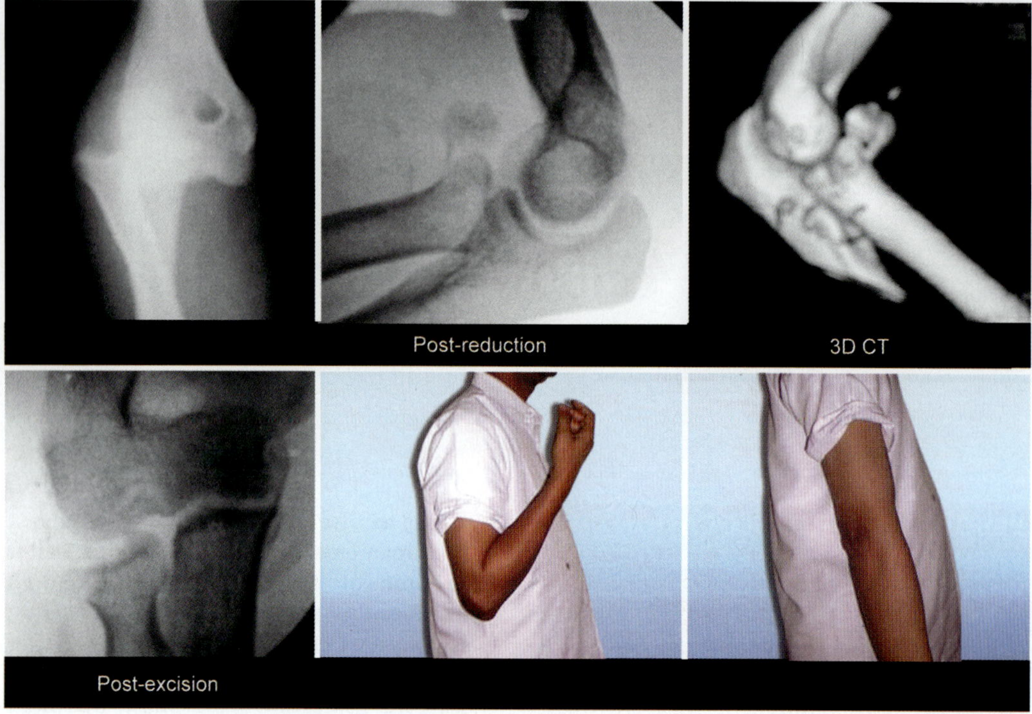

Figure 10.1 Fracture dislocation of elbow

- Use of oral indomethacin is said to reduce incidence of myositis ossificans. Static arm exercise and grip exercise for the forearm encourages good return of muscle tone and power (Fig. 10.1).

CHAPTER

11

Fracture of Medial Epicondyle of Humerus

Injury is commonly seen in children as a sports injury.

CLINICAL PRESENTATION

- Pain/swelling, more on the inner side of the injured elbow
- Elbow joint movements and pronosupination possible with some pain
- In a case presenting few days later, medial bruise may be seen.

A good AP and lateral X-ray examination is necessary. X-ray films of poor quality must be rejected and a repeat film be ordered. It is the clinician, who is responsible for the management of the case. X-ray of the opposite elbow be always taken to lay down a system for the team.

X-ray Findings

- *Medial soft tissue swelling*: The most important sign!
- Small fragment of the displaced medial epicondyle is seen (The size of the piece seen on operation table is much larger than the X-ray appearance, because on X-ray film, only the ossific nucleus is seen and the size of the fragment is much larger than that appears on the X-ray film).
- It is a necessary step to take an X-ray of the opposite elbow for comparison and documentation and to convince the patient's relatives.

Usually the diagnosis is clear on radiological study, as above. Rarely, a CT scan is needed.

Anatomy: The common flexor origin is attached to this area and pulls it away from the host bone. Unless the fracture is reduced and stabilized by internal fixation, good radiological union does not occur. Being an extra-articular injury, the elbow deformity may not appear in an ununited fracture, unless it is a fracture of the entire medial epicondyle.

The center of epiphysis of medial epicondyle appears at the age of six and fuses at the age of sixteen years. Till then, it is likely to be injured and a fracture epiphyseal separation occurs.

TREATMENT

Open reduction and internal fixation is necessary with K wires. Flexion of the elbow facilitates reduction. As per the size of the displaced fragment, one or two K-wires need to be inserted. The wires need to be of 1.6 and 1.8 mm in diameter. In late adolescence, if the bone fragment is large enough and the epiphysis is about to fuse, a 4 mm shaft screw, with or without anti-rotary K-wire is a good combination.

TECHNIQUE

After reduction being held by a small pointed reduction forceps, two K-wires are inserted. Check under `C` arm. Bend the wire carefully, close to the bone and then cut them off. The bent wire may be rotated, so the tips do not irritate the skin.

Closure and above elbow POP slab for approximately five weeks, which is the time required for union. Thereafter, it is preferable to remove the implants (Figs 11.1 and 11.2).

MISSED FRACTURE OF MEDIAL CONDYLE OF HUMERUS

As discussed above, poor quality of X-ray film, incorrect X-ray reading and ignorance of such injury, may lead to a missed injury. This is important, especially, if the fracture fragment

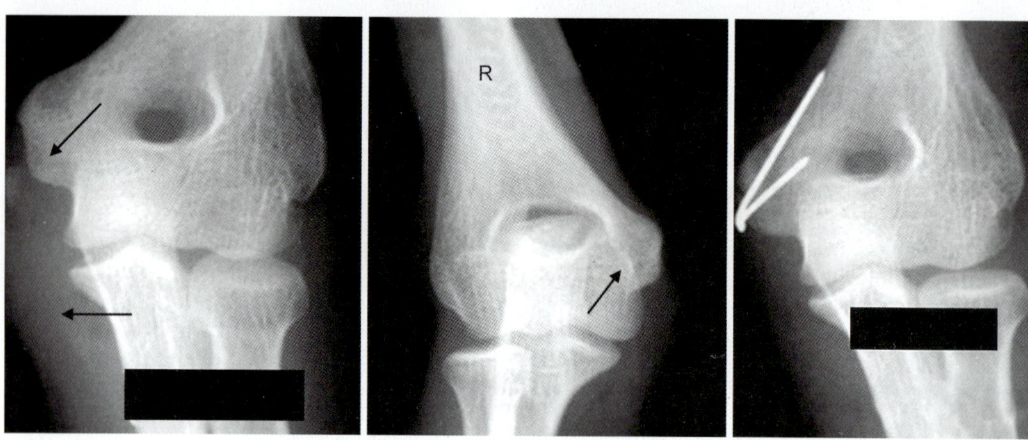

Figure 11.1 X-ray of opposite elbow

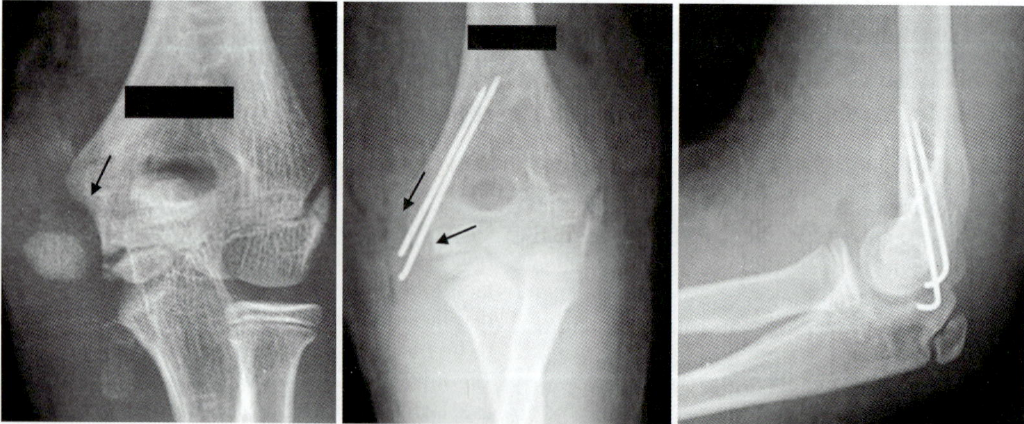

Figure 11.2 Displaced large fragment

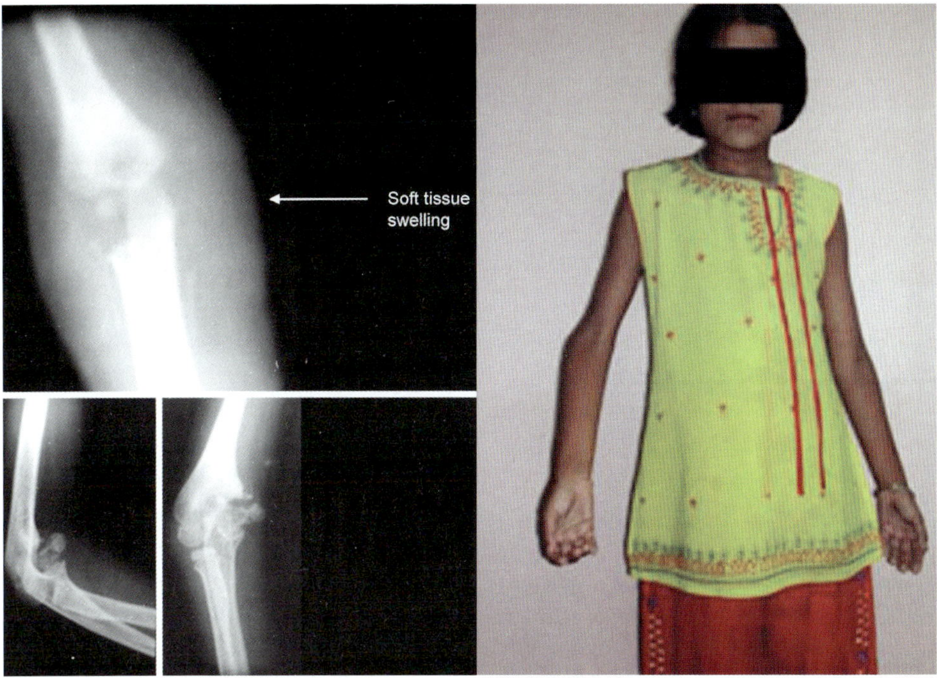

Figure 11.3 Medial soft tissue swelling

is a large one and not just avulsion of medial epicondyle, but includes a part of the trochlea as well.

The growth disturbance leads to elbow deformity, which is disturbing to the patient (and to the treating surgeon later on).

Strong suspicion and information is the key to recognize such an innocuous looking injury. If in doubt, both MRI and a CT scan are preferable rather than missing the serious nature of injury.

As depicted in the photo, it must have been a fragment involving a major part of the trochlea (Fig. 11.3).

CHAPTER

12

Capitellum Fracture

Capitulum forms lateral part of lower end of the humerus. In a lateral view, a line drawn from the anterior surface of humerus is behind the capitellum. It articulates with the head of the radius. This radiohumeral joint has angular flexion and extension, as well as pronosupination movement. Its anatomical congruity with head radius, confers good range of the above movements.

Pathological anatomy: The fracture of capitellum is a shear fracture and the area of bone, anterior to the anterior surface of the humerus, gets displaced. A good lateral view confirms this fracture.

Associated injuries: May be:

- Impacted fracture of head of radius
- Associated fracture of lower end of humerus in the trochlea.

Treatment methods for fracture capitellum, advocated in the past:

Under anesthesia, with elbow extended, a closed reduction by manipulation, by kneading the fragment distally and posteriorly. I had done a successful reduction, followed by above elbow POP slab/cast for 2 to 3 weeks. Careful follow up would be necessary. I believe elbow range of 15 to 100 was restored then, 30 years ago.

CURRENT TRENDS

As per the teaching for an intra-articular injuries, accurate reduction and stable internal fixation is necessary.

Methods: Possible.

- Posterior to anterior 4 mm partially threaded cancellous screw or in any other direction. Often the capitellum is too thin in the central part, for the screw tip to hold it adequately, so that immediate mobilization is possible. Hence there is a tendency to pass the screw obliquely, for good hold, without any benefit. To obtain a good hold on the small fragment, it needs to take purchase on the anterior surface of capitellum, which means, there is a likelihood of irritating head of the radius (Fig. 12.1).
- A patient came for follow up, being operated in other city. Few K wires were inserted and the ends were left long. After a few weeks, cellulitis developed. Eventually restriction of motion was the outcome (Fig. 12.2).

A colleague had fixed the fracture of capitellum, with a screw, passed in an anterior to posterior direction, resulting in restricted range of movement. 6 to 8 years later, patient had another fall, on the same elbow, resulting in fracture of olecranon. This olecranon fracture

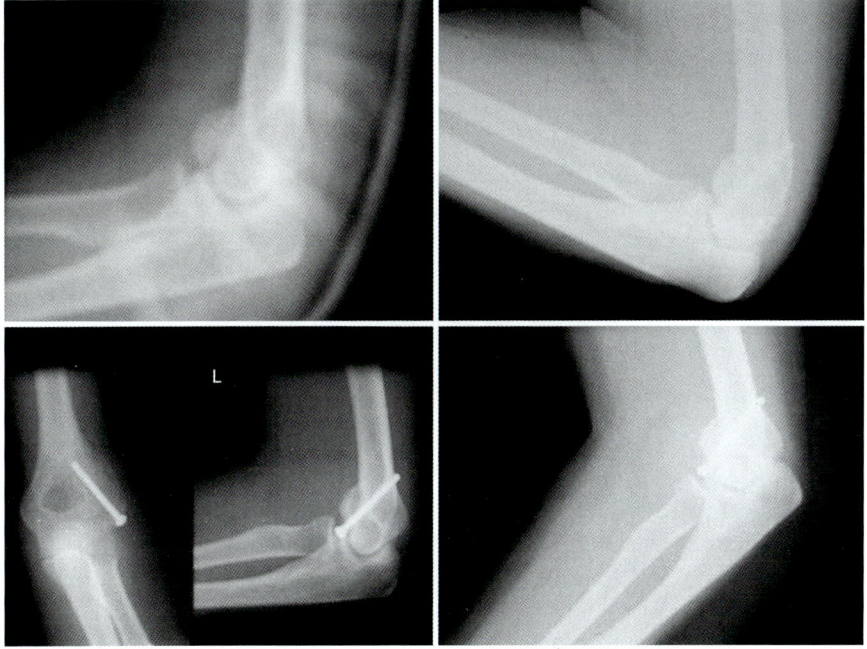

Figure 12.1 Oblique screw

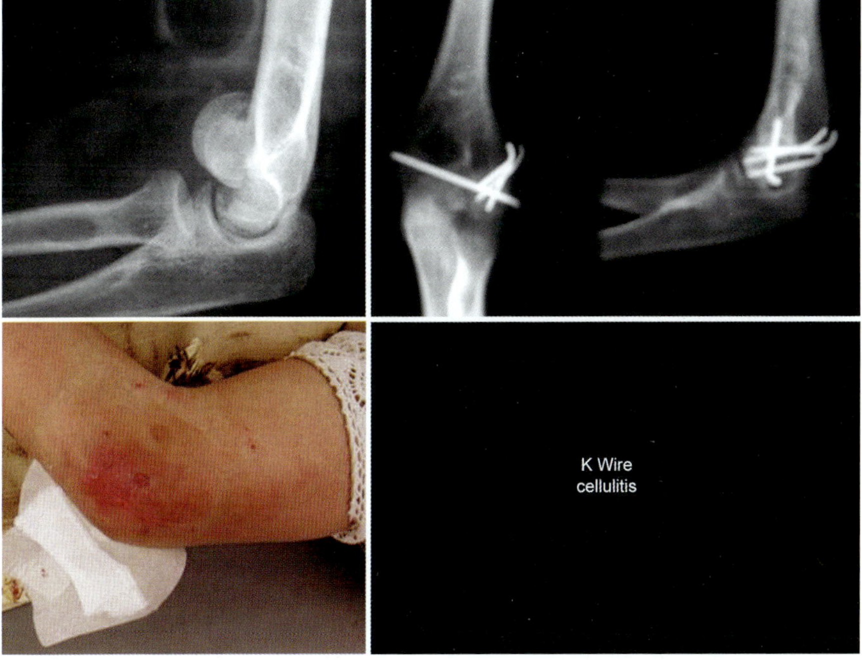

Figure 12.2 K-wire and stiff elbow

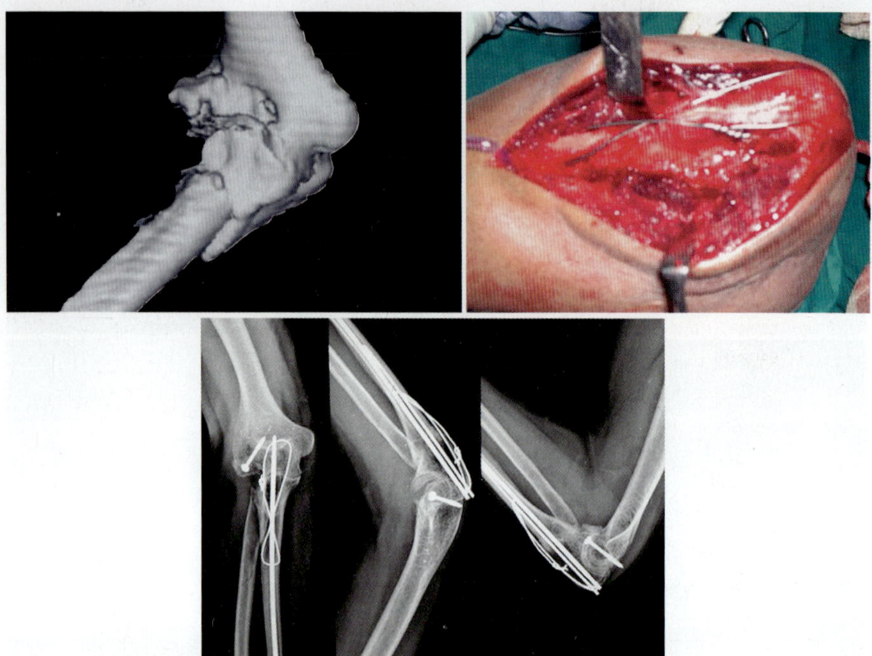

Figure 12.3 Oblique screw. Another fracture

was internally fixed by me. The dynamic X-ray views show the range, which was the same as prior to the second accident, thus restoring the second pre-injury clinical situation (Fig. 12.3).

I have not done internal fixation of capitellum by either a screw or a K-wire. I am yet to see a good result, with a supple elbow and at least 90 % range of motion in any case managed by above technique. But I have seen many cases operated by one of the above methods coming for second or third opinion, with poor range of motion and patient dis-satisfaction.

RECOMMENDATION

Philosophy: In the lateral compartment of the elbow, for comminuted fracture of the head of radius, excision of head of radius has been an accepted method, with a good result in terms of stability and range of motion. Here total proximal end of the radius is sacrificed.

For a shear fracture of the capitellum, I recommend the same and have practised the same, with uniformly good result. The anterior segment of the lateral part of the lower end of humerus is sacrificed while, the posterior part is preserved, Thus, if at all, some instability occurs, it would be in flexion of the elbow only and not in extension. In practical life, this does not affect the elbow function, especially in terms of the stability.

TECHNIQUE

Tourniquet: Lateral approach. The lateral supracondylar ridge is palpated by prono-supination. If the edema is less, the head radius is palpable. The incision is started from above downwards on the supracondylar ridge, till the joint is reached. Head of the radius is palpated, which helps to limit the distal end of exposure and protect the deep branch of the radial nerve.

The displaced capitellum fragment is usually displaced anteriorly. It is visualized and excised. Wash is given, to take away debris if any. Tourniquet is released and closure done.

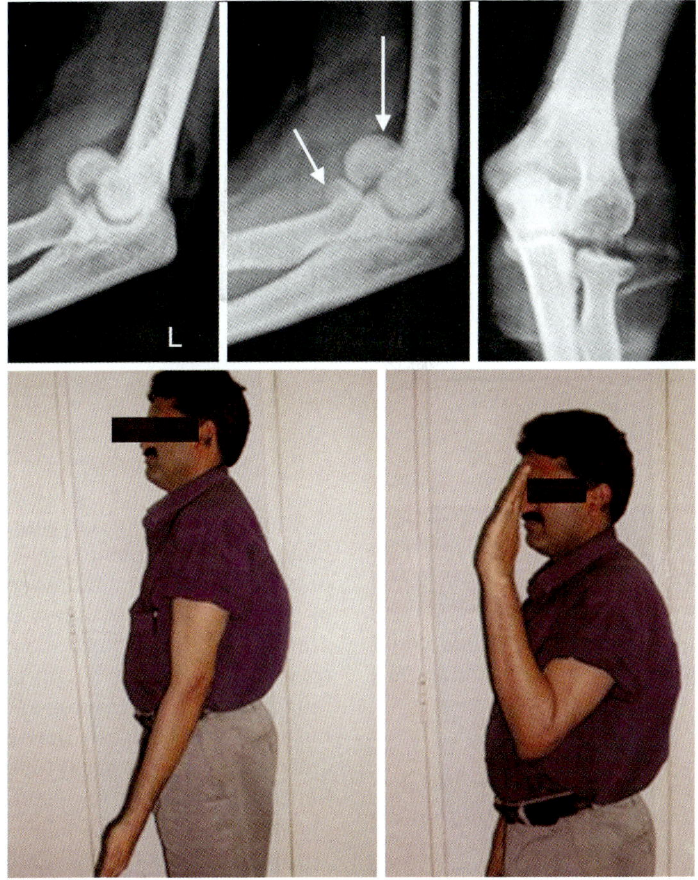

Figure 12.4 Fracture of capitellum and head of radius: Ipsilateral

No drain is necessary: Padded crepe and above elbow plaster slab is given for a week. Then intermittent mobilization by removing the back slab is recommended for a week. Thereafter, only a crepe support is given and active mobilization is continued.

Use of indomethacin is supposed to reduced development of ectopic calcification.

CLINICAL EXAMPLE

A patient had a displaced fracture of capitellum and an impacted fracture of ipsilateral head radius. The capitellum was excised and the head radius was left as such. Mobilization was little delayed for the neck radius to consolidate well. Clinical range is as per the photograph. Note the pronosupination (Fig. 12.4).

MESSAGE

In the years to come, Herbert screw will be useful. Bio-absorbable screws are also available. If it is not available, then it is a safe method to consider the excision, rather than fixation, to regain good range of motion, with a stable elbow.

CHAPTER

13

Radius Neck Fracture

FRACTURE EPIPHYSEAL INJURY TO THE NECK/HEAD OF THE RADIUS IN ADOLESCENCE

The injury to the head/neck of radius could be an isolated injury or a part of Monteggia's injury.

Case 1

Isolated fracture epiphyseal injury of the head of radius:

A tilt till about 30 deg is acceptable with good outcome. Any tilt more than 30 deg needs to be reduced.

Methods available are:

- *Examination under anesthesia*: Manipulation with varus strain and gentle elevation by a thumb/esmarch bandage technique.
- *If this method fails or the injury is old*: Open reduction is done. Though described, humero-radial axial K-wire is not popular due to the possible complications, resulting in poor elbow function in a child.
- Indirect reduction/elevation of head of radius, using an intra-medullary square nail.

The technique of indirect elevation by an IM nail:

Patient position: Supine with the forearm on a side wooden board.

Closed reduction as in case 1 above is done. Radius nail entry point is selected about 8 mm proximal to the distal radius epiphysis. A 2 mm or 2.5 mm diameter square radius nail (with a blunt tip), is selected, as per the medullary cavity diameter. The length has to be slightly longer than the measured radius length. The business end is slightly bent to about 15 deg. The tip of the radius nail is round and blunt and hence it is less likely to penetrate the proximal end of the radius.

The nail is advanced till the head, as assessed by the length of the nail inserted and checked under 'C' arm. The bent end is kept towards the tilt of the radial head. The nail is gently tapped, to elevate the head and confirmed in both AP and lateral views. At times, some degree of rotation of the nail also helps to put the head in proper position. Elbow angular motion and prono-supination is gently checked. The nail at the entry site is cut, with a side cutter, keeping some length on the dorsal cortex of the distal radius. This facilitates its removal later.

- Above elbow posterior POP slab is applied in full supination and maintained for 3 weeks at least. After plaster immobilization, check X-ray on table is taken for record. At the end of 10 days, the sutures are removed and an above elbow POP cast is applied. (The POP slab removed at this time, may be kept aside, to be applied, during mobilization).

At the end of 3 weeks, the plaster is removed and active mobilization of the elbow is started. Initially, it requires perseverance to encourage the child to be able to do active exercises. The exercises and active mobilization of the elbow is done twice a day and POP slab reapplied for the rest of time. Presence of the plaster slab also prevents the child from unnecessary loading the elbow and passive stretching (Fig. 13.1).

Fracture epiphyseal injury head radius, as a part of Monteggia injury:

Case 2

Mild angulation of fracture of the ulna at upper/3 with tilted head radius:

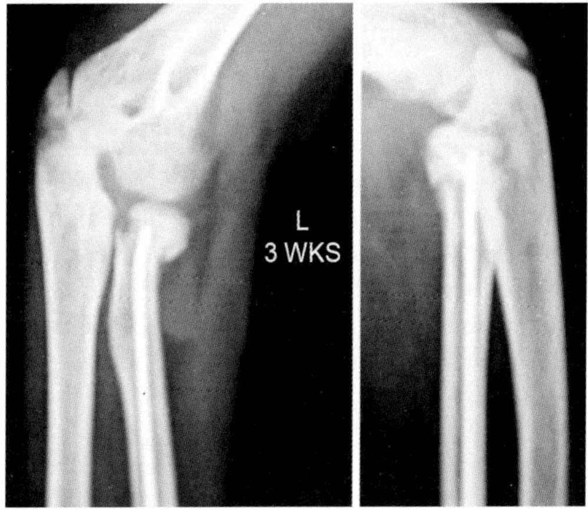

Figure 13.1 Three weeks radial head elevation

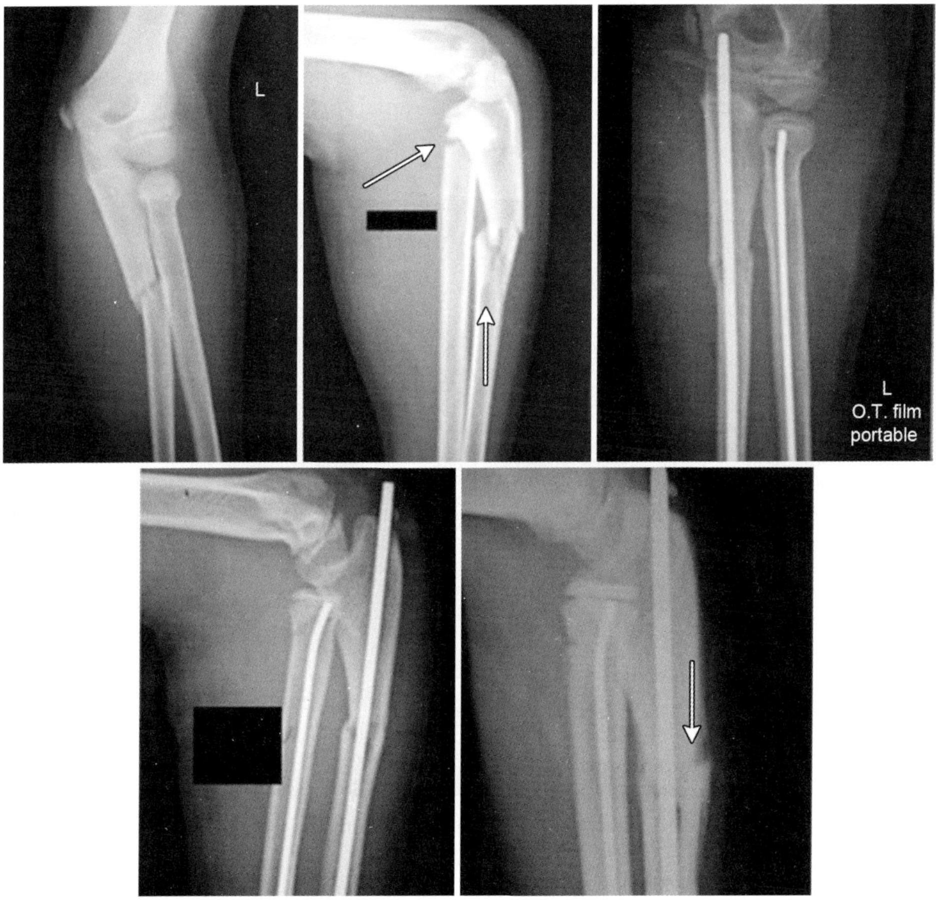

Figure 13.2 Monteggia injury

The Technique

Patient position: Supine. For ulna nailing, arm taken over the chest, supported by the assistant. First closed ulna IM nailing was done. This restored the forearm length and then some varus strain can be given to reduce the head radius.

As per above technique, head of the radius was reduced and then the reduction was maintained by an IM radius nail post-operative AE POP slab and protocol as above was observed (Fig. 13.2).

Case 3

Minimally displaced fracture epiphyseal injury to olecranon + displaced fracture epiphyseal injury to the head of radius.

The head was tilted by 90 deg laterally. A CT scan with 3D reconstruction was done for this severe injury. The elbow was swollen. No neurological deficit was observed.

Technique

- With mild varus strain, gently the rim of head radius was palpated and checked under 'C' arm. It was elevated and reduced by manual leverage by the tip of the thumb. In a fresh case usually 80% reduction is obtained. The 'C' arm image at this stage indicated that the proximal fragment of the head was thin and IM radius nail technique would not work. Besides the tilt was nearly 90 deg. and the tip of the nail would not be able to elevate and elevate the periphery of the head of the radius.
- Hence a 1.8 mm K-wire was taken and inserted under image control in the fracture line, parallel to the upper surface of the head. The wire was then elevated like a joy stick and reduction was confirmed under 'C' arm. The K-wire was then slightly advanced using a power drill, to engage the medial radial cortex for stability.

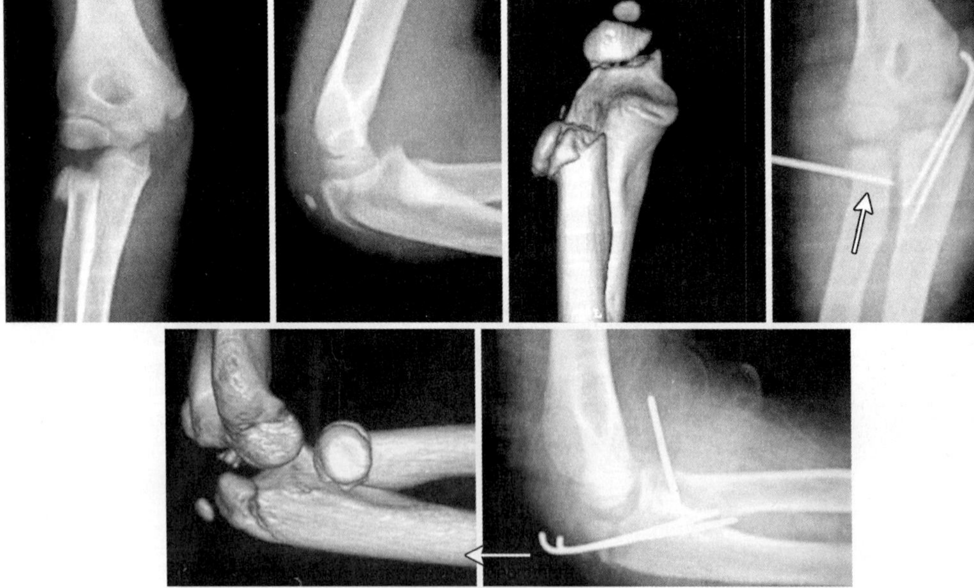

Figure 13.3 Monteggia injury

- While the K-wire is levered upwards, the skin is folded and needs a small incision to prevent pressure necrosis. It is a good idea to pull down the skin and then insert the K-wire, to avoid its infolding. Gently angular, pronosupination movements and stability are checked.
- The olecranon fracture displacement was minimal and hence through a small incision at the tip of olecranon, 2 × 1.8 mm K wires were passed obliquely to stabilize the olecranon. Confirmed under 'C' arm.

Postoperatively: Padded plaster and synthetic posterior slab was applied. Check X-ray through slab on table taken. Limb elevation/exercises for fingers was carried, as usual.

Edema settled in 5 to 7 days and at the end of a week, dressing was changed and X-ray

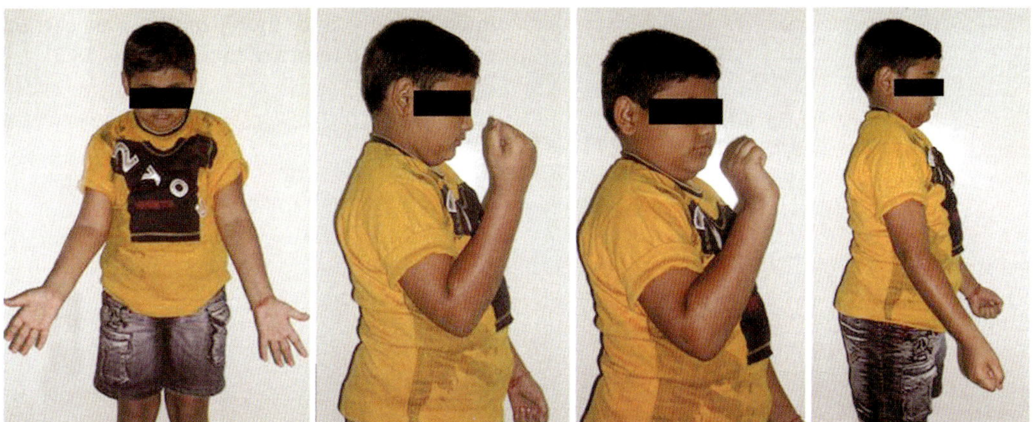

Figure 13.4 Monteggia injury: Clinical result

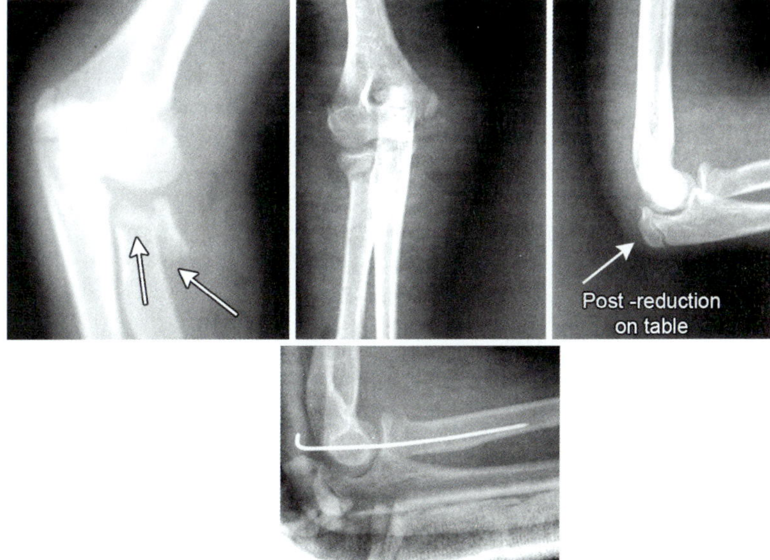

Figure 13.5 Humero-radial K-wire

repeated. At the end of 2½ to 3 weeks, the radial neck K-wire was removed under anesthesia, by rotatory motion, keeping a thumb pressure on the head radius, to maintain its good position.

After 4 to 5 days intermittent mobilization of the elbow, grip tightening and pronosupination exercises were started.

For a good elbow function, pronosupination is more important than the final angular range. As in any elbow injury, only active exercises were encouraged (Figs 13.3 and 13.4).

Case 4

This boy had a displaced fracture of the head radius, with a tilt of 80 degrees. It required reduction. Hence under anesthesia, closed reduction was successfully carried out and an X-ray film exposed for documentation. To offer stability for the reduction, a humero-radial K-wire was inserted and above elbow POP slab applied for 3 weeks.

At this time, the axial K-wire was removed. Thereafter, the plaster support was removed intermittently and mobilization was carried out, with good return of function (Fig. 13.5).

CHAPTER

14

Forearm Fractures

FRACTURE OF RADIUS AND ULNA

For internal fixation of either bone, both a plate and a nail have their own place. Each implant has its advantages and disadvantages. It is difficult to compare and contrast them.

Technically, using a plate as an implant is more demanding. Plate fixation needs more precision, adequate training, observation and a wide range of precision implants, including power tools. Learning curve is a long one. If a precise, technically and mechanically sound procedure is not done and peri-operative care is not correct, a plate would avulse out (Fig. 14.1).

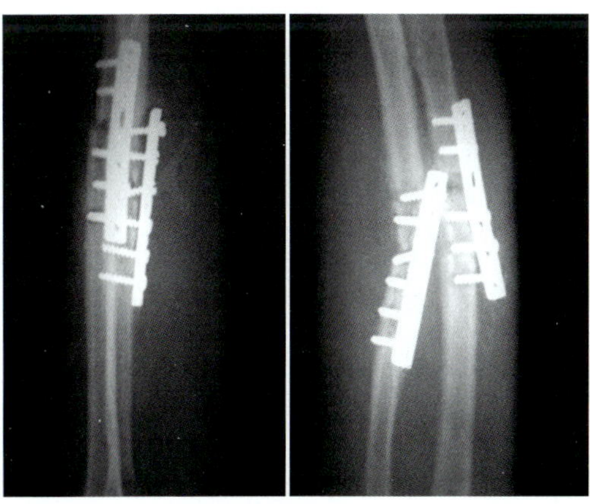

Figure 14.1 Radius and ulna plate avulsed

GENERAL COMMENTS ON PLATE AND IM NAIL AS AN IMPLANT

Should any problem or a complication develop after a plate fixation, its management is more difficult and the outcome less satisfying, compared to a case, where a nail as an implant has failed.

Bone healing and outcome, in general, is better in the adolescent and the young than in the elderly.

In juxta-articular areas, a plate has more mechanical advantages than a nail:

- The short fracture segment in juxta-articular fracture is better held by a plate. On the shorter segment, may be only two screws can be inserted. Still, it will offer a good stability, especially, when a compression is generated across the fracture area.
- The medullary cavity is more wide towards the end of a bone and the nail would have less purchase on this fragment.
- If a nail is to be inserted from this short fracture segment, then the nail entry site is very close to the fracture, as in lower end of the radius. (This is because the nail entry is from a side of the radius, as in the tibia).
- A nail can be passed by a closed method, while a plate cannot be fixed by a closed method.
- In a procedure of nailing in general, and in a closed method, in particular, the soft tissues

around the fracture ends are not disturbed and hence the external callus is more with an intramedullary device. Thus, assessment of a fracture union is easy with a nail as an implant.

Spectrum for use of a plate and a nail:
A plate and a nail as internal fixation device, are complementary to each other. In femur, one has used an intra-medullary nail and in addition a de-rotation plate also. This adds to the rotary stability of the fixation.

PLATE AS AN IMPLANT

- A plate can be used nearly in any part of an entire length of a long bone. A nail is not suitable for metaphyseal injuries.
- A well-indicated and well-executed internal fixation by plating leads to primary bone union. Early mobilization after the surgery is possible (except in a Monteggia or a Galeazzi injury, where the associated joint injury needs to be considered and appropriate external immobilization is necessary).
- Radius being a curved bone, varying at different levels, a plate needs to be contoured very carefully. If not so done, the radial bow flattens, and may reduce the range of motion. This loss of radial bow is also seen after an IM nailing of the radius. (In clinical practice, this is not significant in terms of clinical range seen at the end) (Fig. 14.2).

Radiological Assessment of Fracture Union

After anatomical reduction and fracture fixation by a compression across the fracture, it is difficult to say, when the fracture has united beyond doubt, on an X-ray film. Hence, one has to go by calendar to permit progressive loading on the limb, as permitting to ride a bike, resuming sports activity, etc. After internal fixation by a nail in both the radius and ulna, X-ray appearance is quite clear to indicate if there is a radiological union, which occurs by an external callus and disappearance of the fracture line. When a plate is used on both the bones, especially at the same level, it is difficult to see the fracture area clearly, as, a plate on one bone overlaps the other bone. It makes X-ray reading very difficult (Fig. 14.3).

Stability of Plate as an Implant

Factors and steps contributing to a mechanically sound plate fixation:

- *Sharp drill bit*: Avoids bone heating and necrosis while drilling.
- Sharp tap helps to cut precise threads.
- The drill bit and the tap should match to each other and with respect to the screw to be used. Screw thread, whether cortical/ cancellous is decided, as per the structure of the bone.

Figure 14.2 Radius plate not contoured

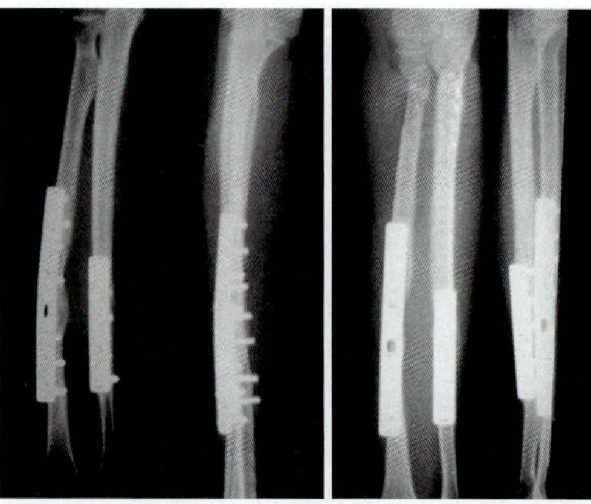

Figure 14.3 Plates overlap

- Prebending the 3.5 mm DCP to bring the opposite cortex under compression.
- Provisional fracture reduction.
- 1st screw close to the fracture on one side: The side on which it is to be inserted first is governed by the fracture geometry, especially in an oblique fracture. Not to tighten it fully.
- Reduction of a transverse fracture, with some manual axial compression. This is important, prior to application of a self-centering forceps on the other fragment, where the 2nd screw is to be inserted in eccentric mode through the oval hole. If the bone ends are held well against each other, then further compression achieved by the sliding hole geometry is utilized for bone to bone compression and not merely to bring the bone ends together.

Thus a screw close to the fracture site is inserted on one side first and then on the other side a screw close to the fracture is inserted in eccentric mode. (In practice, it is possible not to tighten the first screw fully and move the plate over the first screw, while drilling a hole on the other fragment, so that, even the first screw is also placed in an eccentric mode). Both the screws are then alternately tightened. Then screws are inserted alternately on each side of the fracture line in neutral mode.

There is other philosophy as well, especially for a transverse fracture. Use a midway screw in each fragment and load the fracture in eccentric mode as usual. At this stage, usually the ends of both the fragments are slightly away from the plate. Now when one inserts the screws close to the fracture in neutral mode, the bone ends are slightly brought close to the plate and the fracture is further compressed.

Quality of the implants and instrumentation: Must be assured and preferably from the same manufacturing company, to match the drill bit, tap, sleeves and the plate.

Small fragment system: 3.5 mm instrumentation is required. A cordless power drill is a great asset for this technically demanding procedure.

Appropriate education with standard equipment is a necessary a part of training, because it involves soft tissue respect and atraumatic technique. This is better observed and learned than can be described.

Those who innovated tension band plate fixation recommend bone grafting as a necessary part of plate fixation procedure, in fracture of the femur at least. The fracture healing occurs where there is bone to bone contact opposition between the fragments. Bone stabilized by a plate cannot throw a callus. While with an intra-medullary nail as an implant, there is controlled micro-motion and hence some external callus is observed. Therefore, where there is a crushing of bone, comminution or bone loss and a plate fixation is to be done, complementary bone grafting is necessary. This step in the operative procedure is necessary and does not add to the magnitude of the procedure. The quantity of bone graft required is small, and hence, the extent of exposure at the donor site as well. This complementary procedure is far acceptable than having to do secondary procedure of bone grafting, at a later date.

On arrival, one should study the X-ray film, to assess the diameter and uniformity of the medullary cavity. At times, in a lateral view, the radius and the ulna so overlap that one cannot assess the diameter correctly. In such a situation one must insist on another view, so the medullary cavity can be well assessed from one end to the other and surprises on the operation table can be avoided (Fig. 14.4).

Some bones have very narrow and irregular medullary cavity and hence even a narrow nail cannot be passed. In such a situation, a surgeon who prefers a nail as an implant has to keep the alternative of a plate, ready (Fig. 14.5).

If the medullary cavity of one bone is narrow and that of the other acceptable, then:

Combination: Plate for the radius and a nail for the ulna or vice versa also can be practiced and leads to a successful result.

Due to stress shielding, the bone segment under the plate thins out. Hence after removal of a plate, one needs to take extreme care, regular follow up and radiological examination, prior to permitting unrestricted activities. After

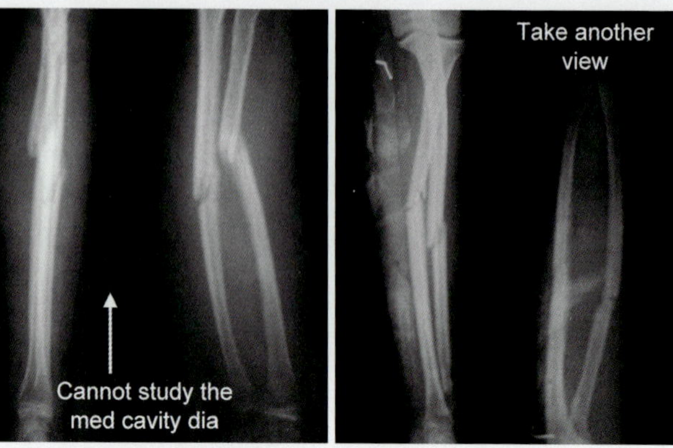

Figure 14.4 Narrow medullary cavity: Diagnosis

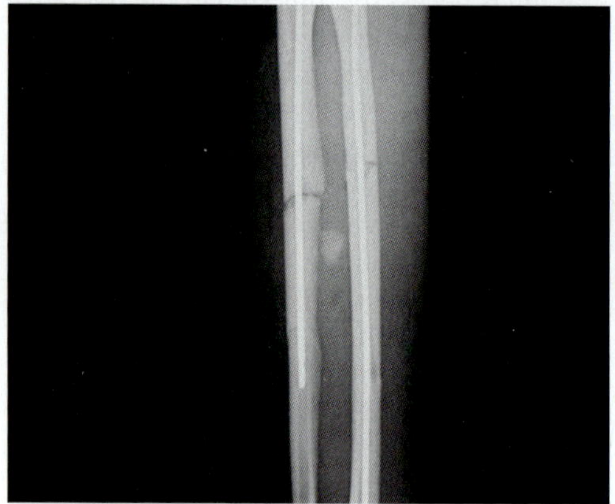

Figure 14.5 Narrow medullary cavity

removal of a nail, such precaution is not that necessary, because a stress shielding does not occur, when a nail is used as an implant.

After a fracture union with a plate fixation, and while the plate implant is in situ, if one has another injury to the same limb, there is a likelihood of a fracture developing adjacent to the plate. This is due to the difference in modulus of elasticity between the part of the bone under and beyond the plate. If this occurs, the management of such an injury is rather difficult. Therefore, after bone union, beyond doubt, it is recommended to remove the plate, at an early opportunity. Removal of the plate permits restoration on the bone elasticity and regaining the bone strength. This is important in adolescent and young persons (Figs 14.6A and B).

As seen in the mentioned figure, in a fracture of the ulna, with a triangular large 3rd fragment, a closed nailing is a good procedure. However, if one has to do a plate fixation, due to some other injury at the proximal end, a carefully done plate fixation, preserving the soft tissue attachment, especially to the 3rd fragment also leads to a good outcome. Often the fragment geometry is such that the plate needs to be on the entire length of the 3rd fragment and one can insert a screw through the plate only, to stabilize it. However, presence of the plate reduces the soft tissue attachment to the fragment and hence the blood supply.

UNUNITED FRACTURE OF RADIUS AND ULNA AFTER PLATE FIXATION FOR BOTH THE BONES

Using a plate as an implant for both the radius and the ulna is a technically demanding procedure. Soft tissue care, anatomical reduction and stable fixation, using a correct implant is very necessary step of the procedure. If the fractures are at the same level, then the wound closure without tension is rather demanding. If the bone union fails to occur, the blood supply to the bone ends is compromised and a revision procedure, if necessary, needs an additional procedure of bone grafting.

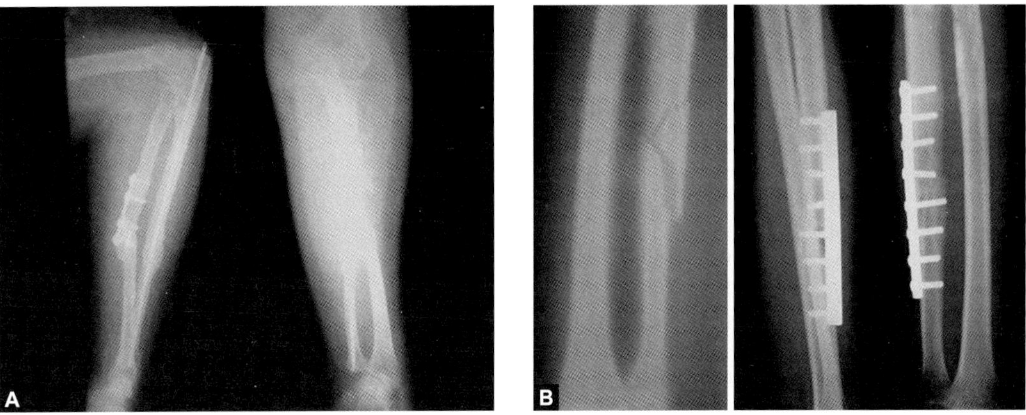

Figures 14.6A and B (A) Plate juxta-fracture; (B) Ulna 3-part fracture: plate

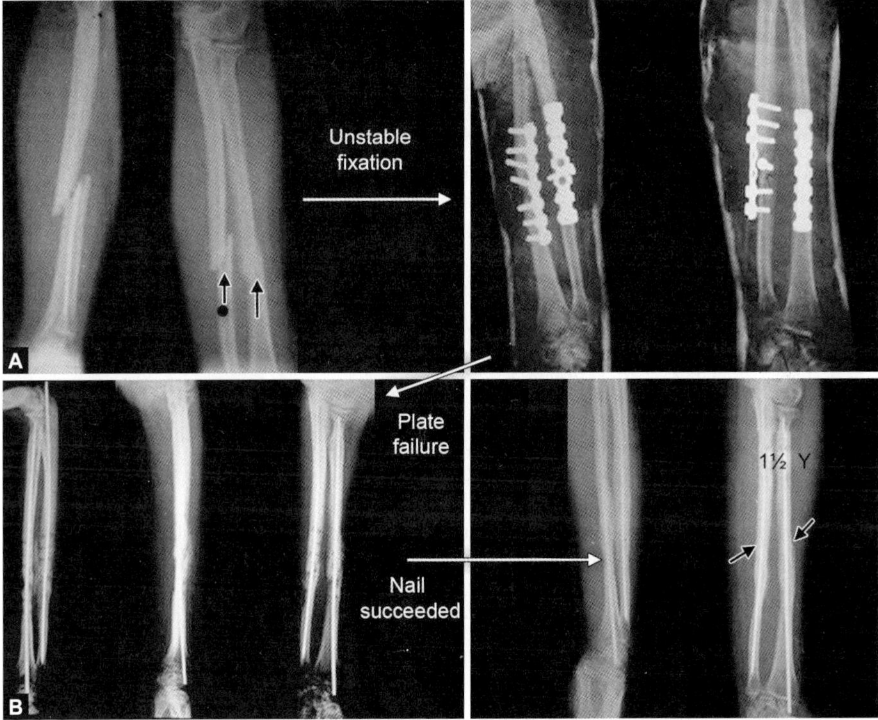

Figures 14.7A and B Plate failure—nail succeeded

In a case, a reconstruction plate and an IFS was used by a colleague. Continued to be ununited with abnormal mobility. I was consulted at this stage. Plate removal, IM nailing and bone grafting led to good union (FIgs 14.7A and B).

Failed Plate Fixation in Radius

A Galeazzi fracture dislocation was treated at another hospital. Surgery of radius plating was done at the same place. The plate fixation failed due to screw avulsion. The team revised it to a duel plate fixation, without bone grafting and immobilization given by a below elbow cylinder cast. (Mechanically, such an immobilization does not give external immobilization, but adds to the stress on the fracture area). One can well imagine the extent of soft tissue stripping required, when two plates are used, which would lead to avascularity of the bone ends. The short forearm cast this way is half hearted immobilization, as shown in the photo. It should be above elbow cast in supination. A position of full supination and mild dorsiflexion at the wrist maintains reduction of the inferior radio-ulnar injury also. I wonder if this dual plate fixation is a biomechanically good alternative. The fracture area is not visible in the X-ray and one cannot make a decision, if it has united beyond doubt (Figs 14.8 and 14.9).

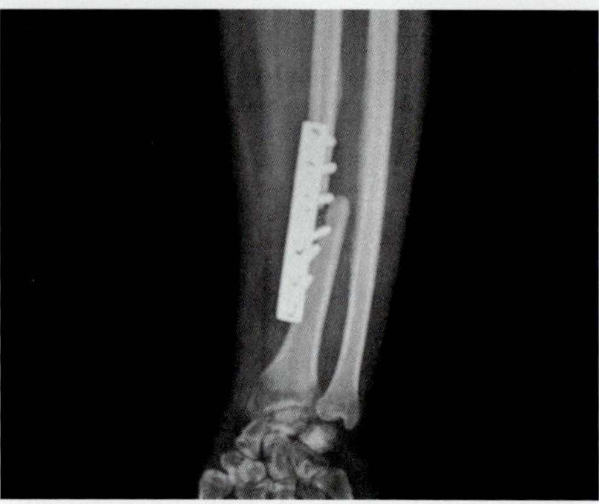

Figure 14.8 Failed radius plate I

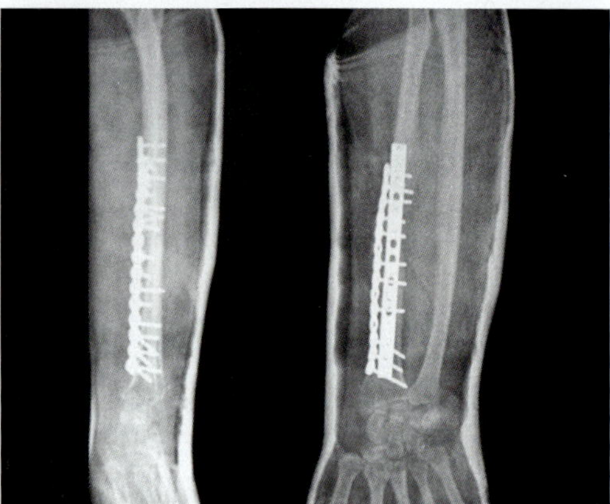

Figure 14.9 Failed radius plate II

BIOMECHANICAL DIFFERENCES IN A PLATE AND A NAIL

- After a successful closed nailing, the soft tissue envelope around the fracture is well preserved, with good blood supply to the bone ends.
  - Biologically, due to undisturbed soft tissues and hence the periosteal blood supply, the fracture healing is rapid, in a successful closed IM nailing. If an open nailing is needed, then it would be little slow and after a plate fixation, it would be still slow due to some soft tissue disturbance. However, due to absolute stability achieved after a plate fixation, it is possible to use the forearm for some light activities (Except a Monteggia or a Galeazzi injury, where external immobilization is required for the adjacent joint injury).
- The nail is a straight and an elastic implant, often taking the shape of the bone, in which it is inserted. In the fracture of upper/3 of radius, often the straight nail reduces the lateral radial bow. However, in clinical appearance and in the final range of motion, this is not noticeable.
- Should a bone grafting be needed for a non-union following a nailing procedure, the surface area available for the grafts to be laid down around the fracture area is much more than with presence of a plate. Besides, the plate is placed towards the skin and hence the bone grafts need to be placed around the plate, preferably on the other side. This increases a chance of cross union.
- During a procedure of plate fixation, in a comminuted fracture, one needs to be more careful. In management of an open fracture, after first aid and initial treatment, one may have to consider plate fixation as a definitive method of treatment. In an open fracture, which is in stage II is treated by a plate fixation, there is more chance

of postoperative infection. With local comminution, small bone fragments often have reduced blood supply. Lack of blood supply reduces the local tissue resistance and local bone ends are more susceptible to infection. Such a situation may lead to further extensive bone loss (Fig. 14.10).

- While a procedure of nailing is planned, at times one finds on table that the medullary cavity is very narrow and even a 2 mm nail cannot be inserted and then one needs to use a plate as an implant. Thus additional range of equipment for a plate fixation needs to be kept ready. At present, 2 and 2.5 mm reamers for either radius or ulna are yet not available. Occasionally, the medullary cavity is so narrow, that as was done in the past, a K-wire is used and this was said to be an internal suture of the fracture. In such a situation, the plaster cast was required for a longer duration. This used to be practised in yester years. Today with availability of precision equipment and implants a plate fixation option is used, which is preferable to a K-wire as an IM implant.
- In an adolescent patient, in some cases after a closed reduction of fractures of both radius and ulna, check X-ray through a cast shows difference in the inter-osseous space proximal and distal to the fracture site. This indicates rotational mal-alignment. To correct this by a repeat manipulation may not always succeed. However, if a nail can be successfully passed by a closed method, rotating the forearm appropriately, the reduction is often successful. The rotational mal-alignment and thus the interosseous space is restored well. This advantage of a closed nailing procedure is not enjoyed by the plate fixation (Figs 14.11 and 14.12).
- In a plate fixation in an ulna, due to less muscle and soft tissue mass over its subcutaneous area, wound healing problem is more likely than that in a radius bone.
- In a child, when soft tissue interposition is expected, open reduction and use of even a 2 mm K-wire will help to keep the bones aligned, in absence of a nail of exact diameter.
- Procedure of a closed nailing requires availability of a `C` arm, while a plate fixation can be done without it.
- A fracture is likely to be distracted after a nail is passed and may remain distracted, in spite of thumping, increasing the chance of a slow union.
  - Following such a situation, if the nail is not changed to another one with less diameter or length or both, the fracture may continue to be ununited and the nail may break at that site. It is observed that when such a breakage of the nail occurs, the fracture ends come in contact with opposition and unite! Of course, such an outcome is not observed in each case of mechanical failure of a nail. When a nail fracture removal of the other segment

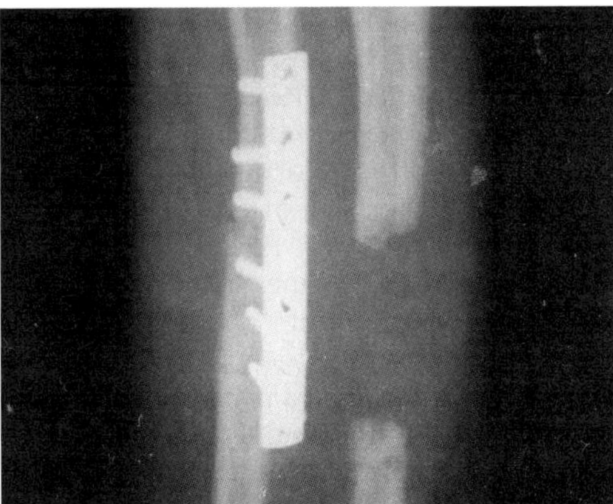

Figure 14.10 Bone loss

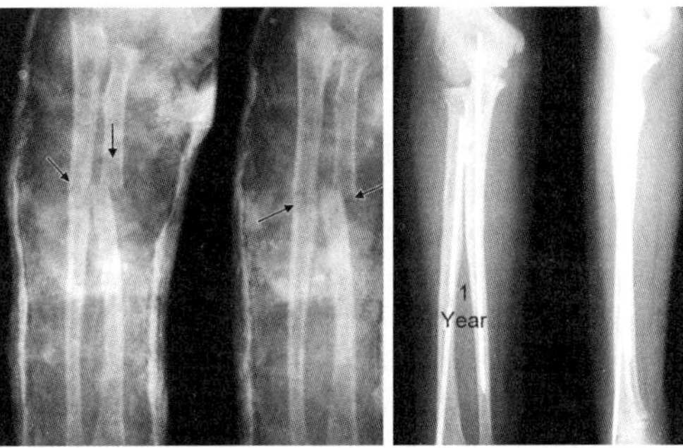

Figure 14.11 Rotational malalignment

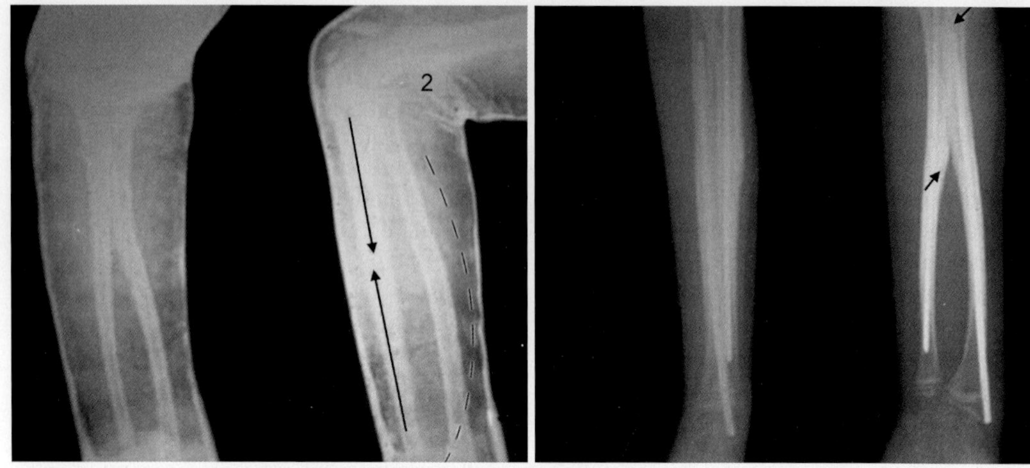

Figure 14.12 interosseous space

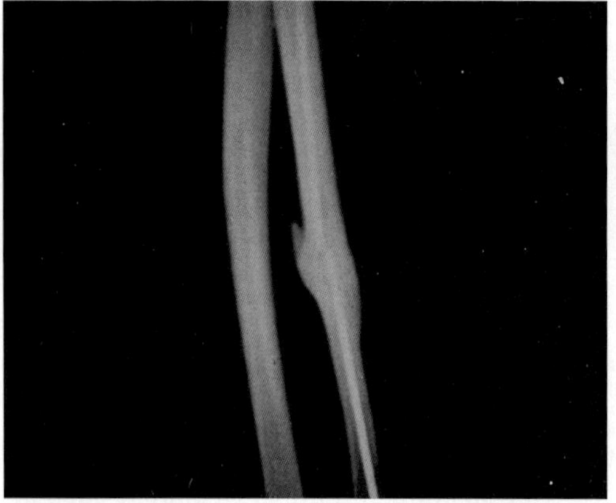

Figure 14.13 Ulna nail broken and fracture united

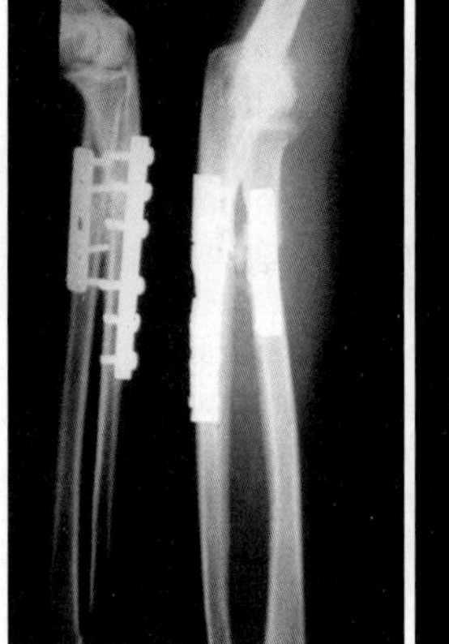

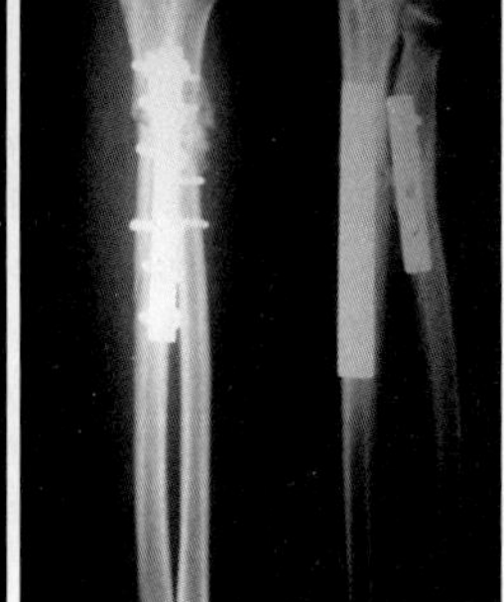

Figure 14.14 Cross union

of the nail is not possible, should a need arise in the future. May be there was some distraction at the fracture site, which kept the bone ends apart. As the nail gave way, the bone ends opposed and the fracture united well (Fig. 14.13).

- Fracture of both radius and ulna in the upper/ 3 level, especially when they are at the same level, demand special consideration. If a plate is chosen as an implant for both the bones and there is a 3rd fragment, one needs to be extra careful, during the dissection/ reduction of both the bones. (At this level of the forearm fracture, if a nail is used as an implant, and closed nailing is successful, it is very satisfying. However, should open reduction is required, due to soft tissue intervention to use a nail as implant, the exposure required is relative less and soft tissue handling too is less. Usually, the nail being elastic, takes the shape of the bone, maintaining the interosseous space. In spite of all the care taken, a chance of cross union is more when a plate is used in both the bones. The radius and the ulna are quite close to each other and hence the fracture hematoma is more likely to communicate with the adjacent bone (Fig. 14.14).

- When a nail is to be removed in time, usually it is relatively an easy procedure and the exposure is at the end of bone only. The scar too is more acceptable.
- After removal of the nail, early return to work.
- After removal of an IM nail there is no stress shielding and hence re-fracture less likely.
- Chance of fracture union is high and that of failure less.
- Often a closed nailing is successful and hence patient is pleased with cosmetic result.

NAIL AS AN IMPLANT

Technique of IM Nail Insertion

Square nail for use in the radius and the ulna has been popularized by late Dr AK Talwalkar. The ulna being a relatively straight bone, the nail tip has a trocar point. The radius being a curved bone, it has to take the shape of the bone, gliding along the endosteum. Hence, it has a blunt, curved chamfer with a rounded tip. (In clinical practice, with some experience, it is possible to use either of the two types in either of the bones, in special situations).

As per the medullary canal observed in ethnic population, the nails are available in 2, 2.5, 3 and 3.5 mm diameter. In some situations, two nails together (stacked) can be inserted in one bone, when the medullary cavity is much wider than the available nail diameter.

The butt end has a threaded end. Unfortunately, there is no standardization in these threads, as manufacturers have their own choice. My suggestion is to have MKS (decimal) system. The diameter and the pitch needs to be standardized, so that it is easy to manufacture a corresponding nail extractor. There should be two types of threads: one for a 2 mm diameter nail and the other for 2.5 and 3 mm diameter nails. The threads pitch should not be too less, as then the hold of the extractor tube on the nail threads is less. This is a practical solution, which everyone should insist.

One should keep a practice of measuring the radius length on the opposite forearm, soon after arrival, to keep the nail of correct size ready. It is measured from ¼" proximal to the tip of radial styloid to ½" distal to the upper end of the radius. The diameter of the nail is visually judged, looking at the analogue X-ray film or on a true size digital film. In an average built person, the radius nail of 8¾ "(22 cm) is required. The ulna nail is also measured and it is an observation that it is usually 2 cm longer than the radius nail.

Having measured the lengths, one should make a bunch of radius nails of 3 diameters in each. This is the length measured. Additional 1 cm shorter and 1 cm longer nails in 3 diameters be available on the trolley. Ulna nails are similarly kept ready. I prefer to have additional 15 × 2 mm ulna nails ready on the trolley, which is used to stack a nail. Nails beyond this range should be sterile and be available. Thus, one knows, what sizes of nails are commonly required and one should maintain the inventory accordingly. It is important and prudent to use a nail of precise length and diameter, for good stability and ease of removal later. If this is not practised, then one has to cut the nail, to make it of a desired length, losing the good extraction threaded end. If the threaded end of a radius nail is cut, the cut end of the nail is sharp, irregular and irritates the tendons, with a possibility of an attrition rupture.

INSTRUMENTS REQUIRED

- Langenbeck retractors
- *Kuntscher diamond awl*: A small version is more suitable. A cobbler awl is useful in adolescent patients.
- Non-cannulated Jacob chuck with a T handle. Non-cannulated is important, because if the accidentally the chuck grip loosens, the nail end will not hurt palm of the surgeon.
- Small Hohmann bone levers
- Small self-centering forceps
- Square punch
- Small hammer approx 200 G
- *Extractor*: Hollow threaded tubes, with a Kuntscher nail extractor
- Small bone scoop/curette

- 2 mm × 180 mm K-wire
- Front and side wire cutter
- Needle nose pliers.

Which Bone First?

- *Displaced fracture radius and undisplaced fracture ulna*: After such a major injury, an undisplaced fracture ulna indicates, possible continuous soft tissue envelope. To achieve a successful closed nail insertion in the radius, one needs to manipulate the forearm, which does cause some angulation at the ulna fracture site. After a successful closed radius nail insertion, the ulna usually remains undisplaced and it is also possible to achieve a closed ulna nail insertion.
- *Displaced fracture ulna and undisplaced fracture radius*: Such a combination is rarely observed. As above, the radius is stabilized first. In an attempt to stabilize the ulna first, there is a chance that the radius soft tissue envelope may get disturbed and then one may have to carry out open reduction for radius. The approach is more demanding and the postoperative scar is also more visible. Ulna being a straight bone, with less soft tissues on the posterior surface, is more amenable to a closed technique. Even if one needs to carry out an open reduction, it is relatively a superficial bone and the scar is not so noticeable, being on the posterior surface.
- *Displaced fracture of both radius and ulna*: Radius is managed first.
- *Conclusion*: Because of different reasons, the radius is stabilized first!

A pneumatic tourniquet is used: General anesthesia/nerve block/IV regional anesthesia have their own merits.

A side table with a radiolucent top and a stand makes it stable. However, the table support leg may come in the way of the 'C' arm tube. Hence, it is possible to use a 12" broad wooden plank, well inserted below the table mattress, after anesthesia procedure is over.

TECHNIQUE OF RADIUS NAIL INSERTION

Preoperative Study

It is necessary to view an atlas of anatomy and study a book on surgical exposure, together. This is more important, in exposure of radius in the upper/3 of forearm. Disregard to this may lead to injury to the posterior interosseous nerve, with a disability, which can be avoided.

Entry in the radius from the distal end: The entry has to be from the dorsal side and the track needs to be oblique. Hence the track has to be slightly wider and longer to get an access in the medullary cavity. Though a point medial to the Lister tubercle is more in alignment with the medullary cavity, I prefer to make an entry lateral to the tubercle. It is easier to access this point because, the space between extensor carpi radialis brevis and the tubercle is adequate. The nail tip lies flush with the bone and does not irritate the tendons. Besides, the nail track and the placement being oblique, the nail tip, due to elasticity, springs back towards the endosteum and remains stable. It thus lies on the dorsal cortex of the radius. Due to the oblique path taken, it does not back out easily, as in the ulna. At the end of surgery, one should mention the point of nail entry, whether it is medial or lateral to the Lister tubercle, in operation notes (and be able to retrieve the notes prior to the nail removal for precise exposure and dissection then).

After draping the limb, sustained traction from the thumb and counter-traction from the elbow is given at least for two minutes. If one can have two assistants, the more trained one holds the fingers, while the other one gives a counter-traction. This helps to align the bones and the soft tissue envelope would fall back in place. Usually the fracture is well-aligned, while the elbow is at 90 deg flexion and forearm in full supination. The 'C' arm is brought in and lateral image, with traction on is studied. The forearm, while maintaining the traction is made slightly prone and the X-ray tube is tilted appropriately, to get the other view of the fracture site. The selected nail is mounted and ready in the T handle. The traction should be released and the nail insertion started. The lateral part of the distal dorsal radius is exposed by a vertical approach and area lateral to the tubercle is exposed. The 1st assistant retracts medially only the skin and laterally the ext. carpi radialis longus and brevis tendons and continues so, till the nail is inserted. The surgeon holds the patient's hand keeping it in palmer flexion and slight ulnar deviation and maintains so, till the nail is inserted till the expected fracture site level. With a small diamond awl, a canal is made first at right angle to the bone and then it is tilted and inclined towards the shaft and inserted along it for approximately 8 mm. Without losing the vision on the field, the awl is kept aside and the nail mounted on the T handle is taken. The chamfer of the nail tip is kept towards the lateral radial bow, to slide easily along it. Backflow of marrow indicates that the nail is in the medullary cavity (Dr KH Sancheti). The two assistants go back to their positions for traction and counter-traction. The surgeon checks the reduction and advances the nail by gentle rotary motion. Usually the reduction is achieved, while the forearm is in supine position. In a transverse fracture, often some translation is noted at the fracture site and the nail can be felt to abut against the wall of the proximal fragment. If so, it is slightly withdrawn. While the traction is continued, some local side to side pressure on the bone ends, aligns the fragments and the nail can be advanced in the proximal fragment. The distance available in the medullary cavity beyond the nail tip and length of the nail outside the entry site are matched to confirm that the nail length is correct. When the nail is for adequate distance in the proximal fragment, the reduction remains stable. Presence of the nail in the proximal fragment is confirmed in 'C' arm, in two views. Now, while the two assistants maintain gentle compression across the bone in supination, the nail is further advanced. Check again in 'C' arm. After having the nail in good position, the forearm is made prone and the wound edges of the nail entry are retracted. At this stage, the tendon of extensor pollicis longus crossing the nail entry area often gets trapped under it. With good retraction and movements of the wrist, the tendon is made free. keeping the tendons retracted, the second assistant maintains the manual compression across the bone, final setting of the nail is done with a square punch. The nail tip is preferably kept 3 mm distal to the edge of the track. This curvature along the length of the nail gives a recoil against the bone and the nail remains well seated in the bone. Due to this mechanics, the radius nail hardly ever backs out, while the ulna nail, being in a straight bone, may back out.

Observation: A transverse fracture is usually easily reduced and the serrated ends offer a telescopic stability. In an oblique fracture, ends tend to stand away from each other. To obtain a good reduction and then entry of the nail tip in the other fragment is difficult to achieve. Often the sharp bone ends penetrate soft tissue around, leading to soft tissue interposition. This makes a closed IM nailing rather difficult.

One should set certain time-frame for a successful passage of the nail in the proximal fragment. It is not prudent to keep on trying too long, with more radiation to everybody. If the closed nailing is unsuccessful, one should not hesitate to do an open reduction.

OPEN REDUCTION

The fracture is exposed by one of the standard approaches, with which one is familiar. One should not try to do an open reduction with a small incision. Though the skin incision may appear to be a small one, often the deeper tissues are too much disturbed, which is not desirable. One should take a moderate length incision for a safe soft tissue handling. On an X-ray film, one should measure the distance of the fracture from the radial styloid and with traction on, measure on the limb the distance of fracture site from the radial styloid and that should be the midpoint of the incision. With availability of a 'C' arm, this is relatively easier to do.

Having exposed the fracture ends, the soft tissue interposition, if any, is removed. The usual practice is to use small size self-centering forceps (in place of yester years' Burn's forceps). (It is possible to reduce the fracture and oppose the bone ends, using an awl. The tip is wedged in between the bone ends and makes a fulcrum of one bone end and levers the other fragment in place.) Having aligned both the fragments, the nail is advanced in the other fragment. This technique has an advantage of maintaining the soft tissue attachments against use of bone holding forceps on either bone ends. One needs to see how it is done and how useful it is.

TECHNIQUE OF ULNA NAIL INSERTION

A selected nail is mounted in a T handle. The assistant holds the patient's hand in one and the lower arm in either hand, keeping the shoulder and the elbow flexed to 90 deg, and forearm across the chest. The surgeon should palpate the olecranon and select a site at midpoint of the olecranon. One should be able to visualize a point, which will be in line with the medullary cavity. A vertical incision exposes the triceps aponeurosis, which is incised, till the flat posterior surface of the olecranon is seen and felt. The entry should be approximately 5 mm proximal to the posterior surface of the shaft, to be in line with the medullary cavity. In adolescent, a small diamond awl and in a child, a cobbler awl is used to prepare an entry point. An entry point from the medial surface of the ulna is also possible, so the nail travels in a curved way and due to the elastic recoil, it remains stable.

The ulna is slightly curved with concavity medially. Hence, the direction of the awl should be maintained accordingly. The awl is exchanged to the nail in a T handle and is passed by manual pressure. As in the radius nail insertion, the nail is never hammered to advance, except tapping for the last 20 mm or so. The fracture is reduced, as in the radius and checked under 'C' arm. A transverse fracture is more amenable to a closed procedure than an oblique one. Having confirmed that the nail is intramedullary, final seating is done and the nail is gently tapped home. While doing the final seating of the nail, the assistant supports the lower arm and with the other keeps the wrist in dorsiflexion and exerting an axial compression. This helps to prevent distraction at the fracture site, while the tip of the nail enters the relatively firm to hard segment near the head ulna.

Nailing and Diameter of the Nail

In both the radius and ulna prograde nailing is the method of choice. Ulna in the proximal part and the radius in the distal part have relatively a wider medullary cavity. It is necessary to have a good fit between the nail and the bone, especially at the fracture site. As is the observation, the radius being a curved bone, the intramedullary nail has a spring-like elastic fitting in the medullary cavity and usually stays as such. As against this, the ulna is relatively a straight bone and the backing out of an ulna nail is more common than that in a radius. Hence, in the ulna, one should prefer to add another nail, in addition to the principal nail. This `stacking a nail` is usually done by a 2 mm diameter square nail.

In a transverse fracture, should open reduction be required, due to soft tissue interposition, then matching of the serrated bone ends assures that rotational alignment is well restored.

In a closed technique, while negotiating a fracture area, especially in an oblique fracture, one should so angulate the fracture area, that the nail tip abuts against the medullary cavity inside the bone spike of the distal fragment and then it is more likely to succeed. If still it does not succeed, it is worth trying to use a narrower nail, which may succeed in negotiating the fracture area and enter the distal fragment. Having thus entered the distal fragment, if needed, one can pass another thin nail as a stacked nail, which is more likely to enter adjacent to the first nail in the proximal fragment.

The Technique of Stacking a Nail

The medullary cavity is studied. If one feels that the proximal segment of the ulna medullary cavity would accept another nail, the first nail is kept approx 2 cm outside the bone at the entry point. Another 2 mm diameter nail is mounted in a Jacob Chuck with T handle and passed adjacent to the first one. The first nail may automatically move further slightly. It is preferred that the length of the second nail be such that, at the final setting, the tip of the second nail should remain in the proximal fragment and should not lie in the fracture area. In fracture of the upper/3 of ulna, the medullary cavity distal to the fracture may accept the second stacked nail. One may pass the nail beyond the fracture site as well. While doing so, the wrist needs to be kept in dorsiflexion and both the elbow and wrist compressed against each other, to prevent distraction at the fracture site. Distraction at the fracture site after a nailing procedure increases a chance of failure of union and/or mechanical failure of the nail. If one cannot bring together the two fragments by manual axial compression, one should not expect to achieve a physiological dynamization as well. Check under the `C` arm that the fracture is well opposed.

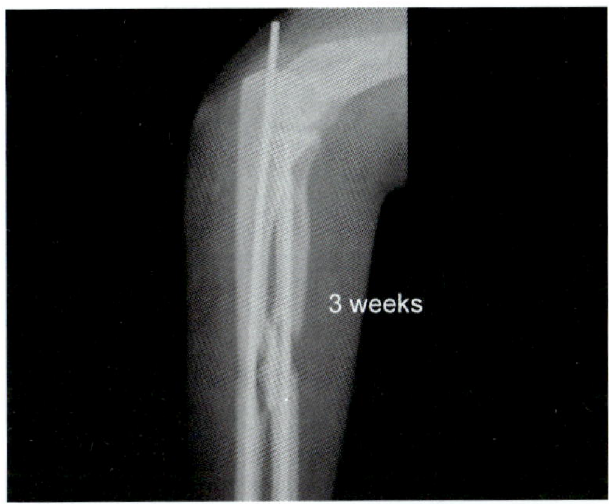

Figure 14.15 Ulna nail backs out

Thus the nail tip of the second stacked nail be either 2 cm. proximal or 2 cm. distal to the fracture site and should not be in the fracture line area. This would also prevent a stress riser effect at the fracture site.

When the second nail cannot be passed any more, it is withdrawn for 1 cm and cut at a point, 1 cm from the bone surface. Then alternately both the nails are gently tapped to set finally. It is preferred to keep 3 mm nail outside the bone surface, to facilitate easy removal later. Thus, the principal nail has threads at the butt end, while the stacked nail may not have the threads, as it is usually cut off. This part of the technique may vary from surgeon to surgeon (Figs 14.15 to 14.17A).

A CASE REPORT

A successful closed nailing in a fracture of radius and the ulna was done by a colleague. During follow up of the case, pain and irritation

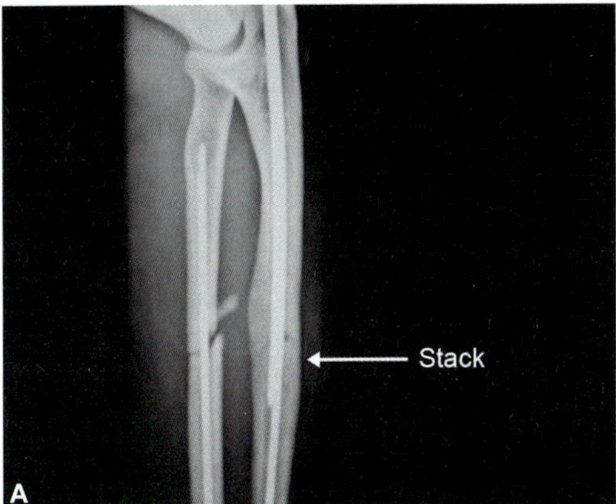

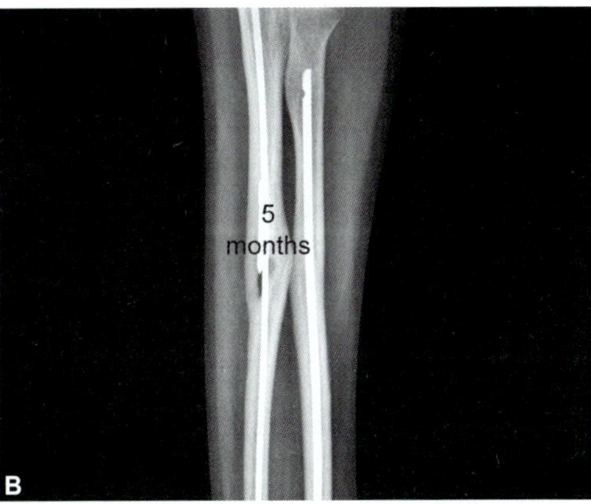

Figures 14.16A and B (A) Stacking ulna nail crossed the FR site; (B) Stack nail tip in fracture line

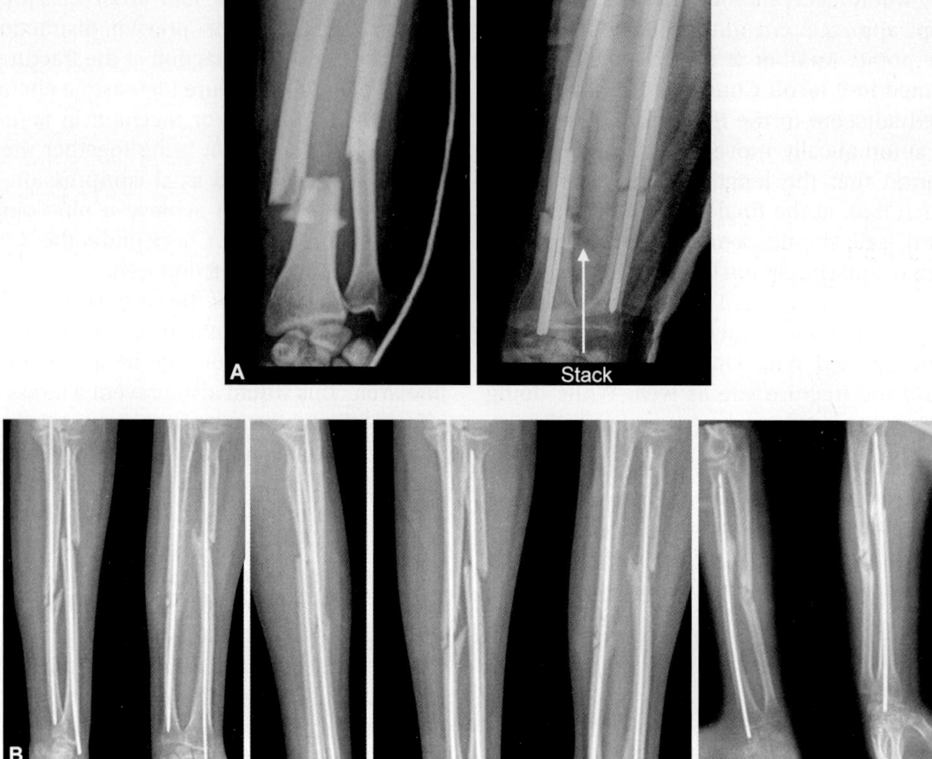

Figures 14.17A and B (A) Stacking radius nail; (B) Early ulna nail removal

at the elbow was observed. This was due to ulna nail tip being too long, outside the olecranon. The surgeon just removed the ulna nail before the fracture united. The fracture failed to unite and presented to me. (The X-ray film was a small one and did not show the olecranon). I feel, rather than nail removal, if the nail was replaced with a short nail and an additional stack nail technique was done at this stage, continued stability would have maintained. The ulna fracture would have united, as the radius did (Fig. 14.17B).

Length of a Nail in Fracture of Radius/Ulna

In juxta-articular fracture, a nail of an exact length is needed. A slightly long nail keeps the fragments well reduced and under tension and stable. However, the tip being locked in the hard end of the cortex, collapse (contact opposition) of the fracture is less likely, leading to delayed union—due to lack of physiological dynamization) (Fig. 14.18).

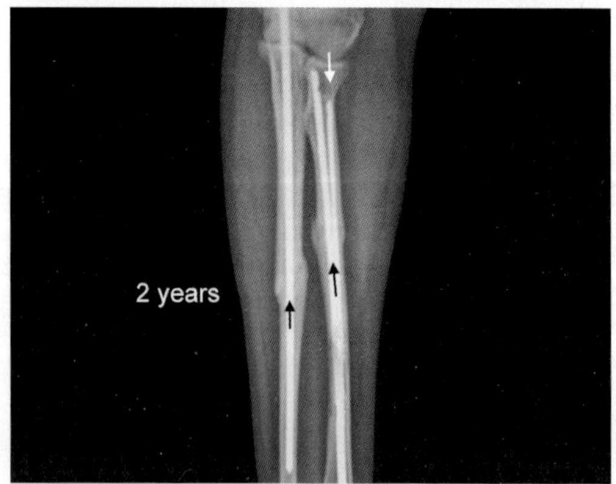

Figure 14.18 Exact length nail: Slow union

Thus, it is desirable to have 5 to 8 mm space beyond the nail tip and end of the medullary cavity. This permits slight axial movement of the nail and better and assured contact opposition between the fracture fragments (physiological dynamization) (Fig. 14.19A).

Trick: If a nail after insertion is found to be little longer than a desired length and if a little short nail is not available in the inventory, two methods can be practised, in such a situation:

- One can cut off a part of the threaded butt end of the nail, which is protruding from the nail entry site.

  or

- One member of the operating team holds the forearm and maintains the reduction, while other person removes the nail gently. The tip of the nail (business end) is cut to the desired length and the same nail is quickly reinserted, without losing the reduction. This has an advantage that the threaded butt end is available for easy removal, when necessary (Dr Anand S Kelkar).

During the ulna nail insertion, the tip outside the olecranon has to be just 2 mm or so. If it is more, after the local edema reduces, the tip irritates the skin and patient is uncomfortable. In the given example, a closed nailing was successful. However, due to the skin irritation at the ulna nail tip, the surgeon just removed the nail and did not change to a one with a short nail. The fracture had not united. In the end, the radius fracture united, while the ulna had a fibrous union, with some abnormal mobility.

The future in this case: As per the observation, the ulna also needs to have a good osseous union, to support the forearm and contribute to load sharing. Now, at this stage of fracture union in this case, one must revise the fixation of ulna and carry out a bone grafting. If this is not done, with a possible another injury, there is a chance of fracture of the radius, as the forearm is supported only by a well-united radius alone.

IMPORTANCE OF ACHIEVING A GOOD UNION IN THE ULNA

Both the radius and the ulna are important to carry out good function of the forearm. Though the ulna has a smaller diameter in the distal half, still it does contribute to the strength of the forearm. In yester years, often a non-union or a delayed union in the distal ulna was not taken too seriously.

Following example will highlight contribution of ulna in maintenance of forearm strength.

A young man had a fracture of the lower/4 of the ulna and a plate fixation was done. Unfortunately, it was infected and the plate was removed. Infection settled. He reported to me at this stage. I recommended revision surgery, to have a good union in the ulna. He

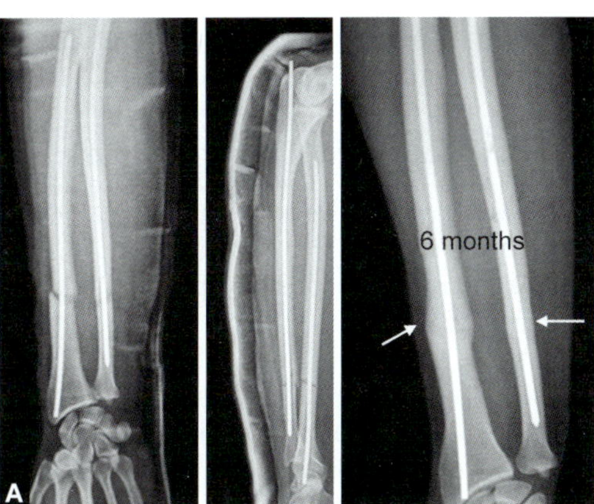

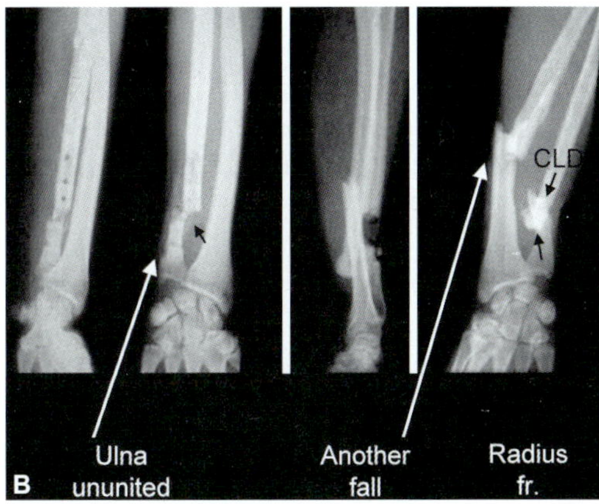

Figures 14.19A and B (A) Good nail length; (B) Ulna continuity important

did not come for follow up. He had another fall from a bicycle and sustained a fracture of the radius shaft. I feel, if the ulna had united well, either after the first injury or after a subsequent procedure, it may have contributed to the forearm strength and the fracture of radius may have been averted. This is just a possibility (Fig. 14.19B).

When the medullary cavity is wide at one end and narrow in the rest of the shaft, the nail which would be accommodated will be relatively narrow for the wider segment. In such a case, if the nail is slightly short, even by 10 mm, the stability is compromised and during mobilization of the fracture, the nail is observed to core the bone around the tip of the nail. This especially, when mobilization is started rather early (Fig. 14.20).

Rarely, during fracture union, one may find massive callus formation in the fracture area. In such a situation, one should consider early nail removal, because the callus often grips the nail so much, that its removal is rather difficult, due to its firm anchorage in the callus mass.

Advantages of a Successful Closed Nailing

- The fracture union is relatively rapid, as the fracture hematoma is not disturbed and remains well-contained in the soft tissue envelope.

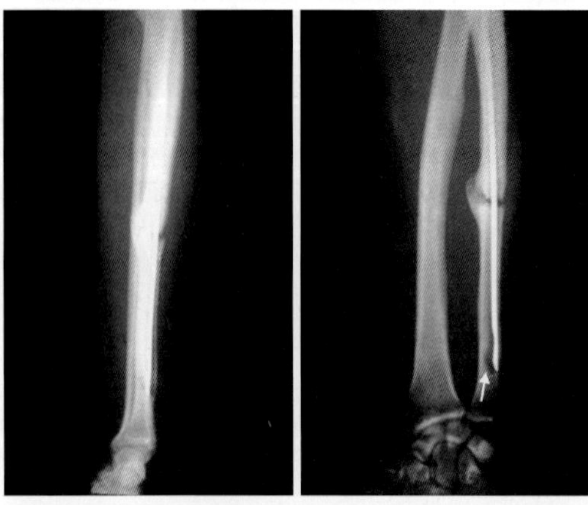

Figure 14.20 Ulna cored by a nail

- The soft tissues around the fracture are preserved.
- Less equipment needed for this procedure.
- The entire circumference of the bone is available for bone to unite. In a plate fixation approx 1/3 circumference is occupied by the plate, has reduced blood supply and its participation in fracture union, would be less.
- No scar at the fracture site and hence pleasing clinical appearance.
- Even in 2 views in a follow up X-ray film, the fracture line and status of union are seen clearly. After a plate fixation of both radius and ulna, especially when fractures are at the same level, even 4 different radiological positions may not give good view of even one bone, to know, if the fracture line has disappeared and the fracture has united beyond doubt.
- In 3- or 4-part fracture of either bone, if closed nailing is successful, the soft tissues attachment to the small fragments is preserved, giving a good chance of primary fracture union. Still, in some cases, the fracture may have a fibro-osseous union. Here few small fragments unite to the major fragments, converting a four-part fracture into a two-part fracture, which is easy to manage as a non-union.

As against this, in a case of plate fixation, due to absence of micromotion, the union between all the fragments may not succeed. Hence, in a 4-part fracture treated with plate stabilization, unless complementary bone grafting is done during the primary surgery, may lead to a slow or a delayed union (Figs 14.21 and 14.22).

Disadvantage of Nailing Procedure

- More X-ray radiation, during a closed nailing procedure.
- Difficult when medullary cavity is narrow/ irregular.
- Loss of radial bow and flattening of the radius (not in clinical outcome).
- Distraction of the fracture in some cases, if due care is not taken.
- Juxta-articular fracture is less amenable to this method.

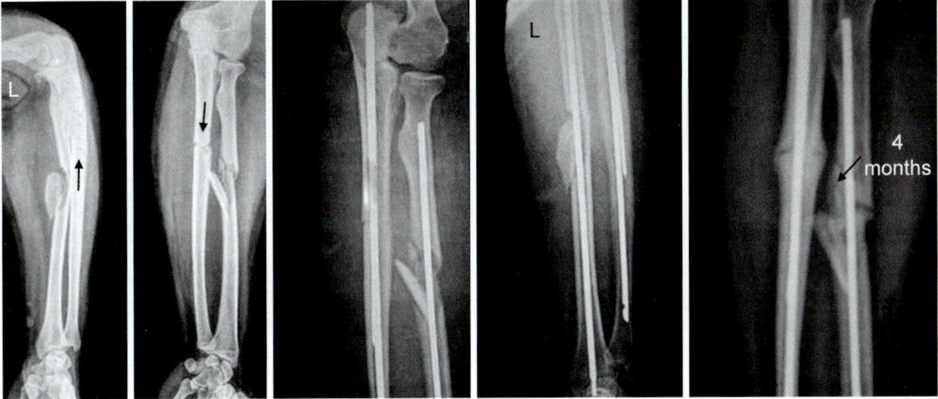

Figure 14.21 3rd fragment successful closed nailing

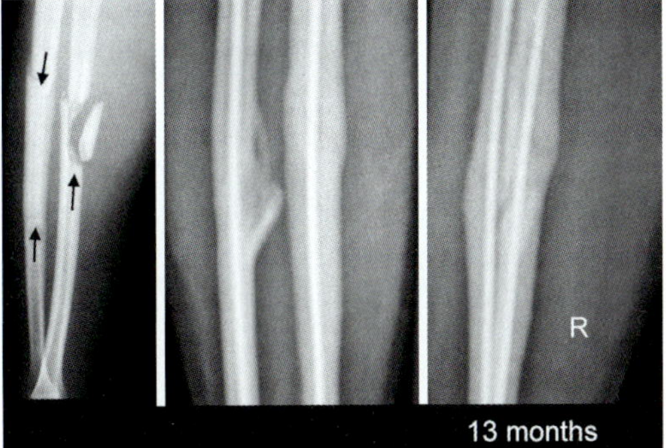

Figure 14.22 3rd fragment successful closed nailing

AFTER A BONE UNION, WHETHER THE PLATE AND THE NAIL NEED TO BE REMOVED

Plate Removal

- As discussed above, after a successful bone union with a plate fixation another injury may cause a fracture through the last screw hole or adjacent to the plate, due to difference of modulus of elasticity in the area below and adjacent to the plate.
- With passage of time, more stress shielding occurs under the plate.
- To remove a plate, all the screws need to be removed. Even if only one screw cannot be removed, then the plate needs to be left as such. In such a situation, the stress shielding is expected to reduce with time, because the plate being disconnected from the bone on one side, may transfer more load along the length.
  - This is mechanically true, if only one screw on any side remains to be removed. If one screw each on either side of the fracture area continues to be present, then stress shielding would continue, because, the plate would still transfer the load.
  - Often the screw head recess becomes round and the screw driver has no purchase on the screw. A screw driver made from a hard material (may be by a reputed manufacturer, usually does not yield, while removing a screw. A good technique is to slightly tighten the screw and then attempt to remove it. Alternate clockwise and anti-clockwise turning of the screw is known to succeed. Certain screw removal devices are available and can be considered as an option and be kept ready. The surgeon needs to be conversant with this procedure. When a screw is removed with difficulty, often the screw track becomes quite wide after its removal. This can lead to a fracture through the screw hole, as the hole acts

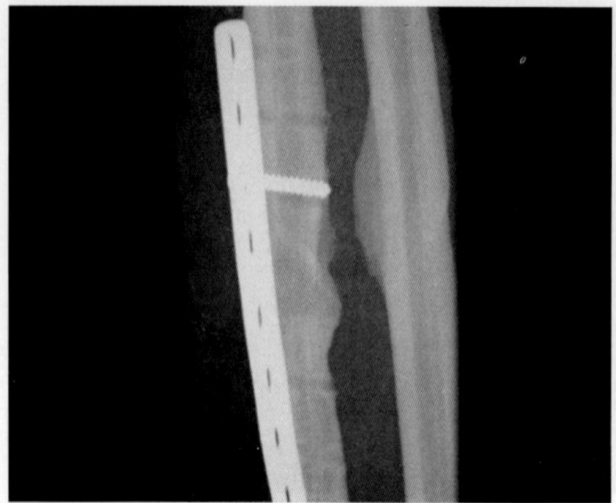

Figure 14.23 Failure of screw removal

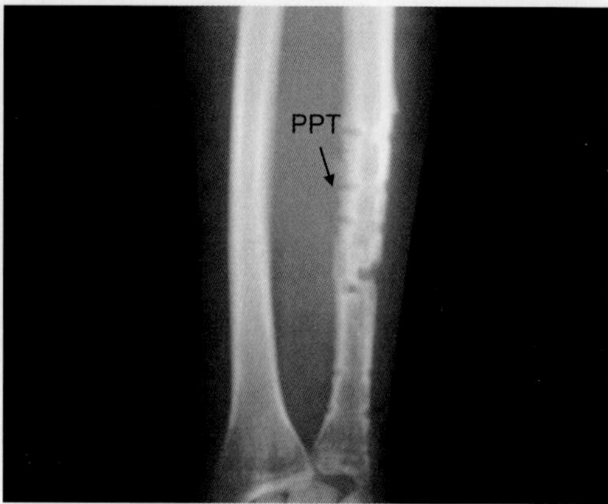

Figure 14.24 Ulna plate bone loss

as a stress riser and even a slight injury can lead to a fracture through an area, which has undergone stress shielding (FIg. 14.23).

- Restoration of the cortical thickness of the bone, the bone elasticity, the trabecular pattern, etc. takes quite a few months, to permit unprotected use of the limb.
- At times in a comminuted fracture, there may be some sectoral bone loss and hence a void in the continuity of the bone. During the primary healing process, the defect may remain as such, after the plate removal. However, if a closed nailing is successful in a case with a local tissue loss, due to crushing, blood supply to fragments is preserved. It is observed, that usually the defect fills up, during the healing process (Fig. 14.24).
- Bone elasticity is reduced and hence resistance to any stress is less. Hence, there is more chance of a refracture with an injury of lesser magnitude, leading to a transverse fracture.
- To prevent such an episode of a re-fracture after plate removal, one may consider to insert a protective nail in the medullary cavity. However, due to the screw tracks at right angle to the long axis of the bone and their lining present in the medullary cavity, passage of a protection nail is difficult.
- *Cosmetic appearance*: The scar after the two surgeries, one of plate fixation and the other of plate removal, is usually quite wide (Fig. 14.25).

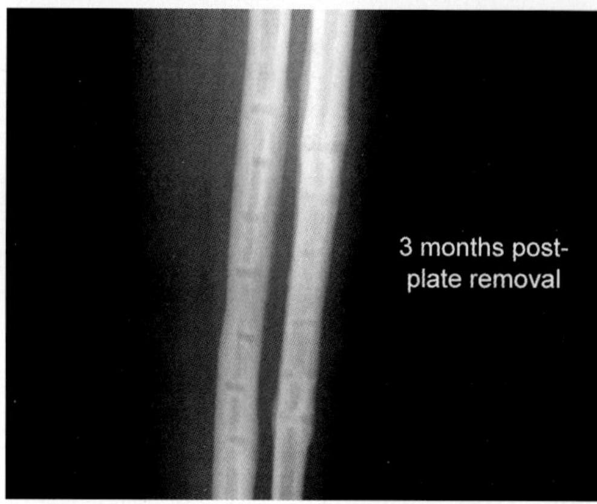

Figure 14.25 Screw tracks

Nail Removal

- An intramedullary nail is a load sharing device, while a plate is not so. Hence resumption of activities like riding a bike/ exercise/sports is earlier after removal of an intramedullary nail than removal of a plate.
- An intramedullary nail is preferably removed approximately six months after good radiological union. During this period, adequate remodeling is expected to occur and should be confirmed.

It is an observation in clinical practice, that in spite of a giving clear advice regarding the timely removal of an implant, very few persons report by themselves for the procedure of implant removal. Often this disregard for the timely removal of the implant is responsible for many problems one comes across during a nail removal after a long interval.

One must have a precision made and good quality nail extraction hollow threaded device. It is necessary to have different diameter of threaded extraction tubes, matching with the nail thread diameter. Usually, with such a device, it is possible to remove an implant safely.

THE TECHNIQUE OF NAIL REMOVAL

Open discussion with the patient and the members of the family, prior to the surgery is important, to explain the procedure and perhaps a likelihood of inability to remove the implant.

My preference is a general anesthesia, as a tourniquet can be safely and comfortably applied. One should discuss with the anesthesiologist, the probable duration expected to be taken for such a procedure, so the type of muscle relaxants to be administered can be well planned.

The time expected for the surgery, position of the patient and draping, etc. needs to be as if the nail is to be inserted, because the procedure at times, may take unexpectedly longer duration.

ULNA NAIL REMOVAL

If the nail tip is palpable or there is a bursa, the incision site is easy to determine. If the nail tip is palpable, on exposure, it is well seen. If the nail tip is flush with the bone, by careful vertical strokes of a knife, one should separate the triceps tendon fibers at the expected place and the shining tip of the nail is located. At times, a 'C' arm is needed to localize it. A 5 mm straight gouge is a useful tool. It is moved around the nail tip, to clear the soft tissues. A threaded extractor tube is slid and threaded over the nail tip. (It is a good practice to have a nail and matching extraction device in the armamentarium, so at the time of removal, the procedure is easy). Having engaged the nail as much as possible, a hook extractor, like a K nail extractor is engaged in the slot. With light blows of the hammer, usually the nail is withdrawn. If, during the procedure of IM nailing, the nail threaded end was cut, then it needs to be held with a narrow nose pliers. Often the pliers slips and the removal is rather difficult. It is at this point of time, that one realizes, why it is necessary to have the entire range of IM nails, in terms of length and the diameter. It is painstaking to maintain the entire range, especially of the commonly required sizes in terms of the length and the width of the nails. However, if one succeeds in maintaining the inventory, then to remove such a nail with threads at the end is far easier.

Often a nail is firmly anchored to the endosteum, by the body reaction. If the end threads are present and the matching extractor available, then the nail is removed with quite some ease (Fig. 14.26).

RADIUS NAIL REMOVAL

At the operation of insertion of a radius nail, I prefer to insert it on the radial side of the Lister's tubercle. However, some surgeons prefer to insert from the ulnar side of the tubercle. It is a good practice to mention this

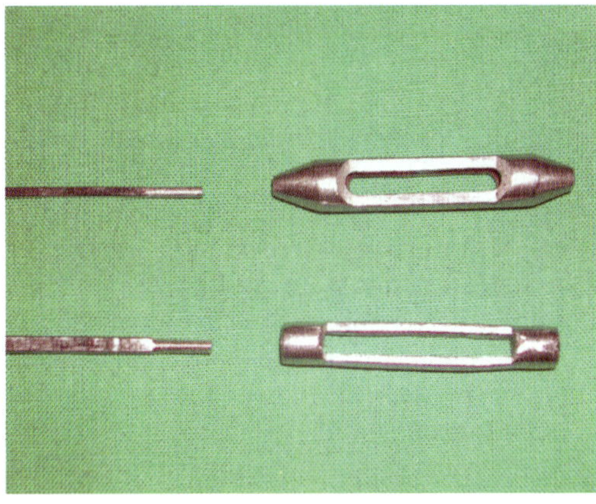

Figure 14.26 Nail extractor

in operation notes, so while the nail is to be removed, one exposes exactly that area. What is more important, is to mention so, at the time of primary surgery and to be able to remember this and retrieve the operation notes of the previous surgery!

The radius nail entry is from a side of the bone, unlike that in an ulna, which is in the same axis. Relatively an oblique wide track needs to be made for the nail insertion. At the end of the surgery, the nail tip rests against the edge of the track. However, due to the nail elasticity and as a bone reaction, the nail may tend to sink in the cavity and some bone overgrowth over the nail tip occurs. This is especially true in adolescent patients.

An incision is made over the previous scar and approach is made on appropriate side of the Lister tubercle. During the nail insertion procedure the tendon of extensor pollicis longus needs to be carefully protected. At the time of nail removal some fibrosis is noted to in this area and one needs to be more careful, to locate the tendon and protect it from the knife edge. Surgeon should hold the patient's hand and move it slightly in palmer and dorsal directions, while the assistant is retracting the skin edges. This helps to see the tendon sheath of EPL easily. The assistant should retract the tendon towards the ulnar side, while only the skin edge towards the radial side. Usually this makes the nail tip visible. Having seen the nail tip, as in ulna nail removal, a 5 mm gouge is used to make a space around the nail tip. In a young person with strong bone, it is possible to lever up the nail tip with the gouge deep to it, so the nail tip stands out. Once this is achieved, the tubular threaded extractor is threaded over the nail tip and the nail removed, as discussed above.

It is a safe practice to release the pneumatic tourniquet at this stage and then close the wounds. After closure, I prefer to add a padded crepe from the wrist to the elbow and a below elbow POP slab, to keep the reactionary swelling/oozing and postoperative pain, especially near the wrist, to a minimum. At the end of three days both the sites are dressed, only the crepe is continued and the plaster support discarded. In removal of only the radius nail, a below elbow crepe bandage is adequate.

NAIL REMOVAL BY A VERTICAL OSTEOTOMY

Looking at an X-ray film one cannot predict, if a nail can be removed with ease. One should also study possible site, where the nail may be jammed in the bone and mark on the film. One should have an open discussion with the patient, the likelihood that the nail may not come out. Many of us have an experience, that a 10-year-ago inserted nail comes easily, while a nail inserted 10 months ago, cannot!

- The nail may have to be left in as such.
- A possibility to remove the nail by a vertical osteotomy should be discussed in advance. After a successful osteotomy, one would need to immobilize the forearm in an above elbow cast for a few weeks and a consent be obtained to that effect. However, even after such an osteotomy, one may not succeed in the nail removal.

THE TECHNIQUE OF VERTICAL OSTEOTOMY

In the last two decades, with availability of a cordless power drill and a saw, this technique has become relatively safe. If the nail cannot be removed even with a threaded extractor, the X-ray is reviewed again and possible site of nail anchorage is studied:

- Expose the possible area, where the nail is likely to be jammed, which is usually the fracture site. The exposure be at least 3 cm on either side of the fracture site, along the length. With a narrow 5 mm osteotome, a vertical line is marked at the proposed site of osteotomy.
- With a 2.5 mm drill bit, serial drill holes are made along this line at a distance of 8 mm. As the drill pierces the outer cortex, it abuts against the nail within and one needs to stop immediately. This step of making multiple drill holes in a line, predetermines the

direction of the osteotomy and prevents any bone splintering in any other undesirable direction.

- Using a 5 mm thin and sharp osteotome, join the holes superficially. If a power saw is at hand, use it after this step, to complete the osteotomy. The blade grinds against the nail.
- With a 10 mm osteotome in the osteotomy, tap and slide it from one to the other end, slightly tilting it, to make the cut slightly wider. To move the osteotome through the entire length, one can hold it at an angle to the bone and with gentle tapping on it, it slides along. The nail extractor tube is attached to the nail and assistant is in readiness to withdraw the nail. The second assistant holds the forearm and stabilizes it. For removal of a nail from the radius, it is kept on the side table, while for removal of the ulna nail, it is held across the chest, as is kept while inserting it. With two osteotomes in the osteotomy cut, the diameter of the medullary cavity increases and at this stage the first assistant, with light hammer blows, removes the nail. With judgement, one can tilt the osteotome, whatever is just necessary. In spite of all this care, at times, a crack is noted, going obliquely from one end of the osteotomy. On a lucky day, the nail comes out after all these efforts.
- Thereafter, the tourniquet is released and closure commenced. Padded crepe and an above elbow POP support completes the procedure.
- *Failure to remove a nail*: Of course, I have faced a situation, when I had to leave a nail in place, even after it moved partly after a vertical osteotomy.

Thus often after removal of a nail after a vertical osteotomy, one may have to immobilize the limb in a plaster or at least delay unrestricted activities (Fig. 14.27).

Fracture of Lower/4 Radius and Ulna

Due to the local anatomy and wide medullary cavity, plating of the radius is a logical method. The distal fragment being small and very close to the radius nail entry site, the nail does not remain in center of the cavity. The medullary canal is also very wide and hence a plate is a better option.

The ulna fracture is conveniently managed by a closed IM nailing technique.

If one decides to stabilize both radius and ulna in the lower/3 area by a plate for each bone, the tissue exposure and tissue reaction is more and wound closure may be difficult. The circumference of the lower forearm is not adequate to accommodate the tissue reaction due to the initial injury and surgical trauma. Thus combination of a plate for the radius and a nail for the ulna is a good method (Fig. 14.28).

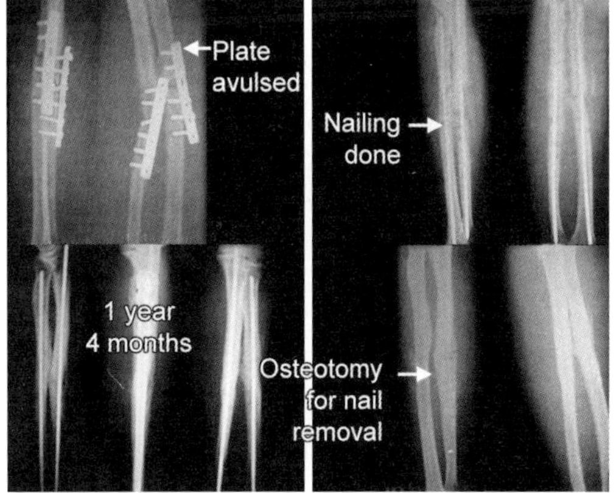

Figure 14.27 Osteotomy for nail removal

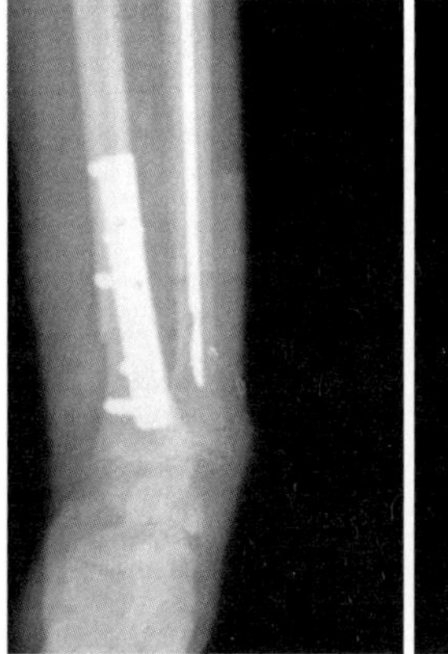

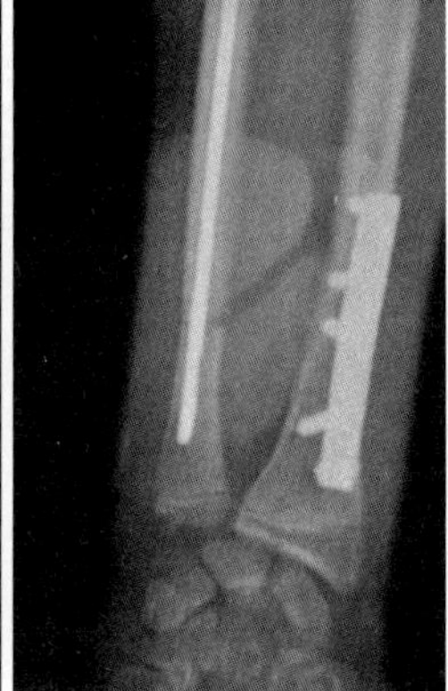

Figure 14.28 Radius plate and ulna nail in L/4

Monteggia Injury

Soon after arrival, this fracture dislocation injury must to be reduced. As per the patient's condition OT availability, etc. one can also plan a definitive surgery of closed reduction and internal fixation, as an emergency procedure. In such an injury, one can adopt technique of stacking the nails, which would offer more stability to the fixation and prevent nail back out.

If the OT facility for a required duration for an emergency internal fixation procedure is not available, one should at least carry out a closed reduction of the dislocated head radius and at a later stage internal fixation of the ulna could be done. This closed reduction of the dislocation, reduces the pain and keeps the tissue edema to a minimum.

Galeazzi injury: Described by Riccordo Galeazzi from Italy in 1930 (Also known as Piedmont injury).

Fracture of radius at the lower/3, with inferior radio-ulnar joint injury. The radius always needs internal fixation. Immediate closed reduction and of the injury in supination and slight dorsiflexion of the wrist reduces the inferior radio-ulnar joint. For internal fixation of the radius, a closed intra-medullary nailing is worth trying and is often successful.

After internal fixation of the radius, one needs to immobilize the forearm in an above elbow plaster cast, in supination of the forearm, with the wrist in slight dorsiflexion. The dorsiflexion keeps the head of the ulna well reduced and one needs to maintain this for six weeks, for good healing of ligaments, which stabilize the inferior radio-ulnar joint. Disregard to this and early mobilization tends to produce a pronation deformity with loss of supination.

Few clinical examples would support this (Figs 14.29 and 14.30).

Variation in the fracture pattern: Few clinical examples:

- *Fracture of the radius in the middle/3 area and segmental fracture of ulna.* In a segmental fracture of ulna, the distal fracture is usually undisplaced. This injury can be managed by closed nailing technique for both the bones. Plate fixation in a segmental fracture of the ulna would be an extensive procedure, compared to a closed nail fixation. At times in a segmental fracture in a long bone, closed IM nailing is successful at one site and may need to open the adjacent fracture site, due to soft tissue interposition. Still, it is biologically safer than use of a plate across both the fracture sites (Fig. 14.31).

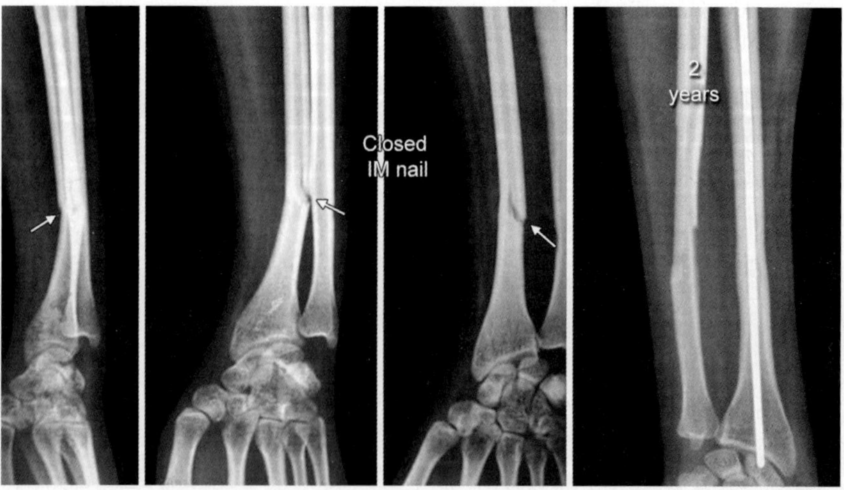

Figure 14.29 Galeazzi injury

- *Fracture of distal/3 of radius and a segmental fracture of the ulna*: The radius medullary cavity was quite narrow, even to accommodate a 2 mm diameter nail. In the ulna, the distal of the two fractures was undisplaced.
- Hence first a closed nailing was done for the ulna, followed by plate fixation for the radius (Fig. 14.32).

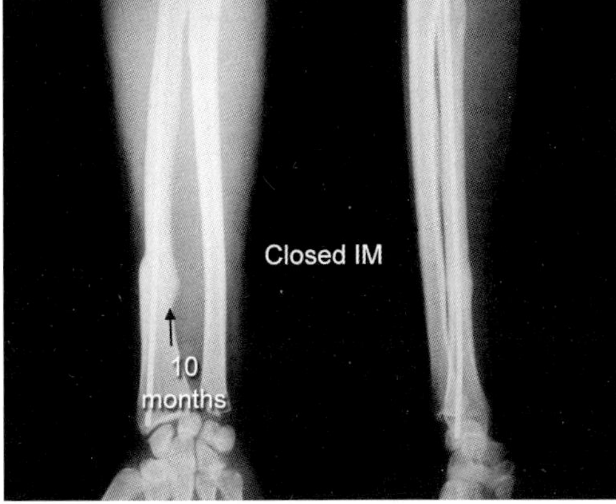

Figure 14.30 Galeazzi injury

- For both the above cases, above elbow cast was given for six weeks and the result was a good union in both the bones.
- Radius fracture with a displaced 3rd fragment and fracture of ulna.
  - *Choice of an implant*: If a plate was used for the radius, one wonders, if it would have been possible to put an IFS maintaining the blood supply to it. May be the fragment may have remained as such only, leading to a delayed/nonunion also and would need later bone grafting.

    Hence a closed nailing for both radius and ulna was attempted and was successful also.
  - The segmental fractures in the ulna united well. Gradually callus was noted at radius fracture, incorporating the displaced 3rd fragment.
  - Postoperative, above elbow cast in full supination was given for six weeks and then a posterior removable slab. This was removed for a bath and exercises. However, at the end, it was observed that the terminal supination was restricted by 10 deg approximately (Figs 14.33 and 14.34).

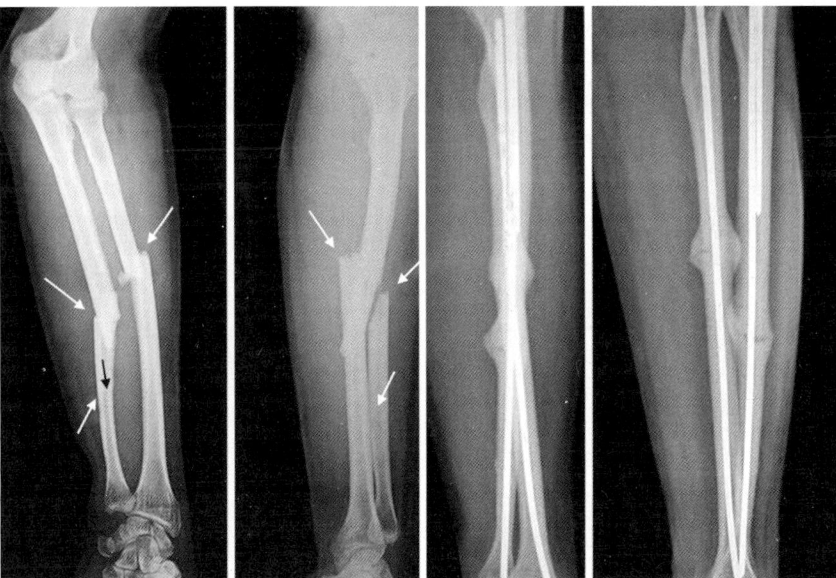

Figure 14.31 Fracture of radius in mid/3 and segmental ulna fracture: Closed IM nail for both bones

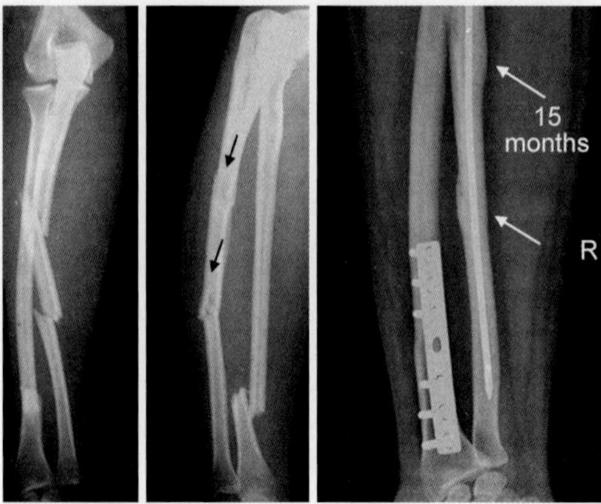

Figure 14.32 Radius narrow medullary cavity and segmental ulna fracture

- *Fracture of ulna in lower/2 area*: Non-operative method of treatment for ulna fracture is known for slow union (Fig. 14.35).
  - Following internal fixation with a nail in either a radius or an ulna or both bones, needs an external immobilization with an above elbow plaster cast for six weeks at least. After this duration, the cast is removed and progressive mobilization of the forearm is carried out.
  - Strengthening the forearm muscles helps further contact opposition of the fractures and their consolidation.
  - Non-operative method of treatment with an above elbow cast for six weeks is possible. However, at this stage, mild local

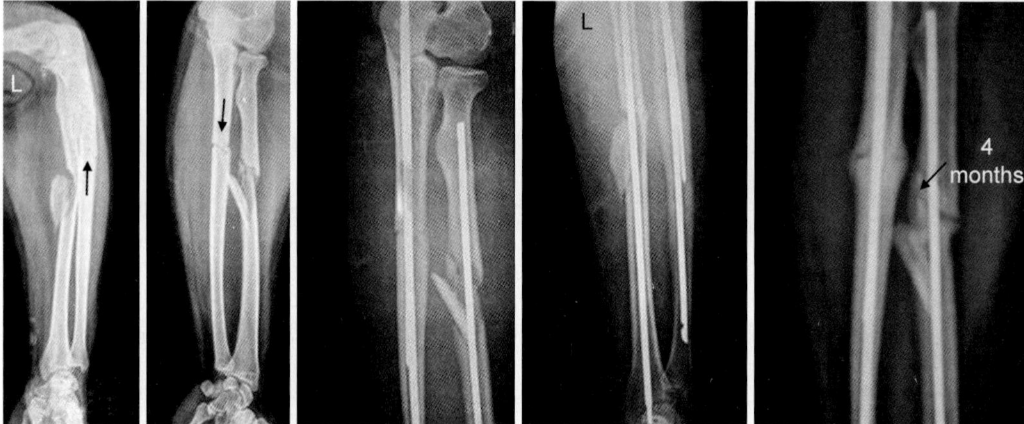

Figure 14.33 3rd fragment in radius fracture

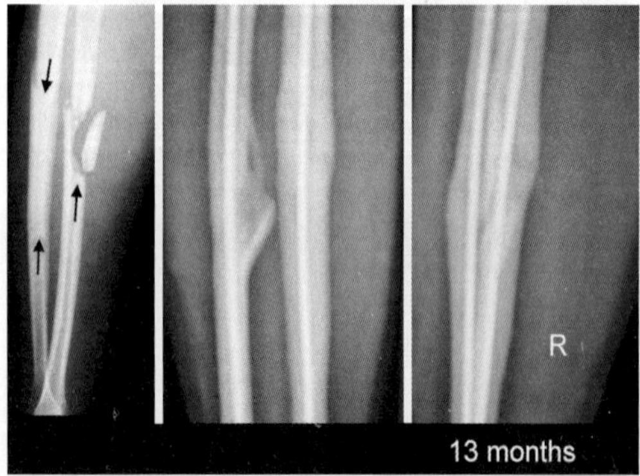

Figure 14.34 3rd fragment in radius fracture

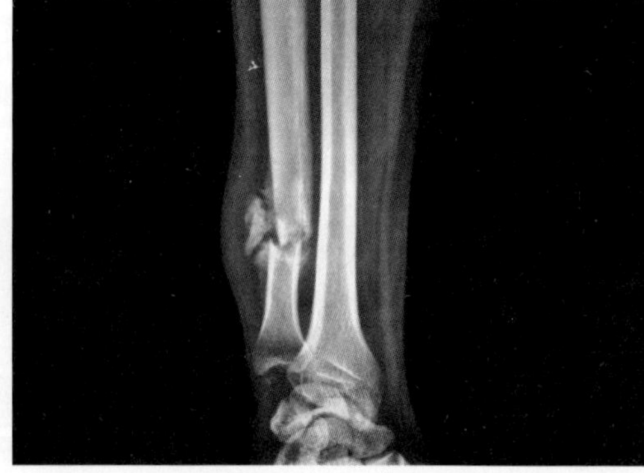

Figure 14.35 Slow union

tenderness and some yield at the fracture site is observed. If immobilization is not continued, the fracture at this stage, at times, goes in fibro-osseous union.

- A closed nailing is usually successful. The medullary cavity in the proximal ulna is much wider than in the distal area. The ulna being a relatively straight bone, back out of the nail is often observed. To prevent this, addition of another short nail in the proximal segment adds to the nail stability in the proximal fragment (Fig. 14.36).

- *Fracture of radius in a case with a malunited Colles' fracture*: In a case of fracture shaft of a radius, the radius nail is passed in a prograde way from dorsilateral part of the lower end of radius. In a malunited Colles' fracture, the distal fragment is so tilted that a nail when introduced from the dorsal side would abut against the anterior endosteal area of the radius and cannot be advanced proximally, along the long axis of the bone in the medullary cavity. In such a situation, the lower end of the radius is exposed anteriorly and a track made just proximal to the articular edge and the nail can be successfully passed along the medullary cavity. The point of this anterior entry is in line with the shaft of the radius. Review of anatomy of this area, prior to a surgery, increases the confidence, during exposure (Fig. 14.37).

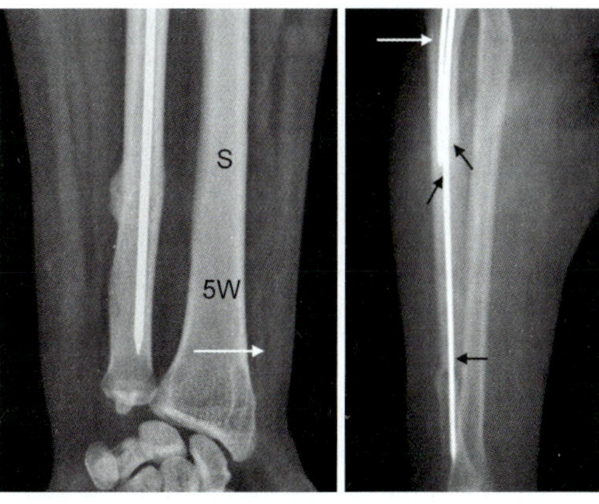

Figure 14.36 Stack nails in ulna

Surgeon who prefers a plate fixation for the radius, may do so, in place of a radius IM nailing procedure (Fig. 14.38).

Removal of a Nail in Adolescence

The radius and ulna gain 75% length from the distal epiphyses, while 25% from the proximal epiphyses. After a successful fracture union after nailing, it is necessary to remove the nails, between 8 to 12 months from the internal fixation.

The radius nail entry is oblique and the nail tip is resting on the dorsal cortex. With bone growth, the bone length increases at this area and the nail tip gradually moves inside the medullary cavity.

RADIUS

Following tips are necessary to know, while removing a nail in patient prior to skeletal maturity:

- Radius nail tip is kept slightly longer and should lie on the epiphysis. It must be contemplated to remove in 6 months. If the removal is not done in six months and if the radius has grown, then the nail tip tends to sink in the marrow cavity and during surgical exposure one cannot see the nail tip, as bone has grown over it.
- After exposure of the area, it is necessary to locate the nail tip. Today, with availability of a `C`, arm this is quickly done. Having located the nail threads, use a narrow gouge to clear bone around it and create a track to accommodate either the extraction tube or pliers tips. If either of the above two methods does not work, one tends to lever out the tip, by pressing down the gouge on the distal end of the radius. This is dangerous, because the pressure on the distal end of the radius is actually on the epiphysis and it may get separated or crushed. I would prefer to use a nose pliers to get a good grip on the nail tip and bend it dorsally, rather than levering it down against the bone.

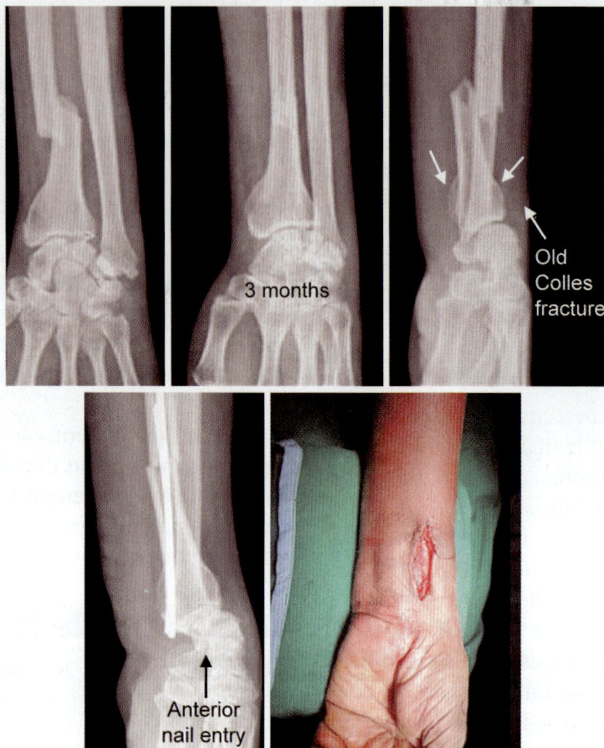

Figure 14.37 Old Colles' fracture and fresh radius fracture: Anterior nail entry

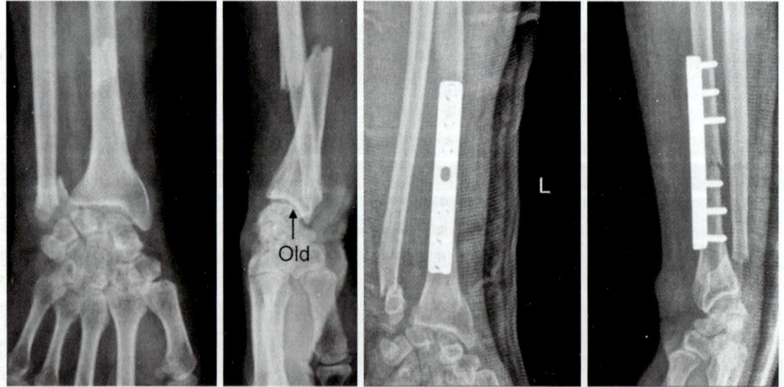

Figure 14.38 Old Colles' fracture and fresh radius fracture: Plate fixation

- Extraction tube is attached and an extractor hook is inserted in the slot, so with few light hammer blows, the nail is withdrawn (Fig. 14.39).

The bone growth is more at the distal end of both the radius and the ulna, and therefore, usually the ulna nail tip remains at the same point of entry in the olecranon. To expose and

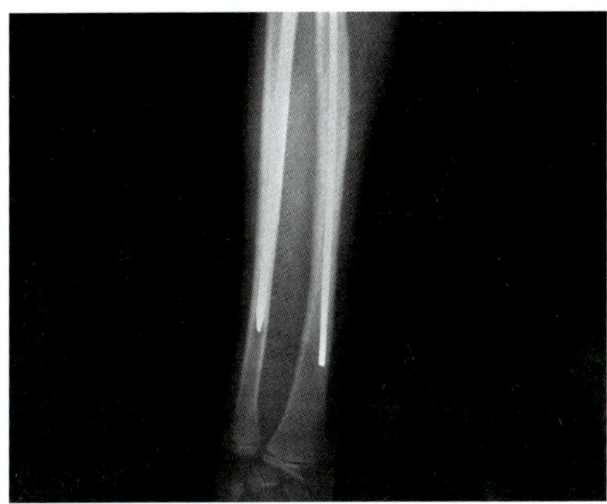

Figure 14.39 Bone over-growth

to hold the ulna nail tip in a suitable extractor is possible.

ULNA

In adolescent patient, take care of the olecranon epiphysis, which it traverses.

Often I put another 2 mm short nail to stack the principal nail and prevent its backing out. Whenever this is done (as a matter of fact in most cases) the nail tip be slightly protruding to facilitate its removal later. Even if it hurts the patient after cast removal, usually a bursa forms and pain is reduced.

The problem of removal of the small diameter nail comes, because it is a 2 mm thin nail and usually cut at a place when it gets locked and the end tends to be smooth without any threads.

If one removes the principal nail first: following problem is likely to be faced while removing the thin and short nail later. In an attempt to locate the tip of the stacked smaller and shorter nail, there is danger of its moving distally and vanishing in the medullary cavity. Hence, following steps:

- Use a gouge and create track around the tips of both the nails. I would not hold tips of both the nails together in a pliers and try to remove. This tends to spoil the threads and attaching a nail extractor is difficult.
- With a needle nose pliers, slightly withdraw the thin nail without threads. See if the thicker nail also comes out partially along with it.
- After the thin short nail is removed, removal of the longer nail is possible with a nail extractor. Having removed the smaller nail, the remaining nail is rather loose in the medullary cavity and can usually be removed by a pliers. The length of the wider nail being quite long, would not migrate distally.

IN GENERAL

- Explain that, when the fracture unites, it is advisable to remove the nails, once both the fractures have united.

  If this not done in time:
  - Bone endosteal growth grips the nail and may make removal difficult
  - Radius bone overgrows and the nail tip sinks in the medullary cavity
- Why is it necessary to remove the nails?
  - If there is another injury to the same limb at a later date, then its management could be difficult. E.g. with ulna nail in place, should there be a fracture of lower end of the humerus, then olecranon osteotomy is not possible.

CHAPTER

15

Bow Fracture of Forearm

BOW (GREENSTICK) FRACTURE OF RADIUS AND/OR ULNA

A greenstick fracture of a forearm, with an obvious deformity, is noted by the child, parents and the CMO on day 1 only. However, a bow fracture is a special condition, with reference to early diagnosis and management and the final outcome as well.

In children between age of 7 to 12 years following a fall, some pain is reported by the child. In the commonly seen greenstick fracture the deformity is quite obvious and hence the child is brought for necessary treatment immediately. However, if the deformity is mild and there is a plastic deformation of the bones, the deformity is not so easily noticed by the parents. Since the bone continuity is maintained, most of the elbow and wrist movements are reasonably good, except rotation - prono-supination of the forearm. The loss of rotary motion is often not realized, both by the patient and the parents as well. The pain and swelling settle in a few days and then an observant parent notices altered shape and restricted rotation of the forearm. By this time, usually 2 weeks have passed, without any treatment.

In such an injury, rotary malalignment needs to be recognized, by the clinician who attends the child first. Restriction of rotation is the important thing to note.

If such a child is brought to casualty/clinic, a senior and experienced clinician should also personally examine the child and submit to an X-ray examination. The anterior bowing, which is common, needs to be appreciated by the clinician.

A CMO, unaware of this injury, may pass it as 'no bone injury'. It is safer to send all such cases by the CMO to the clinician at the earliest, for an opinion at least.

However, to satisfy oneself, to convince a lay person and for purpose of documentation, X-ray of the opposite forearm must be taken, for comparison (Fig. 15.1).

A bow fracture is a plastic deformation in the bone and its correction by manipulation is rather difficult, compared to a greenstick fracture. In the later type, on the convex side, there is a break in continuity and the fracture line is visible on X-ray film and correction of the deformity by manipulation under anesthesia (Reduction) is relatively easy.

UNTREATED/MISSED BOW FRACTURE

All these efforts are necessary to prevent late problems, which include altered cosmetic appearance and loss of rotation. If this is not appreciated and necessary efforts not taken, following example will convince one.

A child had bow type greenstick fracture on the left side over twenty years ago and was

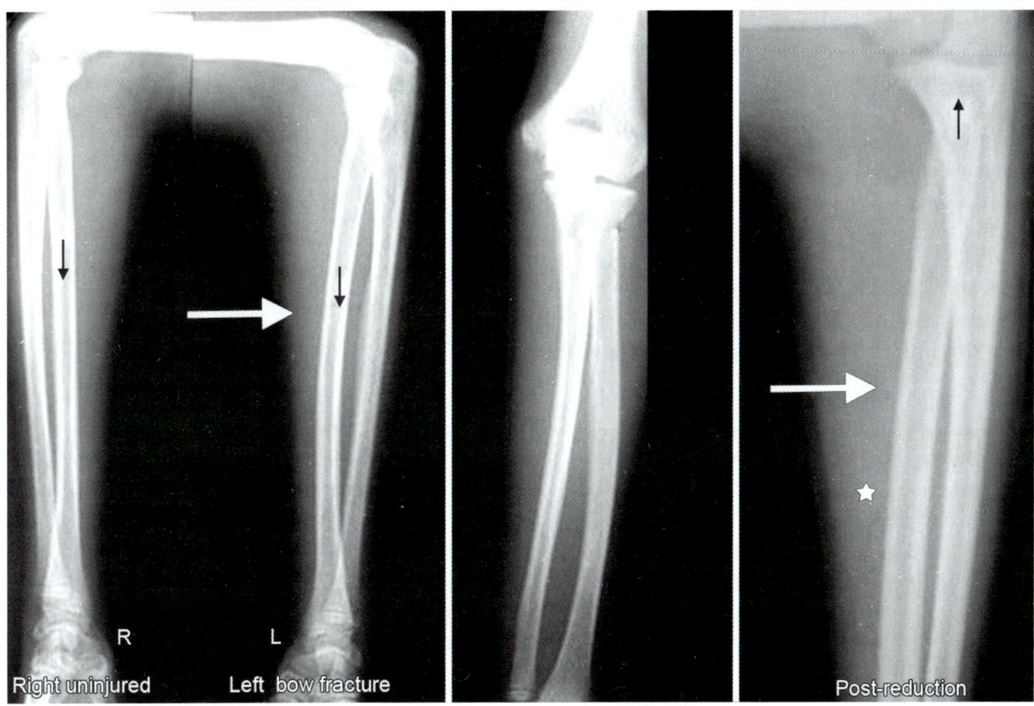

Figure 15.1 Bow fracture

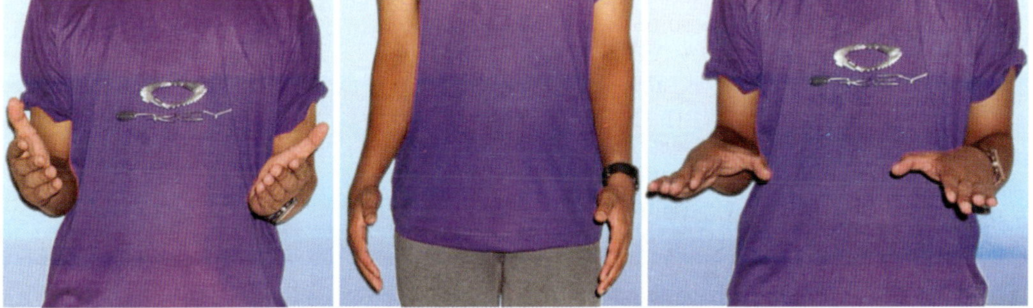

Figure 15.2 Malunited bow fracture

perhaps labeled as a contusion and was left as such. He later on had a similar injury on the opposite side and was again went unnoticed, perhaps in the same hospital. It was at this time, that I saw him for the first time, with deformities, more on the right side, with limitation of rotation, as depicted in the clinical photograph. I have had an opportunity to see quite a few cases of this nature, where in the peculiar clinical appearance, the limitation of rotation of forearm has occurred. Unfortunately, in this child, bow greenstick fracture was missed on both the sides, on two occasions resulting in limitation of rotation on both the forearms.

(The misfortune of this child did not end here. At a later date, he had an anterior dislocation of the head radius and again, it was overlooked. I was consulted for a second opinion. Anterior dislocation of head radius in children is a condition, which may occur without associated fracture of upper/3 ulna. This was diagnosed clinically and on the available X-ray; X-ray of the opposite side was taken for comparison and confirming the diagnosis, beyond doubt. It was appropriately managed).

Any form of corrective osteotomy does not help to improve the prono-supination range of motion (but leaves scars on the forearm).

In general with osteotomy, angular rather than rotational deformity is corrected (Fig. 15.2).

TREATMENT IN A FRESH CASE

Discussion with the radiologist, parents and the family physician is necessary. It is often difficult to convince that there is a fracture and that it needs a surgical procedure of correction (reduction) under anesthesia, at the earliest.

As a matter of fact, often what the family presents as a fresh injury, is usually 10 days old (though the child and the family may not accept the fact) deformity and is difficult to reduce completely and one may have to be satisfied with partial correction only. Any further delay in this procedure reduces further chance of achieving a good reduction.

Few possible end results of a reduction:

- Remote chance of a likely occurrence of a complete fracture occurring at the apex of the bow fracture, while it is reduced.
- The fracture may become a complete one, with some translation and side to side shift, which to a lay person may look worse than the preoperative bow appearance (as if the surgeon has created a fracture, which was not existing prior to the surgical procedure).
- Parents must be informed that after a successful reduction, as the tissue swelling reduces and due to the bone elasticity, the deformity may reappear. To avoid this, one may need to change the cast under GA again, as a stage II of the entire treatment

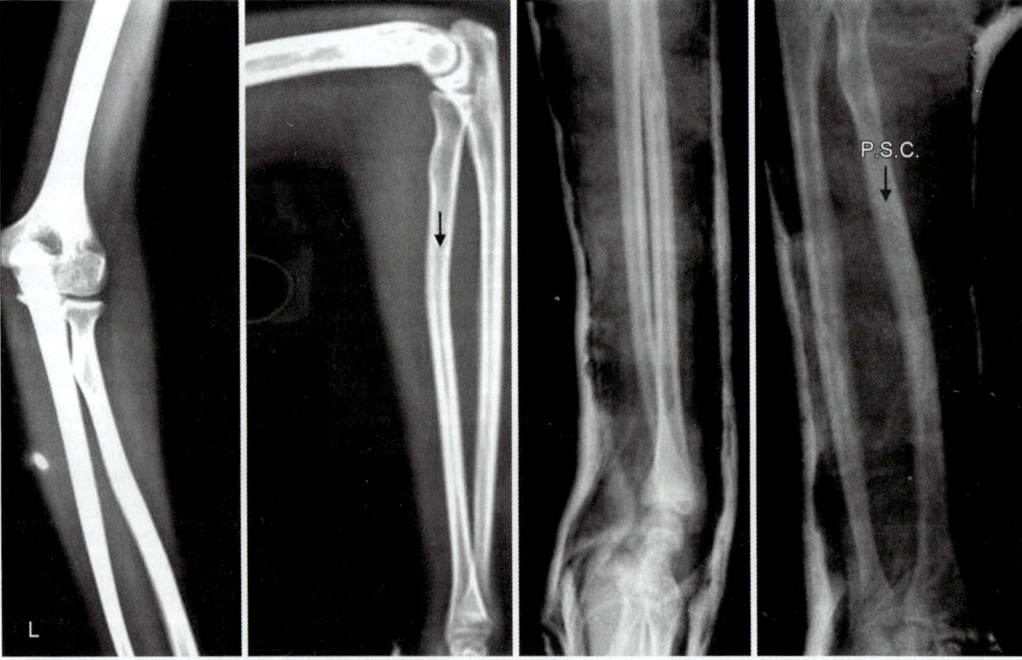

Figure 15.3 Radius upper/3 anterior bow

plan. This would facilitate further correction of the deformity and a good bone alignment can be achieved. A well-molded cast is very important. If this is not well-applied with correct position of the forearm, a well-reduced fracture on the first day may end in a poor final result.

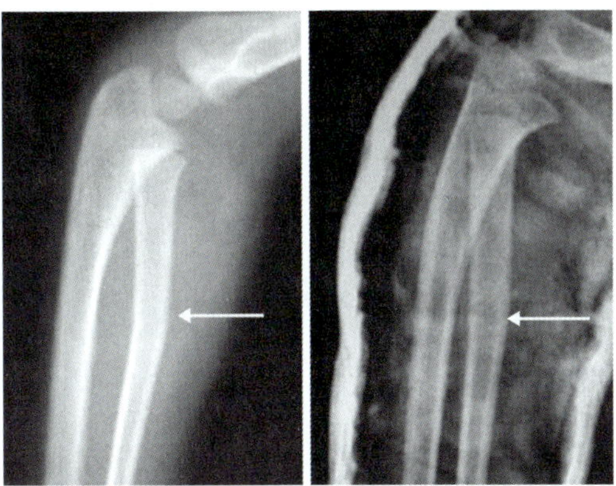

Figure 15.4 Radius upper/4 anterior bow

Any delay in reporting of such an injury, delay in the diagnosis and manipulative reduction, leads to early callus formation, making a good reduction more and more difficult.

STEPS IN REDUCTION OF A BOW FRACTURE

The fracture must be reduced soon under general anesthesia. The radius (which bows more often than the ulna) is quite a strong bone and to manipulate it, to reduce the plastic deformation, is indeed a difficult job. However, with perseverance, patience and reasonable strength, one should be able to reduce the fracture and correct the deformity. Older the fracture, more difficult becomes the reduction, to the extent that one may have to leave it as such/consider open surgery, to restore pronosupination.

Having confirmed the reduction under the `C` arm, X-ray should be taken for oneself and for documentation.

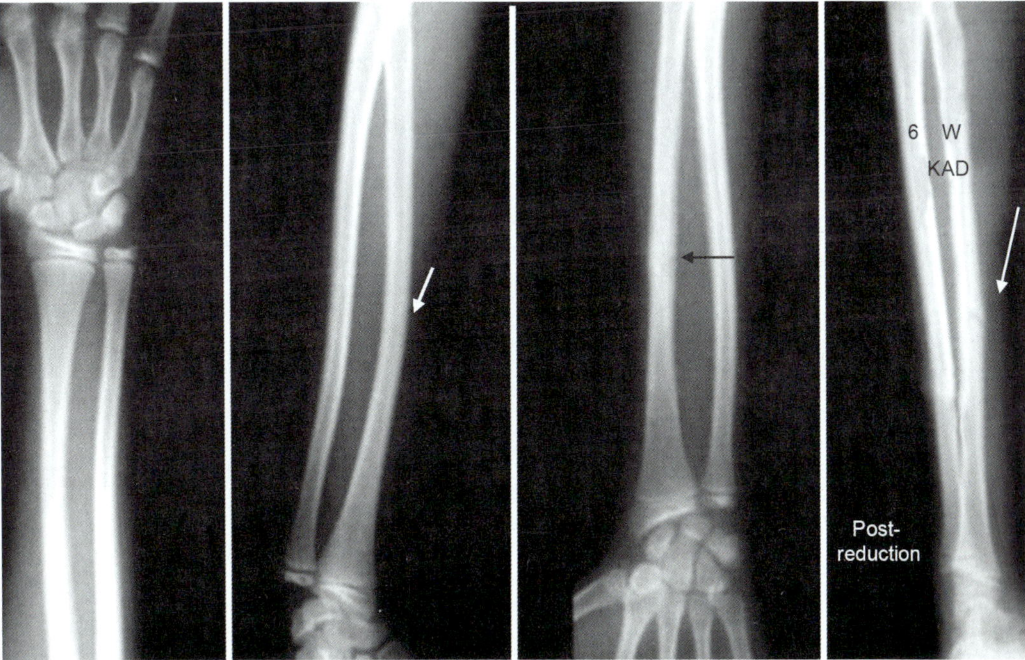

Figure 15.5 Middle/3 anterior bow

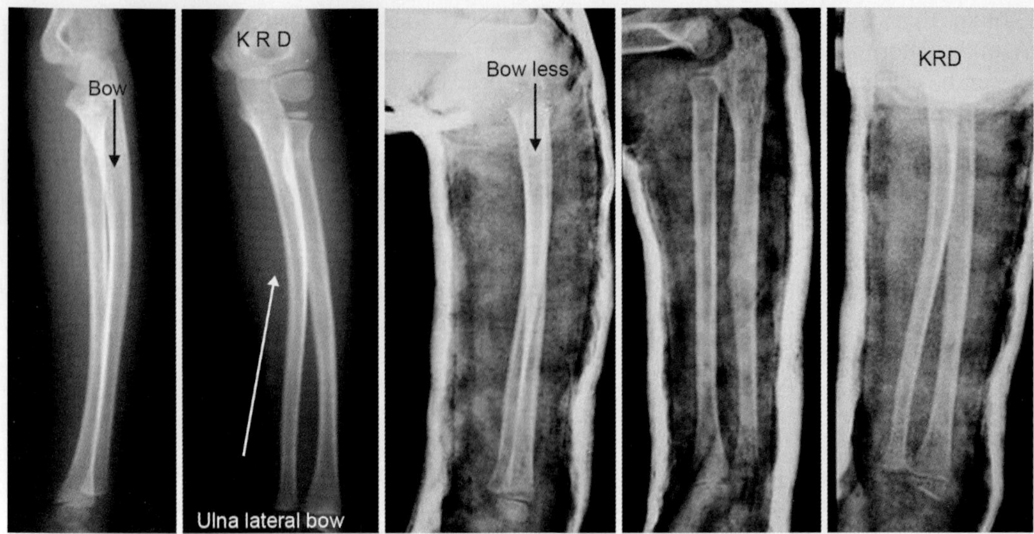

Figure 15.6 Ulna lateral bow fracture

A padded and moulded above elbow POP cast in short of full pronation completes the procedure. (Anterior angulation needs immobilization in pronation). The cast application must be done in two stages: After say 60% of the cast application is over, one should keep differential pressure on the plaster cast, mould it well, to allow the cast to set in the given position and check the alignment under C arm. The cast is then completed. On table X-ray through the cast must be taken. Prior to discharge of the child, a check X-ray through the cast be taken and then, during follow up, X-ray is taken every 5 days on two successive occasions and then every 10 days.

All this is important to offer a full proof treatment, beyond any doubt.

Few clinical examples are shown in Figures 15.3 to 15.6:

CHAPTER

16

Refracture of Forearm

FRACTURE HEALING AND REFRACTURE IN FOREARM BONES IN ADOLESCENCE

A forearm fracture when treated by a non-operative method heals by both external and internal callus. There is a clinical union, followed by radiological union.

The full strength and elasticity of the bone is restored when remodeling and tubulation of the bone is complete. The intramedullary callus should disappear and the marrow cavity must be restored to a preinjury status. Only when this X-ray appearance is restored, a chance of a re-fracture at the same site is less likely.

If the child has another injury, usually a fall on the outstretched hand, before the bone tubulation is complete, there is every likelihood that a refracture may occur. Hence all children and parents should be made to understand this process. One should take an X-ray at the end of 3 to 4 months to confirm that tubulation of bones is complete and then allow any unrestricted activity to play, ride a bicycle, etc. safely.

Case 1

Here though fracture has united, the union is inadequate to allow unrestricted play and danger of a refracture still persists (Fig. 16.1).

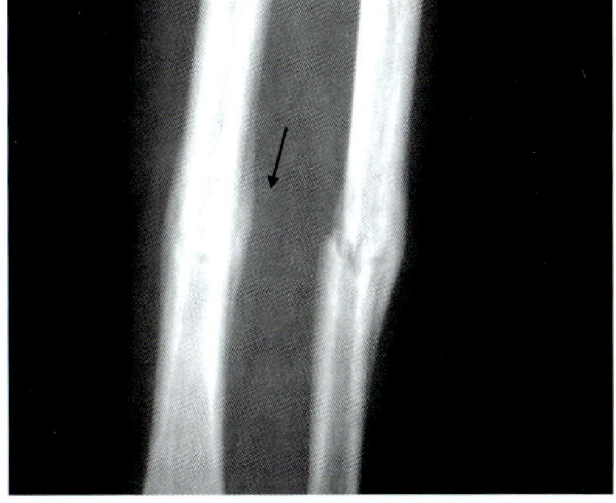

Figure 16.1 Clinical union. No radiological union yet

Case 2

The child had a greenstick fracture of lower/3 radius and ulna and was treated by a closed reduction under anesthesia and plaster immobilization. At the end of two months, the fracture united. However, prior to completion of tubulation, he had another fall, leading to a displaced fracture at the same level. Whenever, a refracture occurs at this stage of union, the local area becomes hard and the fracture is always a displaced fracture. IM nailing is required in such a situation. Due to presence of an internal callus, it requires an open reduction to clear the medullary cavity and to allow passage of the nail (Fig. 16.2).

Post-plaster Removal Care

I believe, though children are very active, they do need specific forearm exercises. The grip strengthening exercises help early and assured bone remodeling and restoration of function.

OBSERVATIONS

- In a primary fracture, usually the fracture is a greenstick one, with angulatory deformity and a soft tissue hinge.
- Before the remodeling is complete and bone elasticity is restored to the preinjury level, the bone union area is rigid, stiff and non-elastic. Any injury at this stage leads to a transverse fracture with displacement. The periosteal soft tissue hinge is absent. Hence

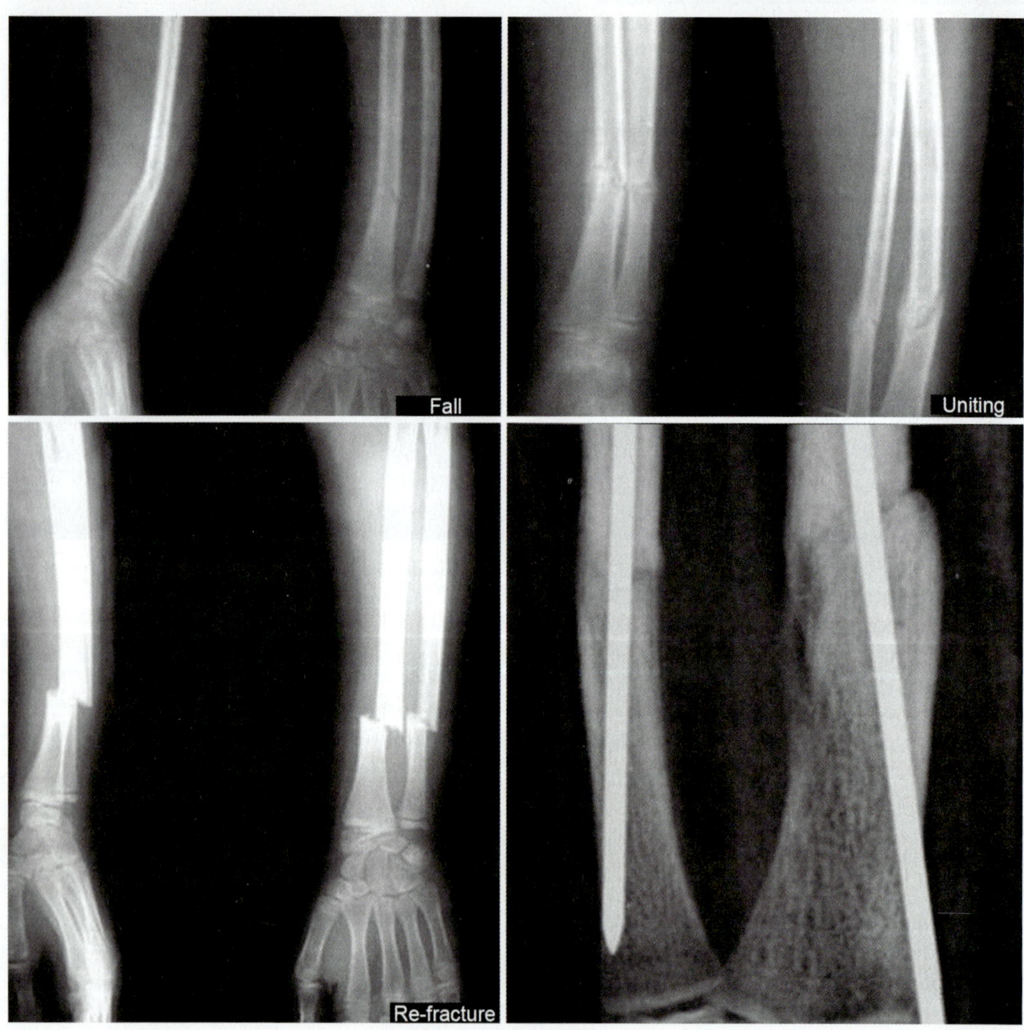

Figure 16.2 Refracture

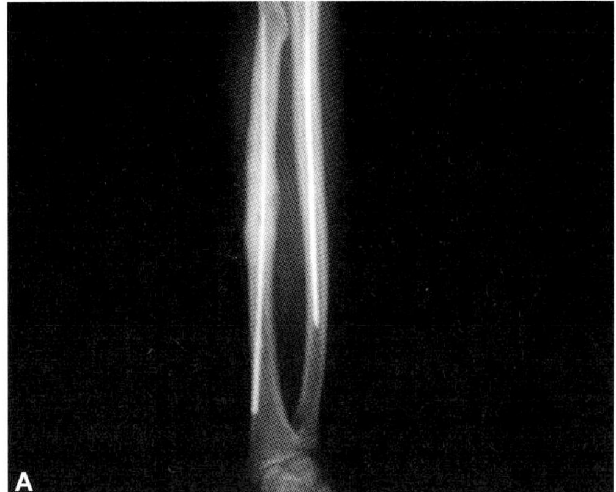

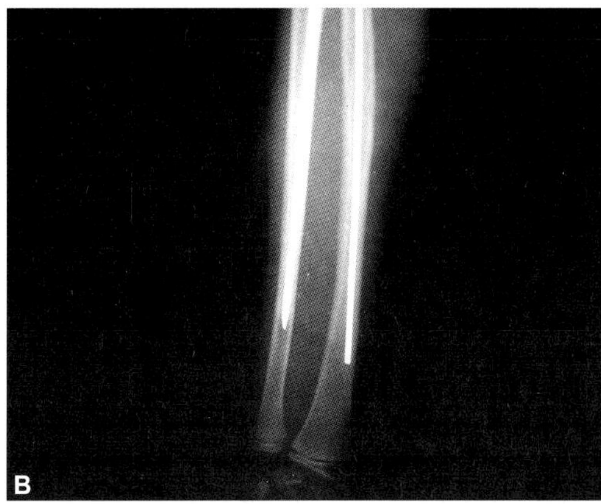

Figures 16.3A and B Bone overgrowth

even if one gets a good closed reduction, redisplacement is very likely.

- One always prefers a closed IM nailing. The surgical scars of nail entry, and if open reduction is required, that on the fracture site are much smaller and acceptable than that after a plate fixation.

After internal fixation with a plate or a nail, the implant removal must be done by the end of a year. If a plate is used to stabilize the fracture, due to stress shielding of the bone, the bone underlying thins out. Hence, after removal of a plate to protect the forearm and prevent another injury, a plaster cast for few weeks is essential.

Intra-medullary implant is a load sharing device and there is no stress shielding effect on the bone. Hence, a refracture after removal of an intramedullary implant is uncommon.

The bone growth is more at the distal end of radius and ulna and, hence, if timely nail removal is not done, the bone overgrows and the threaded end of the radius nail tends to sink within the medullary cavity. This is observed in a radius and then removal of a radius nail is extremely difficult.

In case of an ulna nail, the growth at the proximal end of ulna is less and the ulna nail tip continues to be where it was, at the time of surgery. However, it is desirable to remove both the implants within 8 to 12 months, to prevent them being anchored by intra-medullary bone growth (Figs 16.3A and B).

CHAPTER

17

Monteggia Fracture Dislocation

TRANSVERSE FRACTURE OF OLECRANON WITH FRACTURE OF HEAD OF RADIUS AND ASSOCIATED POSTERIOR DISLOCATION OF ELBOW

Case I

Had sustained fracture of the olecranon, undisplaced fracture of head of radius with posterior dislocation of the elbow.

Elbow needs to be immediately reduced. In spite of care exercised during the reduction, often the undisplaced fracture of the head of radius gets displaced. This possibility must be discussed with relatives, prior to the emergency procedure of closed reduction.

Immediately after an emergency closed reduction, padded crepe bandage and a posterior plaster slab was given. Elevation of the limb was carried out.

If the patient is fit, OT along with necessary equipment is available for the required duration, then the initial closed reduction and definitive procedure can be done at the same time.

However, the time lapsed between injury and surgery should not be more than 3 hours. Beyond that, local tissue edema increases and the patient's discomfort with dislocated elbow is high. In such a situation, carry out initial closed reduction immediately and plan the definitive surgery after 3 to 4 days. This duration allows the edema to settle as well.

Operative Details

Lateral position. Tourniquet. The upper arm was rested on a bolster, with a free elbow movement. Surgeon standing on the front of the patient.

A posterior lazy S incision was taken on the olecranon. Thick flaps were raised. Laterally the muscles from lateral surface of the ulna were erased and one could see the head of radius. The head fragments were removed and assembled to confirm that all fragments were removed.

Then fixation of olecranon by a TBW was done. A transverse 2.5 mm drill hole was made in the ulna shaft, distal to the fracture site, at twice the length of the proximal fragment and a 1 mm soft bone wire was passed through it. Then the fracture of olecranon was reduced and 2 × 1.8 mm K-wires were passed from the olecranon across the fracture.

Figure of 8 loop was completed by passing the wire deep to the triceps tendon and the K-wires. This was confirmed in both AP and lateral images in `C` arm, that the K-wires were in the medullary cavity and the wire loop was deep to the K-wires near the tip of olecranon. The figure of 8 circlage was loaded with a tractor bow, with the elbow in extension.

Stability of elbow was checked: Tourniquet was released.

Drain: closure.

Sterile crepe bandage was applied with elbow at 100 deg flexion. At this stage, one must again confirm that the elbow is well located. When head of the radius is excised, often at this stage of dressing, crepe application and plaster application, the dislocation of the elbow recurs of which, one is unaware. After the completion of POP slab application, it must be checked in a 'C' arm image and X-ray picture must be taken, on the operation table, for documentation. The ulno-humeral relationship is confirmed.

It is disheartening to see in a follow up X-ray taken 10 days after surgery that the elbow is dislocated.

It is a known thing that after a procedure of excision of the head of the radius for a comminuted fracture of head of radius (even without elbow dislocation), X-ray taken after POP slab application shows posterior dislocation of the elbow. (May be at the time of injury, elbow was dislocated, which got self-reduced, before an X-ray was taken on arrival to the hospital). Hence, in all cases of injury associated with elbow dislocation or after excision of head of the radius, the elbow needs to be flexed to 100 deg, and then the dressing is applied, preventing any chance of dislocation. When the elbow is flexed to 100 degree, the taught triceps splint maintains the position and prevents a redislocation.

Follow-up Care

At the end of 8 days, intermittent mobilization of the elbow/shoulder and grip exercises are encouraged, twice a day. After the mobilization, the posterior slab is reapplied for rest and is continued for total 3 to 4 weeks, as per merit of the case. This support helps to reduce the tissue reaction and assists healing.

When to start intermittent mobilization? This varies from a patient to patient, depending upon the initial soft tissue injury and swelling prior to surgery, fracture morphology, stability of fixation, etc. The elbow dislocation needs 8 to 10 days of rest after the reduction, for the soft tissues to heal and continue to maintain the relocated elbow in a stable position (Fig. 17.1).

Case 2

Comminuted fracture of olecranon with fracture of head of radius, without dislocation of elbow.

On arrival padded crepe + AE POP with Fiber plaster posterior slab and elevation given. Had associated ACL injury, for which MRI was done.

Elbow operated 3 days after the injury. As per the previous case, excision of head of radius and internal fixation of olecranon was carried out. The olecranon fracture was comminuted and hence, in place of K-wires, I preferred a square nail for more rigidity and stability of fixation. Not many surgeons prefer square nail to the K-wires for a fracture of olecranon. I feel it offers good rigidity and resistance to angulatory forces, yet allows fracture contact opposition. All cases, where an IM ulna nail was used, have done well (Figs 17.2A to C).

Case 3

Comminuted fracture of olecranon and dislocation of head of radius.

Pre-operative Planning and Technique

The olecranon had an intra-articular fracture with small bone fragments, within the substance. To maintain the reduction of ulna, head of radius needs to be well reduced and stay opposite to the lateral humeral condyle. To facilitate this, the length of the ulna has to be maintained. In fact, both are interdependent: the restoration of length of ulna also helps to keep the head radius reduced well and in its place and vice versa. To maintain the ulna bone length, a rigid implant like a nail is required, rather than few K-wires. The nail tip, while engaging in the head of ulna, restores the bone length and the olecranon fragments fall back in place. This restoration of length, reduction of the fracture, and resistance to angular stresses are better achieved by the use of an intramedullary

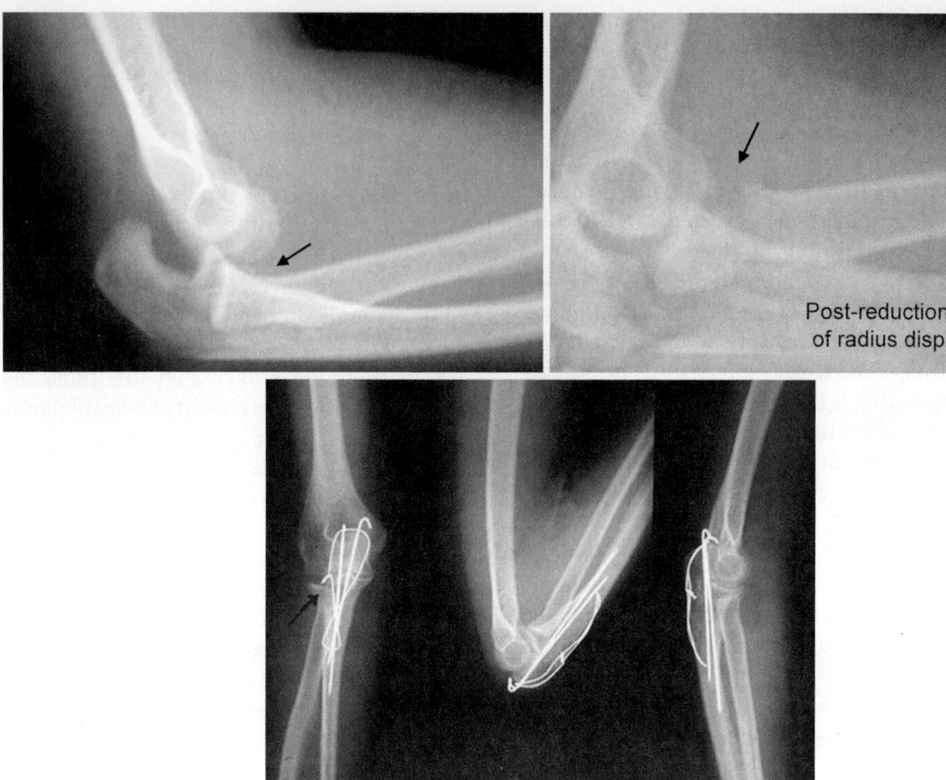

Figure 17.1 Fracture of olecranon, fracture of head of radius with dislocation of elbow

nail in the ulna than by the K-wires. At the same time, it allows axial contact opposition of the ulna fragments. Addition of bone grafts leads to contact opposition and fills up all the voids in the olecranon. This additional procedure of bone grafting, adds to duration of surgery, but assures good union in an expected period.

Early surgery is necessary and was carried out. Closed reduction was done in supine and confirmed under the `C` arm. Then lateral position was given, with elbow on the bolster, while the forearm was hanging down. Surgeon was on front of the patient. Cautery and suction units at the foot end of the table, so that if needed, the `C` arm unit can be brought from the opposite side, i.e. from the back of the patient. Draping should be such so that the iliac crest is accessible to remove bone grafts.

Posterior curved incision was taken on the olecranon. Thick skin flaps were raised. Muscle attachment to bone fragments was maintained, as much as possible. Provisional reduction with traction was done and studied. The fracture had few vertical fragments, which may angulate, when axial loading by TBW is done.

As a preparation of the circlage wire, approximately 3 cm distal to the fracture area, a transverse drill hole was made with a 2.5 mm drill bit and a 1 mm soft wire passed through it and ends laid aside. (The drill hole cannot be made after the IM ulna nail is in place).

Once axial stability is achieved by an IM nail, then passing circumferential wires around the ulna (at right angle to the long axis of ulna), is difficult and may harm the soft tissue attachment to the bone. Hence prior to the fracture reduction and alignment, the fracture was slightly angulated and 2 strands of 1 mm soft bone wires were passed deep to the fracture site—one proximal and the another

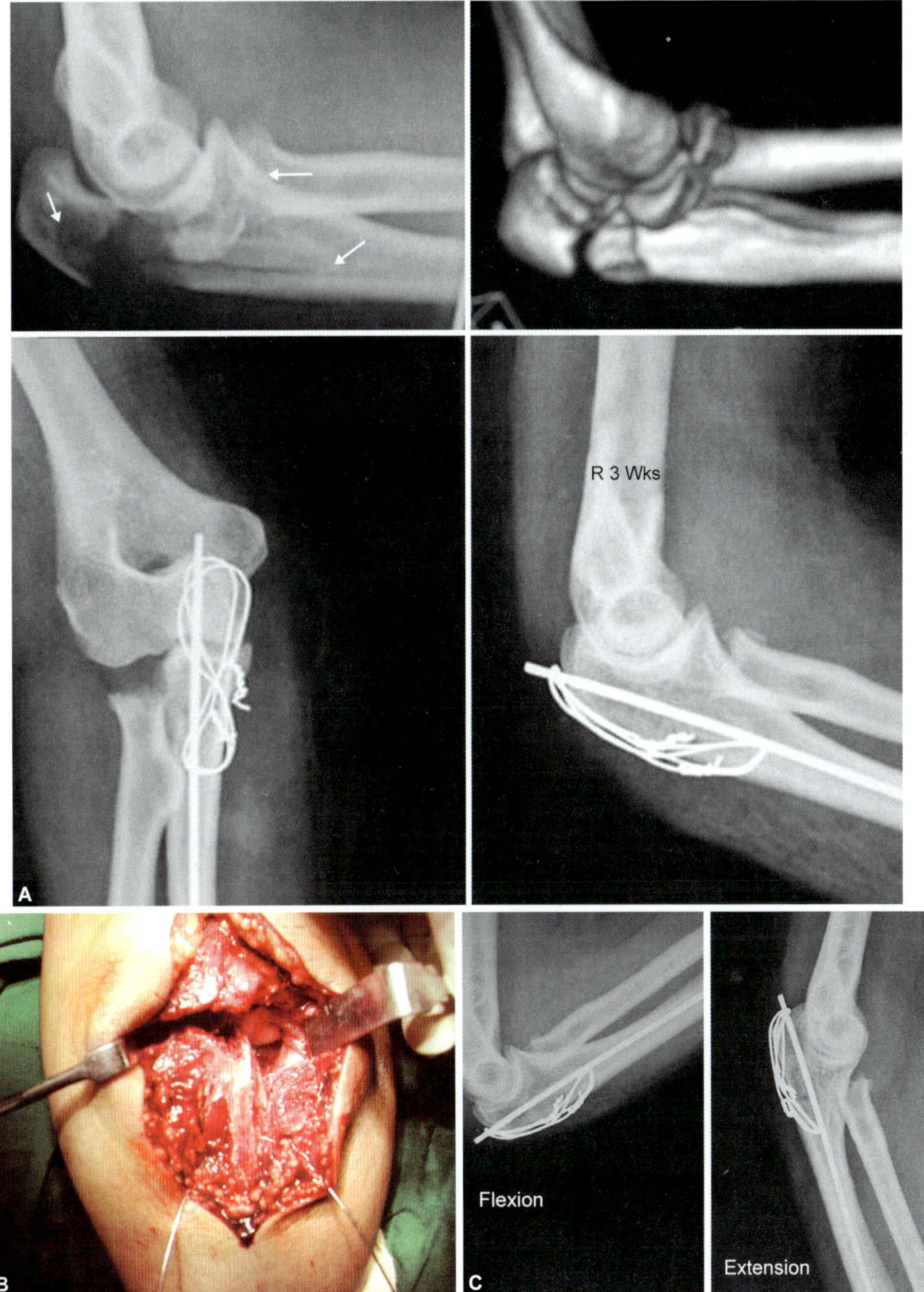

Figures 17.2A to C (A) Comminuted fracture of olecranon and fracture of head of radius without elbow dislocation; (B) Operative exposure and head of radius; (C) Final union and range

distal to the fracture and ends were tagged by hemostats. This was just passed by hand and slided. The ulna fracture ends were devoid of soft tissue attachment to the fragments and this was possible. (If the soft tissue attachment was present, then it should be passed by a round wire passer). The ulna can be easily angulated to achieve this.

Iliac crest bone grafts were taken and laid on the anterior endosteal surface of the ulna. Once the IM nail is in place, one cannot lay grafts anterior to ulna, where they should be placed. Grafts thus laid have a soft tissue bed and get blood supply from the deeper side and help rapid union and consolidation of bone. Few strips were also laid, within the marrow cavity. Such laid bone grafts achieve good bone consolidation.

The surgeon so far was in front of the patient and the first assistant close to the surgeon supporting the limb by the arm and the wrist, with elbow at right angle. The second assistant retracts the soft tissue and now the surgeon moves on the other side of the patient with the trolley. From this place, it is easier to make a track in the tip of olecranon and then pass the nail. Surgeon instructs both the assistants to align both the fragments (fracture reduction) and advances the nail. Retrograde flow of bone marrow from the distal fragment indicates that the nail is in the marrow cavity (DR KH Sancheti).

The circumferential wire around the shaft of ulna was held by its ends in two pliers, crossed across the fracture area and manually loaded, to keep all the fragments with the grafts in place. Wire ends were then twisted, cut and bent. Instead of manual traction, use of a wire tractor bow can be done, to give just the necessary tension in the wire. The second circumferential wire too was tied around the ulna.

Then the tension band wire loop (which is passed through the distal fragment is passed deep to the tendon of triceps and the nail tip, as close to the olecranon as possible. With a tractor bow, the figure of eight wire loop was partially loaded, with the elbow extended. While the tractor bow was in place, the reduction was checked under the `C` arm. Position of the circumferential wires was also confirmed. Now, final tapping of the nail was done and fixation completed by finally loading the wire. Since there are few vertical fragments, load should not be as much as in a transverse fracture. The circlage wire ends were cut, bent and buried well.

Angular elbow and prono-supination movement was checked. Tourniquet was released/pulse checked and closure carried out. Padded crepe and above elbow posterior POP slab given with the elbow at 100 deg flexion. It is necessary to flex the elbow to 100 degs, prior to application of a padded crepe bandage, because usually the elbow flexion angle tends to reduce by few degrees, by the time the dressing and application of crepe is over.

One should confirm in the ‘C’ arm, both before and after plaster slab immobilization and take an X-ray film after the plaster slab immobilization. This puts on record, that the ulno-humeral and radio-humeral alignment was correct at the end of the procedure.

Elbow can be mobilized after 5 days. The posterior plaster slab is removed, while the padded crepe bandage is kept in place and active mobilization carried out. After the active exercises, posterior plaster slab is reapplied. This ritual is carried out twice a day. In such an injury, it is safe to mobilize the elbow under supervision. If one applies a cast and the limb is left as such for two weeks, then restoration of elbow motion is rather difficult. During the first postoperative week, continuous elevation of the elbow, grip tightening every hour, while awake and static arm exercises, is the key to success. Use of oral indomethacin is said to prevent development of myositis ossificans.

Advantages of an im Implant

- Maintains the length of ulna.
- No erasing of soft tissues around the fracture area, especially of small vertical splinters, which are required for a plate fixation.
- More surface area is available for bone bridging across the fracture area. As against

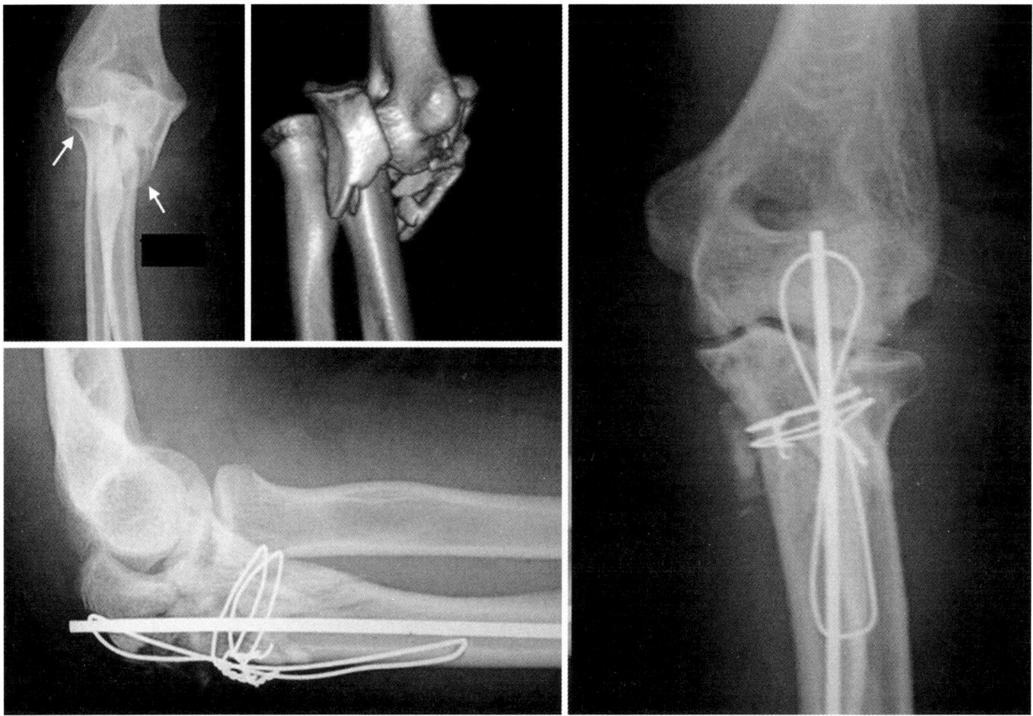

Figure 17.3 Comminuted fracture of olecranon and dislocation of head of radius

this, if one considers use of plate as an implant, it needs soft tissue erasing from the ulna on the dorsal surface, much beyond the fracture site, to have at least three screws on either side. This partly devitalizes the local area and reduces the surface area available for bridging callus. The span of a nail is much longer than that of a plate and the construct is rather elastic. This allows some micromotion, leading to a good fracture union (Fig. 17.3).

CHAPTER

18

Lower/3 Radius and Ulna Fracture in a Child

FRACTURE OF LOWER/ 3 RADIUS AND ULNA IN A CHILD

The Description Applies to a Child between Age 7 and 10 Years

During this second growth spurt, remodeling is good and it is possible to manage a forearm fracture by a non-operative method, with a satisfactory outcome.

Displaced Fracture of the Radius with Greenstick Fracture of Ulna

Here is an example of displaced fracture of the radius and a greenstick fracture of the ulna with anterior angulation. Radius fracture was oblique, was reduced under anesthesia and the fracture ends were hitched. Fortunately the radius was stable after reduction, with some acceptable translation. Padded above elbow POP in pronation was given and could be maintained well.

The anterior angulation is a supination injury and hence the forearm needs to be immobilized in a position short of full pronation, with correct molding.

Lesson: If the fracture can be locked against axial displacement, it would remain stable (Fig. 18.1).

Greenstick Fracture of the Radius and Displaced Fracture of the Ulna

Then fracture had an anterior angulation (indicating a supination deformity) and hence was reduced, with forearm in pronation. A moulded above elbow POP was given. Position maintained well and healing occurred in good position (Fig. 18.2).

WHICH MATERIAL FOR THE CAST?

In such a forearm fracture, I prefer a plaster of Paris material over a synthetic material, because of the following advantages:

- It is soft and relatively slow-setting
- One gets adequate time to mould the cast and hold it well, while it is setting. While it is setting—hardening—one can have a look under the 'C' arm, to confirm the position and if some angular adjustment is needed, it is possible to carry out the same while the cast is setting hard.
- The cast edges, especially at the palm, are soft and do not bite in the skin. When the limb edema settles and a change of cast is needed, one can slit the cast with plaster shears and remove it gently, without possibility of loss of the fracture position. When a synthetic cast is to be slit with a power saw, it needs to be slit on either side and then separate the

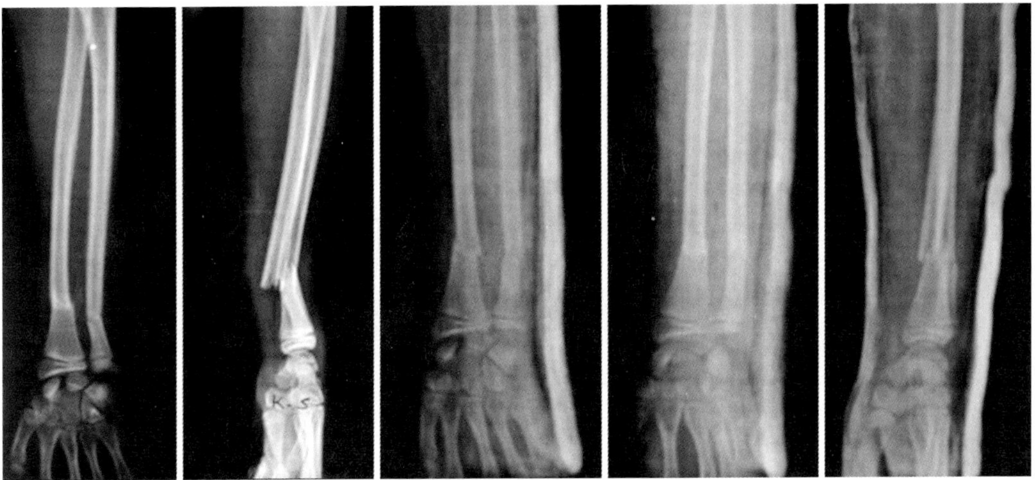

Figure 18.1 Displaced radius and greenstick ulna

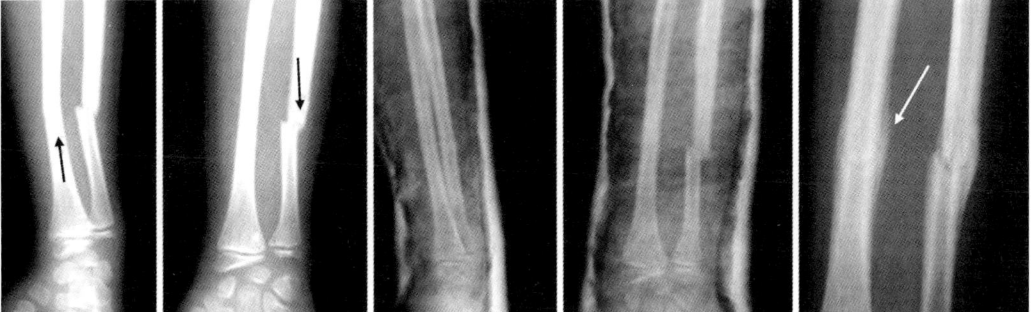

Figure 18.2 Greenstick fracture of radius and displaced fracture of ulna

two shells and take the limb out of it. When this is done after fracture has united, it is safe. When this is to be done, before even clinical union, I feel there is a danger of loss of fracture alignment, while the limb cast is bivalved and the limb taken out of it.

- Some children do not take a good care of the cast and cast becomes soft. In such a case, one may add a 'synthetic cast roll', over a well-molded cast to add strength and resist plaster chipping off. The basic molding must be made by the POP cast and the synthetic add-on roll adds to the cast strength.

CHAPTER

19

Lower/4 Radius and Ulna Fracture in a Child

CASE 1: TRANSVERSE DISPLACED FRACTURE OF THE RADIUS AND ULNA

This is a common injury in children. This injury should be reduced immediately, like a supracondylar fracture humerus before edema appears.

If one follows the following technique, usually a nonoperative method is successful and open surgery can be avoided.

General anesthesia and good muscle relaxation is necessary. Sustained, prolonged traction and counter-traction for at least for 3 minutes by clock, is given and then the displacement is slightly exaggerated to remove any soft tissue interposition. Then maintaining the anterior angulation, traction is given and both the bones are simultaneously reduced. First the side to side displacement is corrected and then the fracture step is corrected by sliding the proximal ends of the distal fragment on the distal dorsal cortex of the proximal fragments, keeping the angulation at 30 degrees. Gentle, purposeful traction and hitching of the bone ends usually offer a good reduction. A clinical indication of a well-reduced fracture is that the index finger looks to be hyperextended at the MCP joint. Clinically, telescopic stability is checked as we used to do in pre `C` arm era. The reduction is checked under 'C' arm. Maintaining the reduction, it is necessary to rotate the 'C' arm tube, rather than rotating the forearm, to get an image in two planes. (If one rotates the forearm, to get another view under the 'C' arm, the reduction is likely to be lost).

Plaster Immobilization

Having confirmed the reduction, the limb is vertically suspended by the first assistant holding the thumb in one hand and the index and middle finger in the other hand. The wrist is held in slight palmer flexion and ulnar deviation. Mid-prone position is a safe one. An above elbow padded cast is given in two stages. In the first stage, a below elbow cast is given, molding it well around the wrist. Slight palmer flexion and ulnar deviation makes the extensor tendons acting as an internal splint to maintain the reduction.

After the below elbow portion is set, it is checked under 'C' arm. Gently, the forearm is made vertical in midprone. Since the below elbow portion has hardened, one can hold that portion as well. Above elbow cast is completed and checked again under 'C' arm.

While applying a cast in a fresh fracture, I prefer to use a cotton roll made from large cotton pack, personally. Such a woolly cotton roll offers more cushion effect than a commercially available compressed cotton roll.

Check X-ray on table is necessary for record. During follow up, check X-ray be taken every 5 days on the first two occasions and then at interval of 10 days. If one finds that there is a change in bone alignment, during the follow up X-ray, then immediately, it is corrected, preferably under anesthesia. A transverse fracture usually has a telescopic stability. Should the radius fracture be oblique, it is more likely to get displaced.

This re-displacement of the fracture has prompted many surgeons to carry out percutaneous K-wire fixation for the radius on day 1 only. The K-wire is trans-epiphyseal in the radius and usually causes no harm to the epiphyseal plate. I prefer to avoid this procedure as far as possible and believe in a close follow up, after a successful closed reduction. Even if a second procedure of re-reduction is needed, I would prefer it to a trans-epiphyseal K-wire.

Information to Parents to be Given on Day 1

- As the swelling reduces, there is likelihood that one may need a change of the plaster cast, may be under anesthesia.
- The cast is usually needed to be maintained for a total of 6 to 7 weeks, as per the age of the child and severity of the injury.
- After removal of the cast, the family has to take all efforts to refrain the child from playing, riding a bicycle, etc. to prevent another fall. This care is important because there is a chance of a re-fracture at the same site.

After Removal of the Cast

- A crepe support and a wrist splint offers support and prevents immediate sports activity. I prefer to make an anterior below elbow cock up slab made of plaster of Paris material. This offers support to the wrist and prevents unguarded wrist movements and thus the pain. Such a splint helps the family to prevent the child from playing/riding a bicycle, etc.
- The POP cock up slab can be removed for bath: After bath, grip strengthening and wrist mobilization exercises are done and the cock up slab reapplied. The grip exercises help restoration of muscle and thus bone strength. It takes at least six weeks from cast removal for remodeling on the bone.
- No sports/cycling, etc. is permitted for at least two months from cast removal. At the end of this period, an X-ray is taken to confirm that sound bone union and tubulation has occurred. If unfortunately, the child gets another fall during this period, a refracture is known to occur, because the bone is yet to regain natural elasticity. Such a refracture usually leads to a displaced rather than a greenstick fracture (Fig. 19.1).

CASE 2: AN OBLIQUE FRACTURE OF THE RADIUS WITH A SERRATED FRACTURE OF THE ULNA

A good reduction was obtained on day 1. However, in a week's time, due to the obliquity the radius fracture, the fracture 'settled' and was displaced. This required an open reduction and a plate fixation of the radius.

A fracture with oblique fracture line is unstable and is known to translate in course of time. If one expects this on arrival, it is wise to carry out the procedure in the beginning only, as a definitive procedure. This avoids another procedure and the delay of a week or so.

Practical tip: The lower half of the radius has a gentle posterior convexity (anterior concavity). While stabilizing the fracture with an anterior plate, slight precontouring of the plate (anterior concave) to suit this shape is necessary. After fixation of the radius plate, one must confirm with a 'C' arm, that the ulna fracture is in place. In this case, it was found to be too much angulated and hence a closed K-wire fixation was done. The ulna can be stabilized with a K-wire passed from distal end, across the fracture engaging one of the cortices of the proximal fragment. In the hands of some surgeons, it is possible to do a closed prograde ulna IM nailing. The nail length has to be precise. The fracture is stabilized well by the nail tip, just engaging the distal end of the head of ulna. A too long a nail would cause distraction at the fracture site.

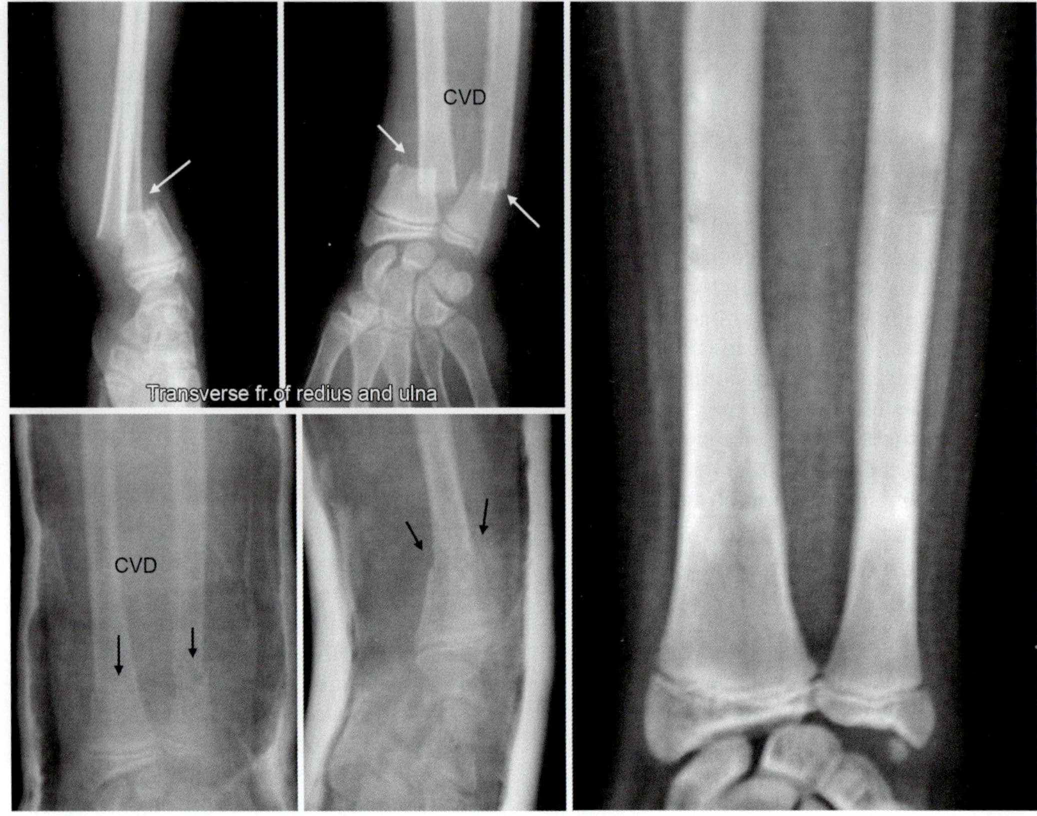

Figure 19.1 Transverse fracture L/4 of radius and ulna

A plate fixation for lower shaft of ulna is possible. However, the distal forearm has a small girth, so the plate fixation on both the bones would cause too much tissue tension, making wound closure difficult. Radius medullary cavity in metaphyseal area is wide and hence a plate fixation is necessary. In ulna, the medullary cavity being narrow, an IM device or obliquely set K-wire is quite effective (Fig. 19.2).

CASE 3: LATE PRESENTATION OF CASE 1

Failed Closed Reduction in a Transverse Fracture of the Radius and Ulna

A child sustained displaced fracture of lower/4 radius and ulna. At a previous hospital, closed reduction was done and check X-ray revealed persistent displacement. (Possibly one did not realize it on table on the first occasion). A second reduction was attempted under anesthesia and was unsuccessful. The child was advised a 3rd procedure of open reduction and a plate fixation.

The child reported to me for further treatment. It was a 3-day old injury. I kept option of open reduction and kept the equipment for open reduction and internal fixation ready and appropriate duration of theater availability was confirmed. Under general anesthesia and full muscle relaxation the procedure was carried out.

Prolonged sustained traction for 5 minutes by clock, followed by closed manipulation and reduction done. Achieved telescopic stability. As the reduction was achieved, the index finger was seen to be in slight extension at MCP joint,

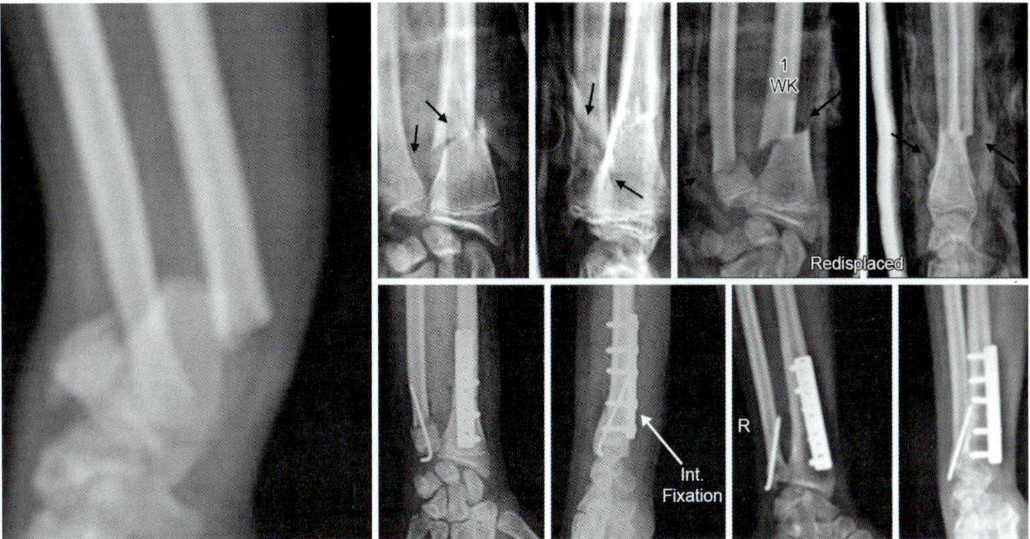

Figure 19.2 Oblique fracture of radius needs ORIF

indicating clinically, good bayonet opposition and restoration of bone length.

Examination under `C` arm confirmed good reduction of both radius and ulna. A padded and moulded above elbow plaster cast was given in midprone. Some palmer flexion and ulnar deviation maintained the soft tissue tension, which maintains the reduction well.

Follow up X-ray every 5 days taken. At the end of two weeks, the radius was in position, while ulna was displaced, maintaining some contact at one cortex. The plaster was changed to a well-molded and less padded one.

Further follow up showed this position was maintained and early callus appeared in due course. Once the callus is seen on X-ray, further displacement does not occur. Bone union was achieved in expected duration. X-ray at six months showed complete union with remodeling (Fig. 19.3).

CASE 4: LATE PRESENTATION OF CASE 2

The boy sustained a displaced fracture lower/4 of the radius and ulna. He attended a peripheral hospital. Closed reduction under anesthesia was attempted on two sequential occasions. Reduction was not achieved. Two weeks after the injury, reported to me. Family was advised, that he would need open reduction of the radius at least.

Being a child, attempt of union had already started and the fracture callus had started to appear. This makes the fracture sticky, preventing a chance of closed reduction. Examination under anesthesia with good muscle relaxation was done. However, end-to-end opposition could not be obtained. Hence, an open reduction of radius was carried out. Stabilization with a K-wire from radial styloid was done. The wire did not penetrate the medial radial cortex, but kept sliding along the endosteum. Due to the elasticity of the wire, fair stability was noted. The ulna was stable and hence was left as such. (It is possible to redirect the K-wire and attempt penetration of the far cortex. However, it may lose the hold on the near cortex and there is a danger to the epiphyseal growth plate as well).

The limb was immobilized in an above elbow POP cast in midprone position. Good union and function noted at the end of 2 months. The child did not turn up for a regular follow up. The K-wire was removed at the end of 6 months (Fig. 19.4).

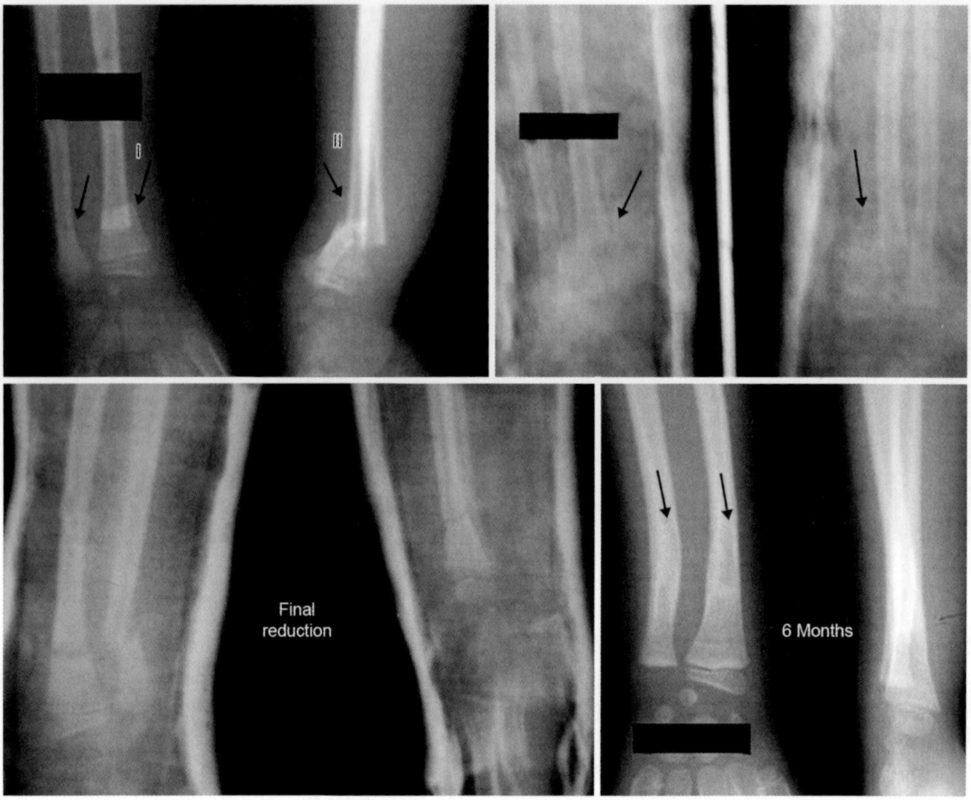

Figure 19.3 Late presentation: Case 1

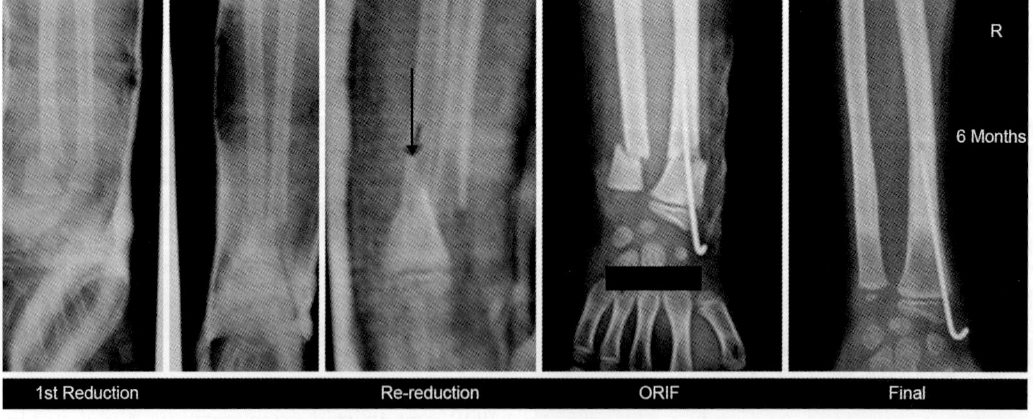

Figure 19.4 Late presentation of case 2

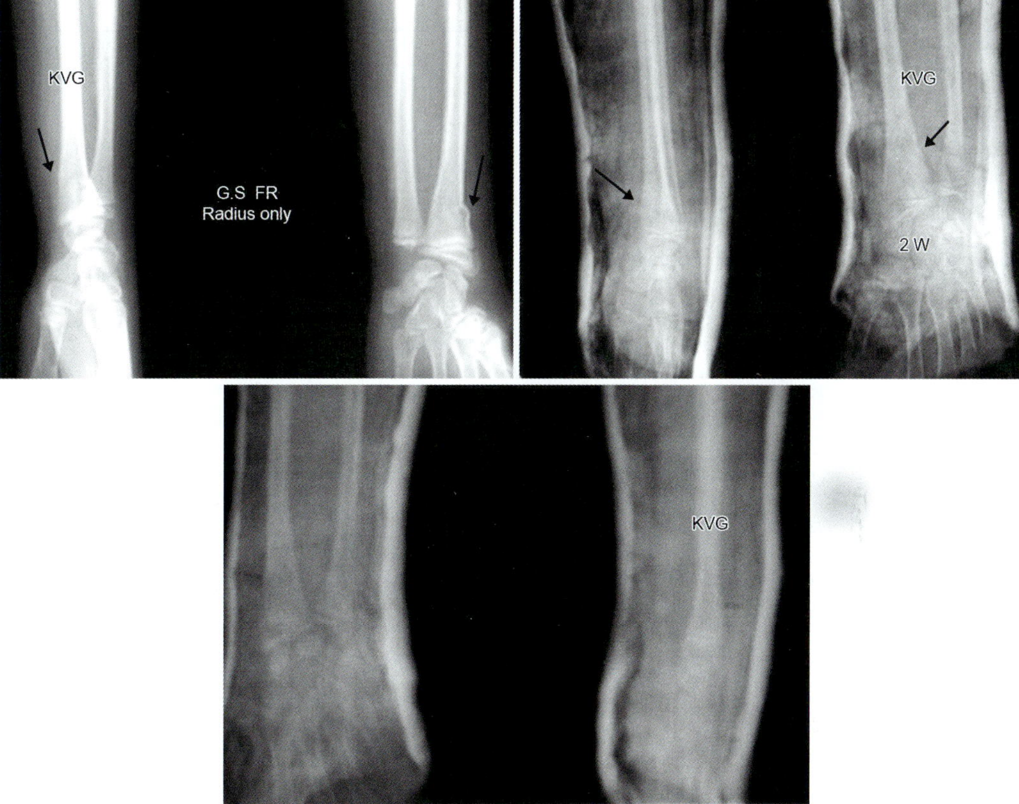

Figure 19.5 Greenstick fracture of radius alone

CASE 5: GREENSTICK FRACTURE OF RADIUS ONLY

A child had a fall and sustained a greenstick fracture of lower/4 radius, with anterior angulation. Under anesthesia, closed reduction was done, with immobilization in mid-pronation, palmar flexion and ulnar deviation. Follow-up X-ray through cast showed good stability. Good outcome. Being only an angulated fracture without displacement, posterior soft tissue hinge persists. Thus re-displacement is less likely and healing is rapid (Fig. 19.5).

CASE 6: GREENSTICK FRACTURE OF BOTH RADIUS AND ULNA

Presented with a greenstick fracture of lower/4 of both radius and ulna. Closed reduction under anesthesia done. Check X-ray confirmed good reduction. Postoperative recovery was uneventful and the position was maintained well.

X-ray after 3 months showed good tubulation was on (Fig. 19.6).

CASE 7: REDISPLACEMENT IN AN OBLIQUE FRACTURE I

A boy had a slightly oblique displaced fracture of lower/4 radius and a greenstick fracture of the ulna. Closed reduction was successful. Careful follow up with weekly X-ray was done.

After 4 weeks, the radius fracture showed radial tilt. It was manipulated under anesthesia and immobilized. Fairly good re-reduction was achieved, with good clinical and X-ray appearance at the end. (As mentioned earlier,

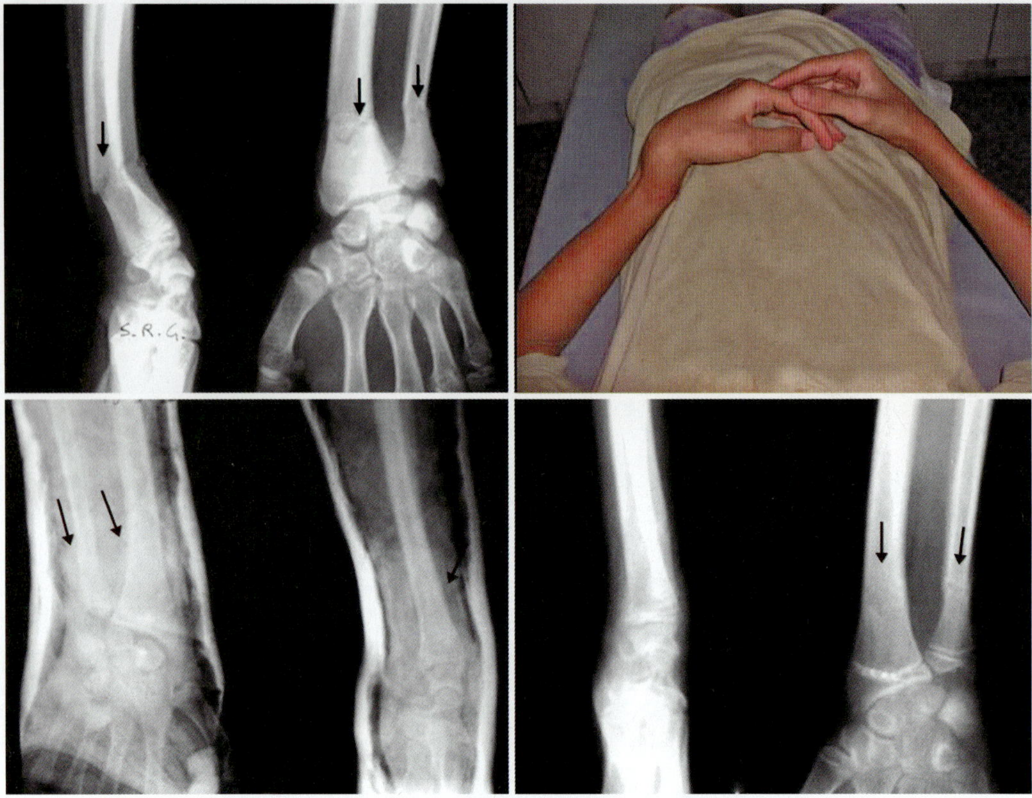

Figure 19.6 Greenstick fracture of both radius and ulna

such a displacement is seen in radius, when the fracture is oblique) (Fig. 19.7).

CASE 8: RE-DISPLACEMENT IN AN OBLIQUE FRACTURE II

A boy of Indian origin, staying abroad, while on holiday in India, came with a displaced fracture of lower/4 radius and a greenstick fracture of ulna. This was similar to the above case. The fracture of the radius had slightly oblique fracture line.

Closed reduction under anesthesia done as per protocol. Regular follow up X-ray taken. At the end of 4 weeks, some angular displacement of the fracture was noted. He was advised for re-reduction and manipulation. He had to return to his country and hence left India. Follow up information received that the fracture led good clinical union and appearance (Fig. 19.8).

MESSAGE

- In such an injury, when:
  - The radius fracture is complete and displaced, while the ulna has a greenstick fracture → the radius is more likely to have displacement at the end of 2 to 3 weeks.

    Reason: Ulna being angulated, early callus formed and the ends are stabilized by the callus. Hence, translation does not occur in the ulna.

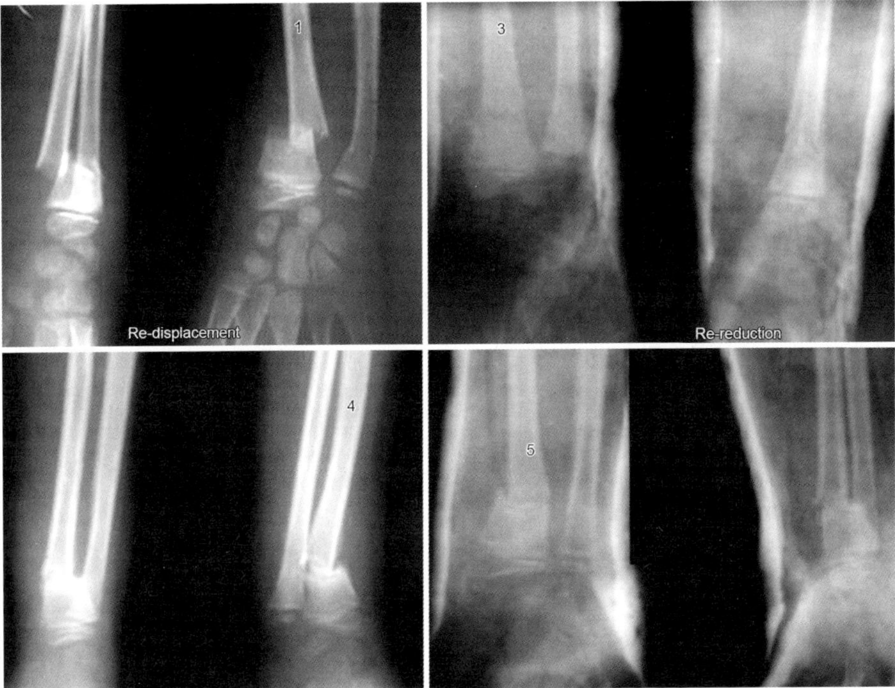

Figure 19.7 Redisplacement in an oblique fracture I

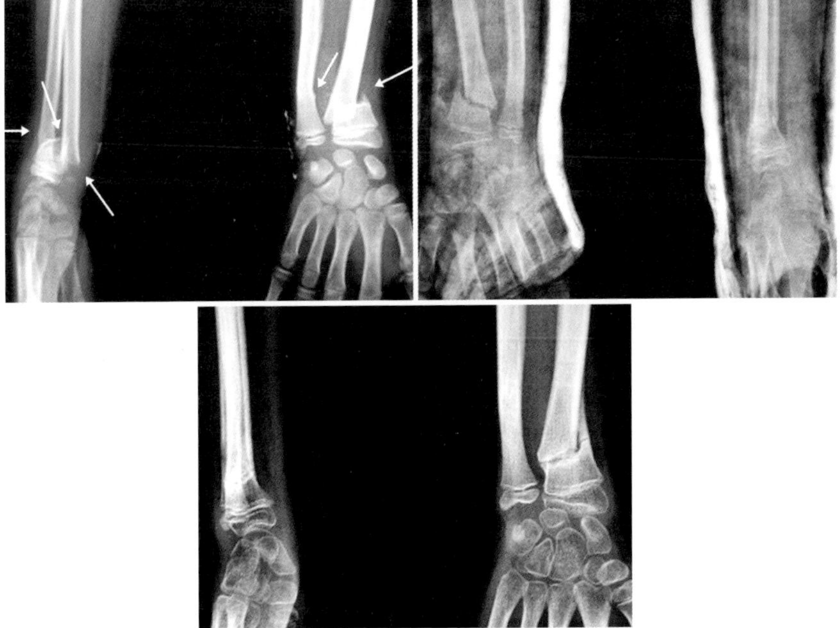

Figure 19.8 Redisplacement in an oblique fracture II

- When both the radius and ulna had complete and displaced fractures, such a late angulation of radius alone is not observed.

  Reason: Both the bones get displaced/ angulated equally.
- If the radius fracture is oblique, it is more likely to get displaced, translated and angulated in the first 10 days. Hence for the oblique fracture of the radius in children below 10 years, percutaneous K-wire fixation and a plate fixation for children above that 10 years of age is recommended.

In a Non-operative Method

- A close follow up and X-ray examination through the cast every 5 days on the first two occasions is necessary, to confirm that the reduction is maintained well.
- Reduction of the limb swelling needs careful change of plaster cast. Great care needs to be taken, while removing the earlier cast, as the fracture may get displaced at this stage. It is possible to carry out this as an out-patient procedure carefully without anesthesia explaining every possibility that, if the child does not co-operate, a general anesthesia would be required.
- When internal fixation is done, early implant removal after fracture remodeling is necessary. Due to active bone growth at this age, often the implant is strongly anchored to the bone, making it difficult to remove it. Besides, when a plate fixation is done, the stress-shielding makes the underlying cortex too thin, which is slow to recover, at a later age.

CHAPTER

20

Malunited Fracture of Lower/4 Radius in a Child

MALUNITED FRACTURE OF LOWER /4 RADIUS

This adolescent boy presented six weeks after a fall on the hand, to the clinic.

Clinically

- Dinnerfork deformity (L) lower end forearm with anterior angulation (Posterior tilt of the fragment)
- Uniting fracture of lower/4 of radius.

X-ray of wrist revealed: Early callus all around the radius with a dorsal tilt of the distal fragment.

How did this occur? (As per the history given by parents).

- After initial closed reduction and immobilization only a below elbow cast was applied and no post-reduction X-ray examination done.
- Follow up X-ray not taken after the reduction.
- When the cast was removed, on noticing dorsal tilt, no specific advice was given in 7 to 10 days and hence chose to consult me.

It is possible that with growth and remodeling, some correction of the angular deformity would occur. However, he was of age 15, towards end of 2nd growth spurt. The patient and parents were very upset, because of the deformity and very keen to have the correction done. Hence I planned open reduction and anatomical realignment as much as possible.

Is it possible to carry out osteoclasis? Yes.

- However, the force required is quite-some and may accidentally injure the lower radial epiphysis.
- The fragments may be well-aligned, but there is likelihood, that some translation would remain, which radiologically may not be acceptable to the parents.
- During follow up, there is every possibility that the deformity may recur, requiring another procedure under anesthesia.

Hence, an open osteotomy was planned, which has all the advantages.

Technique of Osteotomy of Lower End Radius for Malunion

Dorsal Vertical Approach

Plane was developed in between the tendon of extensor pollicis longus and ext digitorum Communis tendons. The sheaths of EPL and communis were incised vertically and the tendons retracted on either side.

Dissected proximally, till the normal dorsal surface of radius was seen. Located the fracture area. The local bone and the callus mass were soft. With a 20 mm wide osteotome, a plane was made in a proximal to distal direction in the old

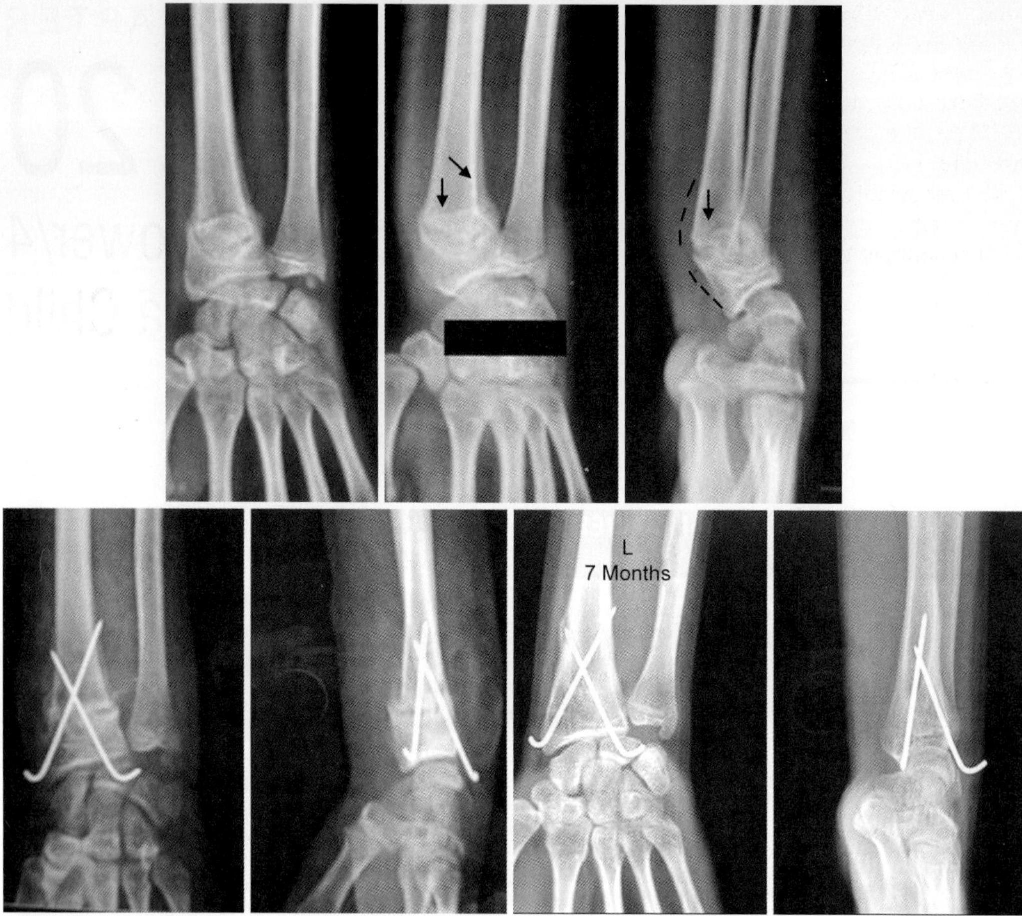

Figure 20.1 Radius lower-end osteotomy

fracture line. By gently tilting the osteotome, fracture was made mobile. One must use a broad osteotome. If a narrow osteotome is used, it may make a notch in the wide fracture surface.

Care needs to be taken, as during the levering of the proximal end of the distal fragment, traction must be given through the patient's hand and this maneuver reduces the crushing of the bone end.

With perseverance and waiting for the soft tissues to get stretched, one can make the fragments mobile. The rotary alignment was restored and the fracture was levered in place.

Checked under the 'C' arm. Pronation of forearm was maintained and cross K-wires of 1.8 mm diameter were inserted. The wires were bent close to the bone, cut and rotated to bury at a suitable position.

Tourniquet Released

The tendon sheaths need to be just opposed to avoid stenosis.

A padded crepe bandage + AE, POP slab in midprone was given. Check X-ray through the POP on table taken. This makes one sure that the fragments are in correct position.

The plaster was left undisturbed for 2 weeks, till soft callus was formed. Then the sutures were removed and an above elbow cast, in midprone was applied. This was maintained for total six weeks. Under supervision, exercises for the fingers and shoulder were carried out.

At the end of 6 weeks, good external callus was observed. Cast was removed. A below elbow removable cock up POP slab was given. Intermittent mobilization and grip exercises were encouraged.

The below elbow POP slab kept him comfortable and also prevented him from playing/riding a bicycle, etc.

The K wires were kept in the bone, as long as possible, and were removed when uncomfortable to the patient. At the end of 3 months, the fracture was well consolidated. Removal of the cross K-wires done at the end of seven months.

CHAPTER

21

Inferior RU Dislocation in a Child

INFERIOR RADIOULNAR (RU) JOINT DISLOCATION

The head of ulna was dislocated posteriorly. Clinically, the head of ulna was prominent posteriorly, with limitation of supination. If the subluxation is fresh/minimal, then it may be possible to reduce it in the OPD, with forearm suspended and in supination. Final position of supination and gentle pressure on the head of ulna with wrist in 15 deg dorsiflexion, reduces it well.

If the wrist appears painful and the dislocation is locked, then it should be reduced under anesthesia and immobilized in an above elbow well-molded POP cast in supination and slight dorsiflexion for 5 weeks (Fig. 21.1).

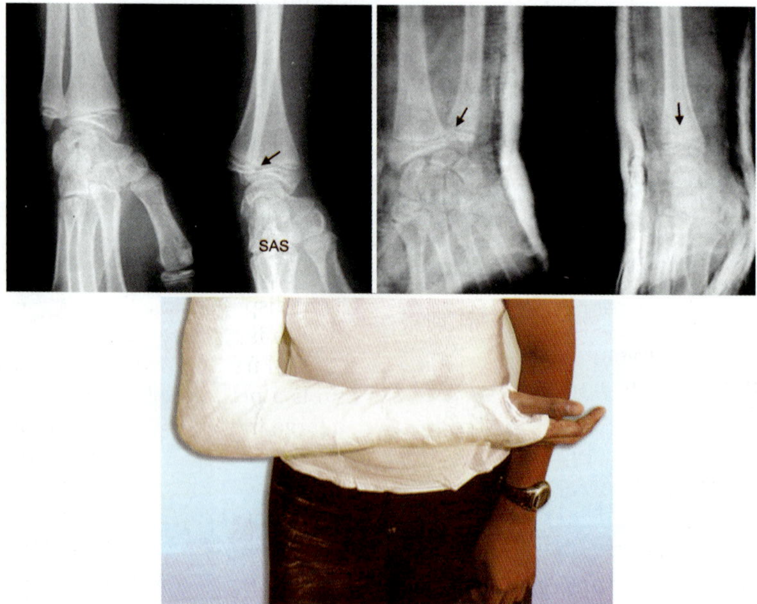

Figure 21.1 Inferior radioulnar dislocation

CHAPTER

22

Colles' Fracture

UNDISPLACED COLLES' FRACTURE

Of late, I have come across more cases of undisplaced rather than impacted Colles' fractures.

It is logical to treat such an injury, without manipulation, with POP cast only. In spite of a well-molded cast with some ulnar deviation and palmer flexion, often at the end of 3 weeks, one finds that dorsal tilt has occurred. The clinician would naturally recommend change of treatment to an operative one, at this stage.

If K-wire fixation was advised on day 1, the patient may have agreed to the procedure. However, at the end of three weeks, the patient may not agree for a closed reduction and a K-wire fixation. Often the patient takes this as failure of entire treatment. Even if he agrees, the fracture has become sticky and a good reduction may not be achieved.

Thus in an undisplaced Colles' fracture, stabilization with K-wires done on day 1, offers stability to the fracture, prevents re-displacement and dorsal tilt at the fracture site.

Recommendation

In an undisplaced Colles' fracture, stabilization with cross K-wires confers stability and prevents any displacement of the fragments. Hence, it is necessary to carry out cross K-wire fixation and BE cast on day 1 and continue the cast, for at least five weeks (Fig. 22.1).

Technique of Cross K-Wires Insertion in a Colles' Fracture

In pre 'C' arm era, K-wire fixation was done, usually, only from the radial styloid area, may be with 2 wires inserted side by side. Before advent of power drill, to hold the reduction and operate the hand drill also was a demanding job. Prior to 'C' arm, one had to do this under image intensifier I an X-ray department. The space available below the tube and the hand to be operated upon, used to be very less, making the entire procedure very cumbersome, though was very desirable indeed.

Now, with advent of 'C' arm, one can do a cross-wire fixation precisely. I prefer to do a cross K-wire fixation to wires only from the radial side. The cross-wire method offers a better stability to maintain the reduction and prevent displacement during follow up.

- C' arm is a good asset for the procedure. In a small frame, 1.6 mm K-wire with a trocar tip is a preferred implant. In a patient with a large frame, a 1.8 mm K-wire is required. A cordless power drill makes the procedure easy. The fracture is reduced by traction, counter-traction and manipulation and confirmed under 'C' arm. The first K-wire is inserted from radial styloid process, anterior to the cephalic vein. The vein may not be visible due to edema. The wire

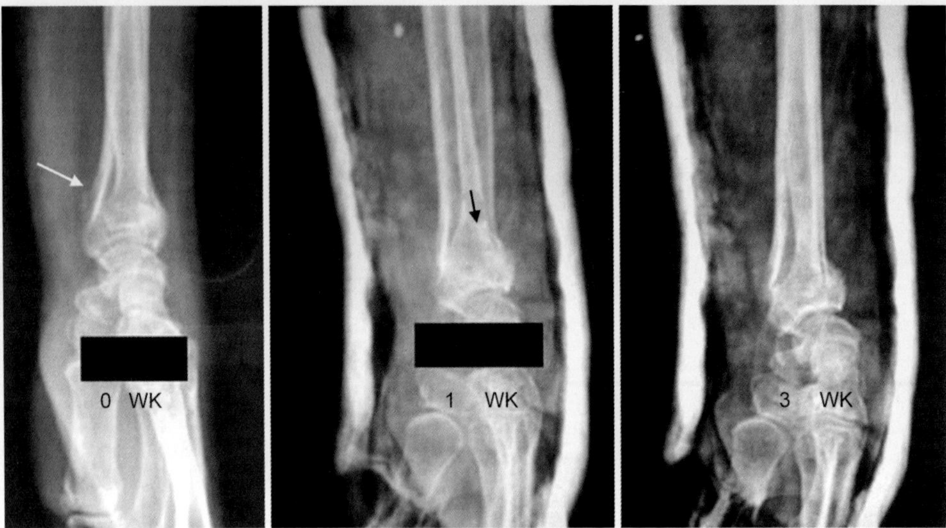

Figure 22.1 Why K-wire

is directed in coronal plane and it exits from the interosseous border of the radius. Confirm under `C` arm. The entry should be in between the vein and the abductor thumb tendon (see your own wrist !)

- The next wire is from the ulnar end of the dorsum of radius and needs to be inserted more vertically, towards the radius, just penetrating the lateral cortex. If one does not increase the inclination, the wire often slides along the dorsum of the radius. If it penetrates the far cortex more than 2 mm, local pain is experienced on the tip of K-wire on the lateral side of the radius, where the wire tip is subcutaneous.

Both the wires need to penetrate the opposite cortex to obtain a good hold and stability. A visual judgment is taken, while holding the hand by the left hand and the point of entry and direction of wire is confirmed under 'C' arm. Then the wire is steadily drilled in one go, till it just crosses the far cortex. *Repeated forward and backward movement of the K-wire is avoided, as it makes the near hole bigger and reduces the hold on the bone.* If this is not practised, loosening and backing out of a K-wire is likely, more so in an osteoporotic bone.

Hence the steps should be:

- Achieve a good reduction. The assistant, who holds the elbow for constant counter-traction, continues to be at the same position, holding the elbow, and the draping is done over the assistant's hand. Assistant holding the elbow is useful to give a counter-traction during the procedure and to supinate the forearm from the upper forearm. He has to wear a lead apron and be here till the end of the procedure.

How to get a leteral view?

- If the forearm is supinated by the surgeon, then during supination holding the wrist, stress is added at the fracture, which may get displaced. Hence, the assistant holding the proximal forearm and the elbow, is to make the forearm supine, by rotation the proximal fragment.
- By palpation of bone landmarks and judgment, insert the radial styloid K-wire through the skin till the near cortex bone resistance is obtained. Check under 'C' arm the point of entry and the direction of the K-wire and drill the K-wire across the fracture in one go.
- Get the feel, that the K-wire has just penetrated the far cortex.

- Disengage the drill and carry out the insertion of second wire, distal to proximal direction, from the ulnar side of the distal fragment. Check the position of this second wire and confirm the position of the first one.
  This reduces the radiation too.
- Check the fracture stability under 'C' arm in both the planes.

Note: It is safer to keep the far end of the wire, slightly, say 3 mm outside the far cortex. (While bending the K-wire, it tends to come back slightly.) The wires are bent, either with a narrow nose K-wire bender or with a metal suction cannula, as close to the bone as possible. It may be further bent by a needle nose pliers and cut at appropriate level. A Maun side cutter is a useful tool for this. If one cuts the K-wire first, then try to bend it, it is mechanically difficult to bend a short segment of a wire! The bent wire end is then rotated in appropriate direction and the skin is manually kneaded, so the bent tip is buried under the skin. If necessary, one should not hesitate to take a small incision to bury the bent end of the K-wire. This would prevent skin puckering by the bent end of the K-wire. After dressing, a padded and moulded below elbow plaster cast is applied, with the wrist in few degree of palmar flexion and ulnar deviation. Thus, usually, while inserting the K-wire, there is no incision, but while removing, one needs to take a small incision.

The extent and type of the below elbow cast:

- I prefer a plaster of Paris material for a BE cast, as it is easy to mold, especially around the thumb. Should some trimming is needed later on, a POP cast is easier to trim with a plaster shears. A synthetic material needs a power saw, which could be dangerous to the patient's fingers !
- Anteriorly, the distal limit of the cast be upto the proximal palmer crease, so that full finger flexion at the MCP joints is possible. The proximal edge of the cast be at such a level, that full flexion of the elbow is possible (Fig. 22.2).

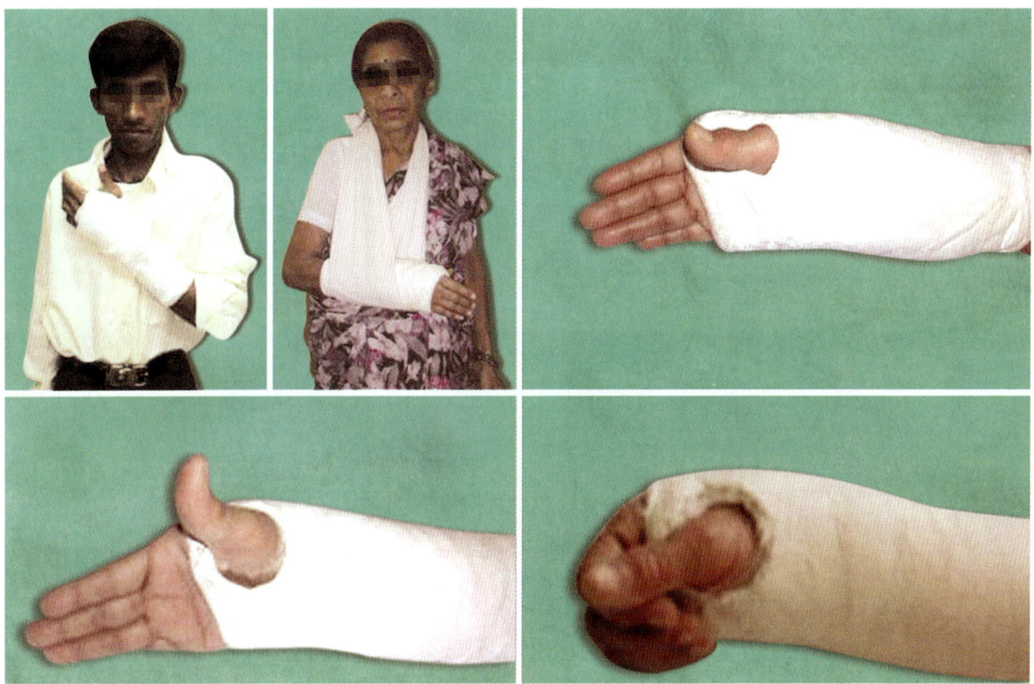

Figure 22.2 Plaster extent

A displaced fracture of ulnar styloid indicates possible instability after such an injury. If the fragment is adequately large, one may consider its fixation to the head of ulna, by a 1.2 mm K-wire, by a closed or an open method. It is observed that in elderly persons, more than age 50 years or so, even if the ulnar styloid is left as such, stability of the wrist continues to be good.

In a Colles' fracture, if:

- The fracture displacement is more
- Some comminution is seen at the fracture site with osteoporosis, not adequate enough to warrant bone grafting
- Late collapse and dorsal and/or ulnar tilt is expected
- Patient is reluctant for an open surgery, including bone grafting—then it is prudent to immobilize the limb, in an above elbow plaster cast in mid-prone position, for 4 weeks. Later it may change to a below elbow POP cast for further two weeks. One observes that with this method, the incidence of late dorsal collapse of the fracture and K-wire back out is less.

Why bury the K-wire tips?

If the K-wires are buried under the skin, after the cast removal, patient can have a bath immediately. The K-wires remain deep to the skin, they can be left as such, adding stability to the fracture area, till consolidation takes place. No dressing is needed and inconvenience of the K-wire tips protruding is avoided.

Patient is informed that, as the local swelling reduces, the wire tips would be palpable, under the skin. If the K-wire tip is kept outside the skin surface, after the cast removal, it needs protection with a dressing and patient cannot have a bath over the fracture area, till the wires are removed (Fig. 22.3).

CT Scan

In certain cases, where the fracture morphology is not clear and for purpose of documentation, a pre-operative CT scan with 3D reconstruction is helpful. This is especially useful in a die punch injury, which needs elevation.

In a three-part fracture, at times, pre-operative decision making could be difficult, as to whether a closed reduction and percutaneous K-wire fixation would be adequate or a plate fixation is needed. In such a situation, equipment for an open reduction, plate fixation and may-be bone grafting is kept ready. Under anesthesia, the fracture is reduced and fracture morphology is studied and accordingly decision is taken.

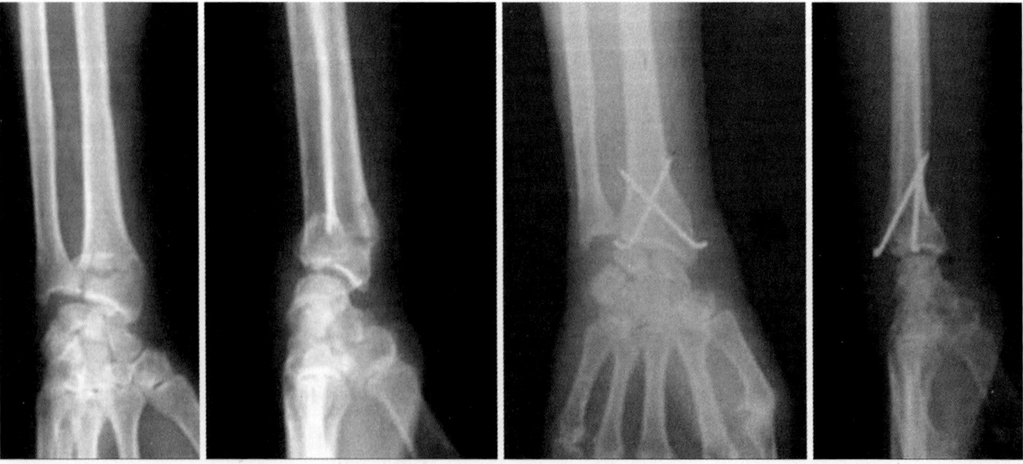

Figure 22.3 Cross K-wires offer stability

Postoperative Important Care

- Continuous elevation of the hand and active movements of the fingers is a must, for initial 3 days at least.
- Active exercise for the fingers and shoulder movements are important, more so in an elderly. In a patient with diabetes, periarthritis of shoulder is a commonly observed complication.
- When a below elbow cast is given, avoid pronosupination of the forearm, as it puts strain on the fracture area.
- The sling should be discarded after 3 to 4 days, after the pain and swelling have reduced. Initially, this is done intermittently. One is encouraged to do light activities, like holding a newspaper, etc. If after discarding the sling, should swelling on fingers reappear, it indicates that the elevation is still needed. Hence, it is wise to continue the sling for a few days more, with emphasis on exercises for the fingers and the shoulder.
- If the swelling reduces too much and the cast is no more a close fitting one, one should immediately change it to a close fitting one.
- *Reflex sympathetic dystrophy*: While the cast is on or after its removal, should fingers swell and range of motion reduces, patient is advised to report immediately to the treating clinician. If supervised exercises are enforced at this stage, the recovery period is reduced. It will also help to control reflex sympathetic dystrophy.

If this complication is observed, after cast removal:

In addition to exercise and suitable drug therapy, a cock up plaster splint support is needed. It keeps the wrist in comfortable position and is the position of rest. This support helps the patient to be able to carry out the finger exercises with ease. Later on, the splint can be intermittently removed and mobilizing exercises are carried out. I find a custom-made POP slab more effective, than a readymade splint. The later even if easy to put on by the patient himself, the former is more comfortable and effective.

In addition to the mechanical support, certain drug therapies, including a short course of steroids help to cut short the recovery time.

In general a little extended and prolonged external immobilization gives a good clinical outcome and keeps a patient more comfortable than early mobilization leading to pain and deformity.

TYPICAL CASES

Case 1: Comminuted Colles' Fracture

Assess

- If the articular surface is intact,
- Study the quality of bone and comminution.

Following action plan method can be considered:

Reserve the OT and plan a procedure for 1 ½ hrs, so should bone grafting is needed, one has adequate time to carry out the procedure peacefully, in the same sitting.

Keep equipment for percutaneous K wiring, iliac bone grafting and external fixator ready.

Discuss with the patient and family likely options of bone grafting and/or external fixator, prior to the surgery, as often the decision needs to be taken on the table.

Appropriate anesthesia is arranged and `C` arm facility must be available. Examine the fracture under anesthesia with traction. This makes the fracture anatomy and dorsal comminution, if any, visible and then decide the procedure to be carried out.

On traction, if one finds dorsal comminution, it predicts likelihood of late dorsal collapse:

Consider closed reduction and dorsal exposure → Iliac bone graft (Synthetic bone substitute) → Cross K-wires and above elbow plaster slab, in midprone for 10 days and then change to an above elbow cast. This procedure needs a total 6 weeks immobilization for the grafts to get incorporated. Bone grafts help to consolidate the bone well, with a minimal late collapse. I feel, this procedure is a safe, of less magnitude compared to plate fixation and/or external fixation and gives a satisfactory outcome. My preference is for autologous bone graft to the synthetic bone substitute, as the consolidation is rapid and assured (Fig. 22.4).

Case 2: Dorsal Comminution

At times, the distal fragment has dorsal comminution, say 2 cm from articular area. Alternatives are an anterior locking plate or a dorsal plate. This case example is from a pre-locking plate era.

Steps

- *Dorsal exposure*:
- Bone grafts are taken from iliac crest and laid in the dorsal void. This is followed by a provisional K-wire fixation, passed from radial styloid, towards the opposite cortex.
- This confers provisional stability. Now, one can fix a plate dorsally. I prefer a reconstruction plate. The provisional K-wire is left as such, as it provides additional angular stability for the fixation and prevents any redisplacement. Above elbow POP slab, followed by a cast, in midprone for 4 weeks is given. This is followed by a below elbow cast for further 3 weeks. One observes a good union, stability and good range of motion.

Even if one chooses to use a locking plate today, the steps would be the same (Fig. 22.5).

Case 3: Only External Fixator Stabilization, without any Internal Fixation

Here is an example, where a closed reduction was done and external fixator was applied. In due course, during follow up, recurrence of dorsal tilt was observed. Thus, an external fixator applied after a closed reduction, would maintain the distraction, but may not maintain the reduction and may later lead to recurrence of the angular deformity.

External fixation merely helps to achieve ligamentotaxis and stabilize the fracture. K-wire fixation across the fracture is necessary to maintain the fragment opposition effectively and prevent late angulation. Both, the K-wires and the external fixator are complementary to each other (Fig. 22.6).

Case 4

Due to the fracture geometry, one finds few large fragments, in the distal fragment, which can be held by K wires. However, still, closed reduction

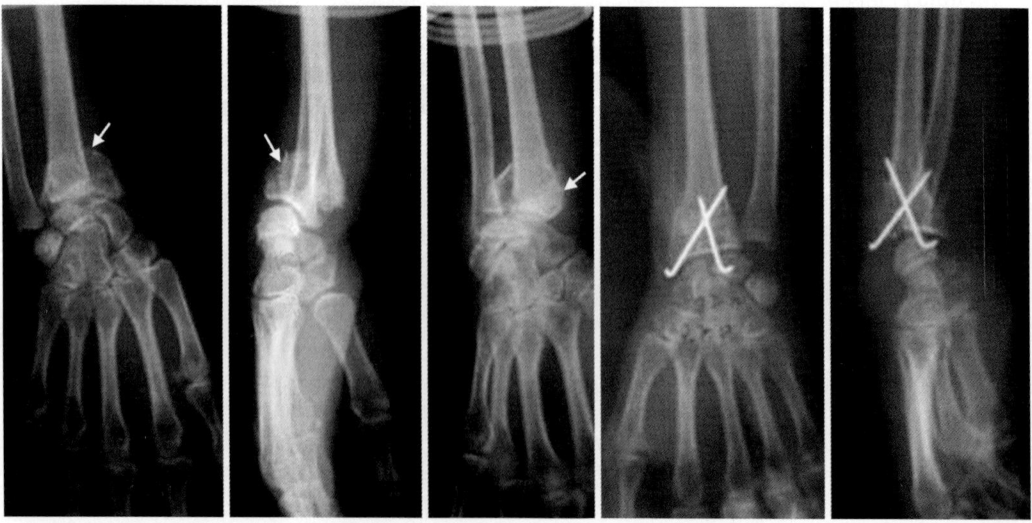

Figure 22.4 Dorsal bone grafting and K-wire fixation

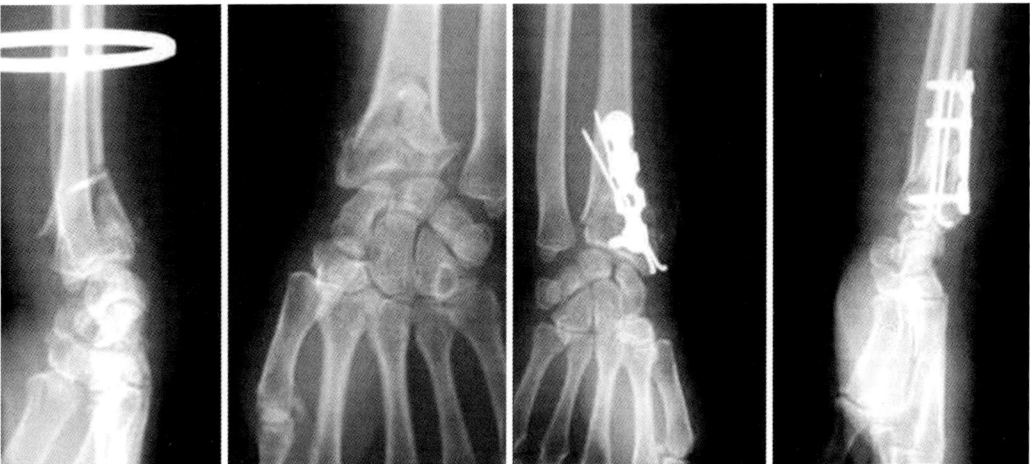

Figure 22.5 Dorsal bone graft and plate

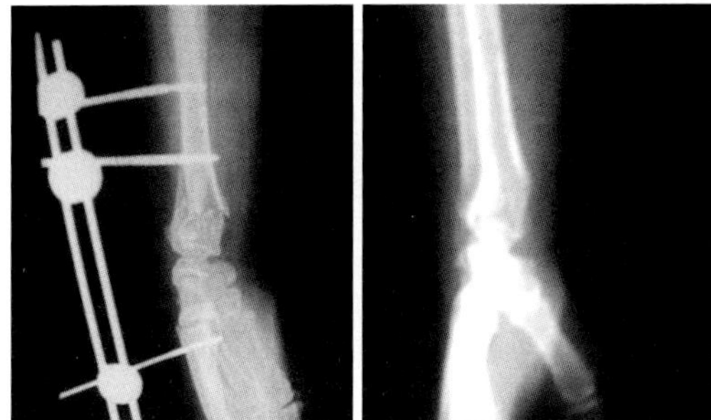

Figure 22.6 Only external fixator inadequate

and K-wire fixation alone may not adequately stabilize the fracture assembly. One needs to add external fixator, to make the assembly more stable. This is a good combination, which would offer optimal stability and good end result and function (Fig. 22.7).

Recommended steps for K-wire fixation + External fixation: Preoperatively should discuss various options like, bone grafting/K-wires/ external fixator, etc. and that the decision may be taken on table after examination under image intensifier and the post-reduction appearance.

Examine under anesthesia and study the fracture geometry. May take an X-ray on table for documentation.

Having decided to carry out this procedure:

- Do a formal closed reduction and study. Mark the sites of Schanz pins and insert them in desired position and direction. Confirm under image intensifier the Schanz pin placement and its hold on the opposite cortex. Do a trial placement of the connecting bars. (The bars may not be passed through the adjustable clamps, but just held over them, to study the alignment.) See below.
- The Schanz pins could be so directed that all the pins are in one line with two bars, one above the other. The other method could be that the pins are inserted at angles and the two bars cross each other. At a point, where they cross each other, they are held together with a clamp, which adds to the assembly stability. The later method is relatively easy to carry out and completes the final assembly rather quickly (Fig. 22.8).
  - When the fixator pins (and hence the bars) are placed medially, the wrist flexion needs to be held, while the position of pins is planned. This is rather tedious.
- After inserting the Schanz pins, a study of alignment is made by holding the connecting bars over the pins. Then the fracture is reduced again. If on image, there appears void in the fracture area, add few cancellous

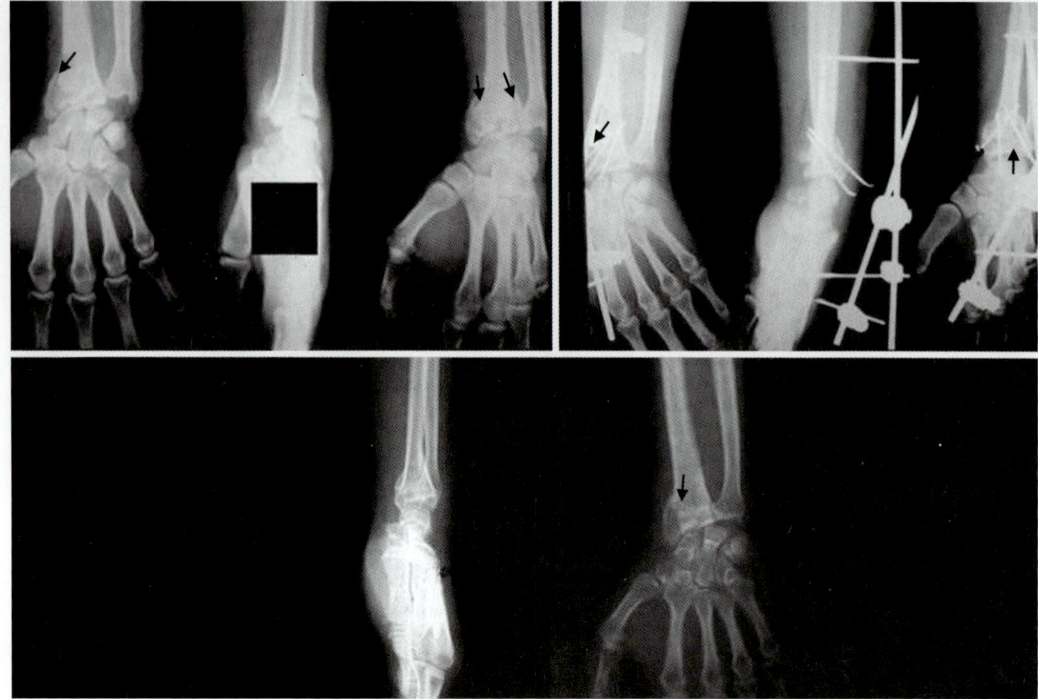

Figure 22.7 External fixator and additional K-wires

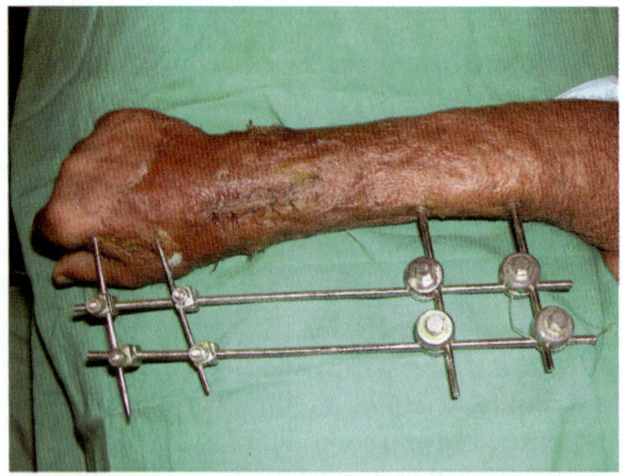

Figure 22.8 Ext. fixator in a line

grafts. Then insert cross K-wires and assess the fracture stability.

- If one does bone grafting and stabilization with the K-wires first and then inserts the Schanz pins, following problem may come: There is a possibility that due to the stress of drilling and inserting Schanz pins, rotation of the forearm, the K-wires which stabilize the fracture, may loosen and the hold in the bone may reduce. This is a precursor of wire back out later. Hence, the Schanz pins are to be inserted first and then the K-wires are inserted. At this stage what is remaining is only adding the connecting bars.
- Add the connecting bars to the Schanz pins, prestress the pins and tighten the nuts over the bars. While attaching the connecting bar, necessary degree of palmer flexion has to be given.
- Postoperative elevation of the hand, immediate finger and early shoulder exercises are important, for restoration of good function of the entire limb as a whole, at the end of the treatment.
- As per the fracture geometry and as per individual case, the fixator is usually kept for 4 weeks, so the fracture has progressed to some degree of union and would not

collapse. The fixator is removed and the cross K-wires are retained. The wrist is immobilized by a below or above elbow cast, as per the fracture geometry, for the necessary duration. This would prevent late collapse of the fracture and uninterrupted bone union.

Case 5: Colles' Fracture with Fracture of Head of Ulna

After stabilization of Colles` fracture, the distal ulna also can be stabilized, by a percutaneous K-wire. It is preferable to immobilize the wrist in an above elbow cast in midprone for 4 weeks, followed by a below elbow cast for further 3 weeks (Fig. 22.9).

Case 6: Fracture of Lower-end Radius– A Large Distal Fragment

In a fracture with a large distal fragment, one can achieve good reduction and internal fixation with 2 cross K wires. However, in young, heavy built persons, K wires alone do not provide good stability, even with additional plaster immobilization. In the given case, one noticed instability later and had to be revised to an additional plate fixation (Fig. 22.10).

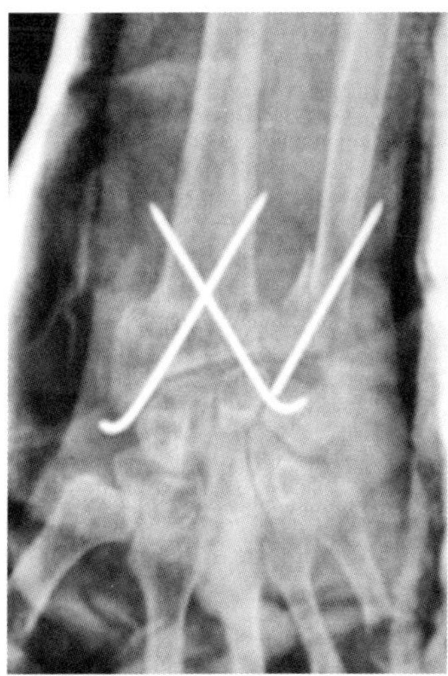

Figure 22.9 Colles' fracture and ulna fracture

Case 7: Malunited Colles` Fracture

Malunion may occur, due to lack of medical aid/associated other major injuries of more priority or a missed injury to the wrist.

This is a case of a malunited fracture, with a severe dorsal tilt in a young worker, who was on Warfarin, for his cardiac condition. He demanded for corrective surgery. A dorsal approach and corrective osteotomy, bone grafting and a plate fixation was done. Postoperative plaster immobilization was given. Good end result (Fig. 22.11).

Case 8: Malunion due to Over-reduction

In a closed reduction of a transverse fracture, over-reduction is possible. Hence, after closed reduction and prior to plaster application one should check the reduction with a 'C' arm. While a lateral projection image is taken, an assistant should supinate the forearm from the upper forearm rather than surgeon supinating by rotating the hand. This helps to maintain the reduction. It is advisable to check again after the cast is set and an X-ray film taken for documentation. If after plaster application, if alignment is found to be unacceptable, it needs to be corrected then only. However, if it goes unnoticed and the cast is in more palmer flexion, the lower radial articular surface tilts anteriorly. Such a position of the reduction if accepted, ends with limitation of dorsiflexion. For a good grip, dorsiflexion at the wrist is essential.

Thus, prior to cast immobilization, while giving a position at the wrist, degree of palmer flexion needs to be corrected. Follow up X-ray examination needs to be done every 10 days. If one finds that the anterior tilt is increasing, it may have to be corrected during the change of cast. This is better done as a definitive procedure, under anesthesia, to get accurate position. Trying to correct the angulation without surgical anesthesia does not work and is not justified.

Similar method is practised in an under reduced fracture as well.

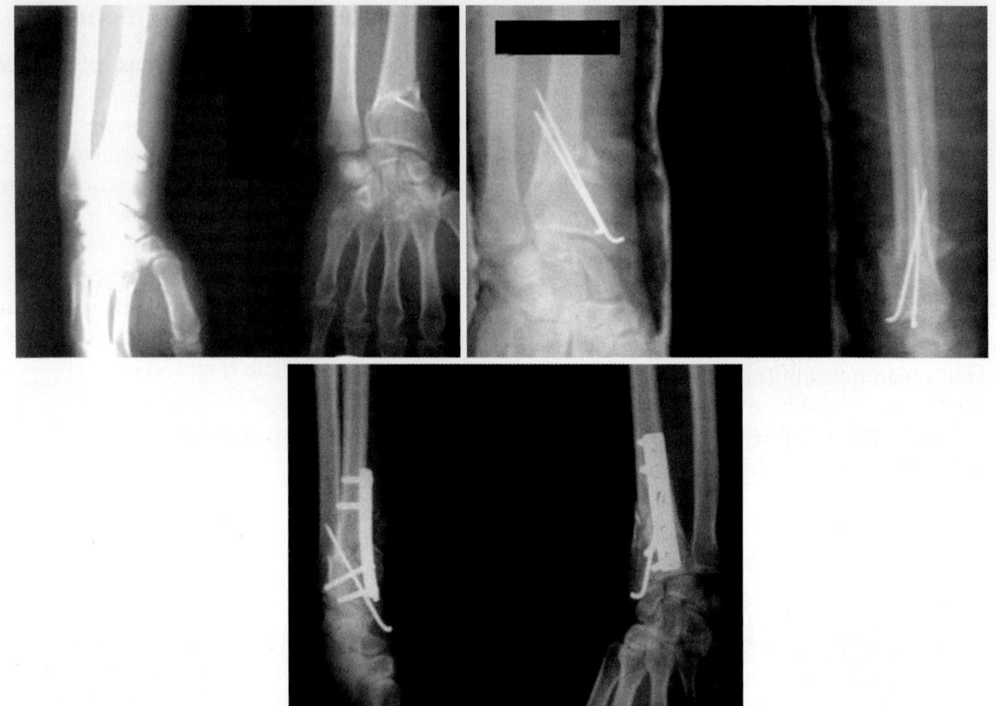

Figure 22.10 Plate is necessary and no K-wire alone

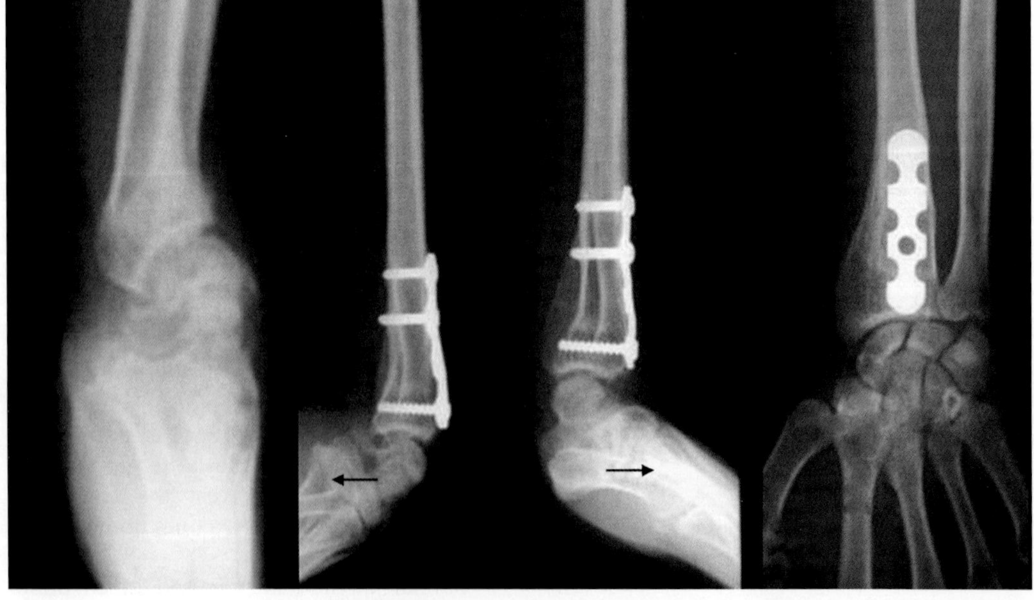

Figure 22.11 Malunion and osteotomy

Why this may have happened?

- May be 'C' arm was not available or failed after the anesthesia was induced.
- Surgeon was too confident of the reduction.
- Did not realize that such an over-reduction can occur!

Message

- Every case is to be looked upon as a case where one should give an excellent result, leaving no stone unturned.
- On table image is important for a good outcome.
- If loss of reduction is noticed during early follow up, it must be corrected soon.
- A Colles' fracture is preferably stabilized with cross K-wires on day 1 only, which is possible today, with advent of a 'C ' arm and power tools (Fig. 22.12).

Case 9: K-wires Backing Out

Why does a K-wire back out?

- Osteoporotic bone
- During insertion of a K-wire, possibly forward and backward drilling was done few times, making the fixation of the K-wire rather loose.

How to prevent?

- Trocar point sharp K-wires
- A correct angle of insertion. Should not be too parallel to the shaft, or else, it slides along the endosteum of the opposite cortex, without penetrating it.

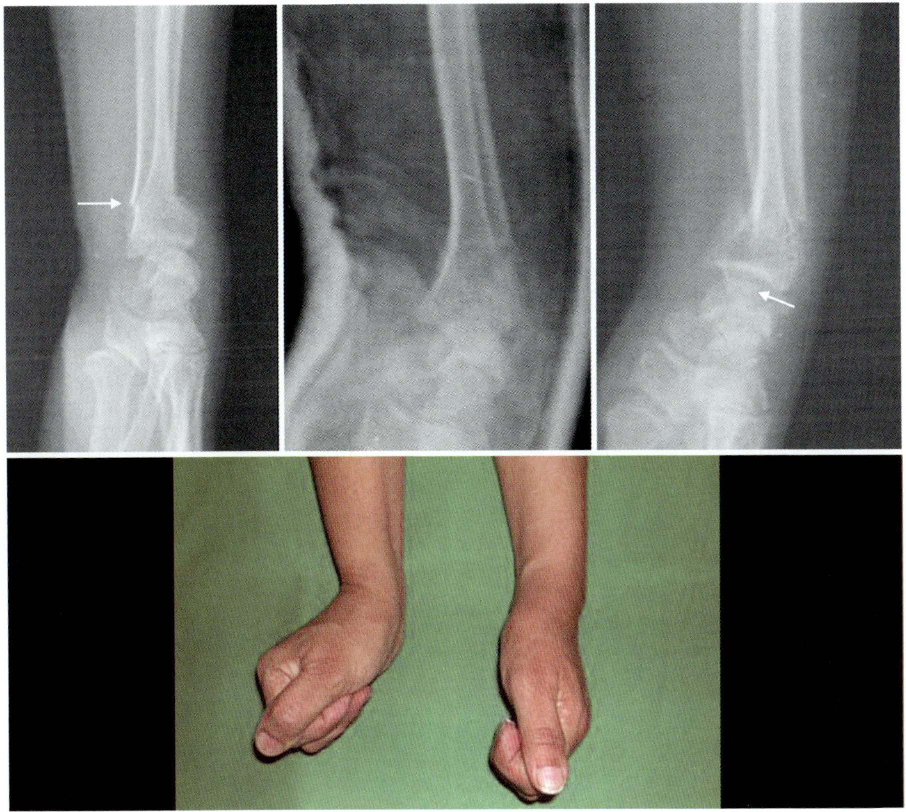

Figure 22.12 Over-reduction

In the given case, cross K-wires were inserted. After a week, patient experienced pain in the wrist within the cast. X-ray through the cast showed K-wire from the radial styloid backing out and had to be removed. Then she was comfortable. Further follow up X-ray showed progressive valgus deformity of the fracture. However, the fracture united. After removal of the cast, rehabilitation was carried out. Gradually the ulnar side K-wire also backed out and a painful bursa formed on the tip of the K-wire. This K-wire was also removed. Patient was comfortable and able to carry out exercises well. Further X-ray showed good union with valgus position with some prominence of the head of the ulna. There was no dorsal tilt and appearance was acceptable to the patient. The patient was rather obese and hence the bony landmarks were not visible.

Message

Only valgus without a dorsal tilt is an acceptable appearance clinically. The head ulna may be prominent, but not that significant (Fig. 22.13).

Case 10: Incorrect K-wire Entry: Anterior Translation

In this case, closed reduction and cross K-wire fixation was done by a colleague. During follow up, he noted that the distal fragment was shifted anteriorly. The immediate post-op X-ray film was reviewed again. The lateral X-ray revealed, the radial K-wire entry was not through the radial styloid tip, and was rather posteriorly. This may have lead to instability, permitting forward shift of the fragment.

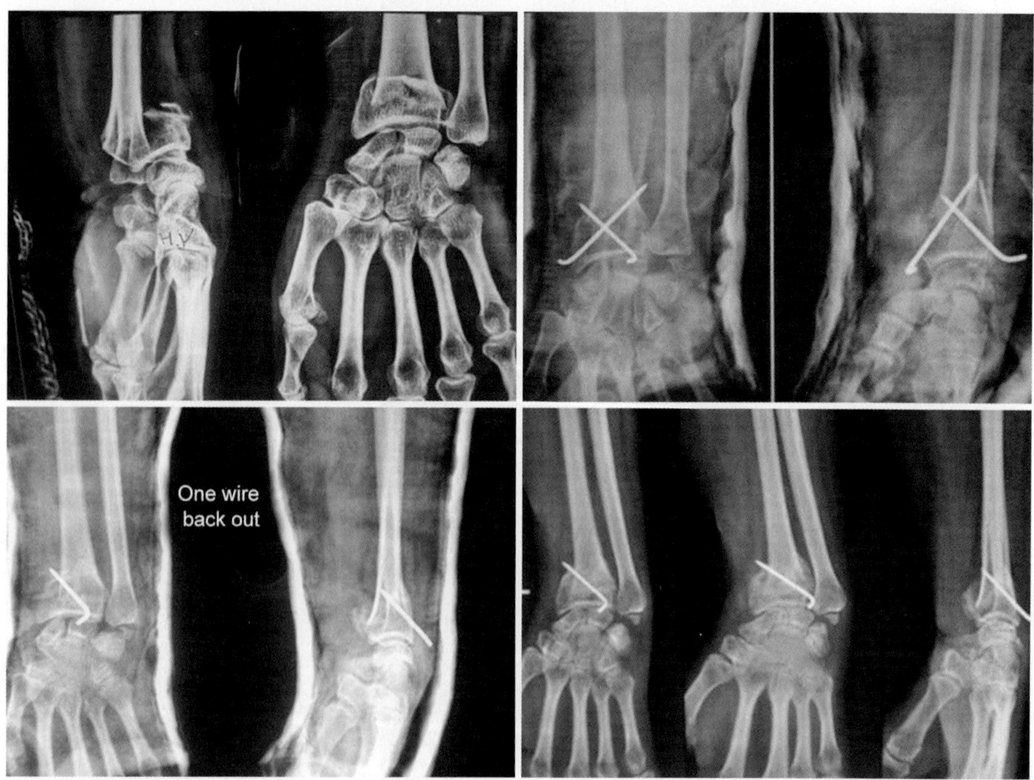

Figure 22.13 K-wire back out

A revision surgery and anterior buttress plate fixation was done. Patient had a good clinical appearance and range of motion.

Message

Every image on the screen, during surgery and every picture on an X-ray film must be carefully seen and studied. In addition to conventional PA and lateral views, both oblique views in the 'C' arm monitor should be studied carefully on table. If the 'C' arm has a facility to record all the exposures made, one should review them all. It is possible to think, if one could have reduced number of exposures made and thus save the radiation hazard (and increase life of the X-ray generator tube, as well) (Fig. 22.14).

Case 11: Transverse K-wire

A 70-year-old gentleman had a fracture of lower end of radius and ulna. Was advised internal fixation for the fracture. Bones were osteoporotic. Patient was not prepared for an open procedure. However, he was willing for a minimally invasive procedure.

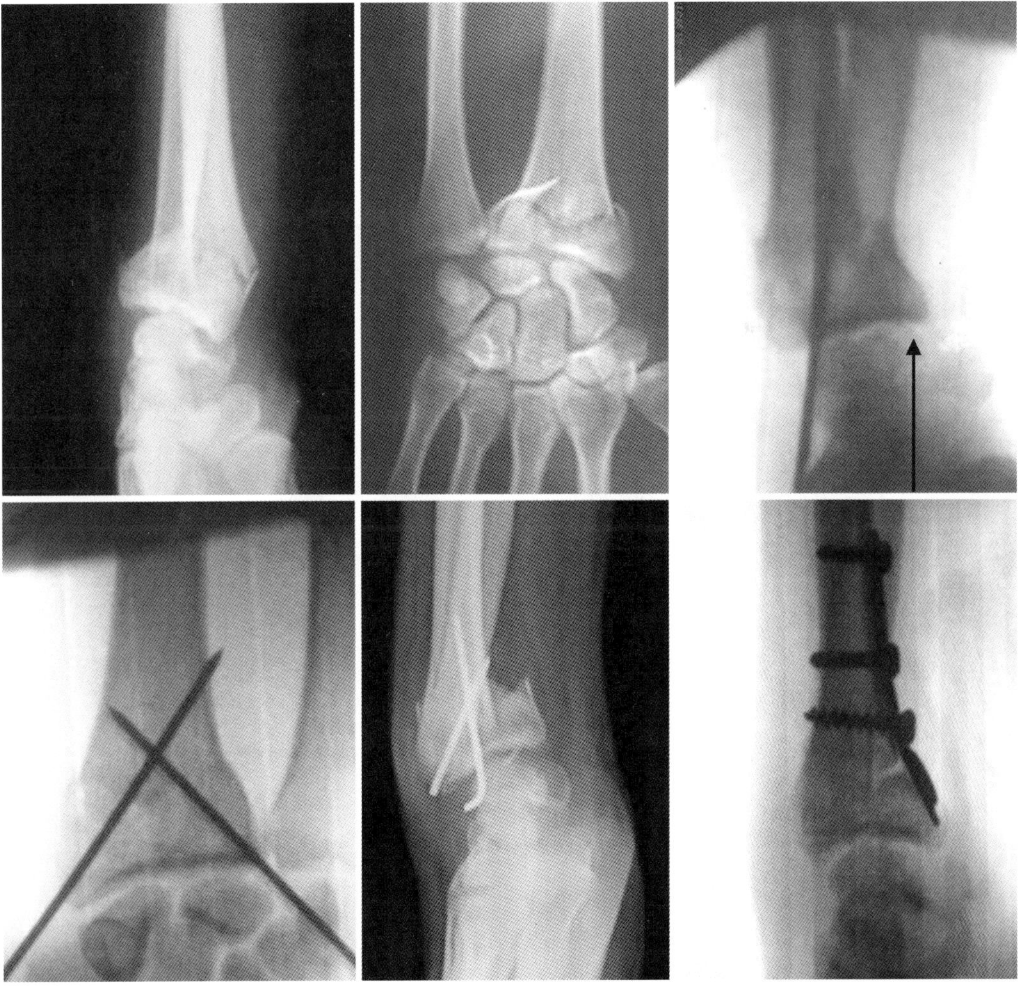

Figure 22.14 Incorrect wire entry

The radius was stabilized with an oblique and a transverse K-wire. In due course of time, due to osteoporosis, as expected, one wire backed out and was removed. The above elbow cast was continued with good union and function (Fig. 22.15).

Message

In such a fracture of both bones, a combination of percutaneous K-wire fixation for alignment and external immobilization by an above elbow plaster cast, for stability, also works well.

Case 12

A middle age lady had a Colles' fracture with multiple fragments with a dorsomedial puncture wound and an ulnar nerve palsy. A CT scan was done. Under anesthesia, one thought, that it would be possible to hold the important fragments with K-wires and was accordingly done. This was carried out and the assembly was found to be stable. For further immobilisation, an above elbow POP cast given, short of full supination. The ulnar nerve recovered (Fig. 22.16).

Case 13

A patient was treated in another city, with K-wire fixation. The K-wire end was kept outside the skin. For further treatment he came to us. The X-ray through the cast did reveal, this end of the K-wire was possibly not buried. On removal of the cast, the wire end is visible as in the photograph. Presence of such a wire, outside the skin, is quite some inconvenience to the patient: needs a dressing all the while, cannot have a bath over the wrist, etc. till it is removed.

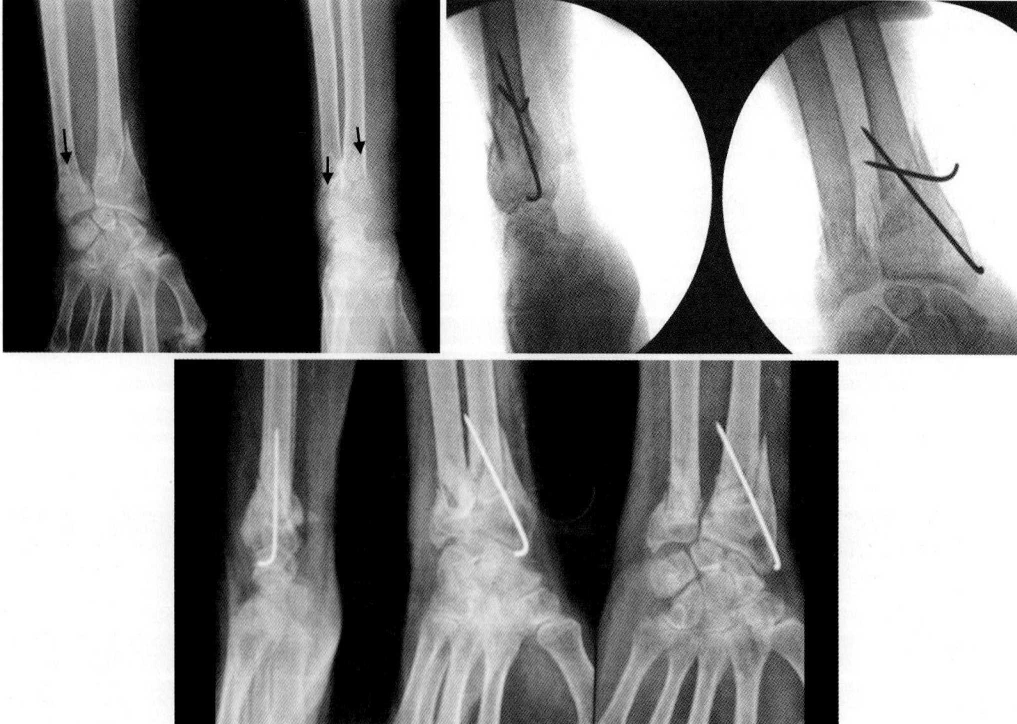

Figure 22.15 Transverse K-wire

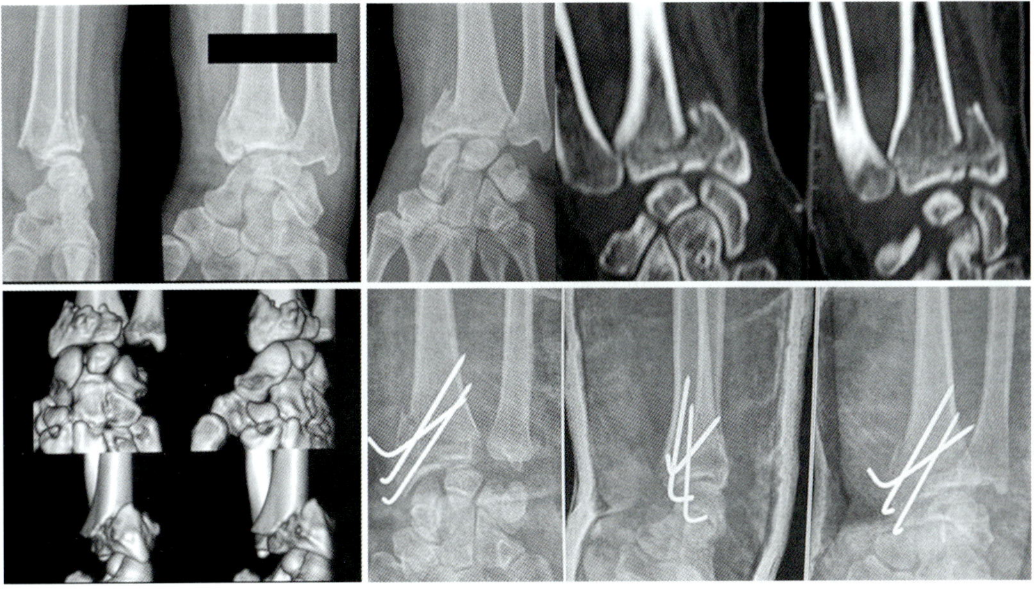

Figure 22.16 Multiple fragments K-wires

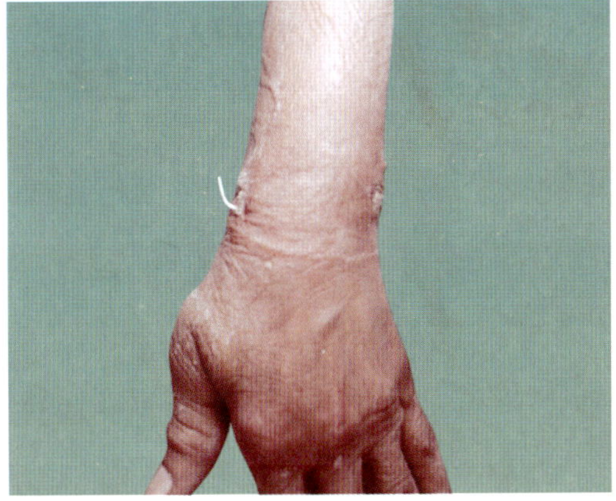

Figure 22.17 K-wire not buried

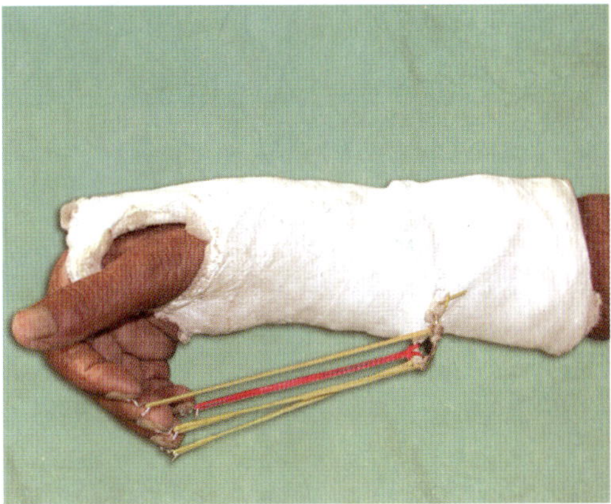

Figure 22.18 Bands for finger stiffness

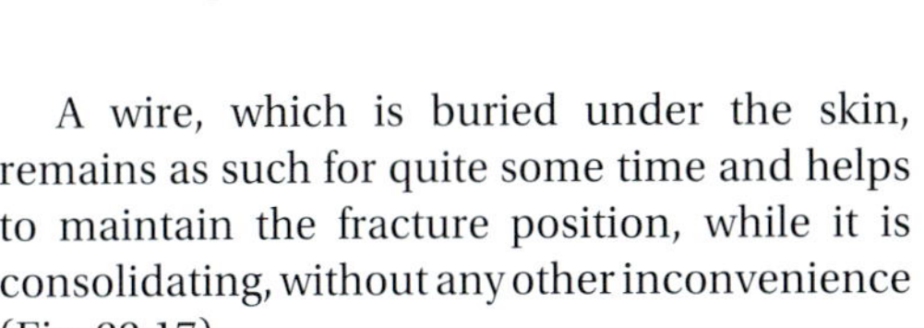

A wire, which is buried under the skin, remains as such for quite some time and helps to maintain the fracture position, while it is consolidating, without any other inconvenience (Fig. 22.17).

Case 14

After a Colles' fracture, during the healing period, one may come across a case, developing finger stiffness, prior to removal of the cast. The stiffness may be resistant to recovery. In such a situation, attaching metal hooks on the nails with an adhesive (or threading a silk thread through the nail tips is another alternative) and anchoring to a band on the cast is quite effective. While at rest, due to the tension of the elastic bands, progressive finger flexion is achieved.

The bands are removed intermittently and finger extension exercises are done (Fig. 22.18).

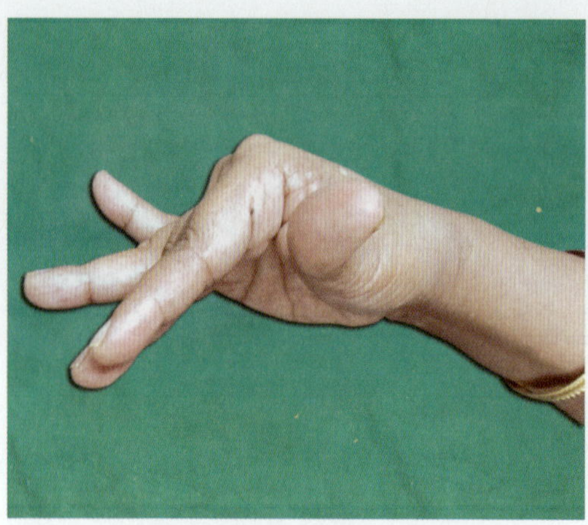

Figure 22.19 Attrition rupture

Case 15

Attrition rupture of tendon of extensor pollicis longus is known since long time. A case of Colles' fracture was treated with cross K-wires with good clinical and radiological result.

At the end of fifteen months after the fracture union, the lady presented with inability to fully extend the index and the middle fingers. Till a few weeks ago, she had full active range of motion of all fingers. This indicates the tendons are not likely to be impaled by the K-wire inserted from the dorso-ulnar side. The attrition may have occurred, due to friction of tendons over the wire tip or may be on the fracture edge, as is described in the past (Fig. 22.19).

CHAPTER

23

Comminuted Fracture of Lower Radius

COMMINUTED FRACTURE OF LOWER END OF RADIUS

A comminuted fracture of lower end of the radius may have fragments on either the palmar or the dorsal side or both the sides.

Why anterior plate?

Anteriorly

- The approach is little easy. The anterior surface of the lower radius has a flat surface, unlike the dorsal surface, which has grooves and tuberosities for the tendons.
- The area is deep to pronator quadratus muscle. The muscle lies well over the plate, while dorsally, the tendons have to slide over the plate.
  Thus there is good soft tissue cover over the plate and the plate is not palpable after the fracture unites.

Anterior locking plate would offer a good stability. However, the plate may not be able to hold the dorsal fragments. Hence, it is necessary to fix both the dorsal radius and ulna fragments with K wires.

Steps

- Examination under 'C' arm and closed reduction was done.
- 1.6 mm K-wires were passed from the radial styloid and the dorsal ulnar fragments across the shaft of radius.
- Anteriorly a buttress plate, preferably a locking plate, was planned. This makes the construct a stable one and late displacement of the fragments is forestalled.
- As a first step, a nonlocking screw was passed through the oval hole of the plate and a drill sleeve was attached to the transverse distal screw hole and one assessed the direction in which the screw tip would go and if it will be well-contained in the bone, not penetrating the articular surface. This helps us to confirm the position of the plate and if needs some adjustment, to move proximally or distally.
- Now, the fixation is completed by inserting the other screws. The obliquely inserted K wires do add to the fracture stability and were kept as such. An above elbow cast completed the procedure.

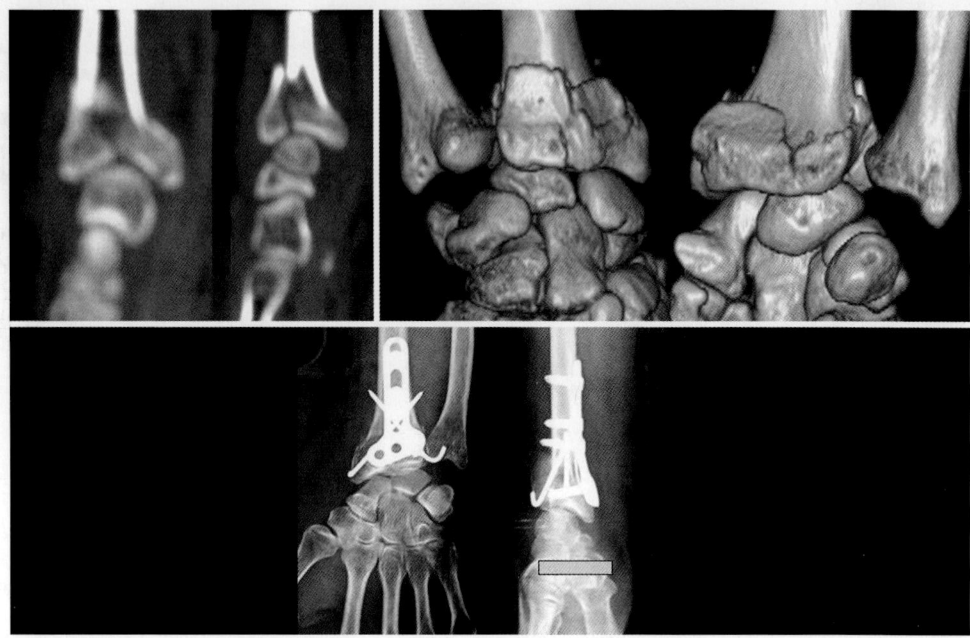

Figure 23.1 Comminuted fracture lower-end radius

- *Observations*: In spite of correct contouring of the plate against the bone, at times, one needs to take the first nonlocking screw 2 mm longer, to have a good purchase on the far (dorsal) cortex. This is done through the oval hole, so that some sliding of the plate for fine adjustment is possible.

If the locking plate is not available, a conventional anterior T buttress plate is used. In addition to the buttress plate, the K wires play equally important role in maintaining the reduction achieved (Fig. 23.1).

CHAPTER

24

Fracture of Neck of 5th Metacarpal

Due to a direct impact on the 5th knuckle, the head of the metacarpal tilts anteriorly, resulting in a posterior angulation. In the past, it was recommended that one should reduce such an injury under anesthesia, with MCP joint fully flexed. Then the proximal fragment of the little finger is pushed dorsally, so the deformity is corrected. Often, one could achieve the correction, only to recur the displacement later. Hence, it has been always an endeavor, to find a technique to stabilize this injury (Fig. 24.1).

In earlier days, when a nonoperative method was carried out, the fracture line would persist at the end of six weeks and active mobilization of the hand was delayed. This may lead to some loss of range of motion.

Here is a method, where the K-wire is passed distal to proximally. However, such a placement of wire, often leads to loss of some motion in the MCP joint (Fig. 24.2).

A better method is to pass a K-wire in the proximal to distal direction, which leads to a good and safe outcome (Fig. 24.3).

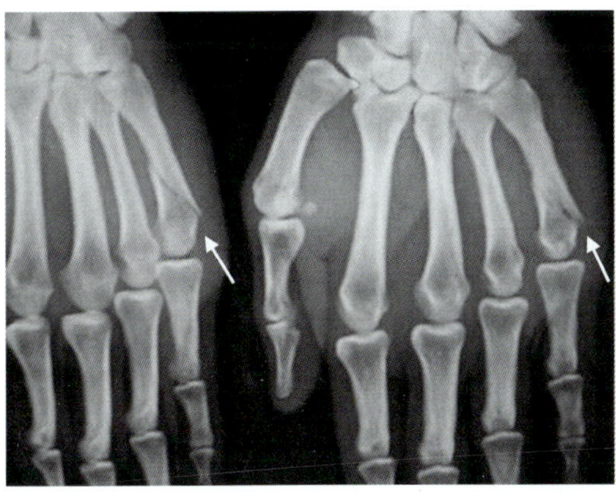

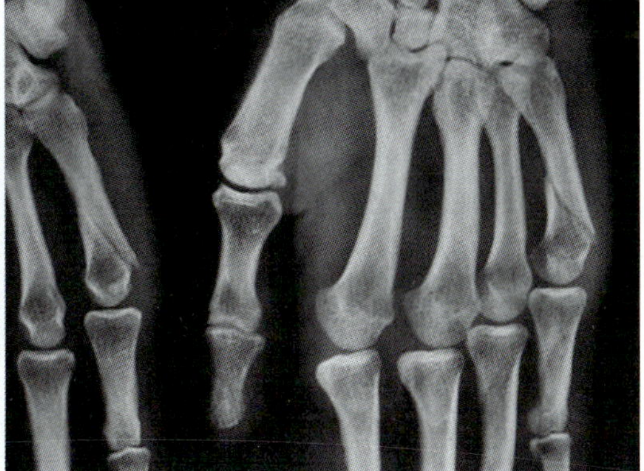

Arrival Non operative method At 6 weeks

Figure 24.1 Non-operative method of fracture of neck of MC5

THE TECHNIQUE

Suitable anesthesia is administered. A tourniquet and a 'C' arm is used. An incision is made dorso-laterally at the base of the 5th metacarpal. Just adjacent to the base, with a cobbler awl, a track is made at right angle to the long axis of the bone. Having pierced the lateral cortex, the awl is withdrawn and reinserted slightly obliquely, along the along axis of the shaft. A 1.2 mm trocar point K-wire is taken and the tip is angulated by 30 degrees, so it slides along the opposite endosteum. The wire is held in a Jacob Chuck with a T handle and by gentle few degrees of rotational movement, is advanced distally. The wire is thin and hence only about 1.5" is kept out of the chuck, to avoid its tendency to bend. As the wire is advanced, one gets a feel of grating, as it slides along the endosteum. The fracture is reduced, checked under the 'C' arm and the wire is further advanced, so the tip is anchored in the subchondral bone.

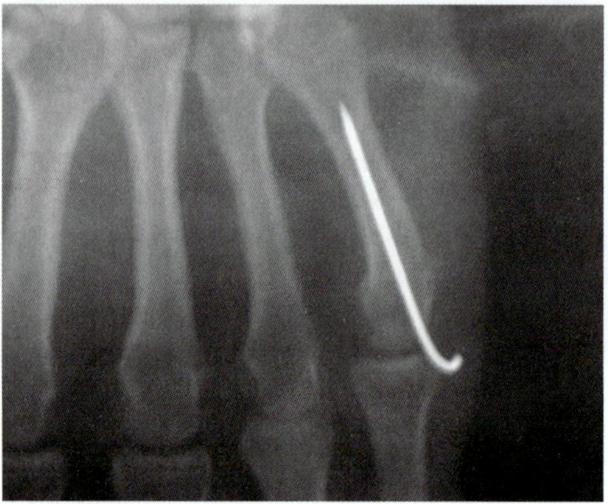

Figure 24.2 Distal to proximal wire

If the medullary cavity diameter permits, one should attempt to pass a second K-wire, for additional stability of the fracture. One should try and rotate the wire after it crosses the mid-shaft, so the tip is directed in another direction, to engage the head of the metacarpal in another sector. This step may not be successful in every case, depending upon the diameter of the medullary cavity.

I prefer to cut off each wire 4 mm outside the lateral cortex, and slightly bend, for easy removal later on. (Similar to treatment given to a K-wire in a Colles' fracture). The tourniquet is deflated.

Some surgeons choose to cut it off close to the bone and leave it as such. I prefer to keep a small segment available, for its removal later on. As in management of Colles' fracture, if the

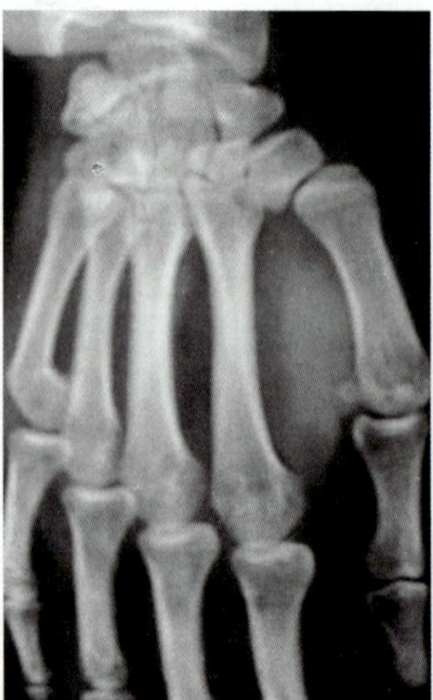

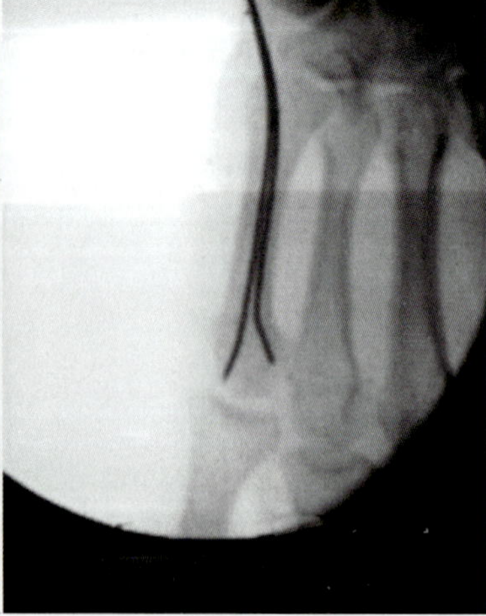

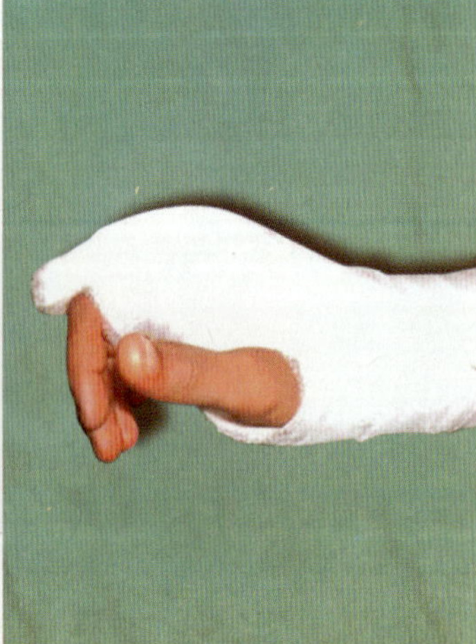

Figure 24.3 Prograde wire fixation

wire end is kept protruding out of the skin, after the immobilization is over, one cannot have bath and the area needs to be dressed all the while, till the wire is removed.

POSTOPERATIVE IMMOBILIZATION

A short anterior cock up POP slab and a dorsal hood slab till the PIP joint, with the MCP joint in 90 degree of flexion—the functional position is applied. The anterior cock up POP slab should be distally till the proximal palmar crease only and not any beyond it. If it is beyond this line, flexion at MCP joint is difficult and the purpose is not served. (The anterior part offers stability to the wrist, while the dorsal hood keeps the MCP joint at 90 degree position). Elevation of the limb is important. It is more important to demonstrate and encourage active flexion and extension of the PIP and the DIP joints, to maintain good hand function at the end of the treatment. If the MCP joint is not maintained at 90 deg flexion, often to regain the MCP flexion is difficult and hence this position is important.

It is worthwhile to practise application of such a plaster support on a volunteer to get a feel of the procedure, so it is carried out efficiently, in an anesthetized person.

CHAPTER

25

Emergency Room Technique

EMERGENCY ROOM CARE

Every injured person should receive a best possible care. Good initial care preserves life and hastens recovery. Aim of this pictorial presentation is to provide knowledge and skill, which would help to build more confidence.

Emergency room care is an important task to be carried out by the hospital staff and the patient as well. The emergency caregivers need to be interested in offering immediate relief to the injured one, as if oneself is in place of the patient. Few simple basic steps often make a vast difference in outcome of a treatment given. Clinical signs, basic care, X-ray positions, technique of first-aid, etc. will help one to understand it. Few cases are presented to make the situation clear and will help to appreciate and understand various presentations. Photographic presentations will make things easy to remember.

Bruise

Following an injury to a bone, the local hematoma takes a specific course, along the tissue planes and is diagnostic of certain injuries. Appearance of a bruise takes about two days to appear, indicating that the injury is at least two days old. It is, therefore, necessary to explain in a fresh case, that such an appearance is expected and need not be a source of anxiety. Failure to inform the patient and the accompanying persons, leads to alarming state in the mind of the patient, who often gives a frantic call to the physician. Having informed this likelihood, increases a confidence in the mind of the patient. Where there is even a slightest pressure of a crepe bandage or a plaster support, the blood does not come to the skin surface, but appears beyond it. Few typical sites of bruise:

- Following a reduction of a Colles' fracture the hematoma tracks, proximal to the cast edge around the elbow or at the base of the thumb.
- In a fracture of neck of the humerus, it tracks along the mid-arm anteriorly. Often in an impacted fracture of neck of humerus, the patient attends the casualty, not for the pain, but because of the frightening bruise on the arm!
- In fracture of the anterior tibial eminence, it tracks towards the anterolateral upper tibia.
- A fracture of head of the radius, due to valgus strain, the medial elbow structures are stretched and a hematoma appears medial to the elbow (Fig. 25.1).

In a case of fracture rib with a small quantity of hemothorax, the blood tracks along the costal margin towards the loin (Fig. 25.2).

On Arrival

In injuries on upper or lower limbs, soon after arrival, all encircling things such as rings, toe rings, ankle bands, bangles, kada, friendship bands MUST be removed. A lady attended my clinic with a below elbow plaster cast had sustained a wrist injury in another city, where a below elbow cast was applied. X-ray was taken through the cast, and to my surprise, a bangle was seen in the cast, which was not removed, prior to cast application (Figs 25.3 and 25.4)!

Hence, whenever, a case with an upper limb injury arrives, immediately all metal or cotton

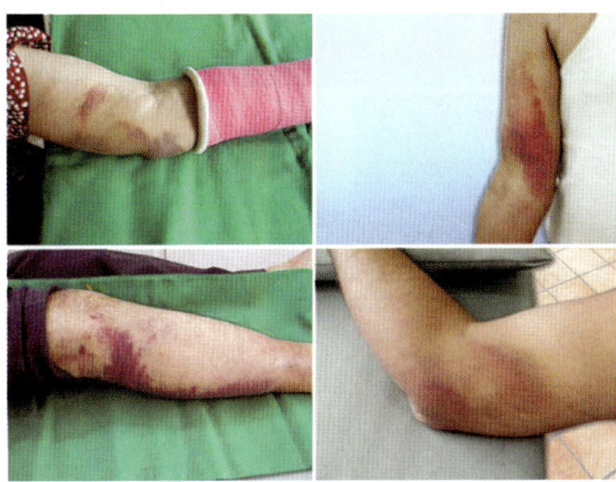

Figure 25.1 Bruise

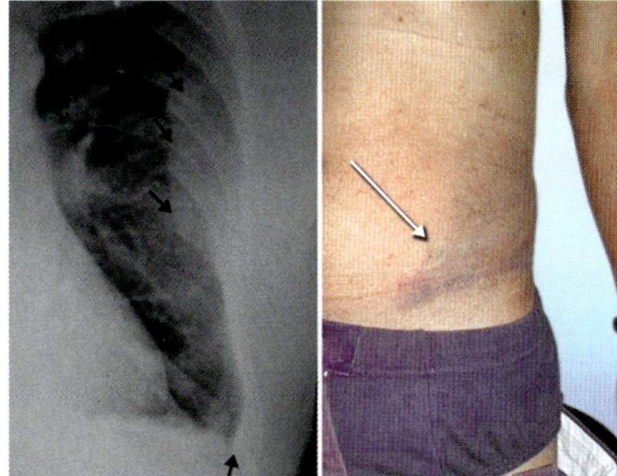

Figure 25.2 Bruise in hemothorax

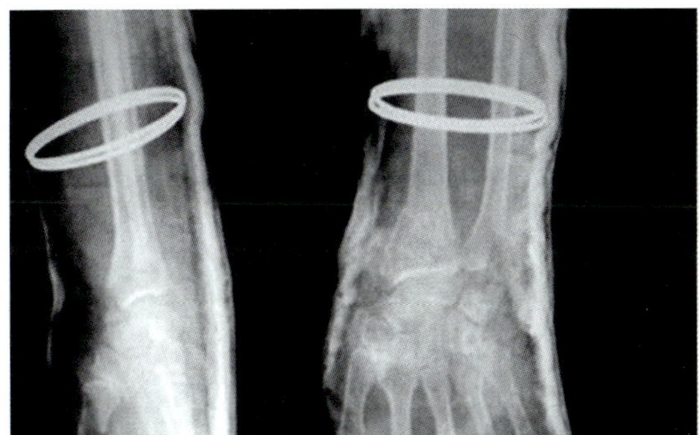

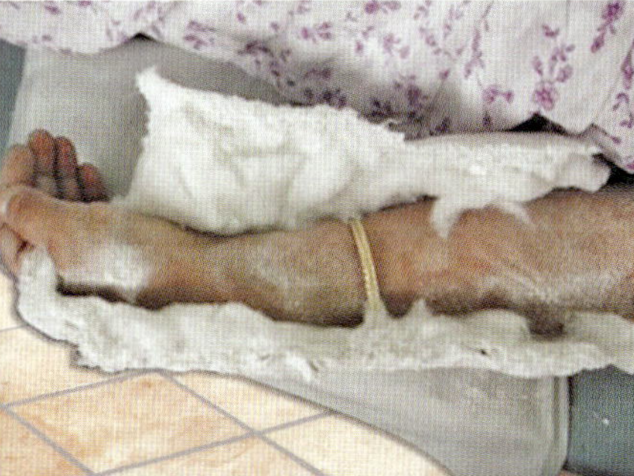

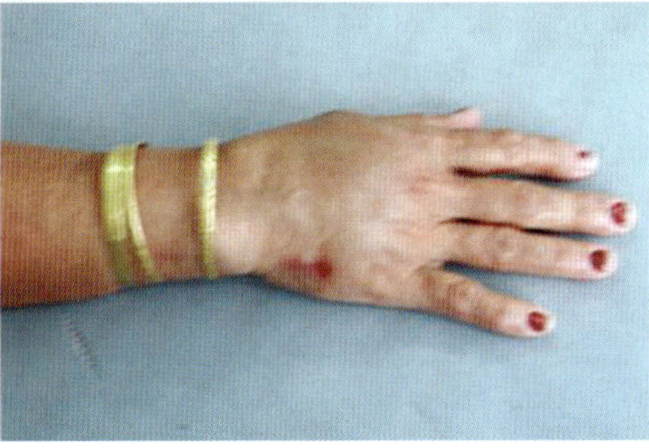

Figure 25.3 Bangle

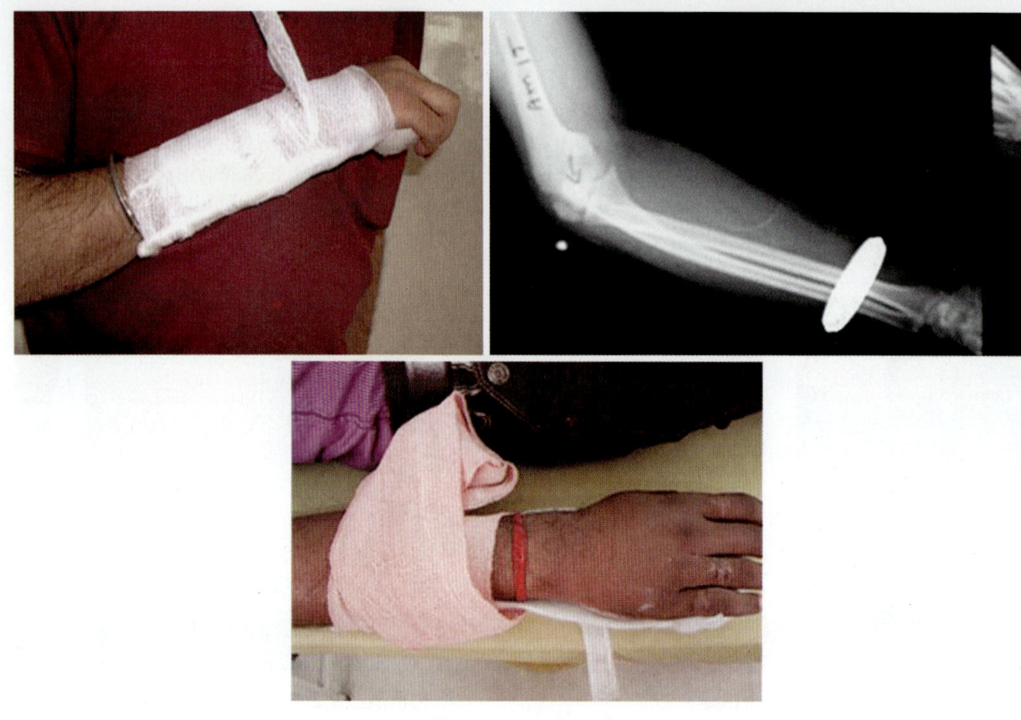

Figure 25.4 Bangle

bands around the limb should be removed. With increasing edema, its removal becomes difficult and the thing needs to be cut. This should be done soon. Various metal cutting tools must be available in ER and need not be sterile (Fig. 25.5).

The X-ray technicians should also be trained to advise to remove rings and bangles, prior to any X-ray procedure. The bone injury may be in one finger and soft tissue injury on the other fingers, still all fingers need to be made free of such things. I happened to see a lady patient, who had an insect bite on a finger, where a ring was on. She did not remove the ring and presented to me. Soon, I cut off the ring and the finger was saved (Fig. 25.6).

Injuries Deep to Skin

Any injury over certain anatomical structure should be taken very seriously. Besides known sites of vessels and nerves, the tendon continuity must be confirmed and documented. Open wounds on hand and foot demand a special attention for any tendon injury. As it is, repair of a tendon injury in any zone, especially in 'No man's zone' is very demanding to manage on day 1 and more so later on (Figs 25.7 and 25.8).

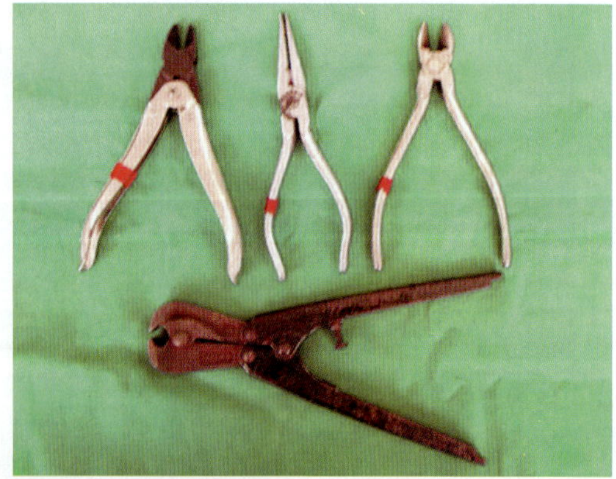

Figure 25.5 Cutting tools

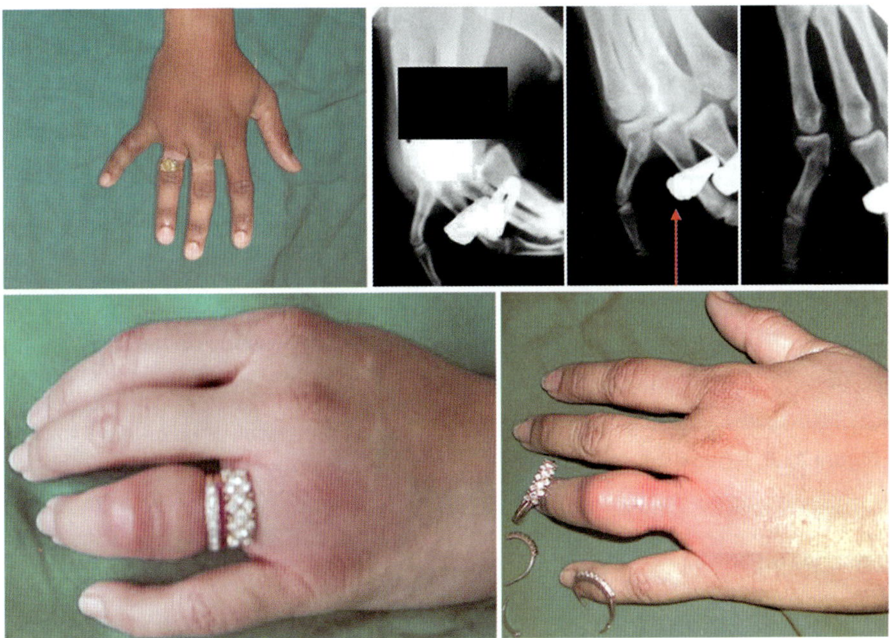

Figure 25.6 Finger rings

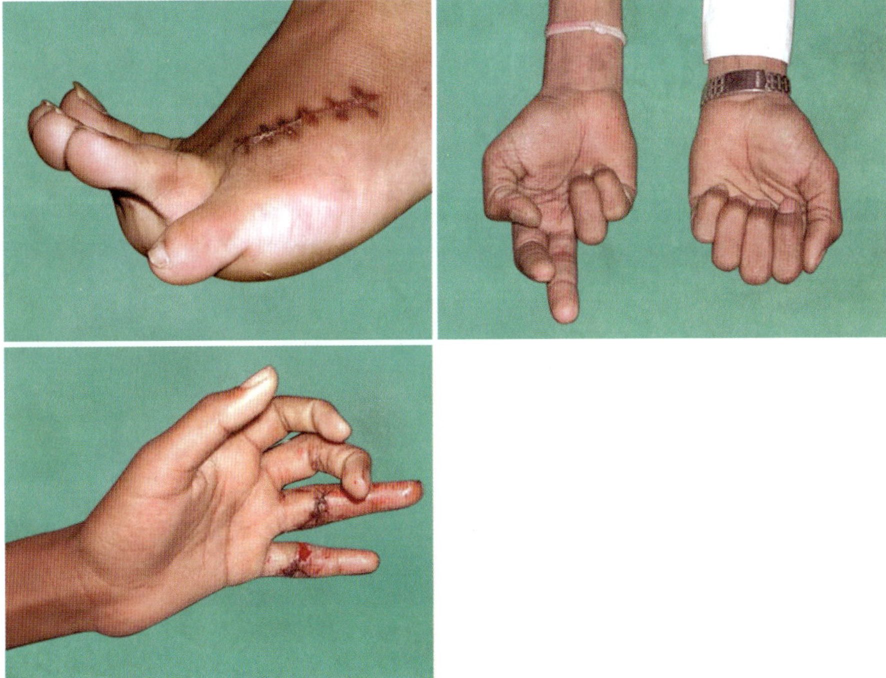

Figure 25.7 Tendon injury at few places

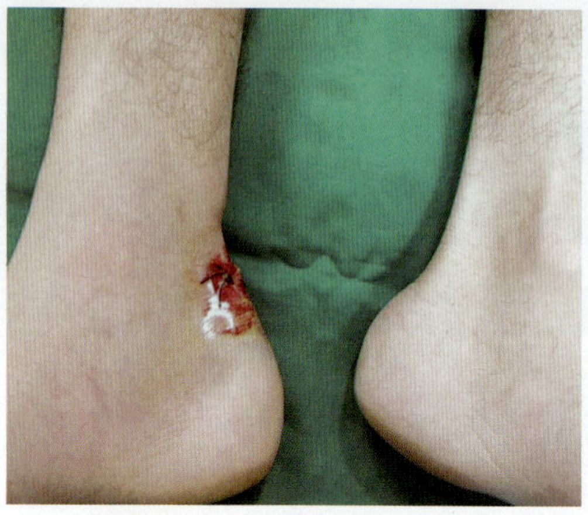

Figure 25.8 Tendo Achilles injury

Dermabrasion

Today, RTA and sports injuries are on increase. A road injury leads to traumatic tattoo of the skin, with deep penetration of dust. Unless immediate care is taken, permanent dark pigmentation is the result. Hence, it is necessary to explain to the patient and family members the need of immediate care to prevent this and must be done on day 1 for optimal result. Under suitable anesthesia, good wound cleaning and dermabrasion should be done, very meticulously. Training by a plastic surgeon will go a long way. Though, it may appear that cost of such a procedure in relation to size of the wound, is rather more, I feel, in the long run, it

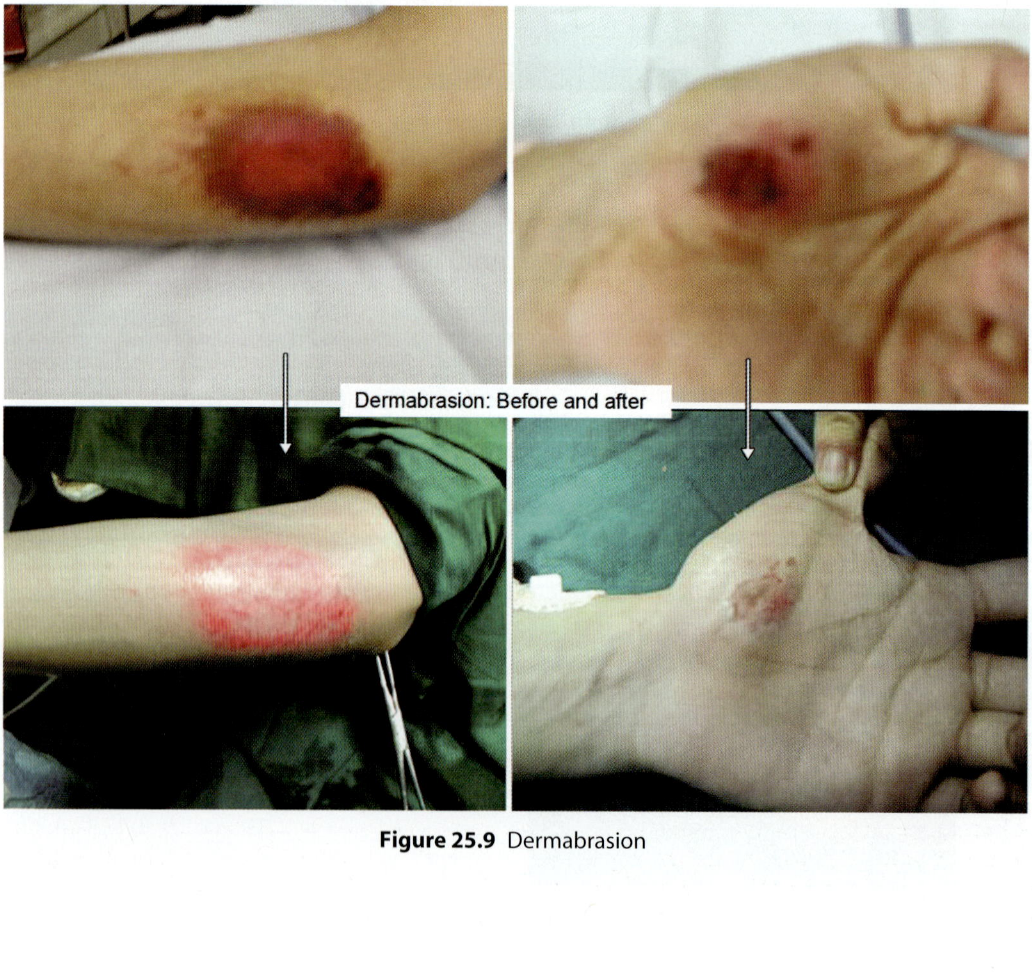

Dermabrasion: Before and after

Figure 25.9 Dermabrasion

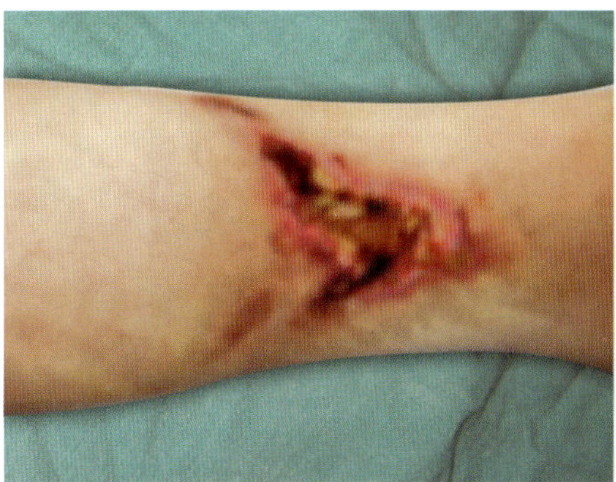
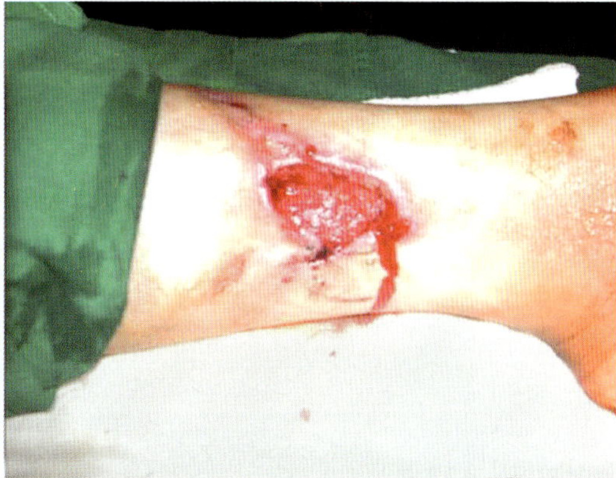

Figure 25.10 Deep eschar excision

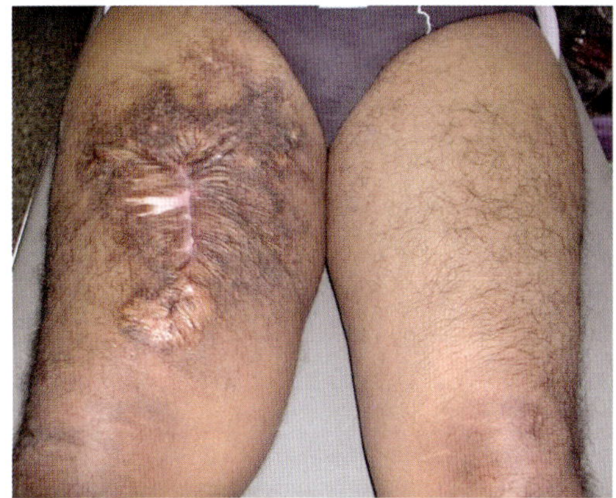

Figure 25.11 Cicatrix formation

is necessary to do this procedure, for cosmetic reasons. Once the initial critical period is over, the result is not satisfying (Fig. 25.9).

Deep Eschar

Due to severe crushing of a skin, without a sharp injury, local skin necrosis is often seen. On arrival, it is difficult for the clinician to assess the depth (as in depth of injury in a case of burns). In a few days, the picture becomes clear. Continued dressing alone, usually leads to an unacceptable scar formation. Such an injury needs to be attended by a plastic surgeon, to excise the eschar and carry out appropriate skin cover procedure (Figs 25.10 and 25.11).

Often abrasions have associated contusion around. Hence thorough cleaning and application of a nonadhesive dressing with padded support will make the person comfortable and the wound heals kindly. In any contusion or open injury, limb elevation and active exercise of fingers/toes is mandatory (Fig. 25.12).

First Aid and Splint Application

In a limb injury, a padded Cramer wire splint is very useful. It offers good immobilization, the length can be adjusted and yet permits X-ray examination through it, to plan further treatment (Fig. 25.13).

Splint and Padding

In a fresh injury, one should expect the swelling to increase with time. Hence, it is very much necessary to add adequate padding, under the splint and then encircle it with just enough pressure. Time and again, one sees, cases coming, well-splinted, but without any padding. This often leads to crippling Volkmann contracture, indeed an avoidable thing (Fig. 25.14).

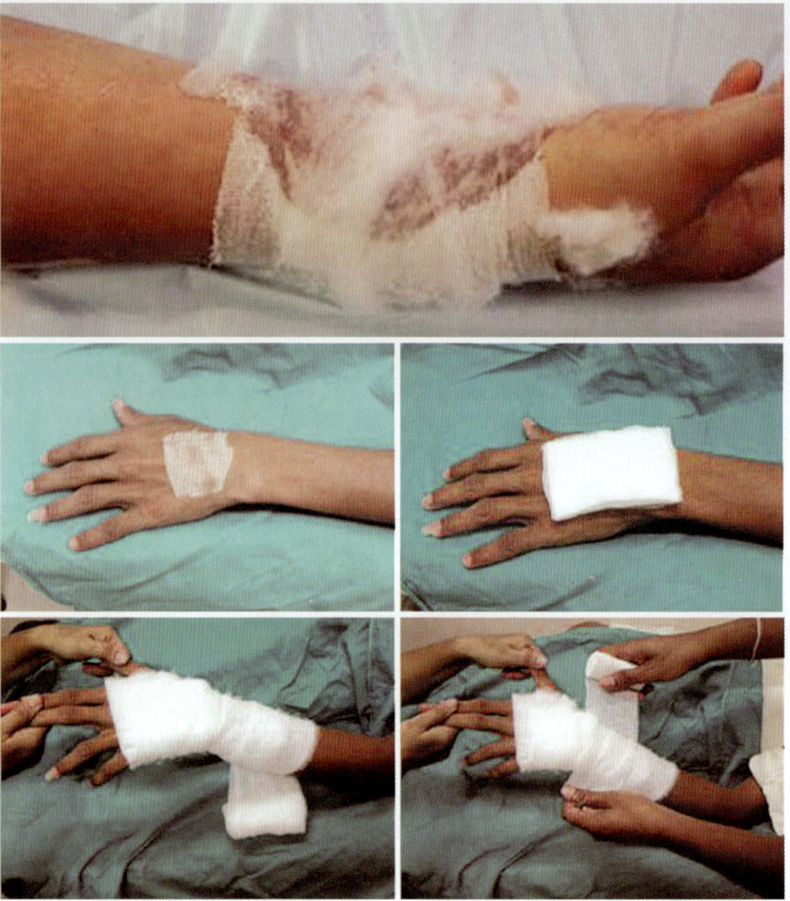

Figure 25.12 Abrasion dressing

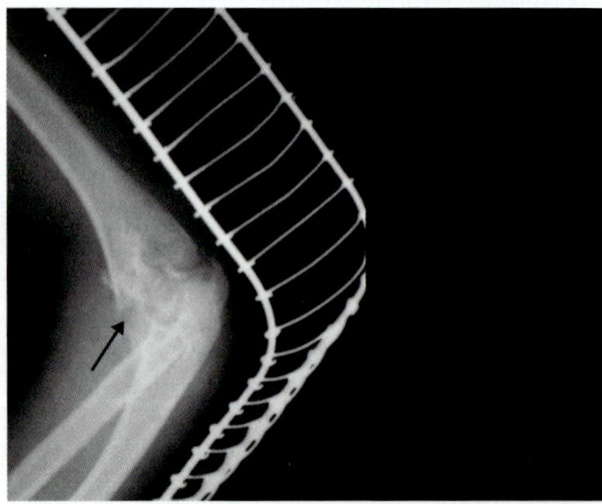

Figure 25.13 Cramer wire splint

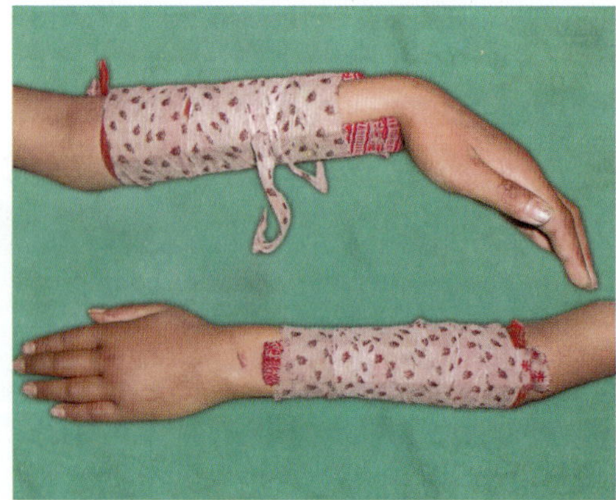

Figure 25.14 Volkmann contracture

Patient Positioning for an X-Ray Examination

- If on clinical grounds, one suspects a fracture, one should take every effort to prove or disprove this. This is very much necessary for an orthopedic resident to learn and understand. Attending the X-ray room in person, to learn the X-ray positioning will go a long way.
- Even after every effort taken, if a fracture is not visible, still, one should assume it to be a bone injury and manage accordingly. This is especially true in a fracture of carpal scaphoid, rib, spine, metatarsal and hip. A few fractures are known to be visible on a film later on. Today, with availability of MRI and CT scan, it is possible to come to an early conclusion. An honest dialogue with the patient and family members will alleviate later problems.
- X-ray of opposite limb, in injuries in children, for comparison has adequately proved this, more in epiphyseal injuries.
- A greenstick bow fracture in forearm, unless diagnosed and treated adequately, leads to restricted prono-supination in later life, which is indeed an unfortunate outcome.
- Whiplash injury to cervical spine needs to be taken very seriously, for obvious reasons.
- Associated injury of organs in various cavities needs a special attention. Availability of USG and CT examination today, has made things rather safe today.

Usually in a suspected fracture of clavicle, AP view is adequate. However, if a fracture is not visible, a tangential view may make it visible (Fig. 25.15).

After a fall, a child's reluctance to touch the foot to the ground is suggestive of an undisplaced fracture of tibia. (Having diagnosed this injury, often it could be quite painful and one may not get necessary cooperation from the child to immobilize the leg. It is justified to do this immobilization under anesthesia) (Fig. 25.16).

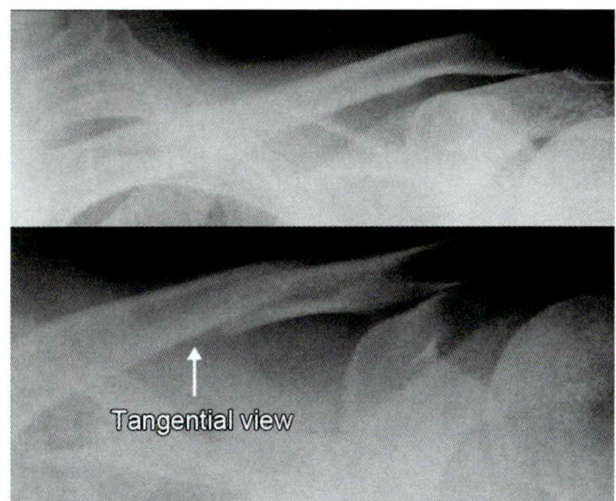

Figure 25.15 Clavicle tangential view

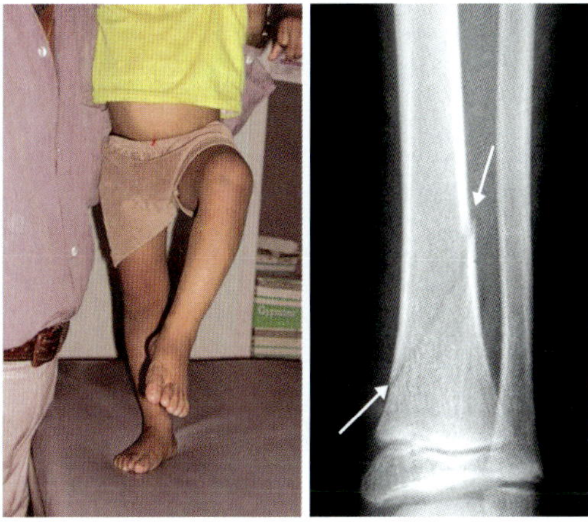

Figure 25.16 Fracture tibia in a child

Injury to the shoulder: X-ray of shoulder must be taken in an anatomical position, i.e. with arm in neutral position. This is easily possible to achieve, if one makes the patient stand with palm facing forwards. Not paying a heed to this prerequisite, usually leads to a missed injury of fracture of the greater tuberosity. In the given example, first X-ray taken in internal rotation does not show a fracture, which the next day, when taken in correct position, reveals it (Fig. 25.17). One should remember the shape of head of humerus in a neutral position and that in internal rotation. (see chapter on Shoulder Dislocation).

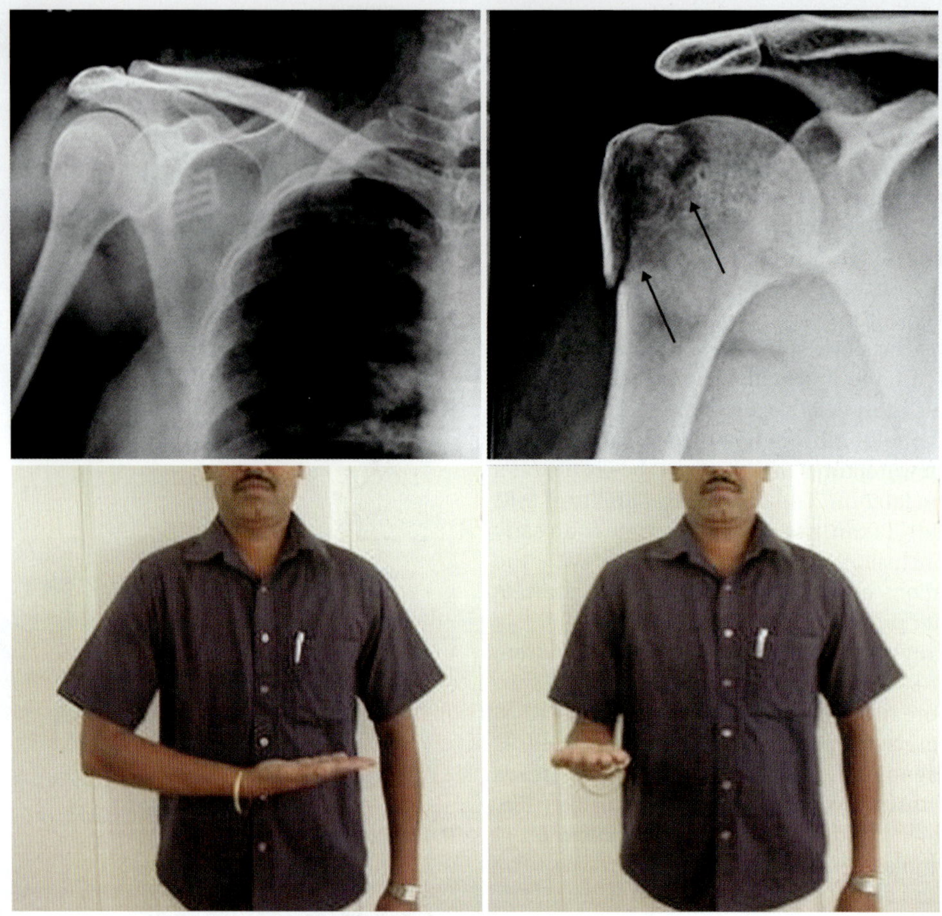

Figure 25.17 Shoulder position for X-ray

Fracture of Ribs

In a suspected fracture of a rib, usually one orders 'X-ray of chest', without mentioning its purpose. X-ray of chest usually means, X-ray for lung parenchyma and is the most common body part, of which X-ray examination is done. It is necessary to specify: 'For ribs'. If the technician does not understand this, ask for X-ray of thoracic spine with the entire chest and one will get a good picture of the chest cage! Often one sees a fracture of the scapula as well, as in the illustration. It is a good practice to mark all the fractures, so during follow up, one can quickly review them all (Fig. 25.18).

In a child injury around elbow needs a special mention, due to the epiphyseal lines and because the epiphyseal centers may not have appeared. Monteggia injury with a green stick fracture of the ulna is often missed. Management in a fresh and an untreated injury is very much different. To mange a missed Monteggia is a pain-taking job and still the outcome is much inferior to that in a well-diagnosed and managed fresh injury.

It is a good idea to call the patient the next day, to be examined by a senior person, to avoid such a situation. It is a safe practice to call such cases the next day, for a repeat examination and assessment (Fig. 25.19).

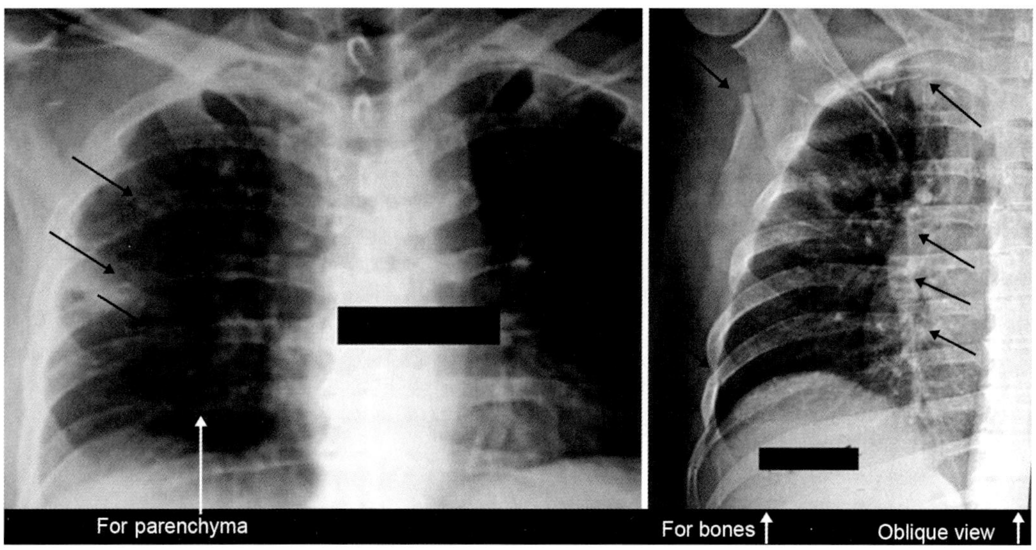

Figure 25.18 Ribs X-ray technique

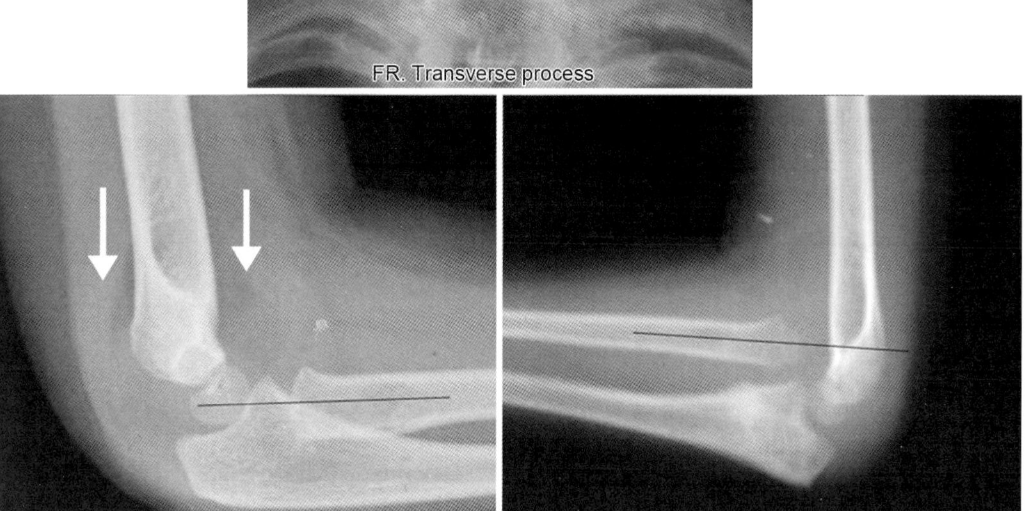

Figure 25.19 Elbow X-ray in a child

Injury to the tibial eminence is often unclear on a plain X-ray and an MRI makes the things clear. This is also true in a cruciate ligament injury (Fig. 25.20).

After a major accident, a patient reports with the back pain and may be able to stand and walk with some support. An X-ray of lumbar spine is taken on arrival. Due to presence of gas shadows, the transverse processes are not well-visualized and injuries are often than not missed. The pain in back is indeed quite severe. Hence, it is recommended to admit the patient and repeat the X-ray. To one's surprise, 3 to 4 transverse processes may be found to be fractured. The patient needs careful indoor management for pain relief. A CT scan with 3 D reconstruction of the spine and rib cage may show the extensive injuries (Figs 25.21 and 25.22).

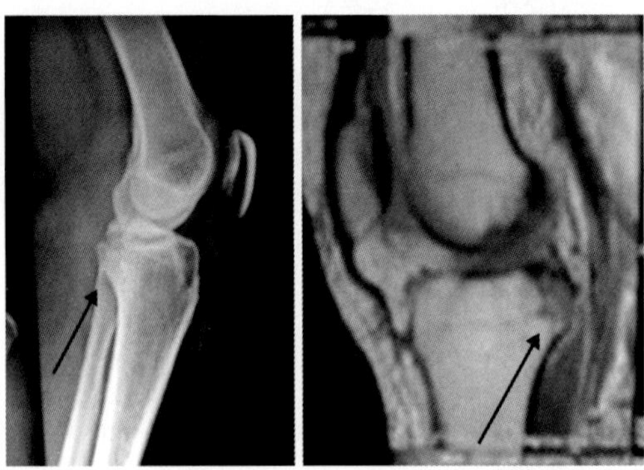

Figure 25.20 Utility of MRI

Knee is a hinge joint and stability in a coronal plane is maintained by collateral ligaments. Medial collateral injury is clinically suspected by varus and valgus stress test and this is confirmed by stress AP views (Fig. 25.23).

In a metacarpal injury, with an oblique or a spiral fracture, there is shortening of the bone. Clinically, it is possible to suspect this by a painful grip, local bony tenderness. In addition to these signs, receding head of the metacarpal is highly suggestive of shortening of the bone, due to a fracture (Fig. 25.24).

Plaster Application

- Application of a plaster slab/cast, for a wrist injury is a commonly done procedure. It is important to keep the distal extent of the support till the proximal palmar crease only and then only, it permits good flexion at the MCP joint. If the plaster edge is beyond this, it needs to be trimmed or else finger stiffness is likely. (However, in a metacarpal fracture treated non-operatively, one needs to extend the edge till little short of the web space).
- Having given a below elbow plaster, a sling is applied for the first 2 to 3 days and be such that the elbow is flexed to 120 degrees, so that the swelling reduces by gravity (Fig. 25.25).

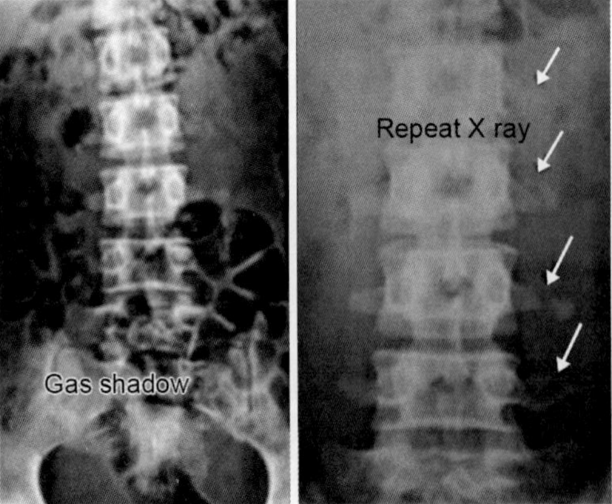

Figure 25.21 Repeat X-ray of spine

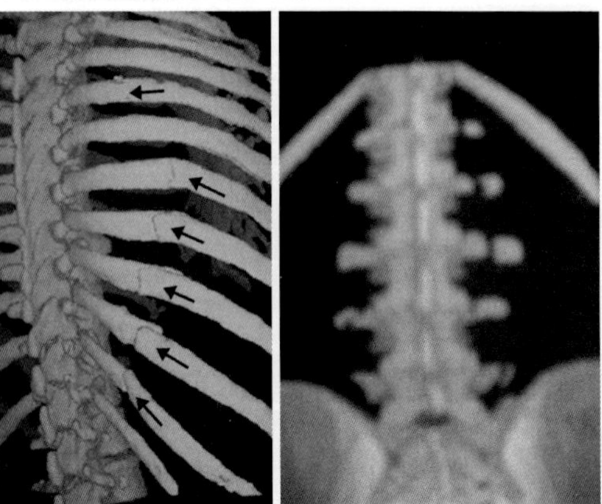

Figure 25.22 CT with 3D reconstruction

- A wrist plaster support should be in 20 degrees either palmar or dorsiflexion. If it is more than that, it is uncomfortable. One cannot do finger exercises well and return of wrist function is delayed (Fig. 25.26).
- Prior to application of a plaster cast (complete POP bandage all around), there should be no form of encircling bandage within. This is important, because should limb swelling occur, the circumferential bandage cannot

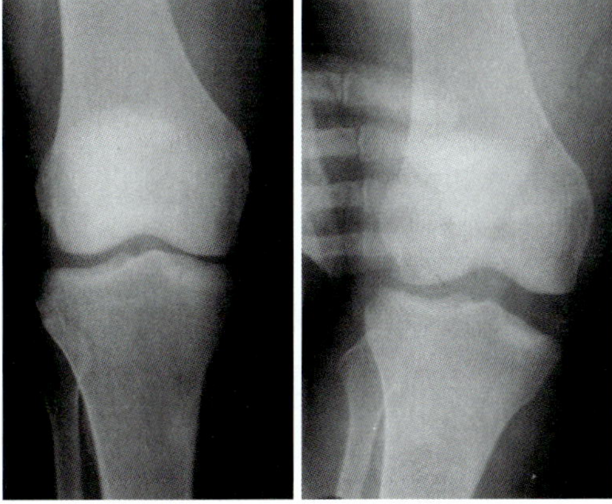

Figure 25.23 Stress view in a knee

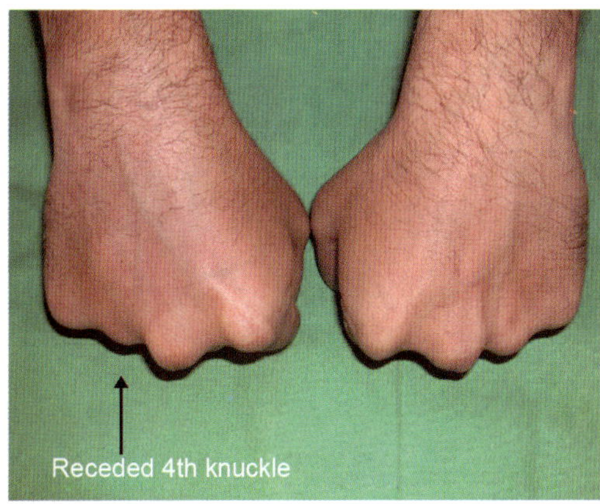

Figure 25.24 Knuckle receded

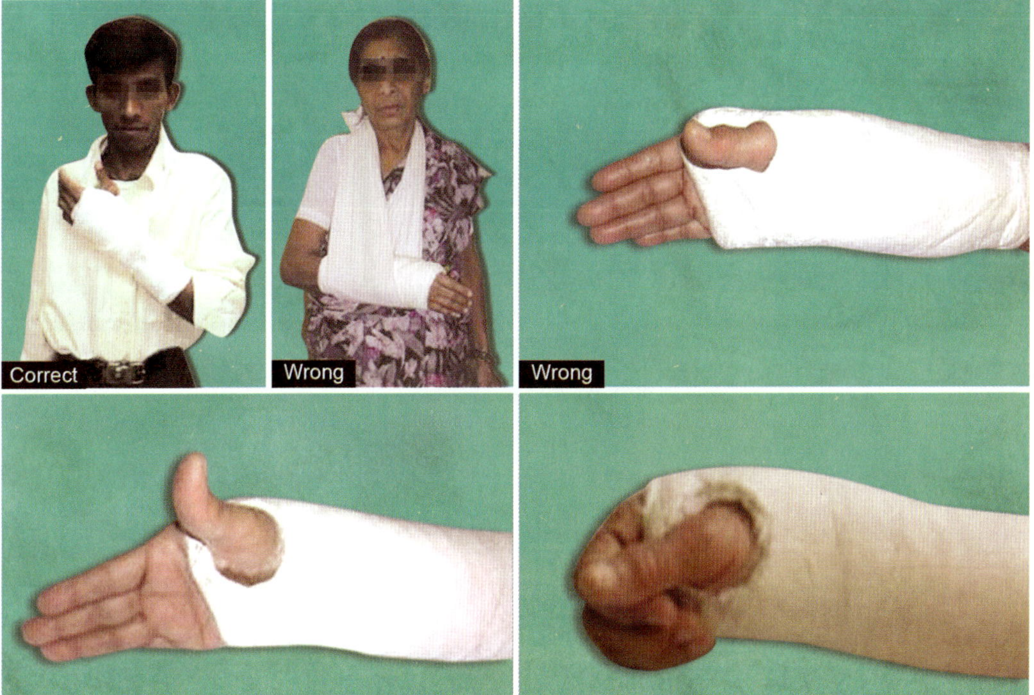

Figure 25.25 Plaster extent

expand and there is a danger of limb ischemia. As is seen in examples, in a few cases it was found to have circumferential bandage and a crepe bandage within a cast, which is dangerous. A joint should be held in a position of final immobilization. In the example, possibly the elbow was held at 70 degrees of flexion and after the cast was applied, the limb was later flexed to 90 degrees, which is known to constrict anterior elbow structures. I have seen a median nerve palsy occurring in such a situation (Fig. 25.27).

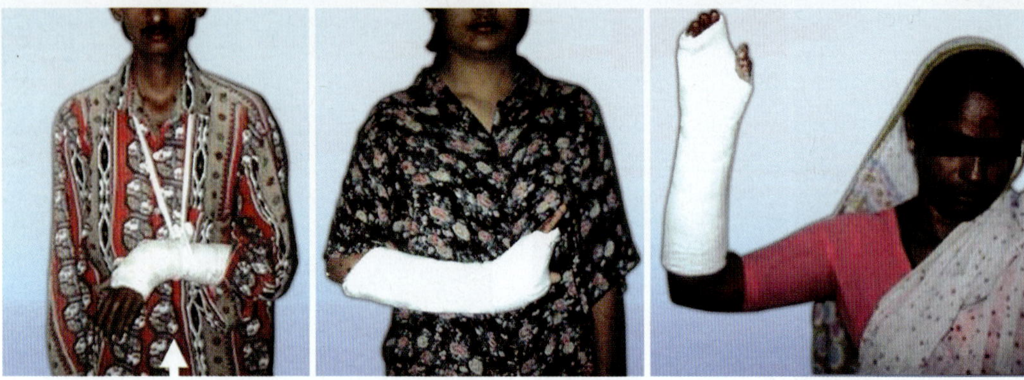

Figure 25.26 Wrist position

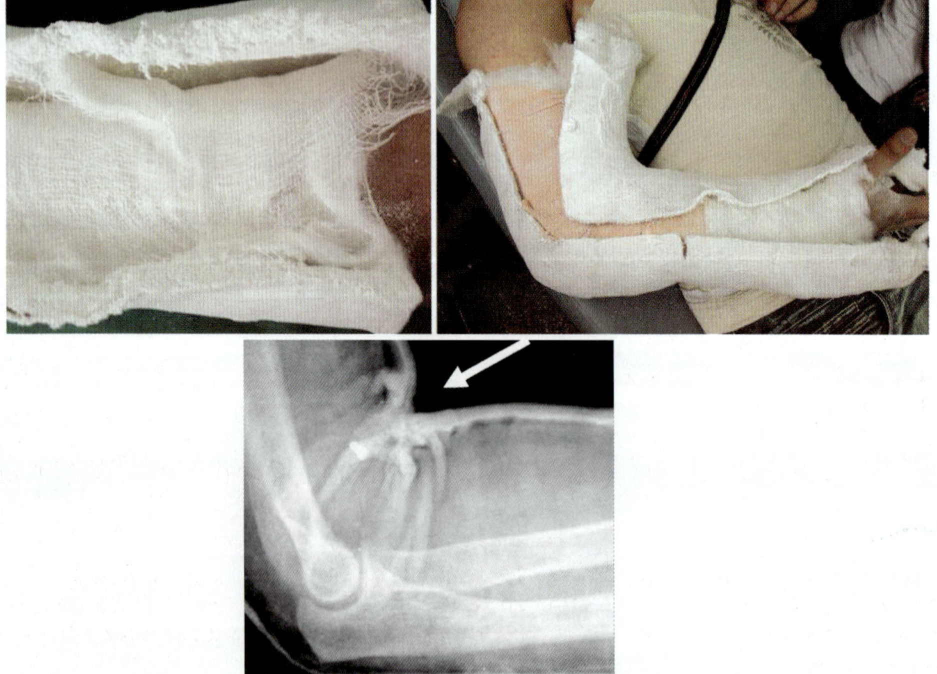

Figure 25.27 No encircling bandage within

Facial Wounds

Wounds especially on a face need a special attention. It is worthwhile to take help of a reconstruction/plastic surgeon on day 1, soon after arrival of the case, to plan a definitive line of action. Good assessment of the wound and possible skin loss, is done and he can accordingly carry out the procedure and offer a best possible outcome. On arrival, wound cleaning and is covered by a tulle gras, till a definitive plan is done. The relative should be explained the philosophy of waiting till the plastic surgeon arrives and that a delay by an hour for wound suture will not change the outcome, but rather contrary to it. (Patient and relatives expect immediate wound suturing, rather than good lavage and sterile cover, till a final plan is done).

Here is an example, with soft tissue crushing and may have had tissue loss from the right upper eyelid. Perhaps, if necessary, care was exercised on day 1, secondary surgery to reconstruct the eyelid could have been avoided (Fig. 25.28).

- Subconjunctival hemorrhage indicates injury to a bone forming the orbit.
- Bilateral subconjunctival hemorrhage and bruise on either side of the root of the nose in absence of an open wound locally, indicates fracture of the anterior cranial fossa (as per a dictum, before advent of a CT scan, etc.)
- Subconjunctival hemorrhage, edema and hematoma of inferior eyelid/lateral hematoma on the cheek and perhaps drooping of the eye-ball, indicates fracture of the floor of the orbit, usually that of zygoma. Today, besides various X-ray positioning, CT scan and 3D reconstruction of the skull, show the fracture anatomy very clear, so treatment can be planned (Fig. 25.29).

Subungual Hematoma

Subungual hematoma in a thumb is a common injury. It is quite painful and needs to be evacuated at the earliest. This reduces the pain remarkably and maintains nourishment of the nail plate and prevents its loss. Under a ring block anesthesia, with a trocar pointed needle, a small hole can be drilled in the nail and hematoma drains away, offering a good pain relief (Fig. 25.30).

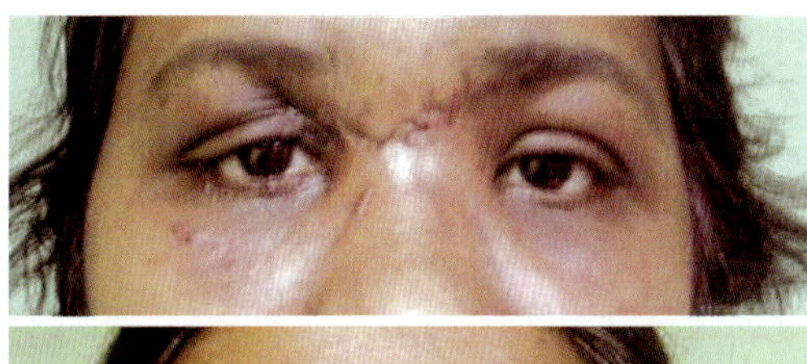

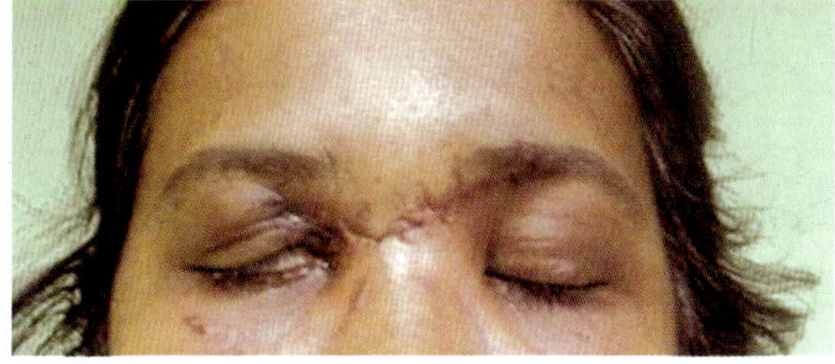

Figure 25.28 Eyelid contracture

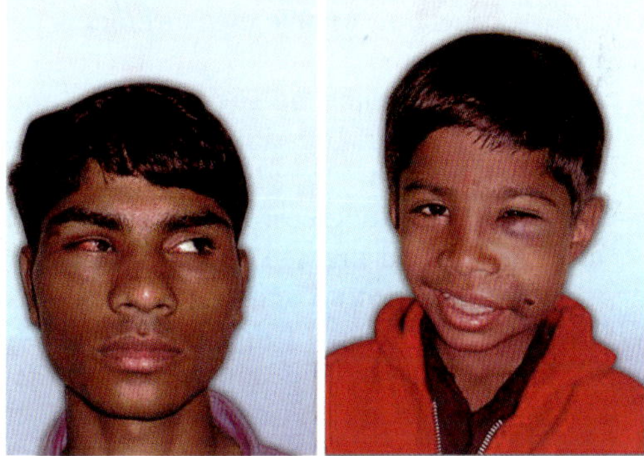

Figure 25.29 Facial bone injury

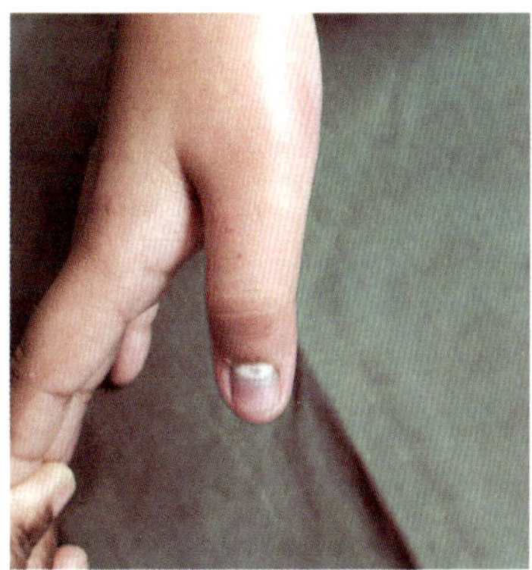

Figure 25.30 Subungual hematoma

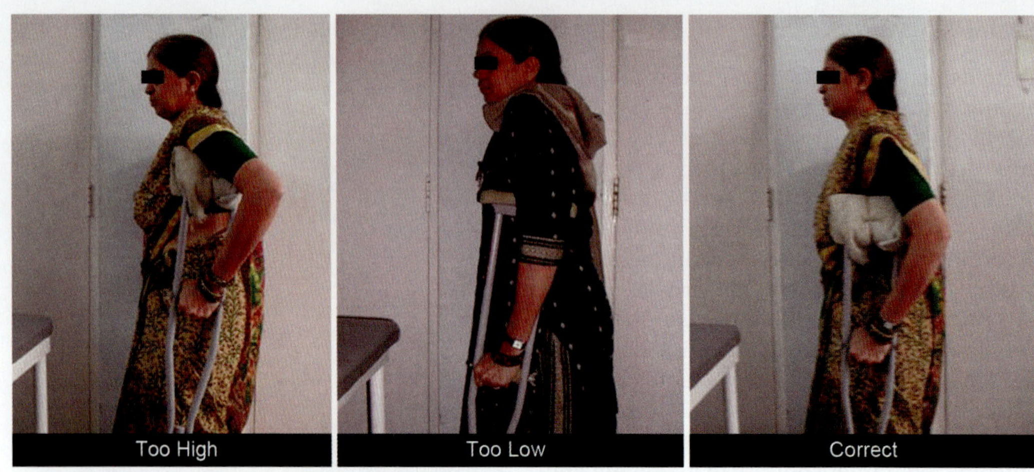

Figure 25.31 Crutch height

Axillary Crutches

One must know how to take measurements for a crutch:

- Height of the crutch be such that, the top should be 3 fingers breadth below the axilla. The hand grip be at such a level that the elbow is flexed 15 to 20 degrees. The upper padded top needs to be pressed against the chest wall by the patient, so that it remains stable. There is a tendency of the first time user, to hang on the padded top and clinician/therapist must explain that the body weight has to be transferred via the hand and not via the axilla. If the total height of the crutch is more, there is a chance of radial nerve palsy. If it is too low, the stability reduces and the person has to bend forwards while walking, which is uncomfortable.
- Same principle is practised when a walker is used. The height should be such that the elbow is flexed to 20 degrees. A walker should have two wheels in front and two rubber shoes on the rear legs. While walking, one lifts the rear walker legs and it propels forward on the wheels and when the rear legs touch the ground, one can safely put weight on the walker and one moves forward, with a stable walker on the floor.

If a walker has wheels on all four legs, it tends to move, when full body weight is put on it, while a walker with all four rubber shoes, needs to be physically lifted at each step, which is inconvinient (Fig. 25.31).

Section II

Lower Extremity and Pelvis

CHAPTER

26

Pelvis and Acetabulum Fractures

In the mid 70s the new classification of fractures came in practice. The difference in the mechanism of injury, classification and principles of management became clear. In the first part, fractures of the pelvis are described and in the second part, that of acetabulum are described. The presentation does not cover every type of injury. The injuries, seen in this geographical area, are described.

Case 1

A person was caught between a vehicle and a wall. Had pain in the lower torso and inability to stand and walk. X-ray of the lumbar spine was taken. A clinician or a radiologist is likely to miss an injury to the transverse processes, so also in the pelvis ring. Some undisplaced fractures or avulsion injuries are likely to be missed. This is because the gas shadows on a day 1 X-ray film obscure the fractures. Hence, it is important and necessary to suspect such an injury and a CT scan with 3D reconstruction should be done. Quite often, one may observe associated injuries in a CT scan with 3D reconstruction, which are not visible or clearly defined in a plain radiograph.

A CT scan in such a case helps to diagnose, plan necessary treatment, predict time required for indoor stay and time taken for recovery. In addition, this investigation is helpful for the purpose of documentation also.

As is teaching, the patient needs to be examined from head to foot. If he has come walking to the casualty department, the gait and spine movements should be noted, before, he is made to lie on examination table. Often, during subsequent examination, few other injuries are also noted, as was a fracture of fibula in a case (Figs 26.1A to C).

Case 2

In a RTA, a young man suffered multiple injuries:

Open book injury:
- Diastasis of symphysis pubis
- Fracture of sacral alae
- Intracapsular fracture of neck of femur on the right side

There was no urinary track injury.

The patient was treated elsewhere and correctly so, by application of an external fixator to stabilize the pelvis and then was transferred to the current hospital, with a Foley catheter in place.

He was assessed and internal fixation of other injuries was planned.

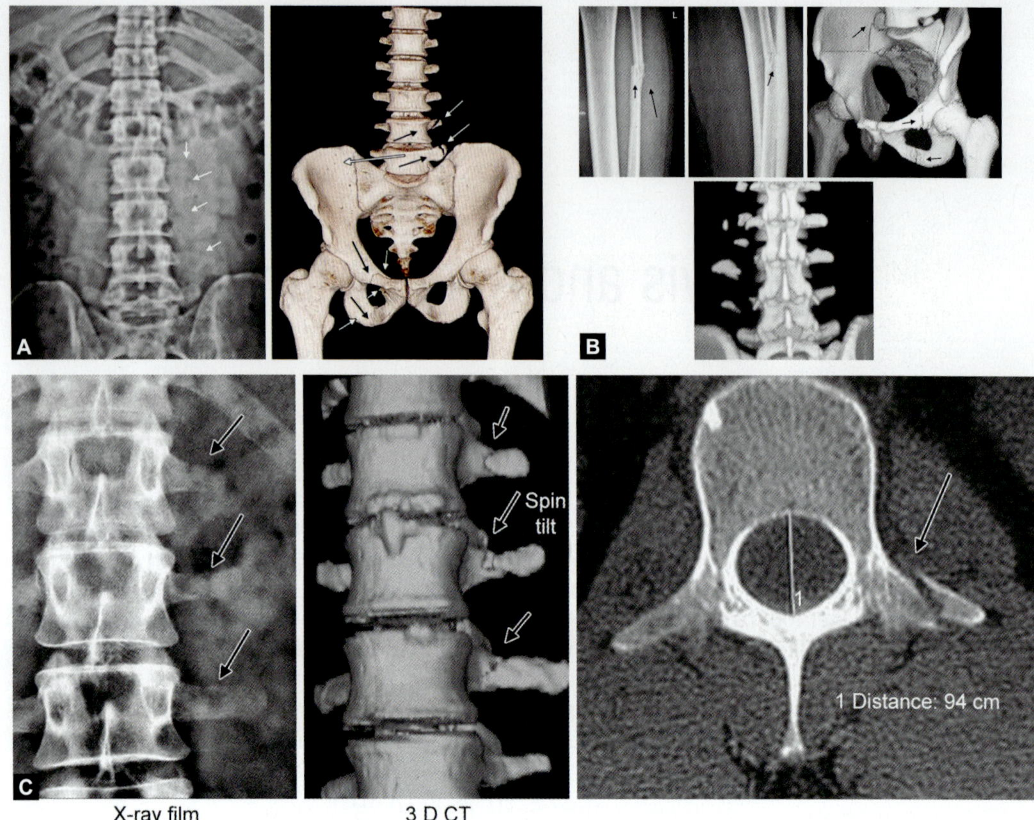

Figures 26.1A to C Importance of CT scan

He was taken on a fracture table. The neck of femur was fixed with a mini SP nail and a plate. 6.5 mm screw and an AM pin were added to it. After wound closure over a drain, the diastasis of pubic symphysis was reduced and fixed, with two plates, one on the superior and the other on the anterior surface. Application of one plate and a tension band figure of 8 loop on the other surface also offers good stability. The external fixator was continued. However, for the posterior injury in the sacrum and the SI joints, rest in bed was continued for the necessary duration. The pelvic ring injuries became pain free. At the end of the three months, the neck of femur fracture line was persistent. Hence, the AM pin and the 6.5 mm screw were removed and a fibula graft was inserted in the neck of femur across the fracture. In few weeks, the neck of femur consolidated well (Figs 26.2A and B).

Case 3

A lady in late twenties, under treatment for rheumatoid disease, had RTA while driving a scooter. She sustained fracture of the right ilium. The ilium was stabilized with few plates across the fracture lines to stabilize them (Fig. 26.3).

Case 4

A person in 50s had RTA and sustained fracture of the left ilium. To treat it non-operatively means rest in bed for 4 to 6 weeks at least. He accepted internal fixation, so that, he could be ambulated earlier (Fig. 26.4).

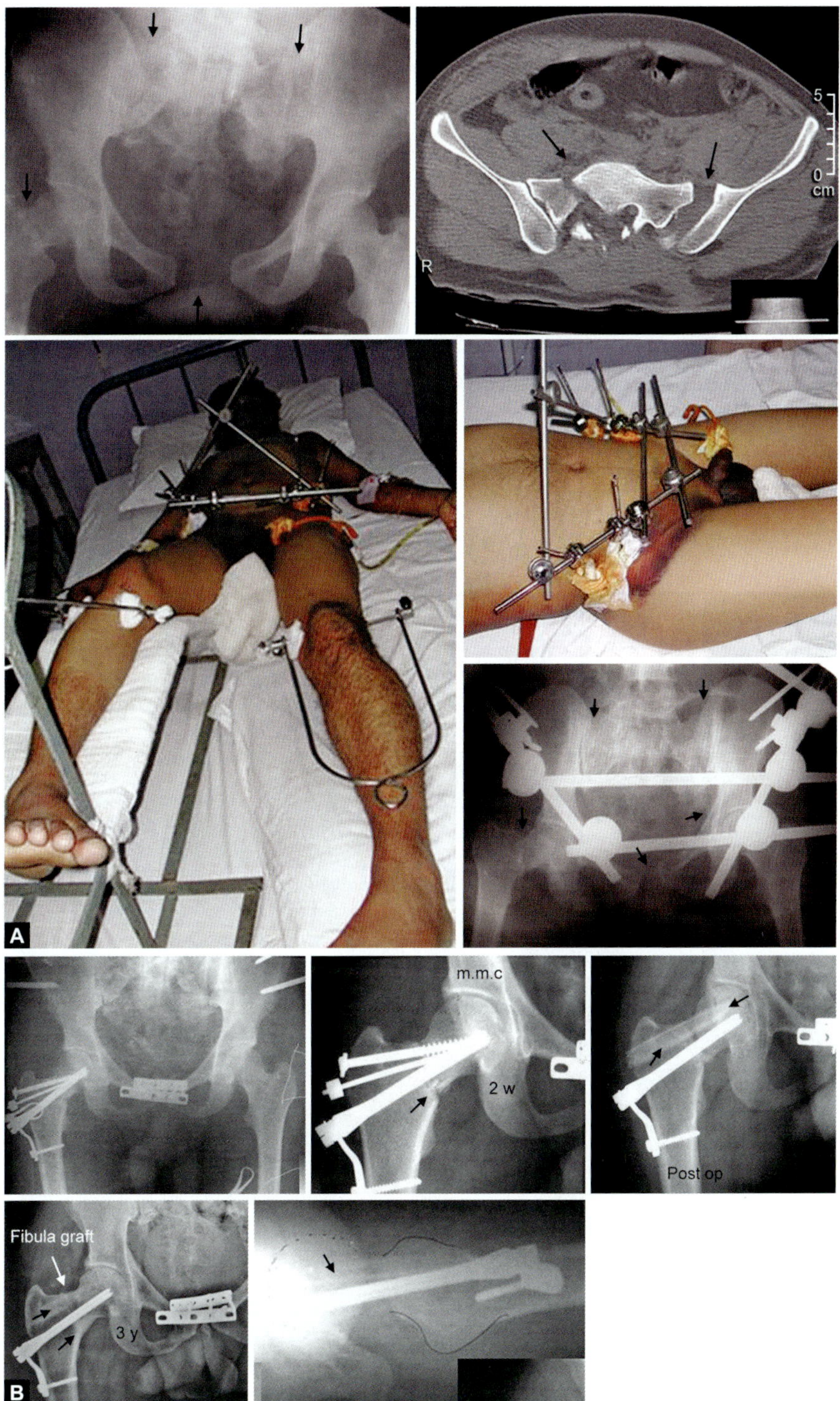

Figures 26.2A and B (A) Pelvis ex fix I; (B) Pelvis ex fix II

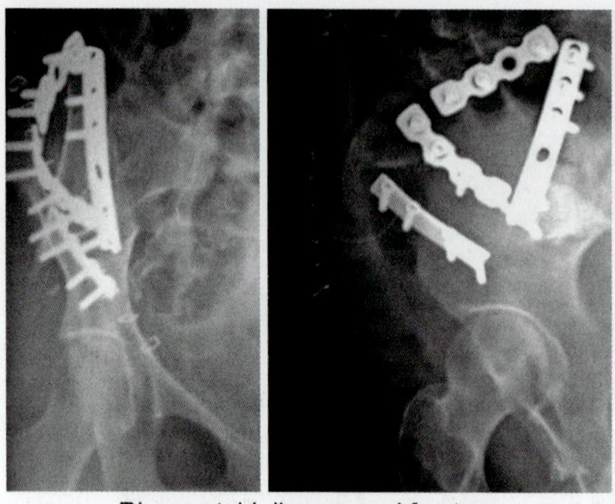

Figure 26.3 Fracture of ilium in rheumatoid arthritis

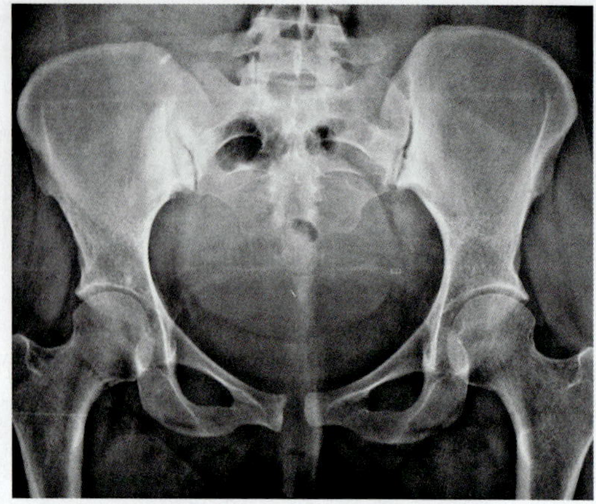

Figure 26.5 Post-partum diastasis symphysis pubis

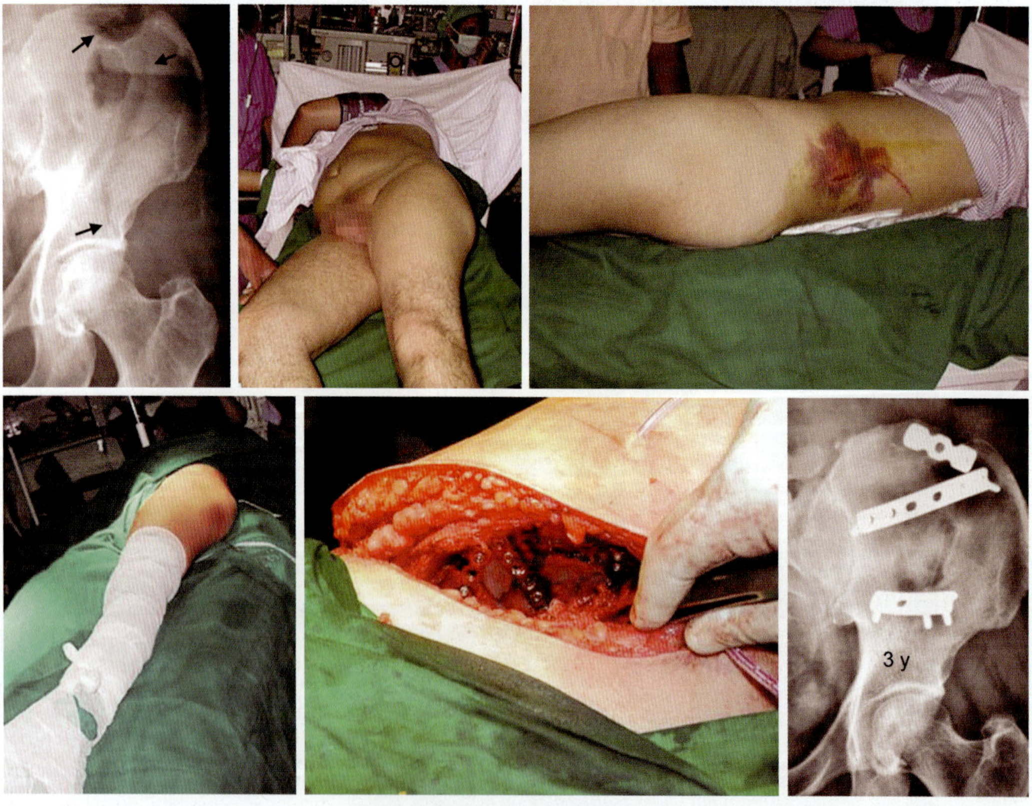

Figure 26.4 Fracture of left ilium

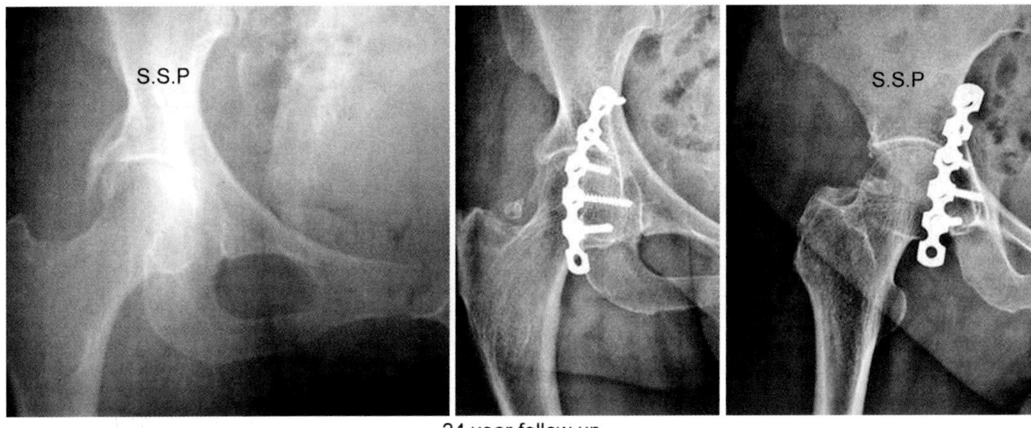

Figure 26.6 Posterior fracture dislocation of hip: 24 years follow up

Case 5

A lady presented with limp and inability to walk well during the postpartum period. Had no H/o fall, etc., but pain during a change of posture/ sitting up to feed the baby and moving about. The symphysis pubis was tender and X-ray examination revealed diastasis of the pubic symphysis.

Such a case needs reassurance and rest in bed as much as possible. With time, the pain reduces. A lumbo-sacral corset offers pain relief (Fig. 26.5).

Case 6

A middle age lady had a car accident, while traveling in a front seat of a car. This has been described as 'A dash-board injury, because the knee hits the dash-board, leading to this typical injury'. She sustained posterior dislocation of the hip with fracture of posterior lip of acetabulum. The fracture was reduced and the lip stabilized with a reconstruction plate. At the end of 24 years from the injury and treatment, she continues to have a good range on motion, with no changes of OA (Fig. 26.6).

Case 7

This elderly gentleman had an accident, again, due to a dash-board injury. The dislocation was promptly reduced and the posterior fragment was fixed. In addition to the posterior lip fracture, there was an undisplaced fracture in the posterior wall of the acetabulum. Both the fractures were fixed and had a reasonably good hip function (Fig. 26.7).

Case 8

A young man had a posterior fracture dislocation of the hip with a transverse fracture of the acetabulum. Both the fractures were fixed with a plate. The plate had to be a long one, to stabilize both the fractures (Fig. 26.8).

Case 9

This elderly person had a rather long posterior lip fracture. Hence, to have access to the anterior end of the fracture fragment, had to do a trochanteric osteotomy, to reach area beyond the anterior limit of the lip fracture (Fig. 26.9).

Case 10

This old man with uncontrolled diabetes had a transverse fracture of acetabulum. On arrival an upper tibial skeletal traction was applied. However, the diabetes could not be controlled. The CT scan with 3D reconstruction indicated that the displacement was not more than 2 mm in any fracture. Besides, the family was reluctant

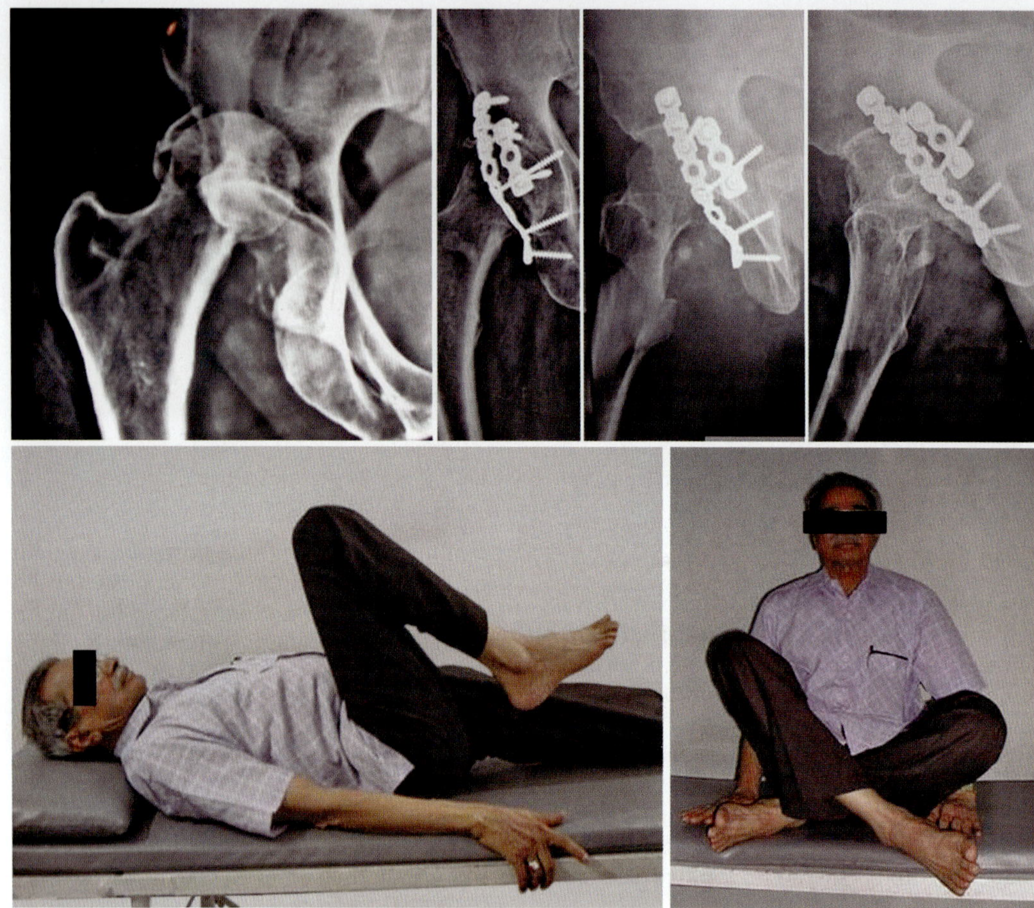

Figure 26.7 Posterior lip and wall fracture dislocation of hip

to undergo a surgery for the injury. Hence the skeletal traction was continued for eight weeks and later mobilized in the bed. Gradually non-weight bearing mobilization was carried out.

At the end of 3 months, gradual weight bearing was started. The pain recurred after six months. X-ray taken then revealed resorption of the weight bearing portion of the head of femur. He did not come for follow up (Figs 26.10A to C).

Case 11

This middle age person had a transverse fracture of the acetabulum and inferior ramus of the ischium. The posterior column was hinged at the ischial fracture and rotated. After exposure posteriorly, the angulated posterior column was reduced. The posterior column fracture had a wide area on either side of the fracture and hence two plates were used to fix it. The stability was good. The preoperative applied tibial traction was continued for further 2 weeks and the intermittent mobilization was carried out. He had good return of pain-free function (Fig. 26.11).

Case 12

This girl in early 20s had RTA and sustained fracture of both columns. There was a large posterior lip segment, with crushing of the base

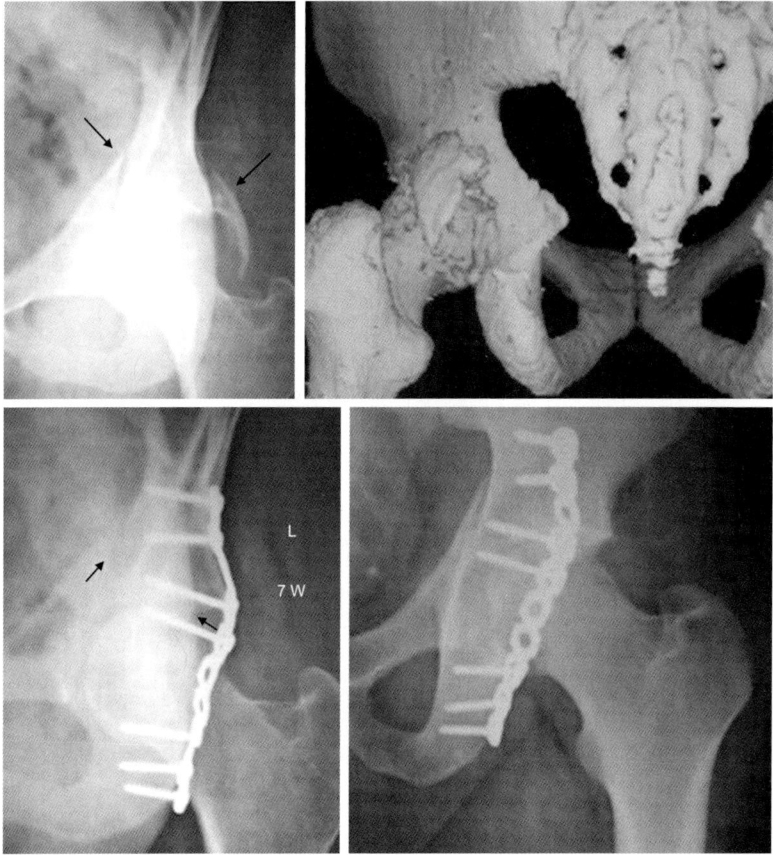

Figure 26.8 Posterior fracture dislocation with a transverse fracture of acetabulum

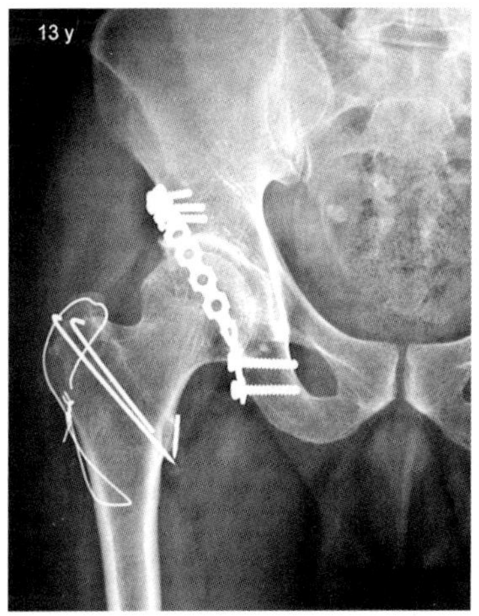

Figure 26.9 Posterior fracture dislocation: 13 years follow up. No OA changes

of the acetabulum. By a posterior approach, the posterior lip and the posterior column were fixed. The approach was carried out by a digastric osteotomy of the trochanter. This helps to maintain continuity of gluteus medius and the vastus lateralis and problem of union of the trochanter is kept to a minimum (Figs 26.12A and B).

Case 13

This elderly person, addicted to ethanol, sustained a fracture of both columns of acetabulum. He would become violent and not maintain the skeletal traction. It was a difficult decision to manage non-operatively, but there was no other option. After fixation of the columns, if he got violent and started weight

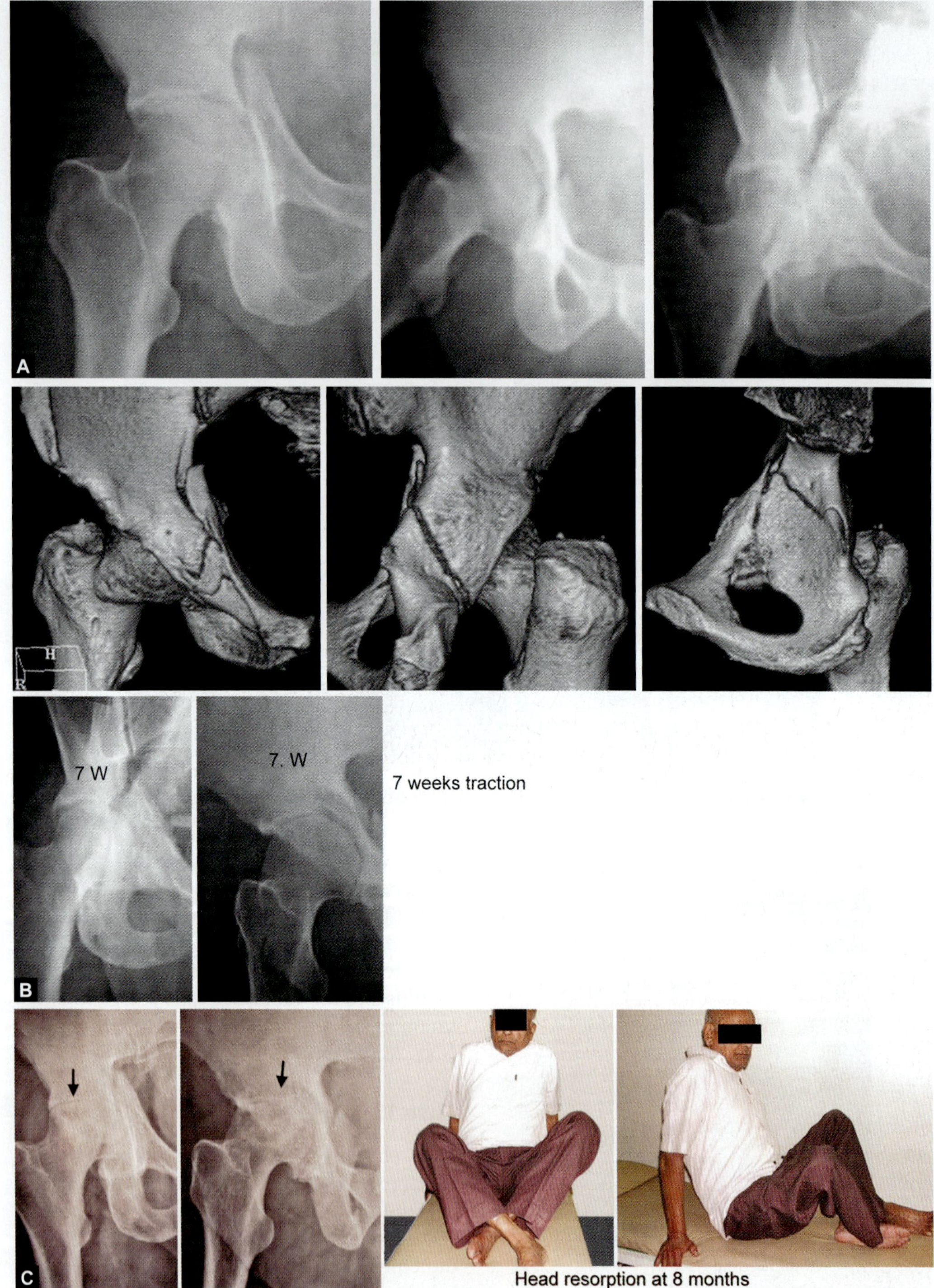

Figures 26.10A to C Pelvis transverse fracture and diabetes

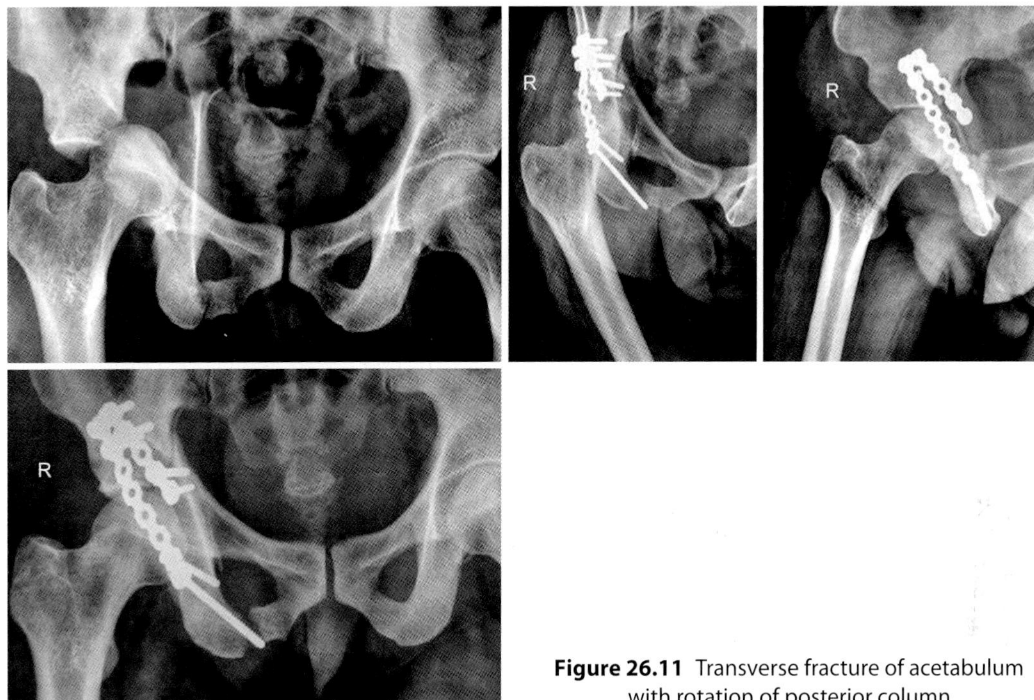

Figure 26.11 Transverse fracture of acetabulum with rotation of posterior column

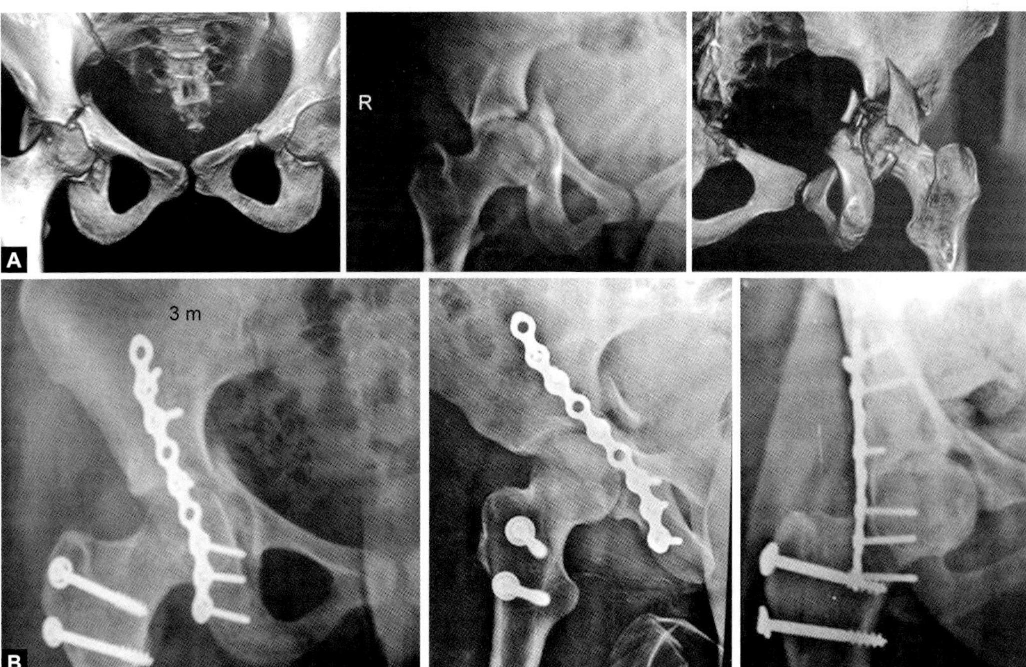

Figures 26.12A and B Both column fracture

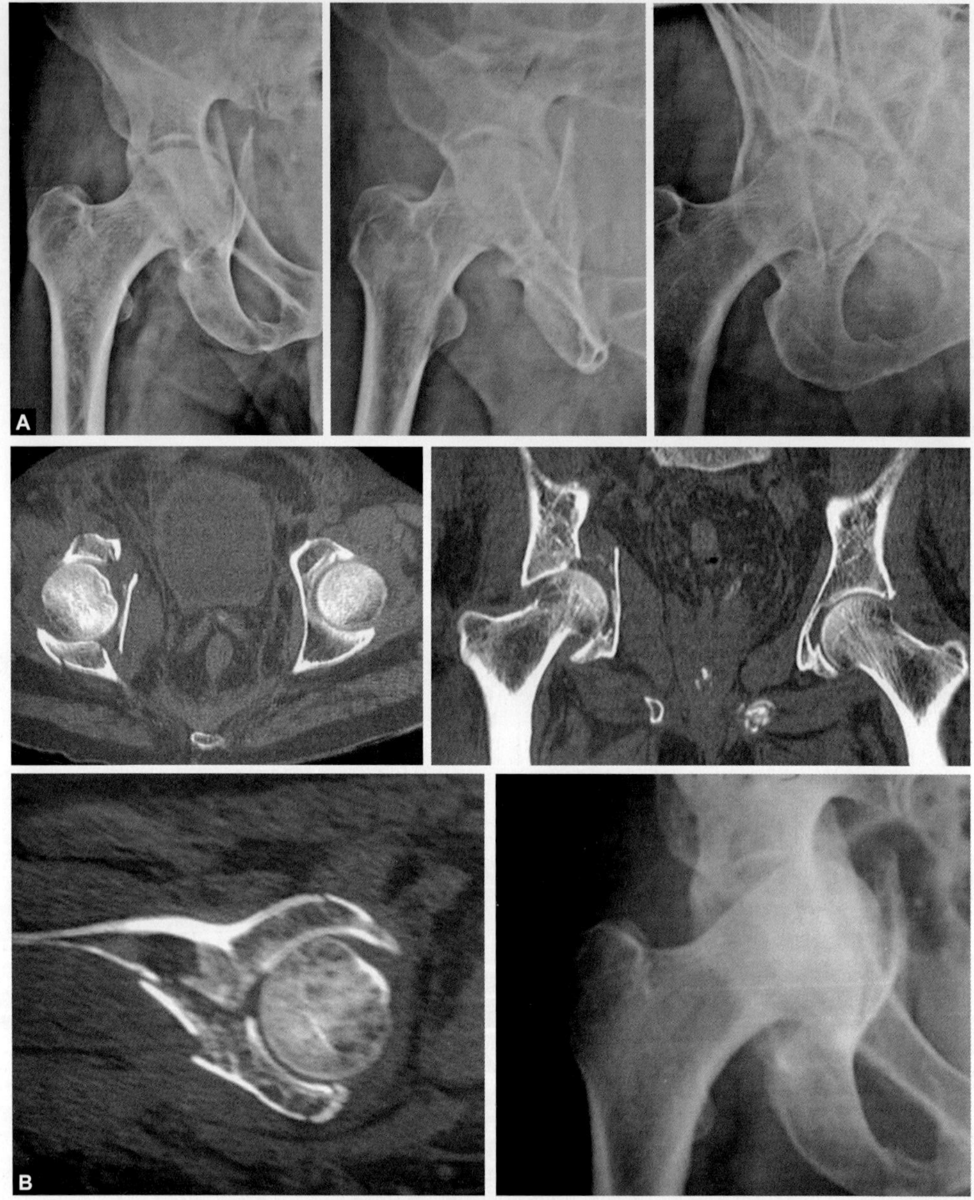

Figures 26.13A and B

bearing against advice, the problem may have been more serious and after discussion with the family, this decision was taken.

The skeletal traction was maintained for six weeks and then a Thomas' splint was applied. This somehow helped to keep him off the weight. He had approx 2 cm shortening, which was managed with a shoe raise. He is able to manage himself (Figs 26.13A to C).

Case 14

A middle-aged lady sustained a transverse fracture of the acetabulum. Soon after arrival, it was reduced and skeletal traction was applied. A CT scan was done and later the acetabulum was fixed with two precontoured plates. This could be done without a trochanteric osteotomy (Figs 26.14A and B).

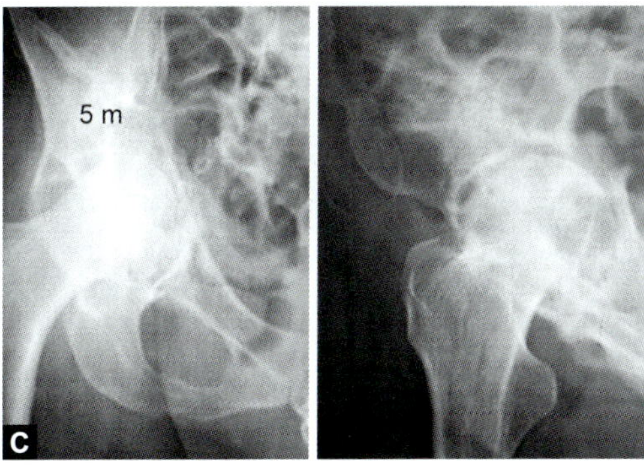

Figure 26.13C

Figures 26.13A to C Fracture of both columns

Case 15

This patient had sustained a transverse fracture of acetabulum. Having done a trochanteric osteotomy, the fracture was being exposed. Just then the contused, probably superior gluteal artery, started bleeding and was taken care of. It was decided on table not to proceed further and skeletal traction was continued. The result was satisfactory. I think, at times, it is prudent to abandon a procedure and have a happy outcome (Fig. 26.15).

This patient had an industrial accident and sustained a bilateral acetabular fractures,

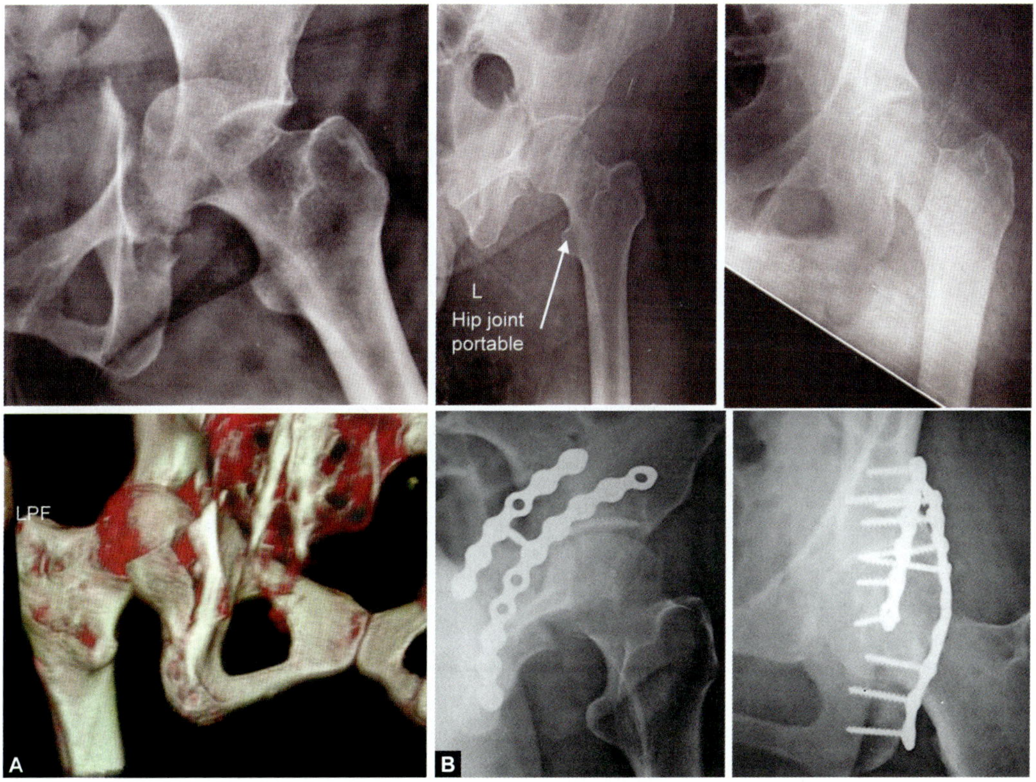

Figures 26.14A and B Transverse fracture of acetabulum

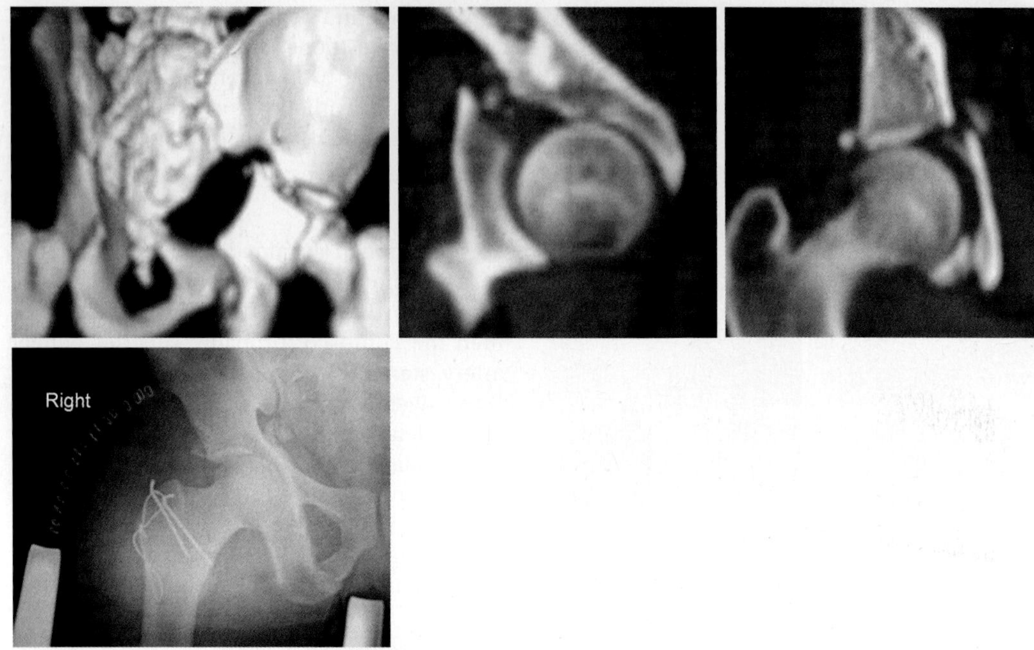

Figure 26.15 Procedure abandoned

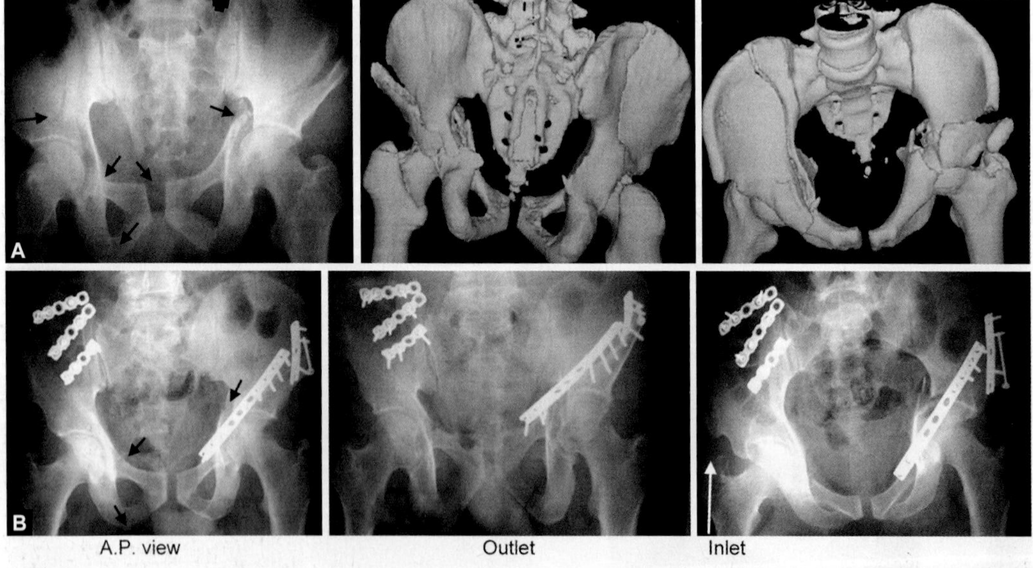

Figures 26.16A and B Bilateral injury

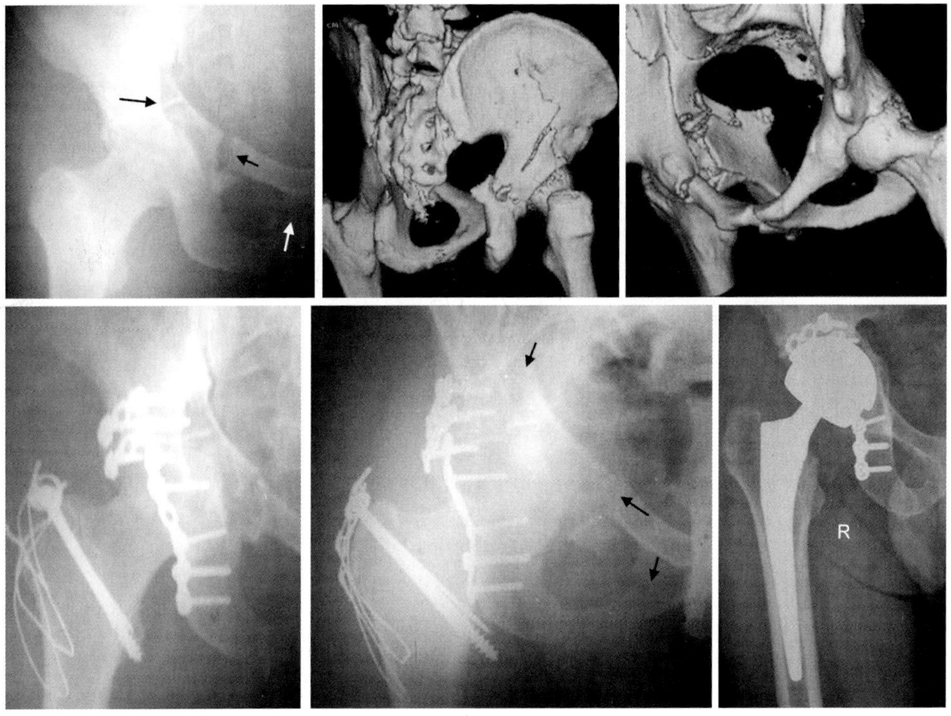

Figure 26.17 Bipolar replacement

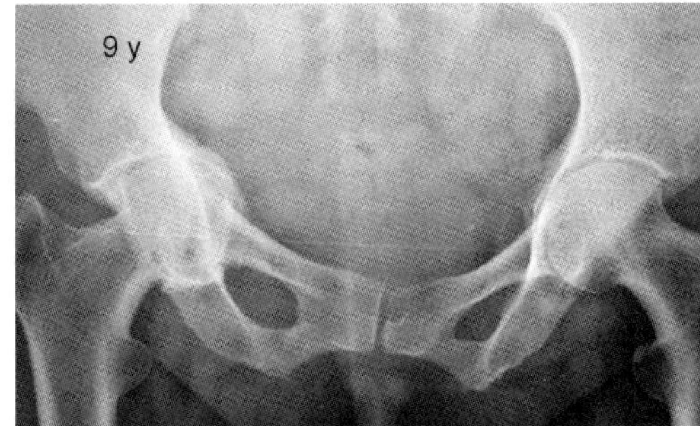

Figure 26.18 9-year follow up. OA changes

without a visceral injury. It was stabilized in two stages. Good outcome (Figs 26.16A and B).

Case 17

A patient in mid 50s, had fracture of both the columns. The posterior part was stabilized. The anterior column was in place and was treated non-operatively. After two years, he continued

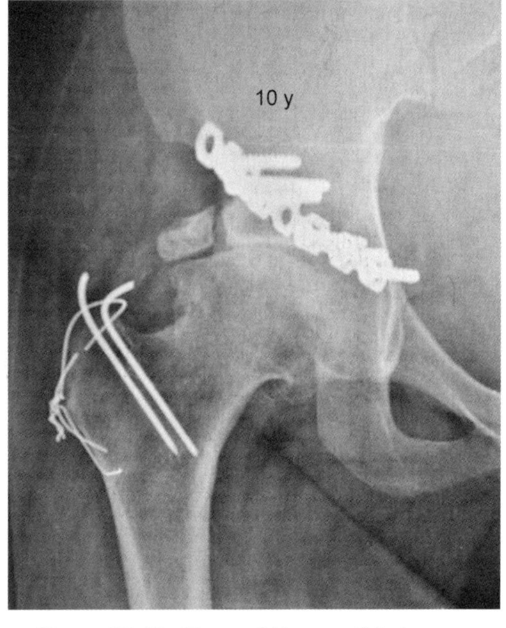

Figure 26.19 10-year follow up. OA changes

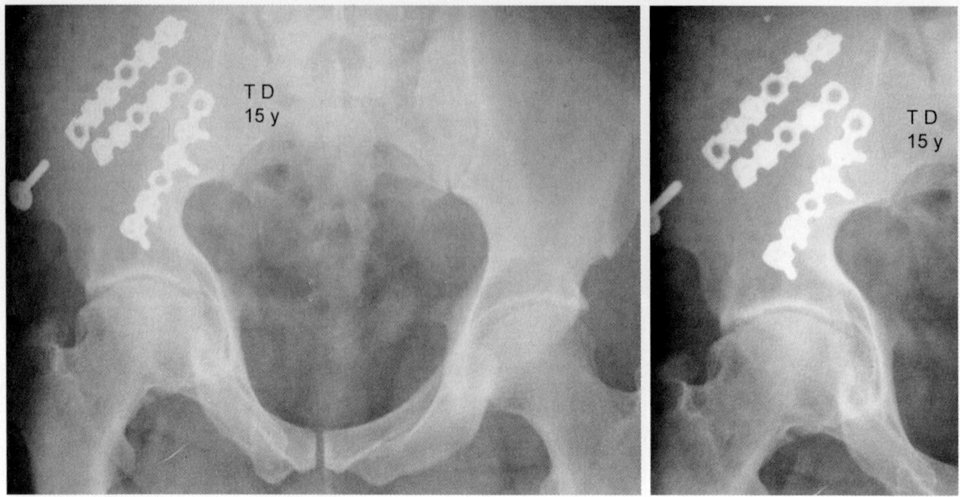

Figure 26.20 15-year follow up. OA changes

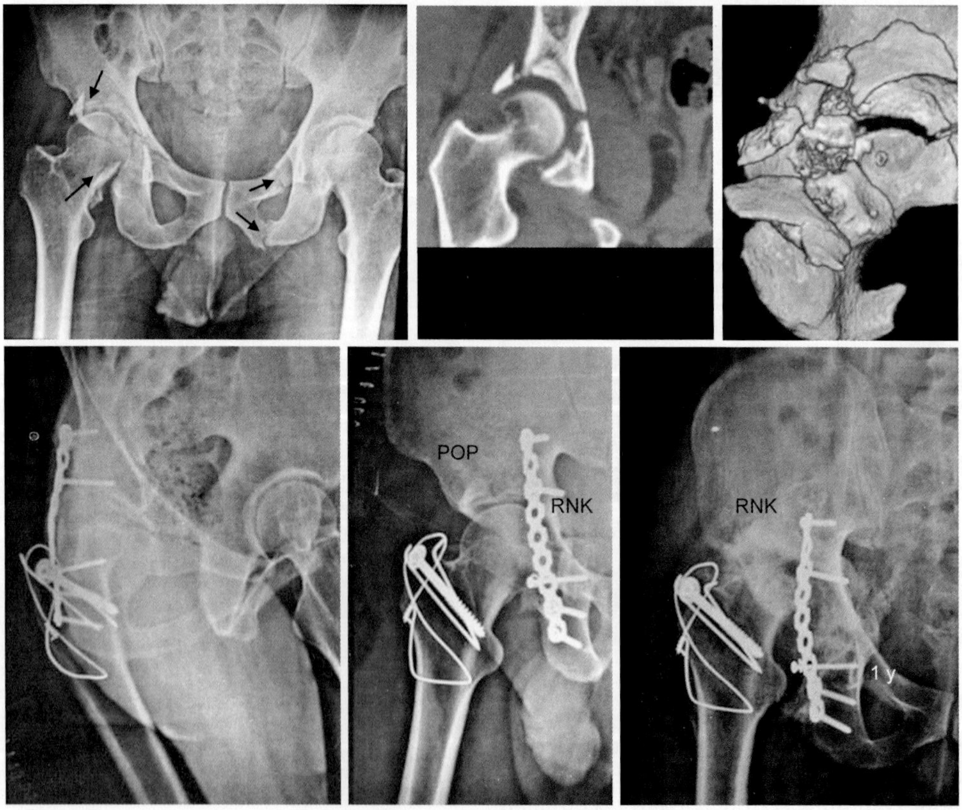

Figure 26.21 Head absorbed

to have pain in the hip. This was due to arthritic changes in the hip. A bipolar replacement was done. He is relieved of the pain and is doing well at the end of 6 years (Fig. 26.17).

Cases 18 to 20: Late OA Changes

A few patients have acetabular fractures in late teens and are stabilized, with a good initial results. However, at the end of ten years or so, have symptoms of OA. In due course of time would need THR (Figs 26.18 to 26. 20).

Case 21

This middle age person had fracture dislocation of hip, fracture of tibia and other injuries. The acetabulum was fixed. He had postoperative psychosis and hallucinations and would not co-operate for necessary care and treatment. Gradually, there was pain and limp in the hip, while the other injuries did well. The head of femur was getting absorbed. There was no evidence of deep infection (Fig. 26.21).

CHAPTER

27

Fracture of Neck of Femur

INTRACAPSULAR FRACTURE OF NECK OF FEMUR

The blood supply to the head of femur is precarious and hence fracture union in general is rather slow and perhaps uncertain, especially after middle age. In the elderly, due to osteoporosis, the implant cut-out is common and hence partial hip replacement is a preferred procedure.

5 to 10% of intracapsular fractures are of impacted and often the diagnosis is late, due to late presentation by the patient.

A variety of implants have been devised to offer good stability of the fracture in the young persons and possibly no definitive solution is still arrived at.

The common sequela of this fracture is nonunion or avascular necrosis. The later leads to arthritis of the hip.

In a high energy injury, fracture shaft of femur is observed to be associated with ipsilateral fracture of neck of the femur. Hence, in every fracture of shaft of a femur, an X-ray examination of hip and the knee is necessary, to exclude any associated injury. A missed associated injury near either end of the femur leads to many problems and a complete diagnosis on arrival is important. Fracture of neck of the femur on the same side, associated with a fracture of the shaft of the femur, is a special situation and treatment planning is important to achieve a good outcome.

At the end of an operation of internal fixation with a K nail (in early days) or an interlocking nails today, one must take an X-ray film of the hip area on the table, prior to closure, to confirm that an intracapsular fracture in the neck is not visible. May be there was an undisplaced fracture in the neck, not visible on day one X-ray film and makes itself apparent at the end of the surgery.

Diagnosis of an Intracapsular Fracture of Neck of Femur

One may have to see a patient presenting with:

- Pain in hip, without any history of a fall/or a jerk, etc. A detailed history may reveal some unaccustomed physical strain in the person. Even an act of standing too long in a social function, to which one is unaccustomed, can lead to an insufficiency fracture.

  In a clinical examination, one should observe the following:

  - Ability to stand unaided. The gait and local bony tenderness on the greater trochanter and anterior to the hip.
  - Has the patient come walking (as in an impacted fracture) or is brought on a stretcher? If on a stretcher, is there an external rotation attitude of the leg?

  - Limb length equality
  - Capacity to do active unassisted internal rotation of the leg
  - Ability to raise the affected leg straight up without any assistance.
- Good quality AP X-ray film with the hip in internal or at least a neutral rotation and a cross table lateral X-ray is important. If no obvious fracture line is visible, one should study trabecular pattern in the neck area, for any disturbance. One may be able to suspect or detect an undisplaced or an impacted fracture in the neck of femur. The X-ray film should be of good quality and the clinician should sit opposite the X-ray film illuminator and study carefully and compare with the hip on the opposite side. If the film does not reveal any evidence of fracture and one still suspects a concealed hip fracture, it is wise to arrange for an MRI scan soon. An insufficiency fracture is detected on MRI and the fracture can be taken care of immediately.

Why is this Important?

In a middle-age and a physically-fit adult, if a fracture line is visible on MRI, it may be possible to save the head of femur by carrying out internal fixation at the earliest. A well-fixed fracture in such a situation is expected to unite and will have a good range of motion in the future. In a displaced fracture of a neck of femur, even after a proper treatment, one cannot predict whether AVN or nonunion can be avoided. In an undisplaced fracture, the chance is less and hence this care is necessary.

CASE STUDY

Case 1

A lady over 70 years of age reported with pain in the right hip area. No H/O fall. However, she was continuously standing a few days ago, for some function in the home. On arrival was able to stand and take few steps with support. Active internal rotation of the hip was painful, but possible, indicating some continuity in the neck of femur. X-ray examination did not reveal a fracture. Hence MRI was being arranged. Just then, she had some pain in the hip and the limb went in external rotation! Immediate X-ray examination was done, which showed a displaced IC fracture of neck of femur. A cemented monoblock bipolar replacement was done. Good recovery and current status at the end of 11 years (Fig. 27.1).

Case 2

A patient over 70 years of age reported with pain in the left hip, without any H/O fall, etc. X-ray did not reveal obvious fracture, but some disturbance of trabecular pattern. Was advised indoor care and MRI examination. Maybe because of ability to move the affected hip to some extent, the patient did not pay heed to the advice given and went away against advice. Returned in 4 days, with inability to move the left hip actively. A repeat X-ray confirmed a fracture of neck of femur (Fig. 27.2).

IMPACTED FRACTURE OF NECK OF FEMUR

After a fall, whenever an elderly person reports, a fracture of neck of femur is to be assumed, till proved otherwise, subsequent clinical and radiological examination, and necessary tests, have been the teaching! A good quality of X-ray and knowledge of possibility of such an injury is equally important!

Case 3

The patient after a trivial fall was able to walk with some support. An X-ray examination was done and sent home, as no fracture was detected in the film. Due to discomfort and some limp, reported again after few weeks. Now, a good quality X-ray film detected some disturbance in the trabeculi and was advised to use a walker to visit bathroom and take rest in the bed. The fracture did not get displaced. Follow up X-ray showed progressive union and relief of pain. (Having diagnosed disturbance in trabeculi, I would like to confirm with an MRI and then manage accordingly) (Fig. 27.3A).

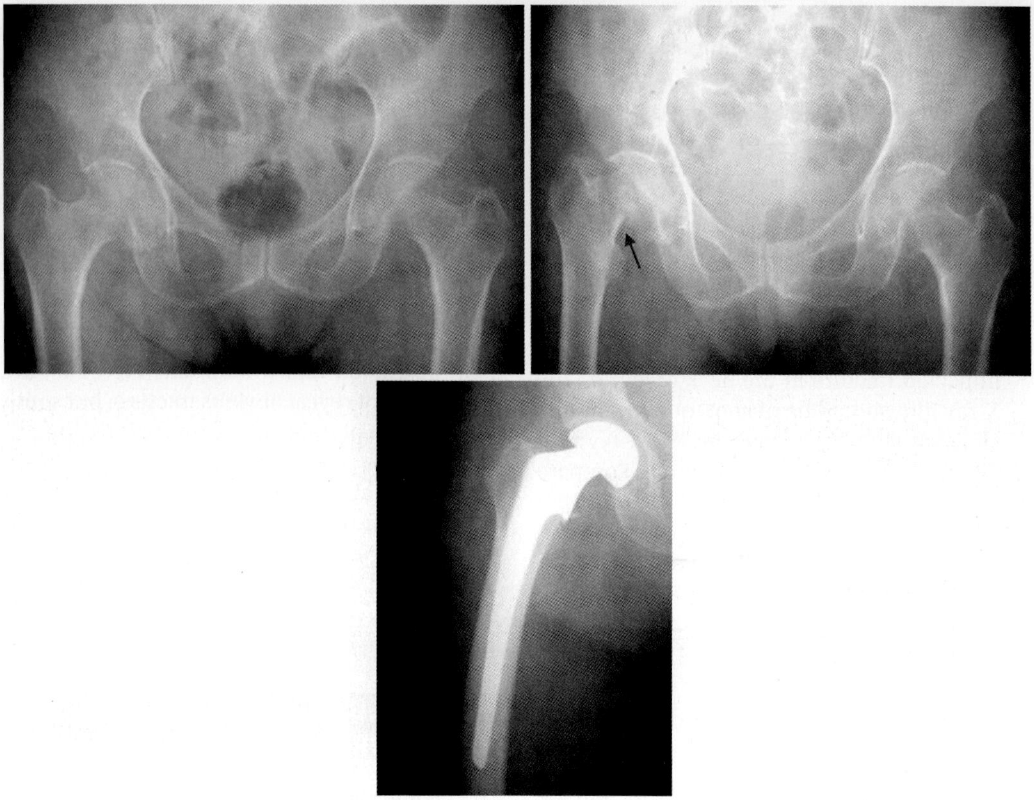

Figure 27.1 Diagnosis I

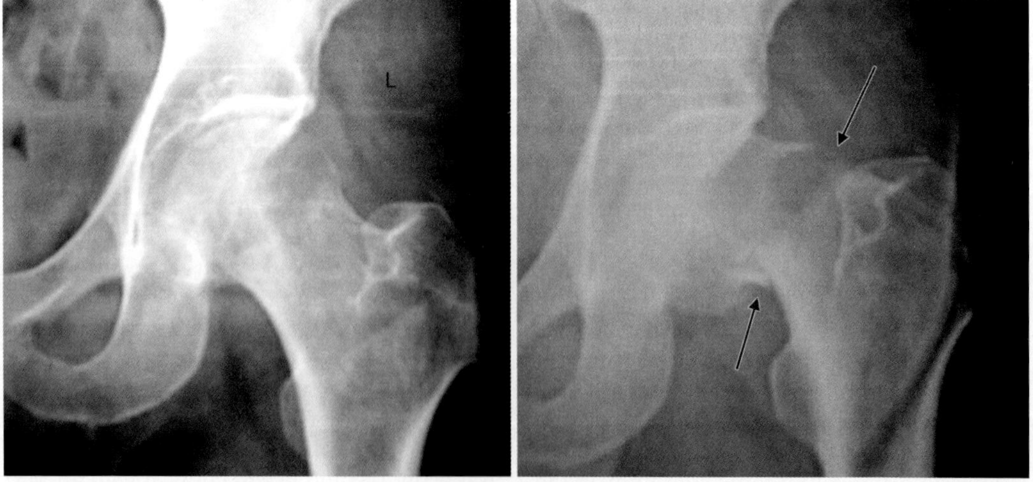

Figure 27.2 Diagnosis II

It is necessary to train the X-ray technician, to take X-ray of every hip keeping it in internal rotation, as much as possible. If this is not practised, an undisplaced fracture can be missed (Fig. 27.3B).

Case 4

The patient presented a month after a fall. Was able to walk, without much pain. X-ray revealed an impacted fracture. Walking with

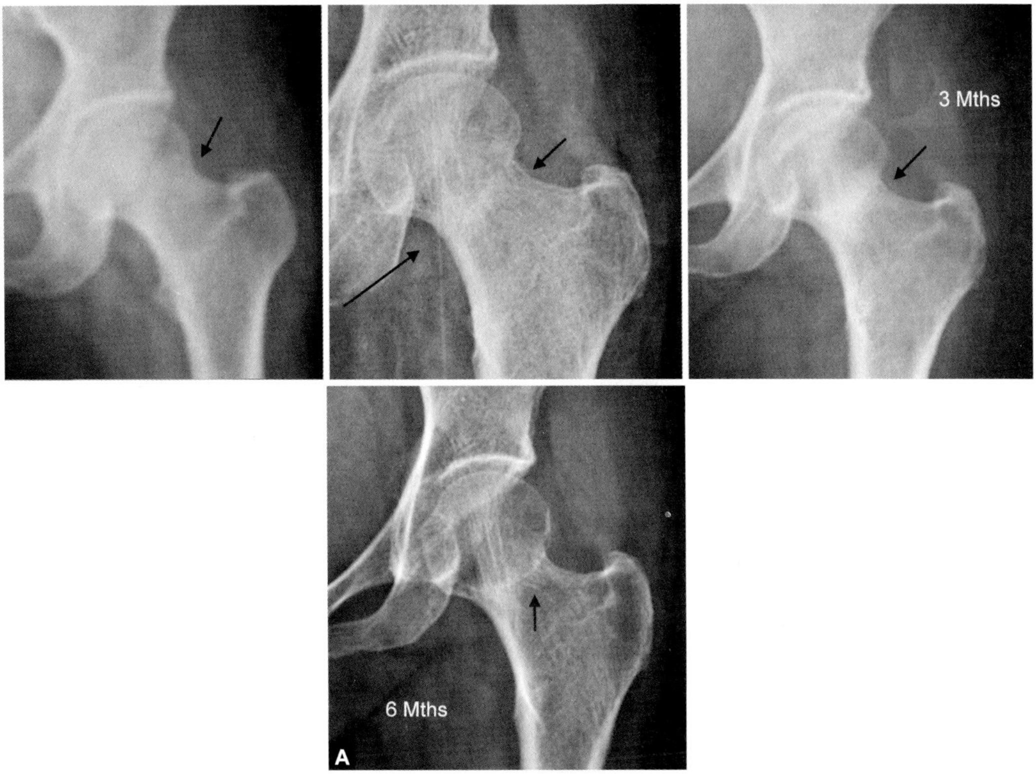

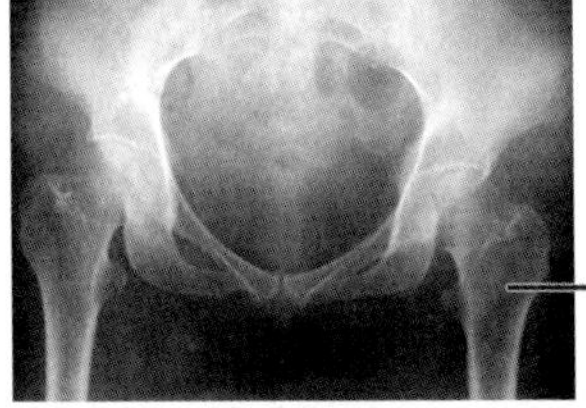

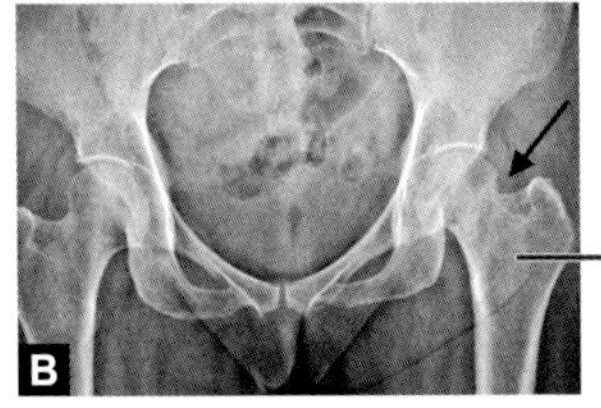

Figures 27.3A and B (A) Impacted fracture: Missed; (B) X-ray in internal rotation revealed a fracture

full weight-bearing, without any walking aid, did not displace the fracture, indicating a stable impaction. Hence, he was treated non-operatively. In such a situation, one wonders, if one should permit continued full weight-bearing or only partial weight-bearing, using a walker. I would prefer use of a walker with a partial weight bearing, for a total duration of two months from the injury, followed by a stick in the opposite side. It is important to explain and alert both the patient and the relatives that due to the mechanism of injury and related fracture geometry, some leg lengthening is likely and that a shoe-raise on the opposite side would be required. (Often patient feels some incorrect treatment has been given, because, usually after any bone and/or joint injury, a limb is known to become shorter and in my case, how it has become long!) (Fig. 27.4).

The fracture has healed well as seen in the X-ray at the end of a year. However, looking at the X-ray at the end of a month, when he presented for examination, I would be tempted to offer internal fixation, with AM pins, to prevent any likelihood of displacement. In such a situation, I prefer smooth pin which is drilled and offers less torque, compared to a screw insertion. A pin, thus, would prevent any possibility of fracture displacement.

Case 5

In a case of an impacted fracture, wherein the patient is able to stand and take a few steps, it is possible that the fracture would unite without getting displaced. Lack of much pain and ability to bear some weight indicates a stable impaction. The fracture is less likely to get displaced, with some movements and only a partial weight bearing. However, one prefers to contribute more stability to it by inserting few AM pins.

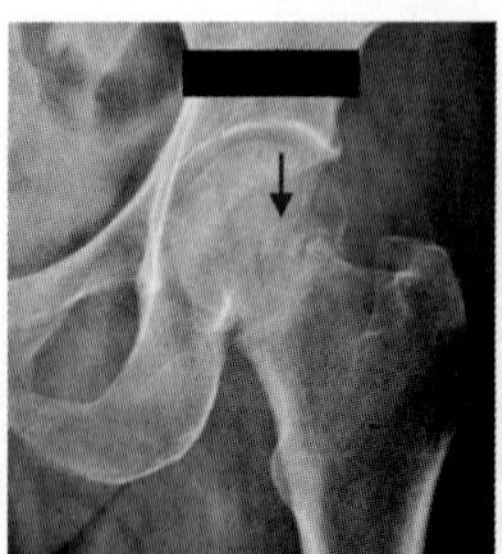

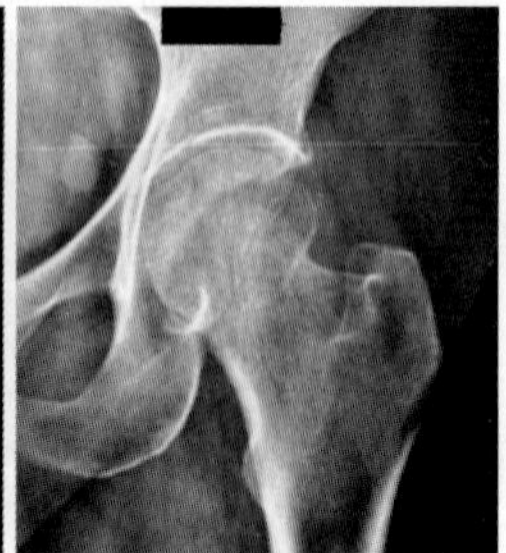

Figure 27.4 Impacted fracture late presentation

Pins or 6.5 mm Screws?

Austin Moore pins inserted in parallel or other mode, add to the stability, without adding stress on the impaction at the fracture site. The butt-end of the pin has threads, which engage in the lateral cortex of the femur. The depth of the threads is not deep, and hence, quite often a pin backs out. Usually a soft bone wire is circled around the base nuts, which help to support all the pins together. Thus, even if one pin tends to back out, the wire holds it in place. This pin design has threads on the butt ends, which get some anchor in the lateral femoral cortex. In Knowel pins, the threads are at the business end, which gets anchorage in the subchondral part of the head of femur. Prior to insertion of either pin, a drill hole is made with a 2 mm drill and then the pin is inserted.

Technique: Using either pin, one should have a full range of the pins. If an AM pin is to be selected, one should decide the length of the pin and select an AM pin which has 15 mm shorter smooth portion. Two nuts should be on the threaded part of the pin and then the pin is drilled in the hole drilled. This way, as the pin is finally drilled in, the threads on the butt-end would engage in the lateral femoral cortex. Confirm under 'C' arm, the depth to which the pin is inserted. Then the deeper nut is tightened over the pin against the lateral cortex and another nut over the first one. This way, when both the nuts are locked against each other, they are unlikely to back out. Similarly, when the threads on the outer portion of the pin engage the cortex, it is expected to remain secure in place. The nut is manually tightened and then with nose pliers, it is finally tightened.

If the pins are inserted, parallel to each other, they would engage in different quadrants and offer more stability to the fracture. A 0.8 mm soft bone wire is turned around the nuts, taking it over each pin and taken deep to the nuts. This way, all the nuts are held and anchored by the bone wire.

What to Avoid

A pin should be drilled in with two nuts on it. If one inserts a pin without the nuts on the threaded part and when one cuts off the extra length of the threaded portion and attempts threading a nut over the cut portion, it usually does not engage over the pin. This is because the cut-end of the pin gets deformed and threads do not accept the nuts.

6.5 mm Screws

While a screw is inserted across a fracture, the torsional force may displace the fracture, as the screw is entering the proximal fragment. However, if a few pins are inserted first, stability is conferred to the fracture and then one may safely insert a screw across the fracture (Fig. 27.5).

IMPACTED FRACTURE IN THE 3RD DECADE OF LIFE

Case 6

At this age, the bone is quite strong. If one chooses to insert two or more screws. One should stabilize the fracture with 2 × 2 mm K-wires, at such a place, that they do not come in the way of the screws. Then first two AM pins are inserted. This stabilizes the head with respect to the neck and then a screw is inserted. Presence of 2 K-wires and two AM pins stabilizes the head of femur, so it is less likely to spin, as the screw threads are engaging in the head (Fig. 27.6).

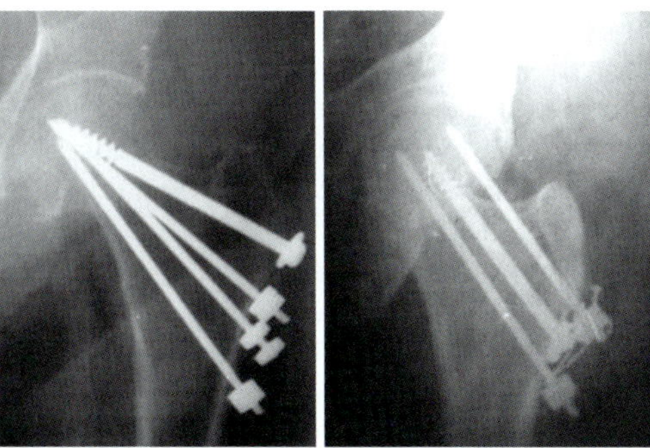

Figure 27.5 Impacted fracture of neck of femur: AM pins

FRACTURE OF NECK OF FEMUR IN THE MIDDLE AGE

Case 7

This middle age gentleman sustained a fracture of neck of femur. The pain was rather less, compared to a displaced fracture. As seen in the X-ray, the superior part of the neck was slightly impacted. Soon on arrival a well-fitting Thomas' splint was applied and was operated the next day.

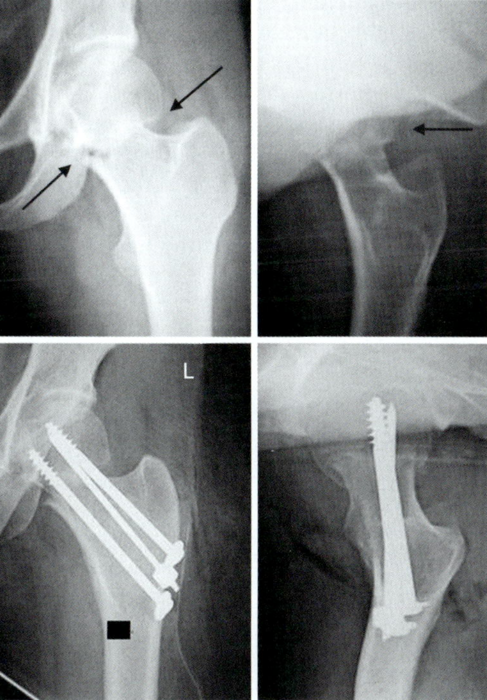

Figure 27.6 Impacted fracture of neck of femur in young

I feel, the DHS available is rather too wide for an IC fracture of the neck and hence I would prefer using a pediatric design of the DHS, as was done in this case.

The Steps

- No reduction of the fracture and the limb is tied as such on a fracture table. The position is confirmed under a 'C' arm.
- Two of 2 mm K-wires inserted: one along the calcar and one very high in the neck, so the DHS and the 6.5 mm screw could be accommodated in the central segment.
- First, the 6.5 mm screw was inserted in the upper segment, so the neck is well stabilized. The screw was not fully tightened. Then the pediatric DHS screw was inserted after tapping. Thus, 2 K-wires and a 6.5 mm screw stabilized the neck well and the head of femur did not spin, while the head of femur was tapped and then a pediatric DHS screw was inserted.
- Final tightening of the 6.5 mm screw was done and the side plate was attached and fixed over the DHS screw.
- In the postoperative period, static quad exercises were encouraged and active internal rotation of the leg was permitted. Straight leg raise is not permitted, because the entire load of the limb comes on the head of femur, which is the fulcrum. It has lost some blood supply and till it is restored again, the head remains soft and hence the care, to avoid any deformation of the head of the femur (Fig. 27.7).

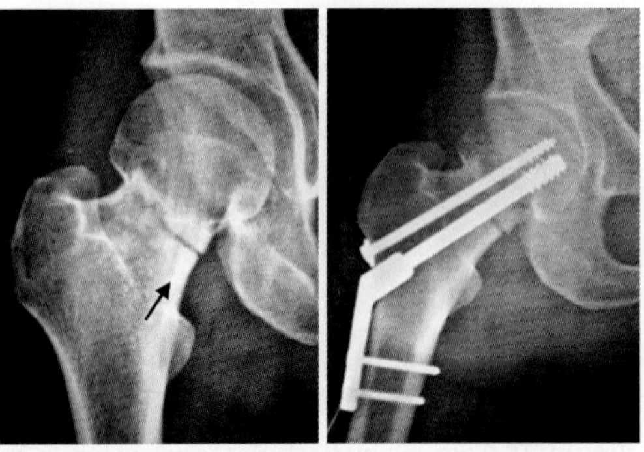

Figure 27.7 DHS and a 6.5 mm screw

Case 8

This old person had apparently an impacted fracture of neck of femur. However, he was unable to bear any weight and had quite some pain in the hip. This indicated that the impaction was not sound. (Internal fixation with pins and a screw could have been done and one would have to wait for few weeks, even to permit a partial weight bearing on the limb). Hence primary partial hip replacement was done with good recovery.

This definitive procedure of a bipolar replacement permitted early ambulation and completed the treatment (Fig. 27.8).

Case 9

This middle age lady had chronic pain in few areas and was in a low physical state. Sustained an IC fracture of neck of femur. X-ray revealed osteomalacia with pseudo-fractures in the pelvis. A bipolar replacement with an uncemented stem was carried out and in due course of time, the bone pathology was also corrected (Fig. 27.9).

Intracapsular fracture of neck of femur is and was labeled as an unsolved fracture. Fifty years ago, a variety of implants were devised to fix this fracture. The revolutionary invention of Smith Peterson nail changed the method of internal fixation remarkably. However, it had some limitations. Then the cross-pinning and a low angle Kuntsher V nail was devised. These devices either backed out or permitted some motion at the fracture area and lost the hold in the bone. In due course, the concept of lateral column fixation came into vogue, which enhanced the stability of the fracture fixation. However, to have a device having a lateral column fixation, yet permitting a controlled collapse is rather difficult. DHS offered a better outcome in such a fracture.

It was realized that the blood supply to the head of femur was precarious. To prevent avascular changes in the head of femur,

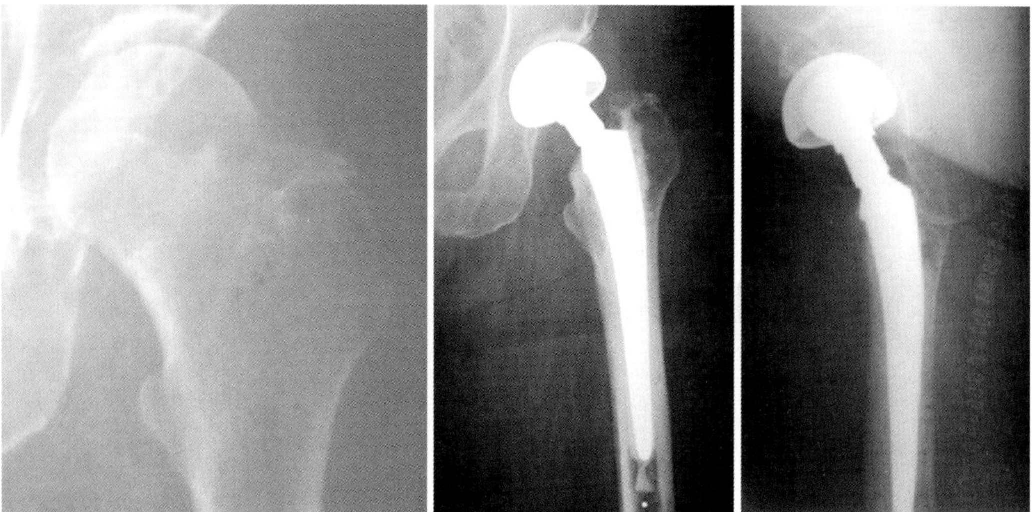

Figure 27.8 Incomplete impacted fracture of neck of femur and pain: Primary hemiarthroplasty

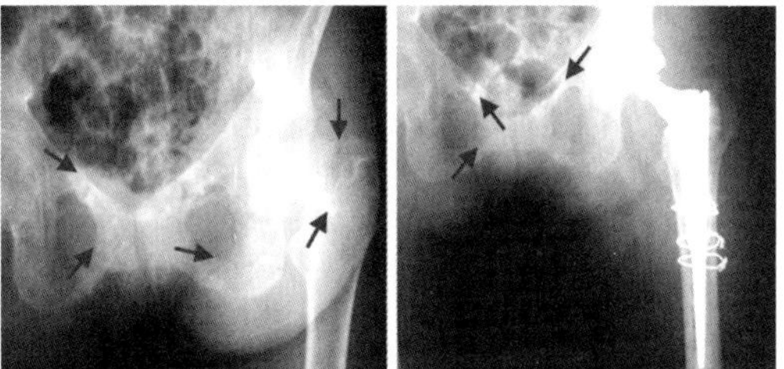

Figure 27.9 Fracture of neck of femur with osteomalacia

a technique of immediate gentle closed reduction and application of a Thomas' splint was suggested. Having done so, early internal fixation was carried out. I feel, this immediate/early reduction of the neck fracture reduces the strain on the vessels and helps to restore the blood supply.

A variety of implants were used and modified, to have better stability and early mobilization. Few of them worked well, because ultimately the fracture union and late outcome is dependent on the blood supply to the head of femur (Figs 27.10 and 27.11).

Then a smaller version of SP nail was developed, which could be passed with relative ease. Being a narrow implant, the distraction was observed to be less. As a complementary fixation, additional 6.5 mm screw and/or AM pin was also used to offer rotatory stability to the reduction. There is always a discussion that a 6.5 mm screw exerts a compression across the fracture area, while the mini SP nail/AM pins just stabilize the fracture. The latter offers more continuous stability. In a 6.5 mm or Asnis screw the shaft diameter is less than the thread diameter. When the thread has created a track of 6.5 mm, the shaft of 4 mm diameter is always loose. Hence, as some fracture resorption

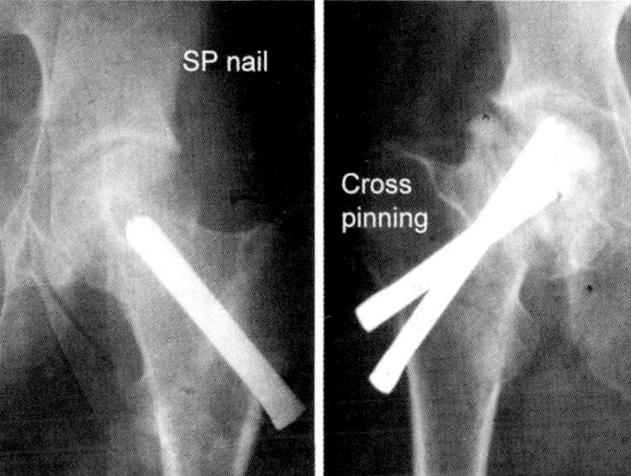

Figure 27.10 Different types of devices

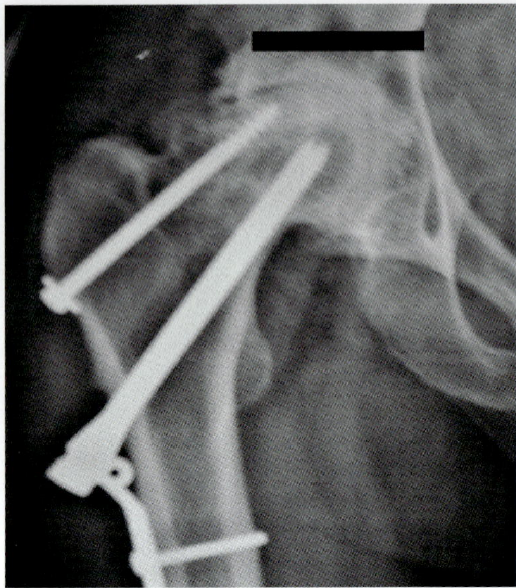

Figure 27.11 Different types of devices

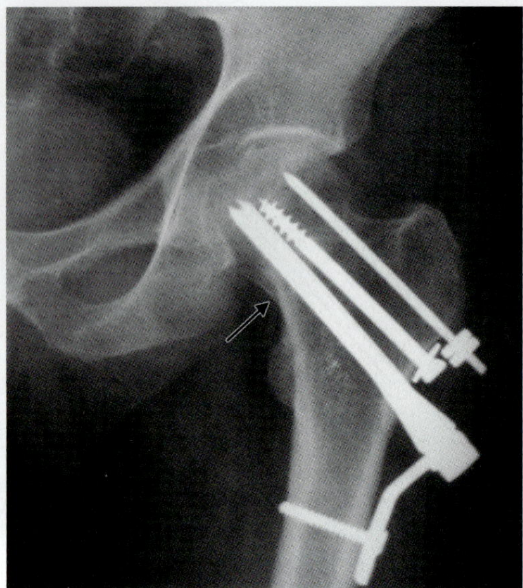

Figure 27.12 Mini SP nail and plate

occurs, the washer and screw head back out from the lateral femoral cortex and then, the shaft of the screw is free to toggle in the track in the trochanter area.

A mini SP pin has a flare in the butt end and is press-fitted in the lateral cortex. Besides, it has a lateral stabilizing plate, which helps the nail to remain in place.

Similarly use of multiple AP pins offers fixation in different sectors of the head of femur and offers stability. Parallel pins and, crossed pins have their plus and minus points. Multiple pins do offer stability to the neck of femur, in spite of the lever load of the entire leg. (The same principle is used, when multiple 3.5 mm raft screws are used in tibial plateau fracture, in a locking plate) (Fig. 27.12).

BASI-TROCHANTERIC FRACTURE

A basi-trochanteric fracture has relatively a broad surface area compared to a transcervical fracture of neck of femur. However, the level of attachment of the capsule is such that part of the fracture is intracapsular, while part of it is extracapsular. Due to the wide surface area, the incidence of fracture union is more than an intracapsular fracture. Since, the bone width and the fracture surface area is more, compared to a transcervical fracture, an addition of a complementary 6.5 screw is possible, which adds to the fracture stability (Fig. 27.13).

At times, due to a high energy injury, one may have a severely displaced basi-trochanteric fracture in the elderly. In such a situation, the blood supply to the head of femur is more likely to be disturbed. Hence, it is worthwhile to carry out a bipolar replacement for assured outcome and is the only surgery required for that elderly person (Fig. 27.14).

A patient from a peripheral area with an intracapsular fracture, often presented a few days after the injury. Often some alternative therapy is also administered and then he thinks of attending an allopathy clinic. This was a common thing of the past. In a person from a peripheral place, to sit cross-legged and to squat is an important part of activities of daily living. Thus, fracture union and preservation of the head of femur is vital, to regain nearly full range of motion. In such a situation, when the patient presents late, one observes that internal fixation with a DHS, an additional complementary fixation with a fibula, adds

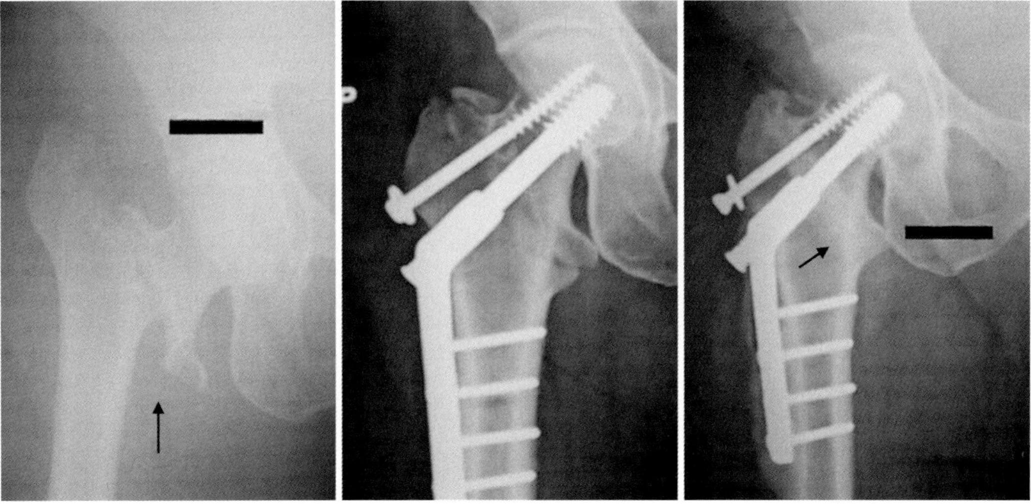

Figure 27.13 Basitrochanteric fracture: Fixation with a DHS and a 6.5 mm screw

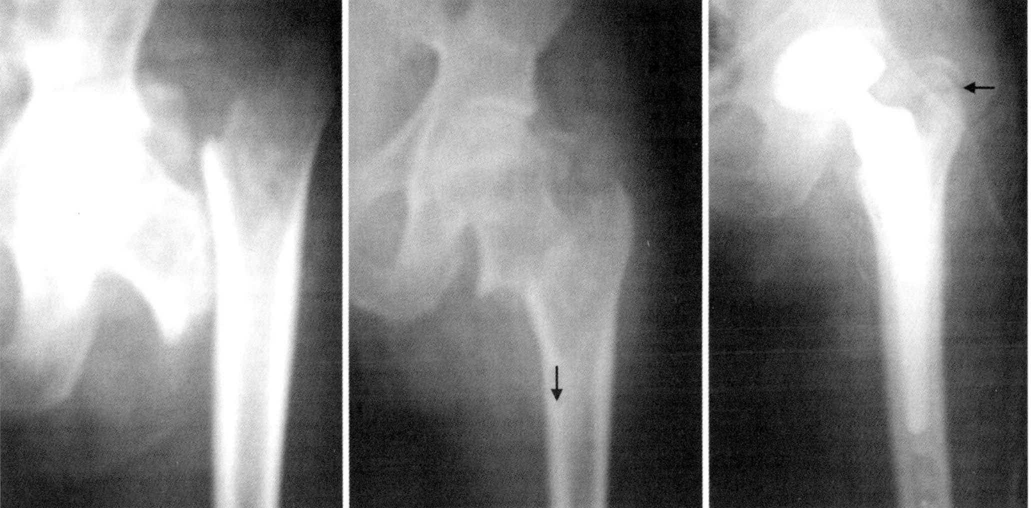

Figure 27.14 Bipolar replacement in a displaced basi-trochanteric fracture

to the mechanical stability and biologically assists fracture union. This combination is known to improve a chance of fracture union. The stability and mobility thus achieved is superior to that after a secondary procedure of joint replacement or after an osteotomy, should the fracture leads to a delayed union (Fig. 27.15).

Case Study

This young man had a pubic diastasis, fracture of both sacral ala (an open book injury), and an intracapsular fracture of neck of the right femur. As a first aid, an external fixator was applied to the iliac wings and patient shifted under my care.

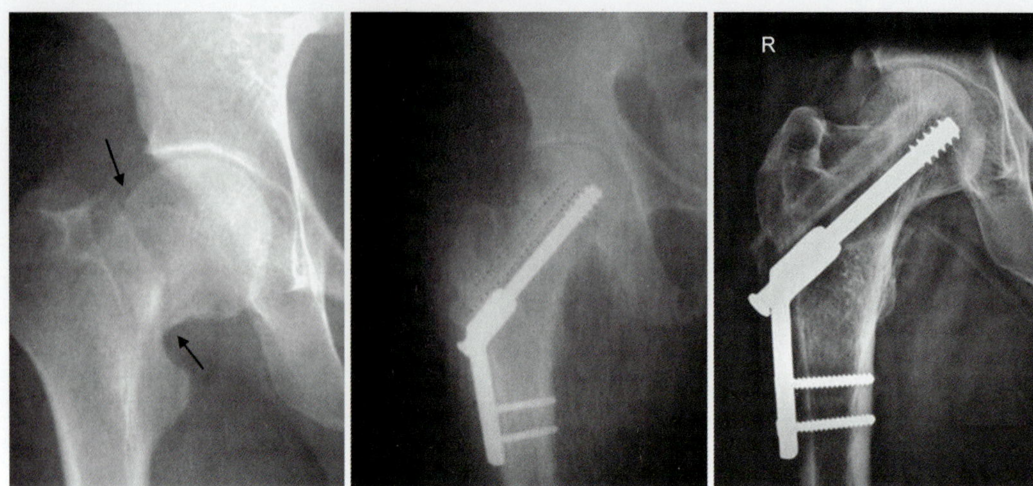

Figure 27.15 Complementary fibula fixation

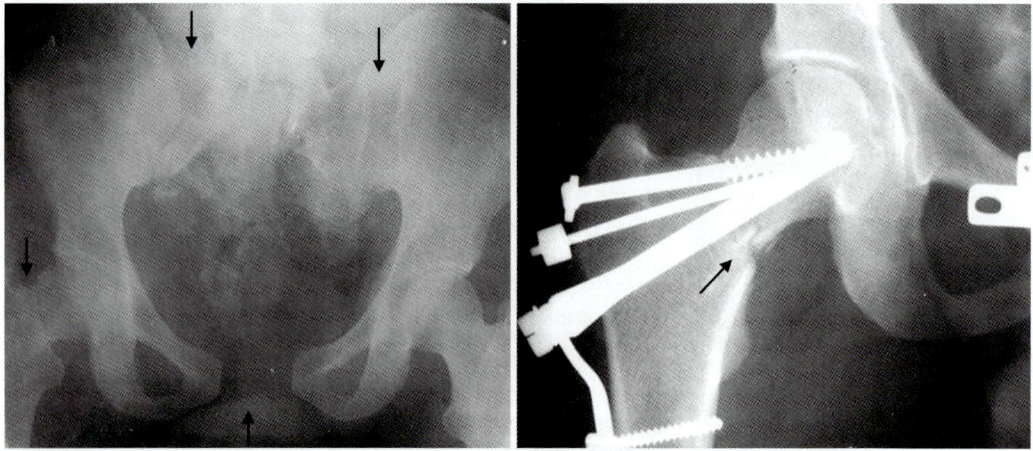

Figure 27.16 Fibula graft

The diastasis was fixed with a plate and the fracture of neck femur on the right side was fixed with a mini SP Nail, etc. The fixator was continued for total six weeks from the injury. The patient was gradually made to sit up, etc. At the end of three months, there was no evidence of union accross the neck of femur. Hence, the AM pin and the 6.5 mm screw was removed. In this area, a track was created and a fibula was inserted across the fracture. In the next 2 months, the fracture united (Figs 27.16 and 27.17).

IPSILATERAL FRACTURE OF NECK AND SHAFT OF FEMUR

The case shown below was managed 18 years ago, when the conventional K-nail and pin fixation for the neck was carried out, and was the method available then.

In a case of ipsilateral fracture of shaft of femur and neck of femur, the later fracture is usually of basi-trochanteric type. Both the fractures were managed on a fracture table. The K-nail was inserted by open method. Necessary

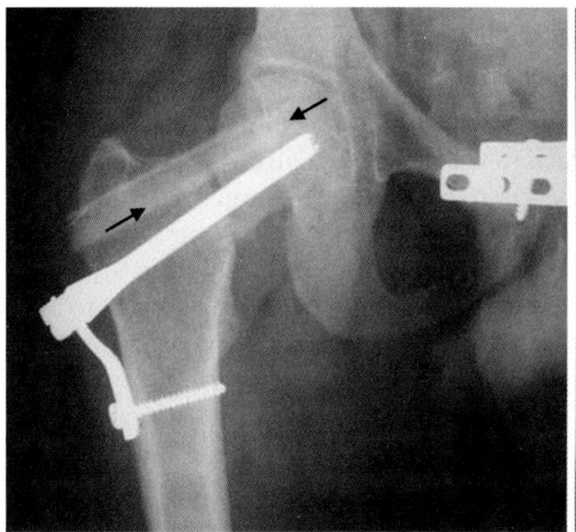

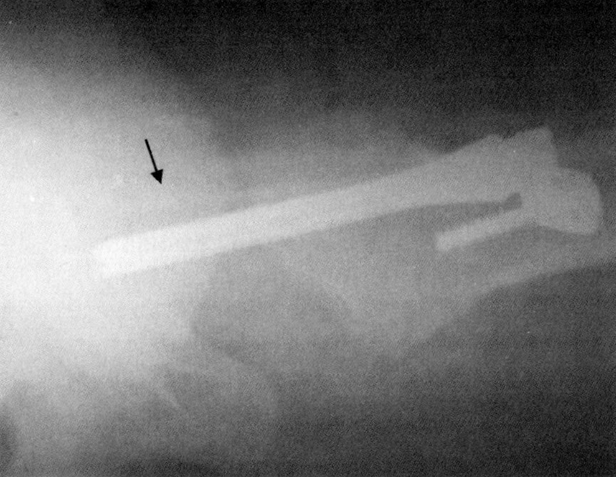

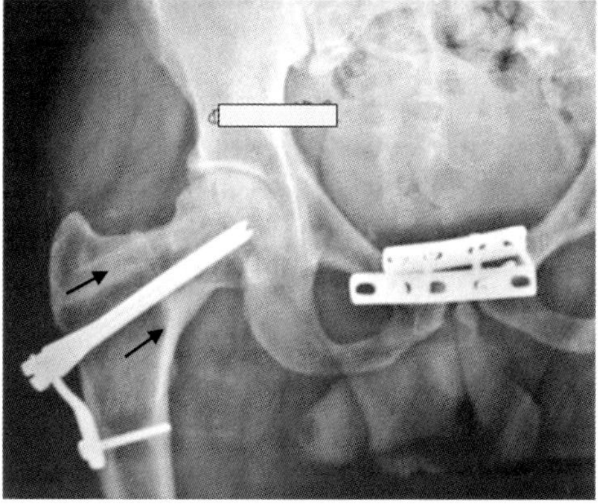

Figure 27.17 Fibula graft

care was taken to have rotational alignment at the shaft fracture site. Since the shaft fracture was managed by an open method, usually, one could achieve this by matching the fracture ends well.

Fixation of the Hip Fracture

The leg was turned to slight internal rotation at the hip. The appearance of the lesser trochanter is the guideline.

Managing the Associated Fracture of Neck of Femur

Usually 3 AM pins could be passed adjacent to the intramedullary nail in the femur. Out of these, two are usually anterior and one posterior to the nail. After insertion of the first AM pin, the fracture was gently impacted with a Bohler punch, to bring the neck fracture surfaces in contact opposition. Then the other two pins were inserted. (currently, it is called a miss, a nail technique). Being a young man, he could tolerate immobilization with Thomas' splint and was applied for six weeks. At the end of this period, the knee was mobilized. Gradually the knee range improved well. At the end of 10 to 12 weeks, there was no evidence of union in the neck of femur, while the shaft fracture was uniting well. The hip fracture required a secondary procedure, to achieve union in the neck of femur:

At this point of time, for the neck of the femur, a revision surgery was carried out on a fracture table, keeping the ipsilateral fibula area also draped and thigh tourniquet in place. The

K-nail was removed. Then the AM pins were removed and a mini SP nail and a plate were fixed. The mini SP nail was in the lower part of the neck. In the upper part, a guidewire was inserted and over it, a track was made with a DHS reamer. The length of fibula required was measured. The middle/3 area of a fibula is of round shape. Appropriate length of fibula was removed from this mid area. The narrow end of the fibula was trimmed like an arrow, for ease of entry and passage in the neck of the femur. The ridge on a side may be made round by a bone file. The fibula thus prepared was gently tapped on the prepared canal. If the resistance required is too much, it should be removed and canal made more wide. At this stage, the neck of the femur has an internal fixation device, while the femur shaft was to remodel completely. After completion of the procedure, the limb was again immobilized in a Thomas' splint for six weeks. At the end of 2 months, good union was observed at both the shaft and the neck. The limb immobilization may be little inconvenient, but assured a good outcome, leading to the fracture union (Fig. 27.18).

Case 10

A patient presented for the fracture of neck of femur, after 4 to 5 days from a peripheral area. The limb was not immobilized till arrival, which may have caused disturbance to the blood supply to the head of femur. The fracture was not reduced, nor immobilized and patient was transported for a long distance. On arrival after the diagnosis, immediate Thomas' splint was applied and surgery was planned. The chance of AVN and perhaps nonunion was obviously more. Hence, after closed reduction, internal fixation with a mini SP pin and a primary fibula grafting was done and the fracture united well. In such a situation, one may also use a pediatric DHS as the neck size was small (Fig. 27.19).

Case 11

A lady of 25 years of age had sustained ipsilateral fracture of shaft and neck of femur in RTA, in some other state. She was treated with a plate fixation for shaft of femur and no primary bone grafting for the shaft was

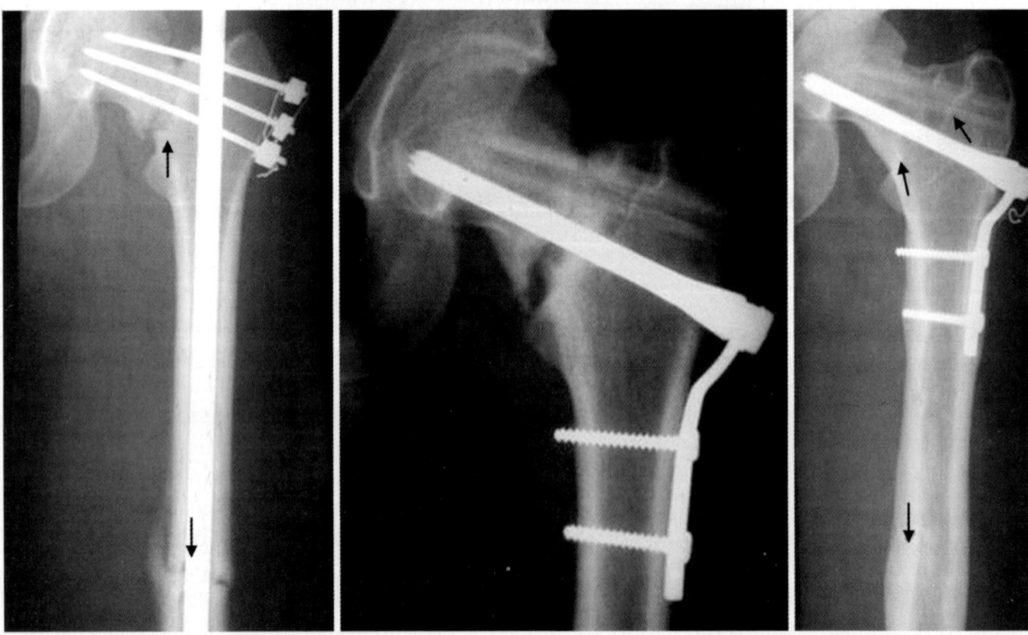

Figure 27.18 Ununited fracture of neck of femur and uniting fracture of shaft

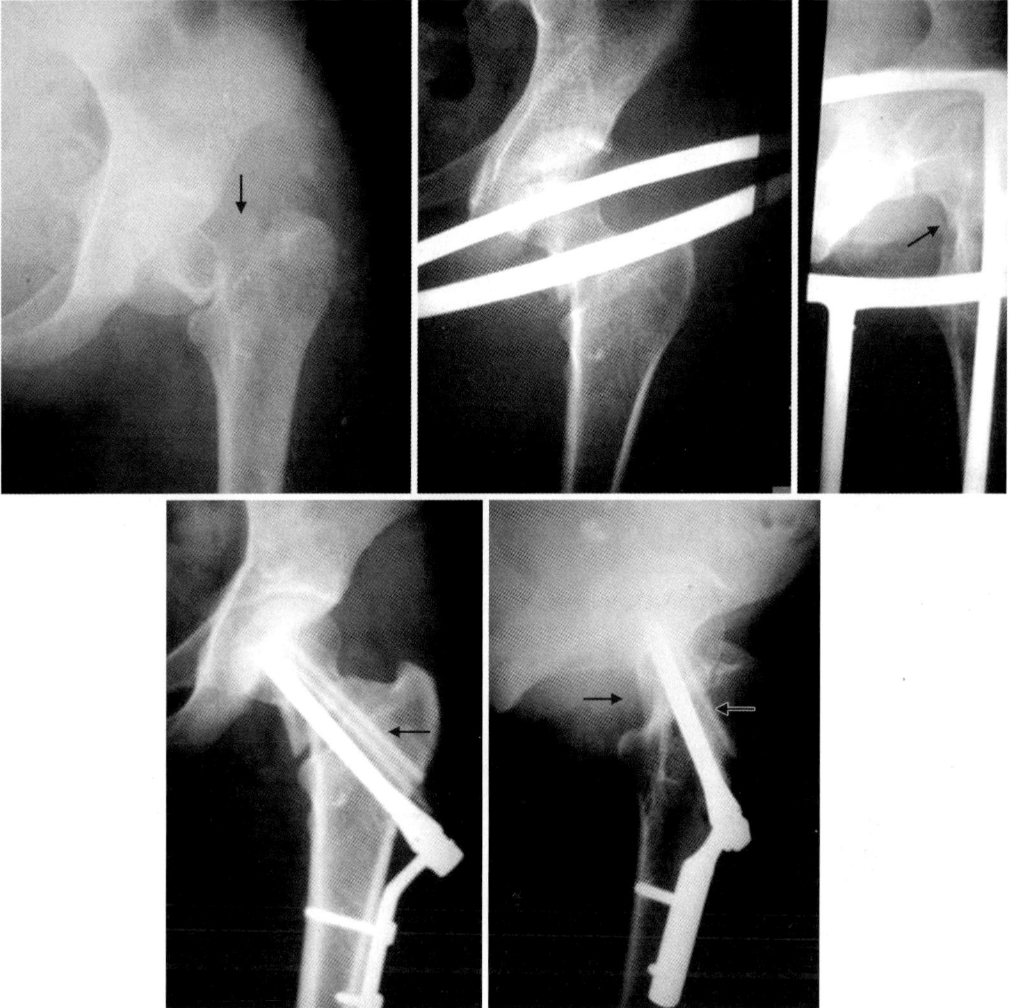

Figure 27.19 Late presentation of fracture of neck femur. Primary grafting

carried out. For the neck of the femur, a 6.5 mm screw and superior to it, a fibula was inserted. No external immobilization was given and she was gradually mobilized and brought to her home town later. This was the time, I saw her. At the end of the four months, the fracture of the shaft of femur continued to be radiologically ununited. The neck of femur was stable and the fracture line was not visible. Hence, for the shaft of femur, decortication and bone grafting was done and it united in due course.

Lesson

It is a teaching that, whenever a fracture shaft of femur is fixed with a plate, complementary primary bone grafting is mandatory. However, this teaching is not always followed and thus a revision surgery is needed, with loss of working days for the patient (Fig. 27.20).

Case 12

A young man had sustained a fracture of shaft, of femur in the mid/3 area. Was fixed with a

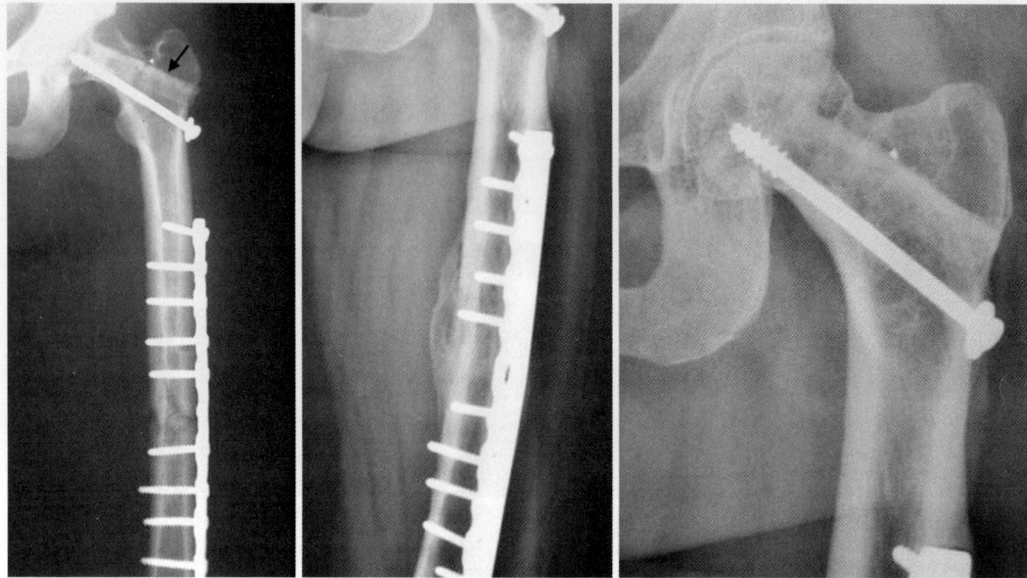

Figure 27.20 Fracture of neck and ipsilateral shaft of femur

plate and the fracture united in due course. The plate fixed on the femur shaft was not removed. Years later, he had another RTA and sustained a basi-trochanteric fracture on the same limb. A repeat X-ray was taken, with a scale by the side, to confirm, if a side plate of the DHS would be accommodated by the short segment, proximal to the previous plate. (Scanogram) The fracture of the neck femur was fixed with a DHS. One should keep one and two hole side plates for the DHS ready on the table and use the one which is accommodated above the proximal end of the femur plate. The fracture united in due course (Fig. 27.21).

Message One Gets

- After fixation of a shaft femur fracture with a plate, one should consider plate removal at appropriate time. After the plate removal, one needs to keep the person off the weight on the operated side and a careful follow up needs to be done till the stress shielding has disappeared and the bone elasticity restored. One needs to follow up and observe the following changes after a plate removal:
  - The cortex thickness under the plate should be restored back.
  - The screw tracks should fade out and the area be filled up with bone.
  - The trabeculi in the area should cross the fracture.
  - The strengthening and mobilizing exercises for the limb are important.
  - Weight bearing is later progressively increased.

All theses steps are necessary to achieve good restoration of bone strength and elasticity and avoid a possibility of a fracture through a screw hole.

There is a possibility of managing such a case of plate removal. After plate removal, one may insert an IM nail, as a protection against a refracture of femur. The nail may be a K-nail and not necessary to be interlocking nail. The latter procedure is more extensive, than a K-nail only. I have no experience of this procedure, but the thoughts are as follows:

- Insertion of a nail would maintain the continuity of the marrow cavity and the marrow circulation would be better. The bone remodeling will occur unrestricted.

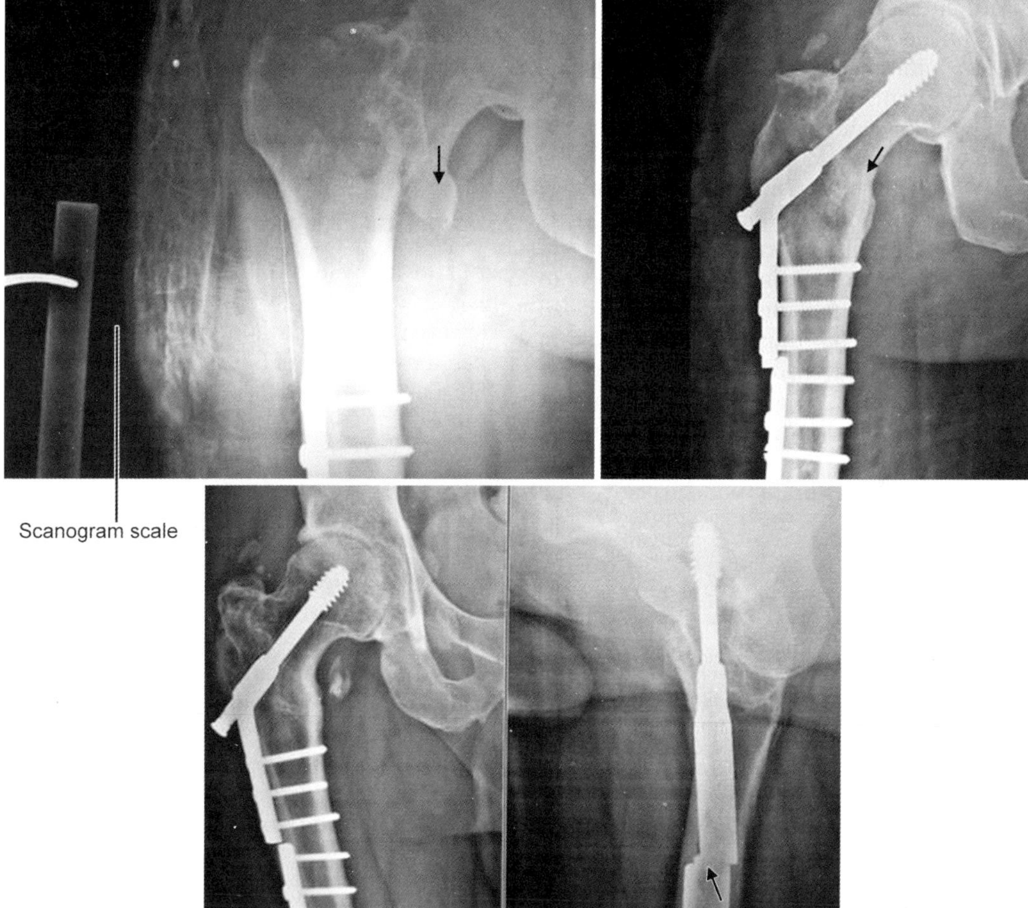

Figure 27.21 Previous fracture of shaft of femur

- Should there be another injury, the bone and the nail may just bend and the bone ends would not get displaced. Managing such an episode would be possible by a closed interlock nailing.
- After removal of the protection nail, there is no stress shielding of cortex and the recovery is relatively quick and assured.
- The important step is removal of the plate and screws, followed by having a negotiable medullary cavity. After a successful removal of all screws and the plate, bone trabeculi form across the medullary cavity along the screw tracks, which resist passage of a nail. Today, flexible reamers are available and the first reamer to be used is a fixed head reamer, with terminal cutting edge. This should be able to negotiate the screw tracks and prepare the canal.

Sequential fracture of neck of femur, following an ipsilateral fracture of shaft of femur:

A middle-age person had sustained a fracture shaft femur and was successfully treated by interlocking nail. The nail was not removed. After about fifteen years, had another fall and sustained an intracapsular fracture of neck of femur on the same side. The nail could be successfully removed and a cemented bipolar replacement was done. Prior to cement insertion short screws were reinserted in the proximal screw tracks from the lateral side, to prevent cement flowing out, during pressurization of cement. (The medial surface was unexposed and due to soft tissue cover, the cement did not flow out) (Fig. 27.22).

We were fortunate to be able to remove the femur interlock nail successfully 15 years after the procedure. Looking back at the above two cases, one feels, it should be a protocol to remove the femur implants, both a plate or a nail after the fracture has united well. However, in spite of advice so given, of all the cases, very few patients are willing for a procedure of implant removal and get it actually removed. Younger the patient, better the recovery, in terms of remodeling and restoration of elasticity of the bone.

Case 13

22 years ago, a young man of 40 sustained an intracapsular fracture of neck of femur on the right side. It was fixed with multiple AM pins and the fracture united in due course. One of the pins backed out, leading to local bursa formation. He also had changes of post-traumatic OA in the same hip. However, he was able to walk and carry on with his profession. Three years ago, he had another fall, sustained a fracture of neck of femur on the left (opposite) side. He was now over 65 years and an uncemented bipolar replacement was done on the left side (Fig. 27.23).

Segmental Fracture of Shaft of Femur

Prior to innovation of a reconstruction nail, plate fixation at both the sites was practised. However, with innovation of the nail, it has been possible to stabilize both the fracture with a nail, by closed technique (Figs 27.24 and 27.25).

FRACTURE OF NECK OF FEMUR IN ADOLESCENCE

Presence of epiphyseal plate makes the blood supply to the head of femur in children slightly different from that in adults. The preferred method of stabilization has been closed reduction and insertion of multiple Moore's pins. Senior teachers have recommended, after internal fixation by Moore's pins, application of a hip spica on table for six to eight weeks. The wound used to be dressed through a window

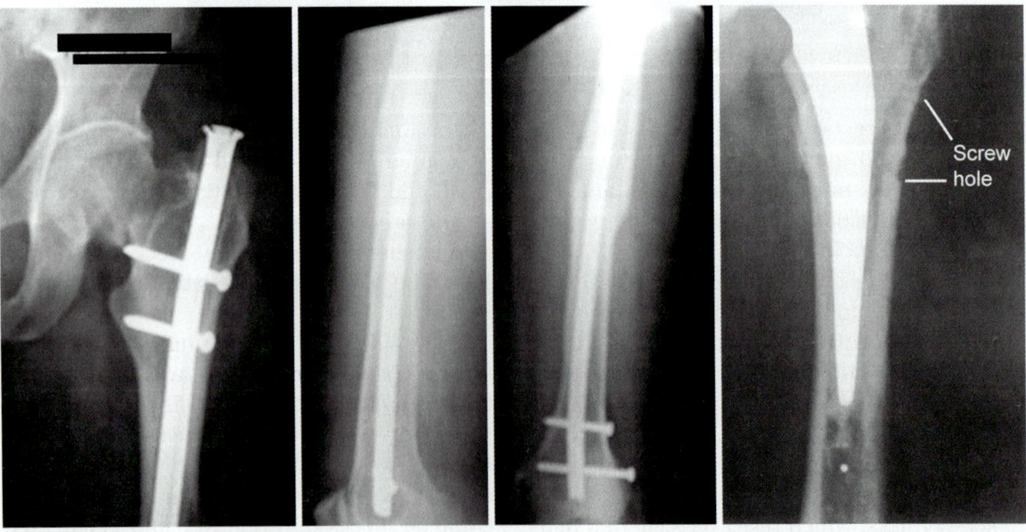

Figure 27.22 Sequential fracture of shaft of femur, followed by fracture of neck of femur

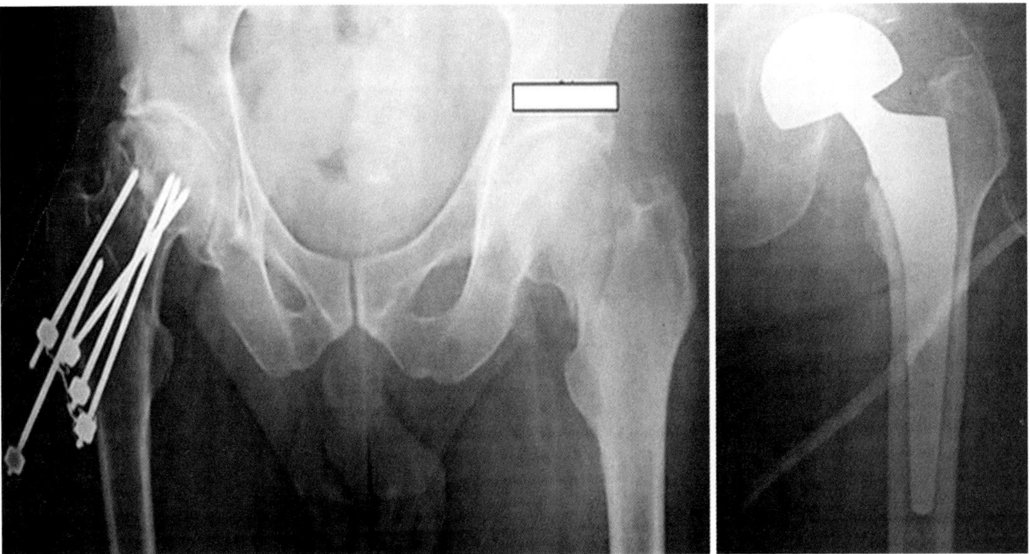

Figure 27.23 Sequential fracture of neck of femur

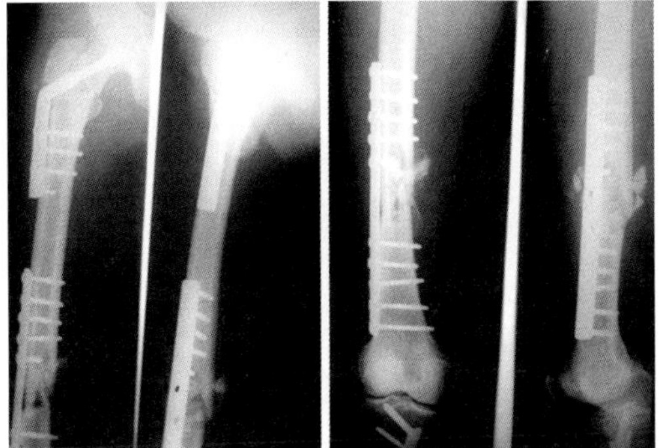

Figure 27.24 Ipsilateral fracture of neck and shaft plating

made in the hip spica. The fracture would unite. However, the long-term outcome would depend upon the restoration of blood supply to the head of femur.

A Moore pin has been a preferred implant. Due to the diamond shape tip, it penetrates the epiphyseal plate and does not cause growth disturbance (Fig. 27.26).

In a few cases of fracture of neck fixed by AM pins and plaster spica, a few cases developed varus and problem of union. Hence, in mid 70s, a trend had come up, to carry out a defunctioning intertrochanteric or subtrochanteric osteotomy. This protected the fracture area from adductor forces and the fracture would unite well. However, there was no control on maintaining the position of osteotomy ends and hence some unwanted displacement also occurred within a spica. My preference would be internal fixation and a spica cast alone, may be for 1 ½ limbs, as used to be done in yester years, with a good outcome (Fig. 27.27).

Currently, more reliance is on cannulated cancellous screws, inserted short of epiphyseal plate.

Today perhaps a surgeon depends upon fixation with cannulated cancellous screws and no external immobilization is given. In due course of time, some bone resorption occurs on either side of a fracture. Maybe, during early mobilization, perhaps some weight-bearing is also done. This leads to loss of hold of the screws on the distal trochanteric fragment and implant back out or cut out is observed. (When a screw backs out slightly, the compressive hold on the bone is lost. The screw shaft on the lateral cortex is contained in a wider track made

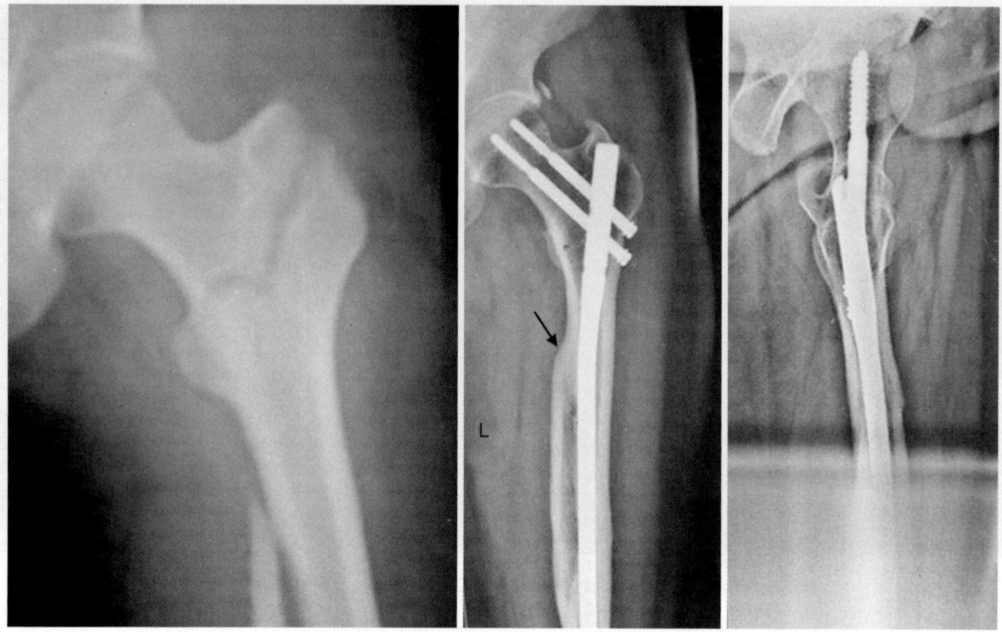

Figure 27.25 Ipsilateral neck and shaft fracture: AFN

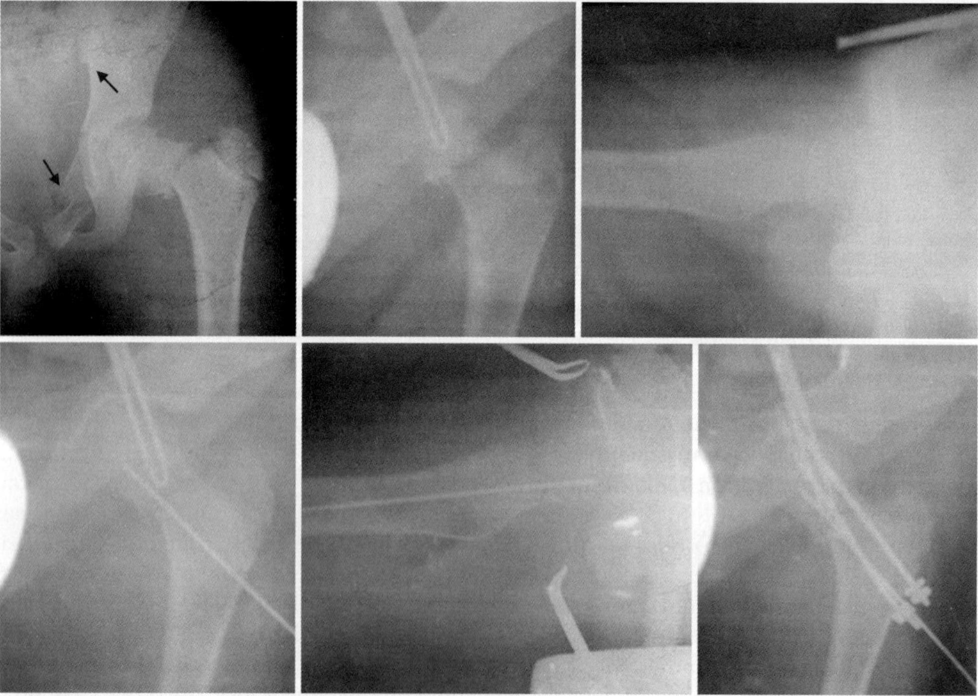

Figure 27.26 Fracture of neck of femur in adolescent

by the threads and the screw is free to toggle). Again, one feels, if plaster spica immobilization is given, on table itself, the fracture would get good rest and protection from external stresses and union would occur in expected duration. Spica for six to eight weeks is a less cost to pay in terms of inconvenience than the management of screw cut out and the status of the hip at the end (Fig. 27.28).

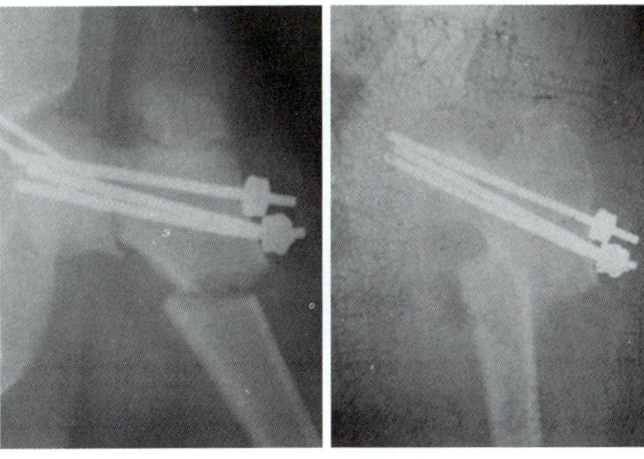

Figure 27.27 Osteotomy getting displaced

OSTEOTOMY IN FRACTURE OF NECK OF FEMUR

For delayed or fibrous union, McMurray's osteotomy is useful. The picture shows few methods of fixation. Knowle pin fixation, osteotomy and spica lead to a good outcome, as shown.

To dispense with the spica cast, Tipmann plate was used. However, the stability of the assembly was only by the top screw, which often gave way. Hence, again a spica cast or a well-fitting and abduction maintained Thomas' splint was necessary.

Subtrochanteric osteotomy with excess valgus osteotomy, often leads to avascular changes and arthritis (Fig. 27.29A).

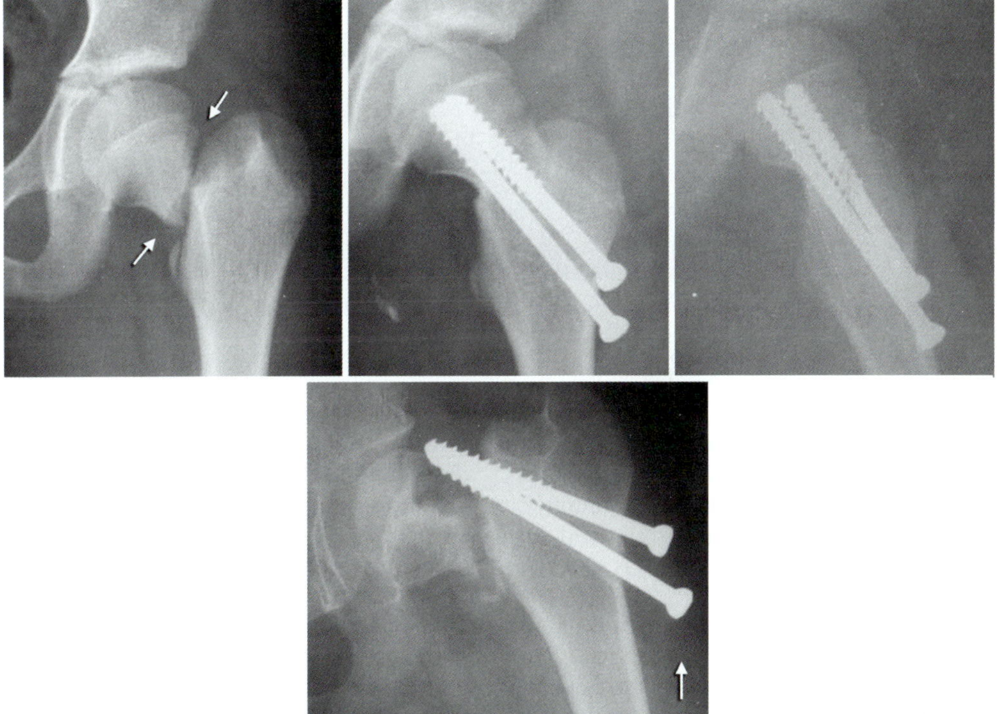

Figure 27.28 Importance of hip spica cast

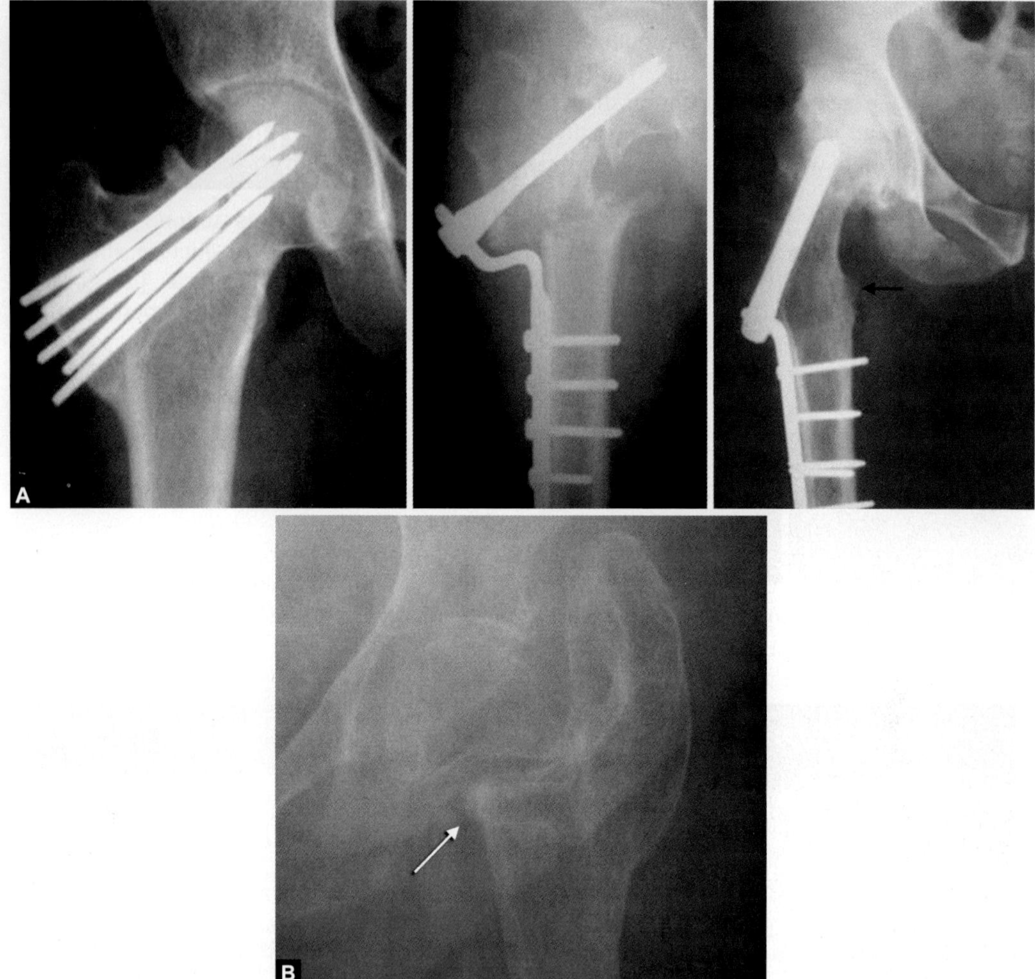

Figures 27.29A and B (A) Methods of osteotomy fixation; (B) Osteotomy without fixation

Prior to fixation of intertrochanteric osteotomy, only hip spica was given and the osteotomy united well. At times, the fracture of neck of femur may continue to be ununited and the angular support created supported the head of femur and the instability was reduced (Fig. 27.29B).

A middle age person had sustained a fracture of neck of femur. Was fixed with a mini SP pin and cancellous screws. However, the fracture displaced and did not unite. He reported at this stage for further management.

Hence, a reposition osteotomy was planned. A fracture table was used. Preoperative drawings were done and the procedure was carried out.

The previous implants were removed. The fragments were stabilized with a K-wire in the superior part of the trochanter and the head femur.

Osteotomy and the wedge was marked and drill holes made along the proposed site of bone cut, to weaken the lateral cortex. The direction of osteotomy was confirmed that it was above the lesser trochanter.

A guidewire was inserted at the proposed place of the 120 degree reposition plate blade component (double angled plate) and a track was made along the guidewire with a seating chisel. It is important to do this step, prior to the osteotomy, when the continuity of the shaft exists. (Once the osteotomy is made, the proximal femur becomes mobile and this step becomes tedious).

The osteotomy was completed with a 10 mm thin blade osteotome, step by step. Both the anterior and the posterior cortices need to be cut or else the corresponding deformity would occur.

The distal fragment was gently displaced medially. At any step, the limb traction was not changed. The 120 degree reposition plate blade was inserted close to the guidewire, keeping parallel to the guidewire. (The illustrated case was done in pre 'C' arm era and hence an X-ray was exposed to confirm the position). The proximal end of the distal fragment was purposefully kept medially. Fixation of the plate was started from the second hole from the lower end. The screw length needs to be taken slightly more, to engage the far cortex. As one proceeds to insert screws from below upwards, sequentially, the uppermost end of the distal fragment comes laterally and interfragmentory compression occurs across the osteotomy, stabilizing the osteotomy.

Finally, a 4.5 mm screw was inserted in the proximal fragment inferior to the blade component, to have a more hold on the proximal fragment.

Postoperatively a Thomas' splint was applied for six weeks and the limb maintained in abduction. The recovery was uneventful and union occurred well. Gradually the post-immobilization knee stiffness reduced, so he

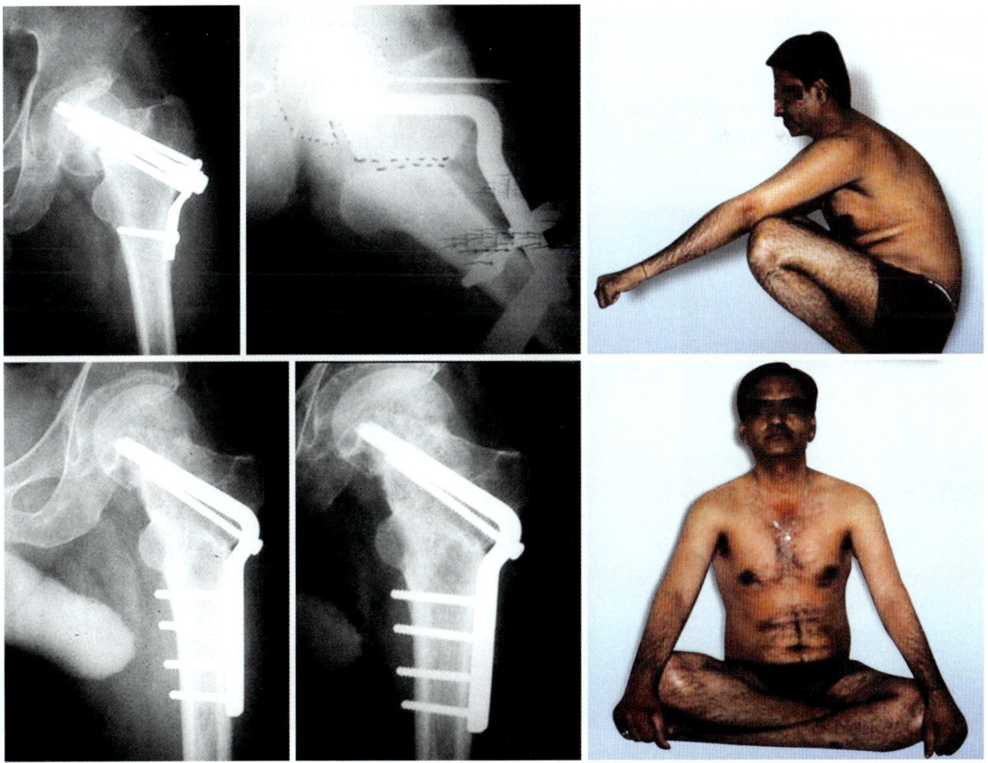

Figure 27.30 Reposition osteotomy

could squat and sit cross-legged as well, in due course of time.

Follow-Up

At the end of 12 years, he was symptom free. However, at the end of 20 years, some pain and limp appeared, indicating changes of osteoarthritis (Figs 27.30 and 27.31).

Postoperative Infection

Infection is an unfortunate complication after an internal fixation, especially in an intra-articular fracture. This young man had an intracapsular fracture of neck of femur and was fixed by a DHS and a 6.5 mm screw. Postoperative recovery was uneventful. During follow up after few months, had pain in the operated hip and X-ray showed erosion in the superior surface of the neck of femur. The lower half of the neck showed good union. Hence all the implants were removed and he was advised not to bear weight on the leg. However, he continued to have pain and the X-ray showed further destruction of the hip area. MRI confirmed the same.

Hence, a staged procedure was planned. The head and the neck were removed, joint clearance was done and an antibiotic impregnated cement spacer was inserted. The hip was immobilized in a Thomas' splint for six weeks. Then markers like ESR/C. Reactive proteins, etc. were studied. In spite of the skin traction, the upper end of the femur migrated upwards, as expected. He was admitted and upper tibial skeletal traction was applied. The proximal end of the femur was thus brought down as much as possible, which would make the surgery relatively easy.

Removal of the spacer and uncemented THR was done. During insertion of the stem, a crack appeared in the proximal femur and a circlage wire was added. He is doing well as of a year after THR (Figs 27.32 and 27.33).

A patient came for a second opinion and the history is as follows: He had sustained injury to the right hip and thigh in an RTA. He was operated and a reconstruction nail was inserted, so both the neck and the shaft could be fixed. The postoperative X-ray shows the shaft femur to be in external rotation, as per the appearance of lesser trochanter. Unfortunately, infection occurred and the surgeon removed the neck bolt. The fracture of neck continued to be ununited. Patient was permitted to move

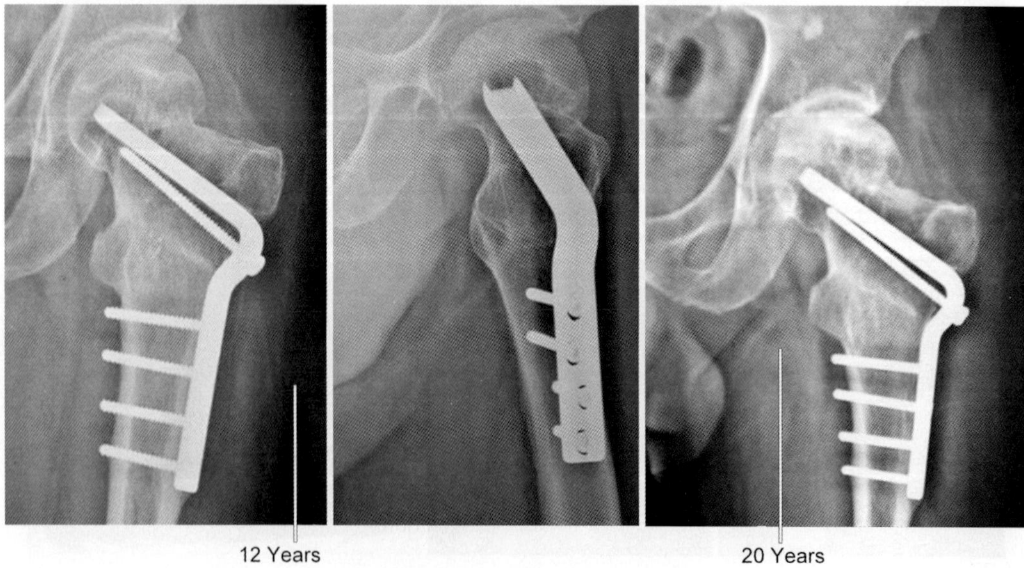

Figure 27.31 Reposition osteotomy

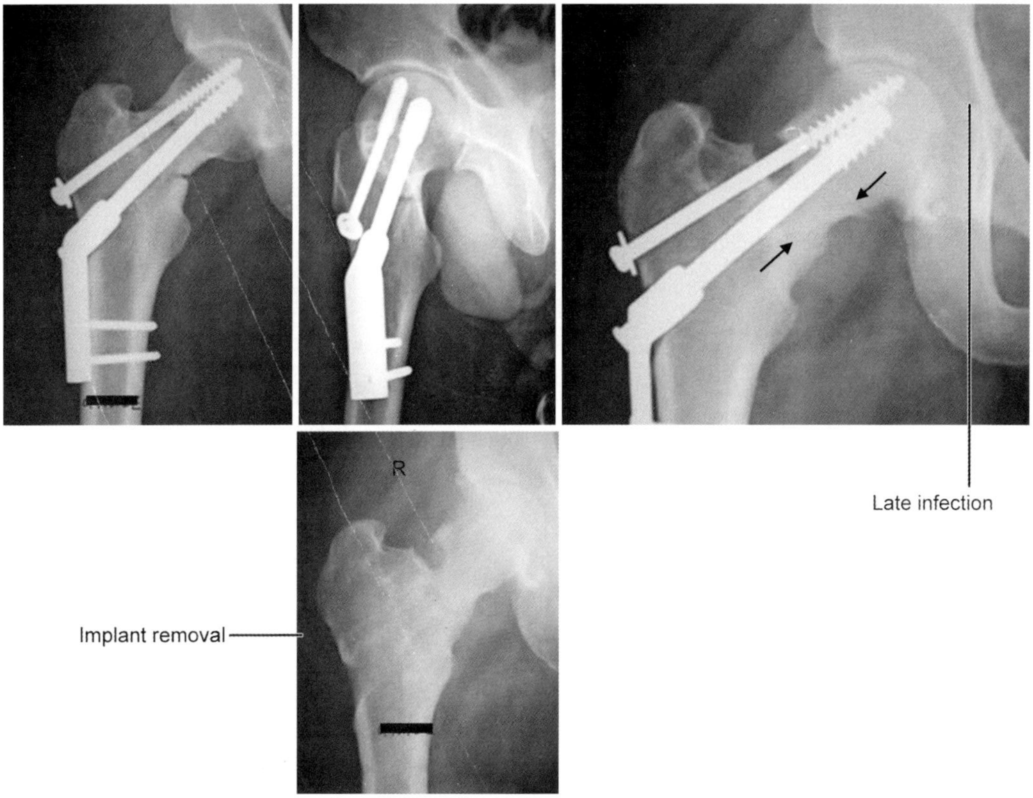

Late infection

Implant removal

Figure 27.32 Late infection

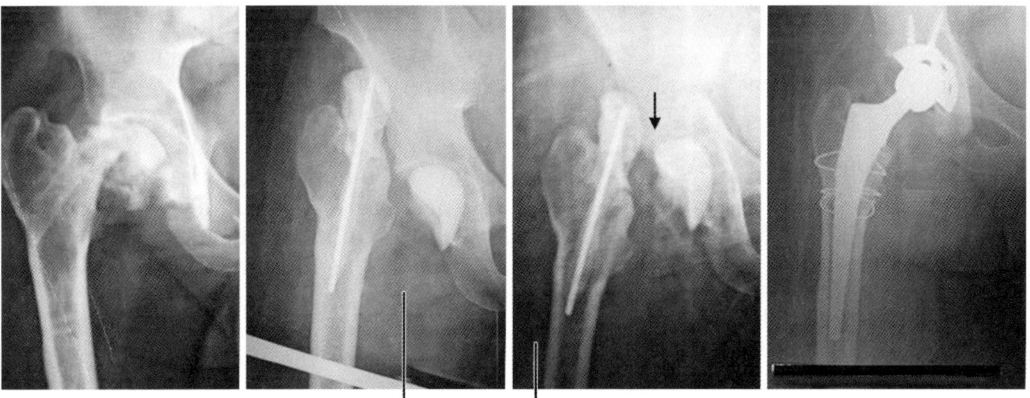

Figure 27.33 Late infection

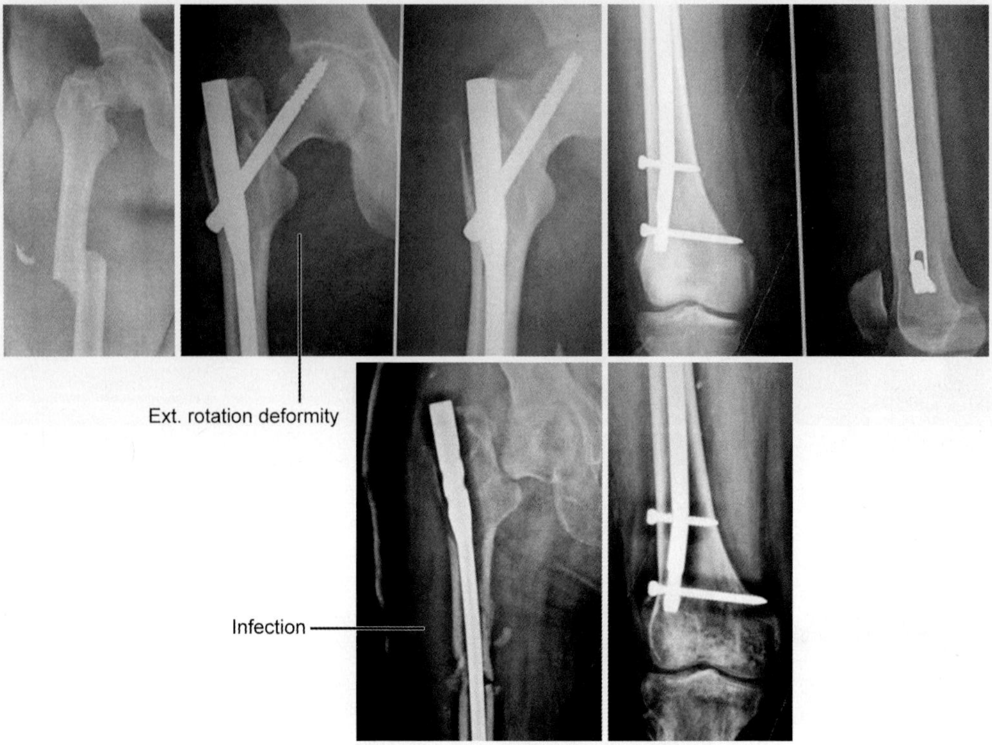

Ext. rotation deformity

Infection

Figure 27.34 Inadequate reduction, followed by infection

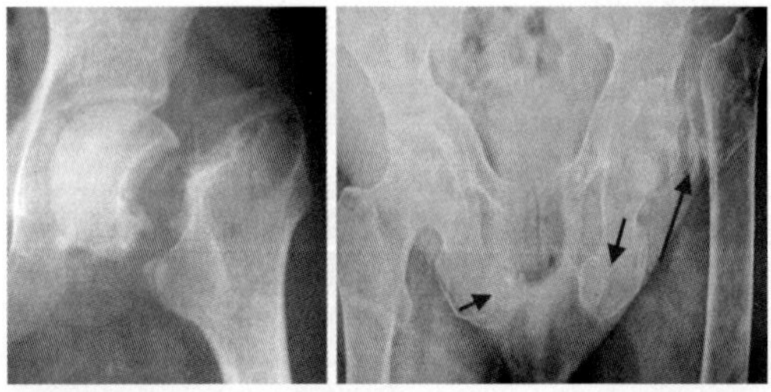

Figure 27.35 Non-union fracture of neck of femur

about with a walker. The fullness around the thigh, X-ray appearance of the shaft of femur indicates continued infection. It was at this stage that he consulted for an opinion. No follow up was informed (Fig. 27.34).

In the Past

Due to lack of medical care in the peripheral areas, a standard treatment was not available, and even if offered, every patient did not accept it. Locally available splints were applied and gradually the hip became pain free. The patient is then gradually able to walk with shortening and lurch and the family accepted the outcome. An intracapsular or a basi-trochanteric fracture resulted in non-union, while a pertrochanteric fracture united with shortening and external rotation deformity (Fig. 27.35).

In the last few decades, the understanding of the fracture treatment has improved and the necessary operative treatment is possible and available. Most of the fractures united and patient returned to the professional activity. However, in few cases, the avascular necrosis of head of femur, or changes of osteoarthritis are observed, which required THR in due course.

Observation

- Whenever, an intracapsular fracture of neck of femur ends with a gap non-union, the head usually remains vascular, as seen on the X-ray film.

- Whenever, one observes a change of avascular necrosis in the head of femur, the fracture in almost all cases has united. The possible causes of increased density in an avascular bone put forth are:
  - Dead bone attracts calcium ions from the adjacent tissues
  - Calcium is deposited in a dead tissue
  - The bone collapses and hence more tissue is per square area (Fig. 27.36).

Some cases of intracapsular fracture of neck of femur, united well, did not have changes of AVN or OA, even at the end of 30 years from the injury, as observed in this case. He has a good function in the injured hip (Fig. 27.37).

STRESS FRACTURE

A young man started preparation for a physical test for entry in police department. He started this very aggressively all of a sudden. The extent of the distance covered and the speed was increased too rapidly and that too on a hard surface. He developed a painful limp on both the sides and presented for treatment. X-ray of pelvis did not reveal any injury and hence a nuclear scan was done. This indicated bilateral stress fracture in neck femora. He was advised to take rest in the bed. However, as soon as the pain reduced, he resumed the practice again, against the medical advice. Within 10 days, he had pain in the hips and presented with a pair of crutches. Repeat X-ray showed an incomplete subcapital fracture of neck of femur on the right side.

The right hip was internally fixed and a Thomas' splint applied, to be sure that he remains in the bed for six weeks. In due course of time, both the hips became pain free and the fractures united (Fig. 27.38).

TYPES OF PARTIAL HIP REPLACEMENT

The hip prosthesis is either a Thompson or an Austin Moore prosthesis. It has different sizes of head diameter, but the stem size and the neck length is the same.

Later on Monk design was developed wherein, due to motion at two levels, the range of motion improved. With innovation of bone cement, stem is fixed in the femur and the incidence of loosening of the stem and related complications decreased (Fig. 27.39).

Approximately since 20 years hence, cement restrictor, indigenous cement gun and restrictor were available. This helped to pressurize the cement in the femoral canal and stem fixation improved remarkably. The incidence of stem loosening and sinking of the stem in the shaft, drastically reduced (Figs 27.40 and 27.41).

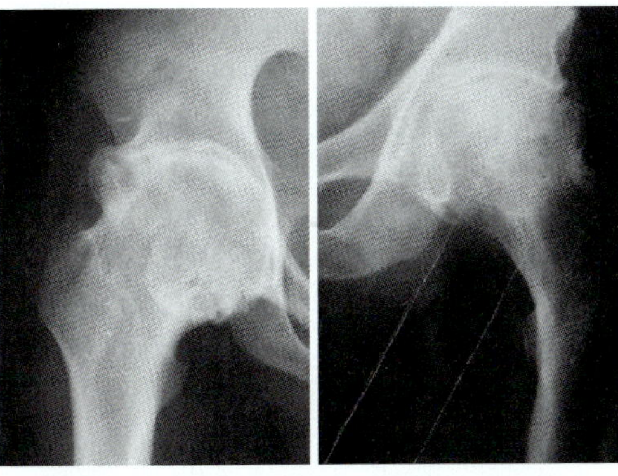

Figure 27.36 Late OA after fracture union

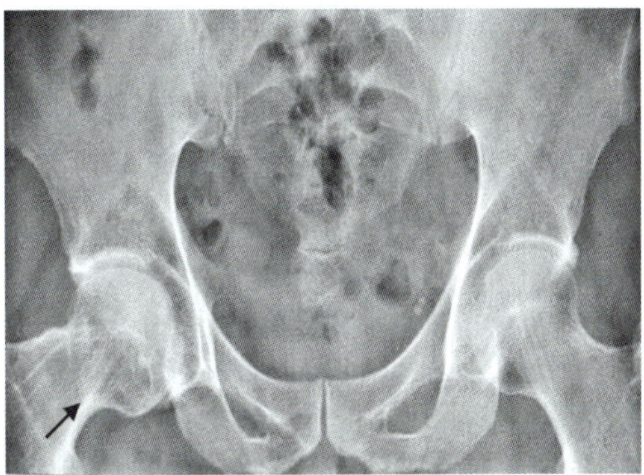

Figure 27.37 United fracture of neck of femur with good function at the end of 30 years

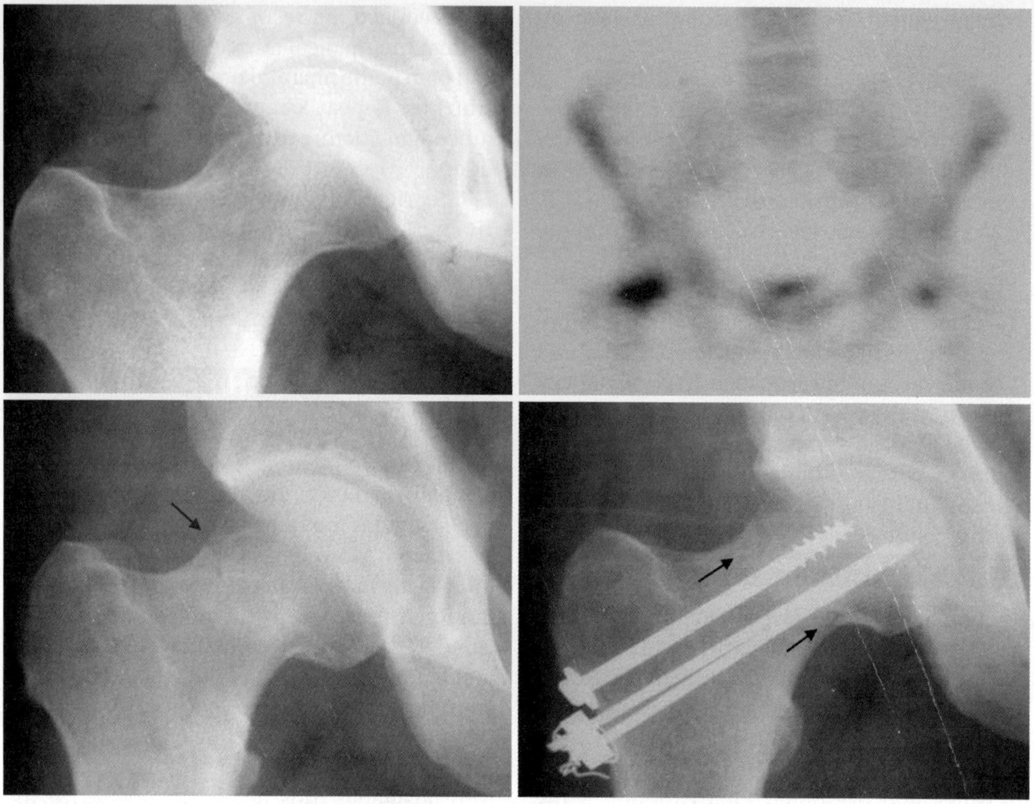

Figure 27.38 Stress fracture of neck of femur

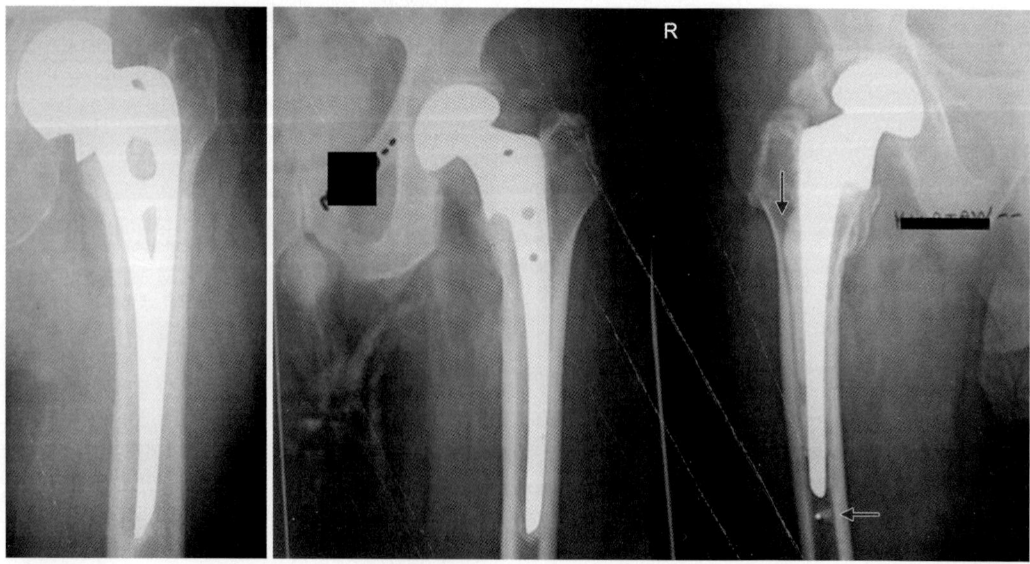

Figure 27.39 Types of prosthesis

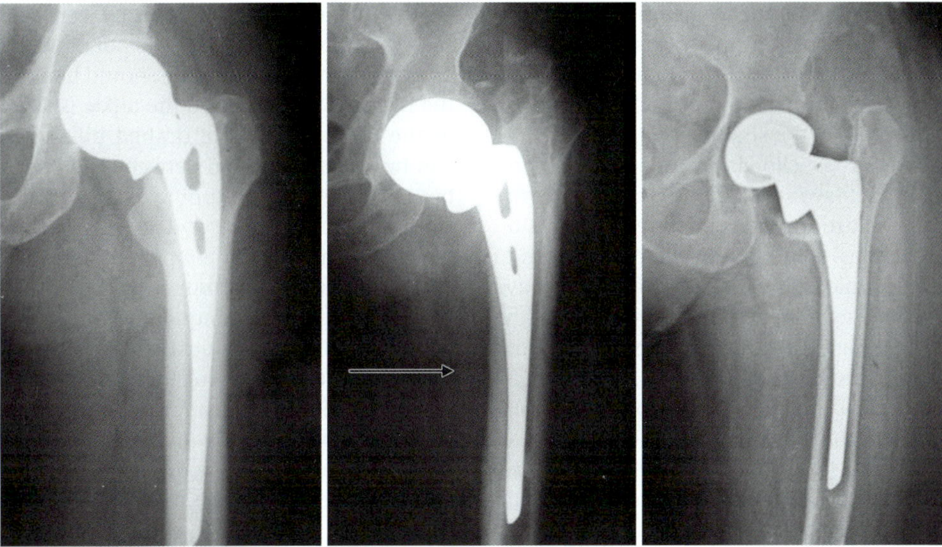

Figure 27.40 Sunk prosthesis

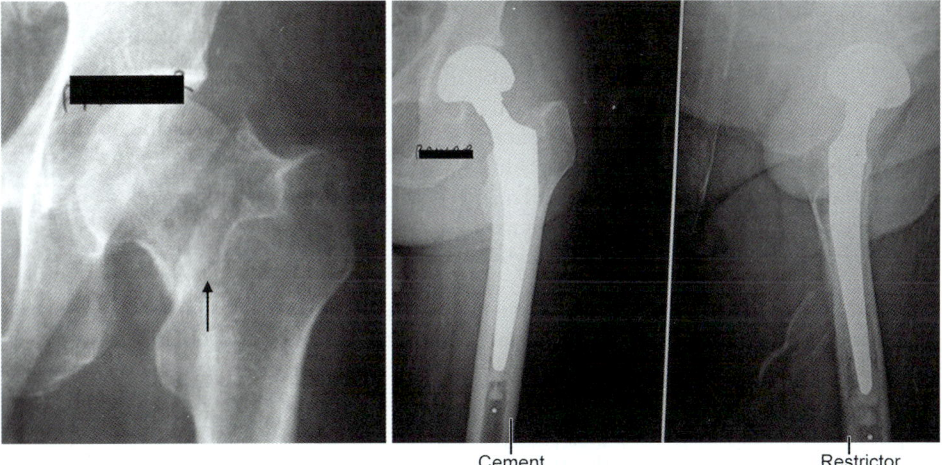

Figure 27.41 Bipolar cemented stem

FIRST AID ON ARRIVAL AND DIAGNOSIS

- *X-ray examination*: AP film as the patient is lying is taken.
- Then, with the traction on the leg on, I would gently internally rotate the leg and take X-ray in this position, to know the length of the neck and the level of fracture.
- X-ray of opposite hip: AP and cross-table lateral X-rays are taken to study the diameter of the medullary cavity, especially to know, if it is too narrow, for even a small stem. Lateral view shows if there is excessive anterior

bowing of the femur in the proximal part. If so, even short stem prosthesis tip may abut against the anterior cortex of femur. The use of a broach then has to be careful, to prevent perforation of the shaft of femur.

Usually the clinician can, gently and gradually, achieve some internal rotation of the hip, to be able to apply a below knee skin traction and a Thomas' splint. Every clinician desires to avoid a possible AVN of the head of femur. I have been trained to reduce a fracture on arrival at the earliest, take an X-ray of the hip on the table and apply a well-fitting Thomas' splint. I feel, with an unreduced hip fracture, there would be excess tension on the vessels nourishing the head of femur and if one has reduced the fracture, further disturbance of blood supply to the head of femur is reduced. One has, thus, taken every effort to maintain the blood supply to the head of femur and offered pain relief because of closed reduction, till further definitive reduction and internal fixation is carried out.

Besides, even if one considers the additional cost of this procedure of closed reduction on arrival, it is quite less compared to the total cost of the treatment. If one takes this effort, one has done everything possible to reduce further damage. (I am aware, few studies do show, that the loss of circulation to head of femur has occurred at the time of initial injury only. However, the pain relief offered by a well-reduced hip fracture is also important).

IMPORTANT STEPS IN A BIPOLAR REPLACEMENT

Few important steps are described and reader should refer to the necessary books for the entire procedure and the technique.

Patient Position

Posterior approach is described here. The surgeon himself should arrange the patient position, to avoid problem and irritation during the surgery. If the operation table has suitable anterior and posterior supports to maintain position they are used. Alternatively wooden supports are used (Fig. 27.42).

The pelvis should be exactly vertical and stable, so after draping, it does not move about. The leg on the opposite side should be flexed in the hip and the knee and the ankle is strapped to the table. To have a draped pillow, which can be later inserted in between the knees is a better option than strapping it to the table. The vacuum suction tube and electrocautery are placed on the front of the patient and the tube and the cable should come from the front of the patient. Wide and adequately long stockinet should be sterile. The stockinet should be folded in a W shape and not rolled, while it is loaded for sterilization. The steam would not penetrate all the way in a rolled stockinet. Indigenously available sterile Y shape drapes cover the area well, followed by sterile adhesive transparent sheet. The expenditure on such disposable articles is well worth.

Exposure

The greater trochanter and PSIS are palpated and marked. Surgeon stands behind the patient, while the assistant on the front. The instrument trolley is towards the leg side, adjacent to the surgeon. This makes it possible for the surgeon to pick up instruments himself and also for the scrub nurse to hand over to the surgeon.

After incising the subcutaneous fat, as one sees the deep fascia, the fat layer is erased from the fascia. This helps to identify the layers during closure. The fascia is incised and usually the trochanteric bursa needs to be excised. The short external rotators and the pyriformis muscle are identified and are tagged with vicryl at two places. The muscles are then erased from the insertion, with an electrocautery and the tagged vicryl threads are taken over the posterior edge of the wound. This improves the retraction and protects the sciatic nerve as well. Often erasing the insertion of ileopsoas helps the exposure. The hip capsule is incised and fracture is identified. The proposed level of the bone cut on the neck is marked with a cautery or a pen. This point is usually 12 mm from the upper end of the lesser trochanter. With a power saw, the cut is made. Saline irrigation is not required, if the blade is sharp. (Irrigation

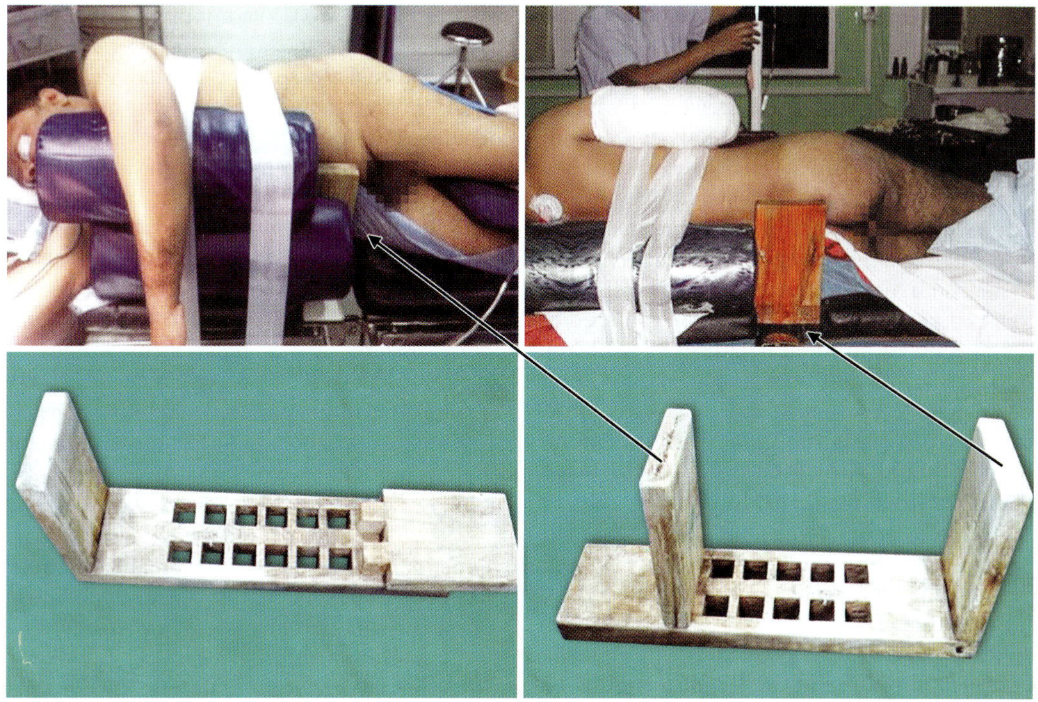

Figure 27.42 Wooden pelvic support

during a saw cut, splashes it all around!) The cut part of the neck is removed with a towel clip. This creates more space to remove the head of femur. Usually a towel clip can catch the head of femur well and remove it from the acetabulum after cutting the ligamentum teres. It is necessary to submit the head for HPE to avoid any surprises later on.

The tissue on the medial side of the greater trochanter is excised, to facilitate insertion of the canal finder/taper pin reamer. The adjacent lateral part of the neck is removed with a nibbler, so a canal finder can be well-aligned, just medial to the lateral femoral cortex. With a taper pin reamer the canal is entered and gently reamed. Though, one has studied the canal width on an X-ray film, this step also gives idea about the canal roominess. (It is necessary to have a true size AP and lateral X-ray of the proximal femur of the to-be-operated or the opposite side, to study the anterior bowing of upper femur, which is common in this area. This has relevance in planning the stem length).

Thereafter, a rasp is used serially from small to large size. It is preferable to insert it in 15 degree of anteversion every time, so the stem will enter in the same direction. At times, a large rasp enters the canal in neutral position, but not in anteversion. In such a case, it is necessary to insert a medium stem, which can be inserted in anteversion. This is important or else, correct anteversion cannot be obtained, with a likelihood of dislocation of the prosthesis. A trial stem mounted on an introducer is inserted in anteversion and gently tapped. Further steps in trial reduction are well known. In a case where the canal is too narrow, it is safe to ream it well with power reamer. This should permit insertion of a small stem in correct anteversion.

The neck offset has to be adequate. If it is less, then during external rotation of the hip, the intertrochanteric crest on the posterior surface of the trochanter abuts against the posterior wall of acetabulum and the degree of external rotation is restricted.

The length of the trial stem is noted. The diameter of a cement restrictor available is suitable for a large femoral canal. In a patient with a narrow canal, the restrictor may get jammed before it reaches down till the desired level. Hence, one needs to cut alternate petals from the root, to make it narrow and supple. In addition, the length of petals may also need to be trimmed. After the restrictor is placed at the desired depth, the introducer is removed. At this stage again the trial stem mounted on introducer is inserted in the canal to confirm that it can freely traverse in the femoral canal till the desired level, indicating that the cement restrictor is seated at the correct level. If this step is not done and if the restrictor had inadvertently tilted and is placed more proximally, then what would happen? After introduction of the cement, while the final stem is being inserted, one may find that the final stem cannot go down till the desired level, due to the placement of the restrictor more superiorly, a disaster indeed!

Cement type: Time taken for curing, etc. One can refer to manual for technical details. The cement curing is related to the temperature at which it is stored prior to the surgery, the ambient room temperature in the operation room, etc.

In early years, one would manually knead the ball of soft cement in the femoral canal. With availability of a cement gun, one can insert the cement from the depth and gradually proximally, filling the canal completely from below upwards. The stage of curing at which one inserts the cement is important. It is put in the cement gun, while in a fluid stage and the nozzle is attached to the gun. The cement is delivered till the gun nozzle tip and the curing stage is checked. When it becomes non-tacky, the nozzle is inserted in the canal and the cement inserted distal to proximally, upwards in the canal. Gradually the gun nozzle is withdrawn from the canal, as the canal gets filled. Then, the cement is manually pressurized, so it enters the cancellous endosteal surface, to interdigitate well. The final stem prosthesis, mounted on the introducer, is inserted along the endosteal surface of the lateral cortex and in correct anteversion. It is important to observe that while the stem is being inserted, proportionate quantity of cement is displaced and there is a backflow from the canal, as the stem is advanced. This indicated that the stem is entering the correct passage in the medullary canal. (See a case described later).

In a case having very narrow medullary cavity, where just a small stem would be accommodated, it is preferable to insert the cement in a rather fluid state. If it is inserted in the usual viscid state, insertion of the stem could be difficult, so much that, one may not be able to insert it fully till the desired level.

After the cement has set well, again a trial reduction is done and final head and neck assembly is put in. At this stage, one should assess the hip stability, while hip is in 90 deg flexion and some internal rotation.

During the exposure of the hip, the capsule and the acetabular labrum is incised. During closure of the joint, the labrum should be sutured back.

If the tendon of gluteus maximus at the insertion was cut for some reason, it is reattached. One should reattach the tagged external rotators and pyriformis to the trochanter. At the posterior border of the greater trochanter, drill holes are made with a 2 mm K-wire. An ethilon loop of 3/0 size on a straight needle is passed through a hole in greater trochanter, picks up the vicryl tagged to muscles. Both the tagged external rotator sutures are thus brought through the trochanter and tied together. This trans-osseous suture reconstructs the posterior structures and enhances the hip stability.

Closed suction drain tubes are inserted and wound closed in layers. Adequate gamjee padding and application of a crepe spica is a method one should try. It supports the posterior structures well, offers good pain relief and the wound remains supple. This support helps tissue layer co-option, reduces dead space if any and prevents hematoma formation in the posterior dependent area. The wound heals more kindly. This benefit is complementary to the closed suction drainage. It is worthwhile trying this technique, by those, who have not practiced it still.

Instruments to be Kept as Standby

- TBW set
- Narrow plate fixation set (may be locking plate as well, should some fracture in shaft occur)
- Straight rigid femur reamers
- Power drill/and flexible reamer set with 6 to 10 mm reamer heads. If the canal is found, to be too narrow, the 6 and 7 mm reamers, which are used in shoulder replacement are useful.
- Size 37 cup and extra small diameter stem. Not all manufacturing resources prepare this, but one should try to make them available.

The dictum: If one keeps everything ready, usually it is not required!

- Preferably take an X-ray of pelvis with both hips, to know the neck shaft angle, the depth of the acetabulum and the lateral curvature of femur.
- Try to have a lateral view X-ray of the proximal femur. A cross table lateral view shows both: the diameter of the canal and the degree of anterior bowing of the femur. The X-ray should be of true size, to calculate the canal diameter.

FEW TECHNICAL THINGS

- In a non-modular design, a trial stem is not available. The level for the neck cut is decided by a visual judgment. If proper lateralization of the canal level of the neck cut is not done, the stem would not sit properly at the correct level in the canal and may continue to be at a higher level than desired. This leads to leg lengthening (Fig. 27.43).
- When the final stem is being inserted and tapped home, one should observe the trochanteric area, to know, if a crack develops in the bone. If a crack appears, a prophylactic circlage wire is inserted around the trochanter. If one takes the loop above the lesser trochanter, it stays there and does not slide down, when loaded or with time. If necessary, a 2.5 mm drill hole is made in the proper area and a 0.8 mm wire is threaded through it. When such a circlage is added, during reduction of the prosthesis, only continuous traction and local pressure on the head is given, to reduce the head in the acetabulum. In a case like this, it is safe to start weight bearing little late, as per the extent of the crack and the stability achieved.

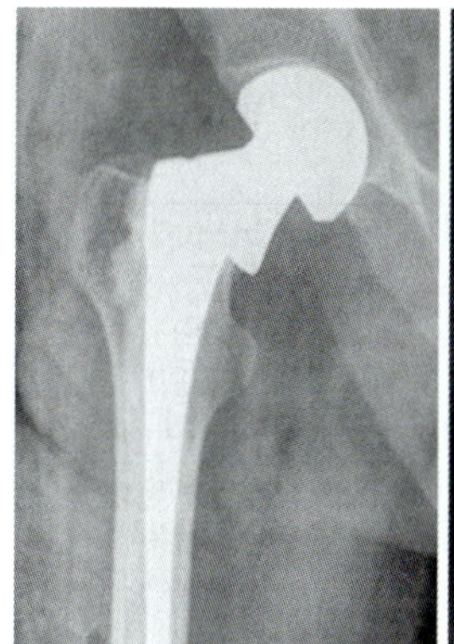
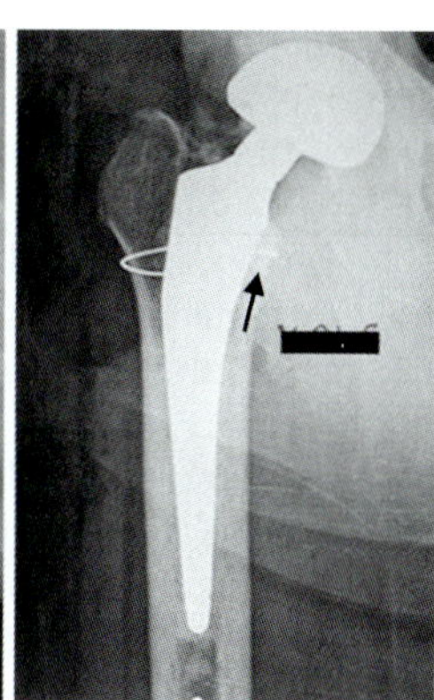

Figure 27.43 Techniques in bipolar

- At times, the patient may present late or surgery needs to be delayed, due to medical problems. When surgery is delayed more than a week, it is preferable to add upper tibial skeletal traction, to keep the trochanter at its place or else reduction of the prosthesis is difficult. Thus, if a patient has to be in supine position, with a skeletal traction on, one should arrange for a water or an air bed, to prevent bedsores. Once a sore occurs, it is difficult to manage it. Besides, it is quite close to the operative field. The patient takes a position in bed, such that the pressure sore always occurs on the gluteal area on the same side as the fracture.

Thus for some reason, if the surgery is delayed:

In such a case, the incision should be generous and may be one has to release the insertion of gluteus maximus and quadratus femoris as well.

One may come across some uncommon appearances of acetabulum or the proximal femur. One needs to be careful in such a case and hence this write up.

A gentleman age 70 years reported with a fracture of neck of left femur. X-ray of pelvis was taken. Both the hips had coxa vara. On detailed interrogation, he informed he had some abnormal gait since childhood. However, the depth of the acetabulum was satisfactory and hence, a cemented bipolar replacement was successful. Possibly, he had bilateral slipped capital femoral epiphysis (SCFE) (Fig. 27.44).

A lady, more than 75 years of age, had sustained a fracture neck of left femur. The X-ray revealed possibly a shallow acetabulum. A cemented bipolar replacement was done. Unfortunately in the postoperative hospital stay the prosthesis head dislocated, which was promptly reduced and she was kept in bed for further three weeks. After the discharge, in her home, she dislocated the hip again. She remained in home for two weeks with the hip dislocated, because of some family matters. Revision surgery planned:

She was more than 75 years of age and bones were osteoporotic.

Plan and what was Done

- Exposure through the previous posterior approach.
  Options →
- If the anteversion is incorrect, change the stem and insert in correct anteversion.
- If anteversion is correct, change the head to one with more offset.

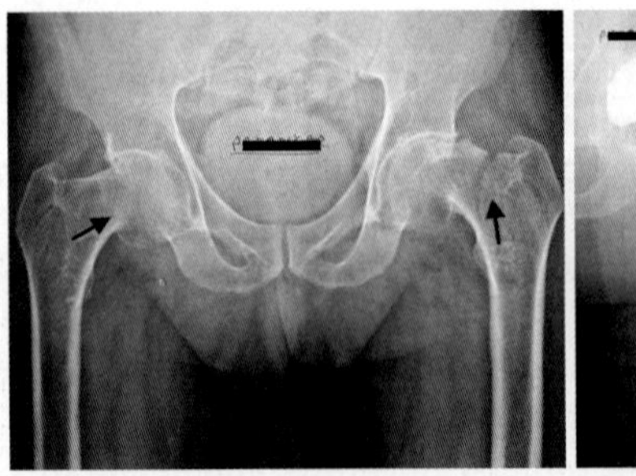
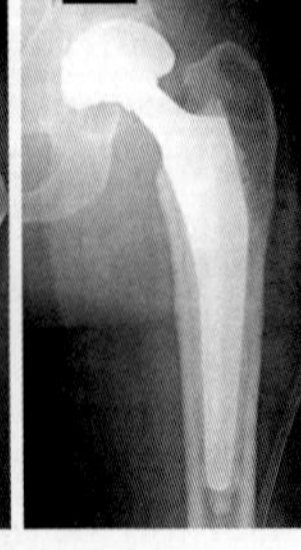

Figure 27.44 Bilateral SCFE with coxa vara

On exposure, fibrous tissue was found to be covering the cup, due to the time lapse.

The press fit cup could be removed. While it was removed, the stem also came out. The stem was of medium size, as per the documentation and was again confirmed, when removed. The acetabulum was found to be indeed quite shallow.

The anterior capsule was contracted and was carefully excised, to avoid impingement. While removing the cement, pieces started falling in the cement mantle itself and were difficult to retrieve. Hence with a power reamer, the mantle was attempted to be broken down, but failed.

Then with a cork screw extractor, one could penetrate the terminal part of the cement mantle. A medium stem could not be inserted. Hence a small stem in anteversion was inserted for trial.

An uncemented cup was planned. Acetabular reaming, trial and final HA coated cup and the screws were inserted. Posterior stabilized liner was inserted.

Cemented stem: Due to presence of the cement mantle, the cement gun nozzle may not enter the femoral canal. This was confirmed. The syringe nozzle was made slightly flat, with a nibbler, so that it could enter the canal. The cement was inserted with a cement gun, in the femoral canal, while it was in a fluid state. The cement was pressurized with hand. A small stem was then inserted in proper anteversion. Trial reduction was carried out and the final head was inserted. Hip was found to be stable.

Postoperative recovery was uneventful.

What One Learns

- Especially in women with a wide pelvis and a shallow acetabulum, this episode may occur.
- Cement mantle may be reamed, but removal of the cement fragments and the cement sand is tricky.
- In the presence of the cement mantle, one has to use a stem, which is one size smaller,

to insert it in proper anteversion and that such a smaller stem should be available.

- In elderly person with osteoporosis, removal of the cement, by making a window in the shaft and closing it again with cables/ circlage could be avoided. Instead a 'Cement in cement' technique can be used.
- In such a case, it is necessary to wear a lead apron, prior to the surgery, because, one may have to take an image at any stage of surgery and protection of the team is of vital importance (Fig. 27.45).

A case presented to the clinic for further treatment. The X-ray films were arranged serially and studied. The case gives us many messages, worth remembering, in a day-to-day clinical and operative work.

An elderly person sustained a hip injury and reported to a hospital in another city. The X-ray film was not clear, as one can see. A partial hip replacement was planned and carried out in the same hospital.

- The postoperative films show, AM prosthesis with a fracture around the trochanter. The day 1 X-ray film is unable to show the fracture morphology. There was perhaps loosening of the stem and hence the limb was put in a traction on a Bohler frame.
- The surgeon, perhaps having realized that the stem is loose, changed it to a cemented bipolar prosthesis. Postoperative X-ray film was not available for me to see. He was kept in the bed and not permitted to be ambulated. After few weeks X-ray of the hip was taken, showing the femoral stem was outside the canal and the canal was occupied by a cement restrictor and a mass of cement above it.

How this may have had happened? There was a fracture fragment with its distal end near the subtrochanteric area. The cement was inserted in the medullary canal. Then while the modular stem was being inserted in the medullary cavity, the tip of the femoral stem went out of the femoral canal through the gap in between the displaced fragment the proximal end of the trochanteric fracture.

The important step is to confirm on table, the track, which the stem tip is following was perhaps not done. Obviously the backflow of cement from the femoral canal must not have occurred, which was not realized by the team (Fig. 27.46).

The Patient Reported at This Stage

Obviously, this had to be revised.

Removal of the stem and the cup, removal of the cement in the canal, followed by insertion of a long uncemented stem was done. The femur shaft was reconstructed with cables and circlage wires. On table X-ray, two views were taken to confirm that the stem is well within

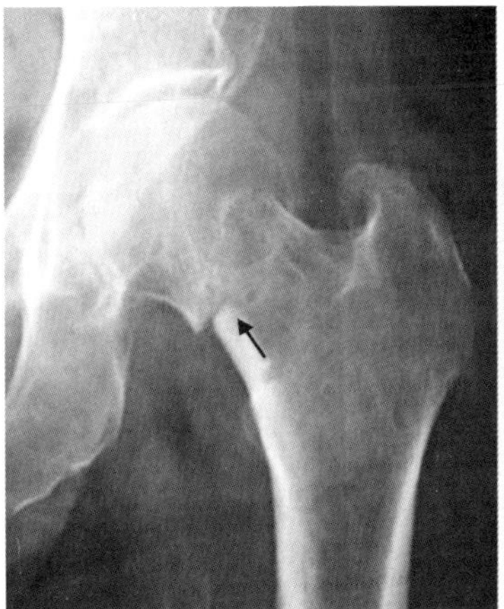
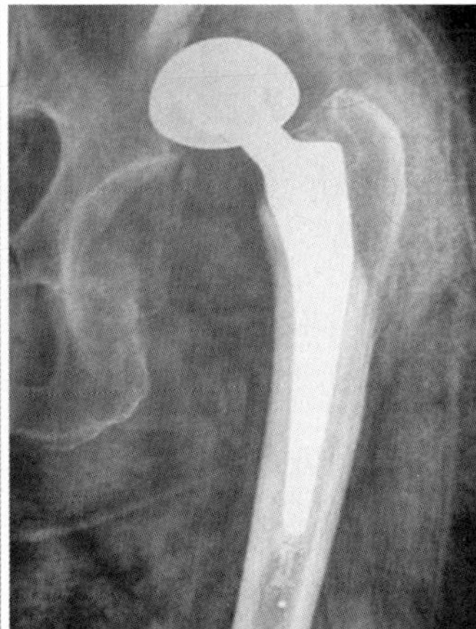
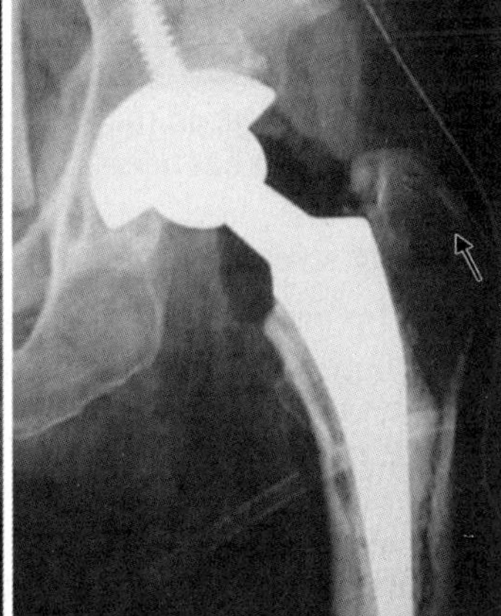

Figure 27.45 Shallow acetabulum

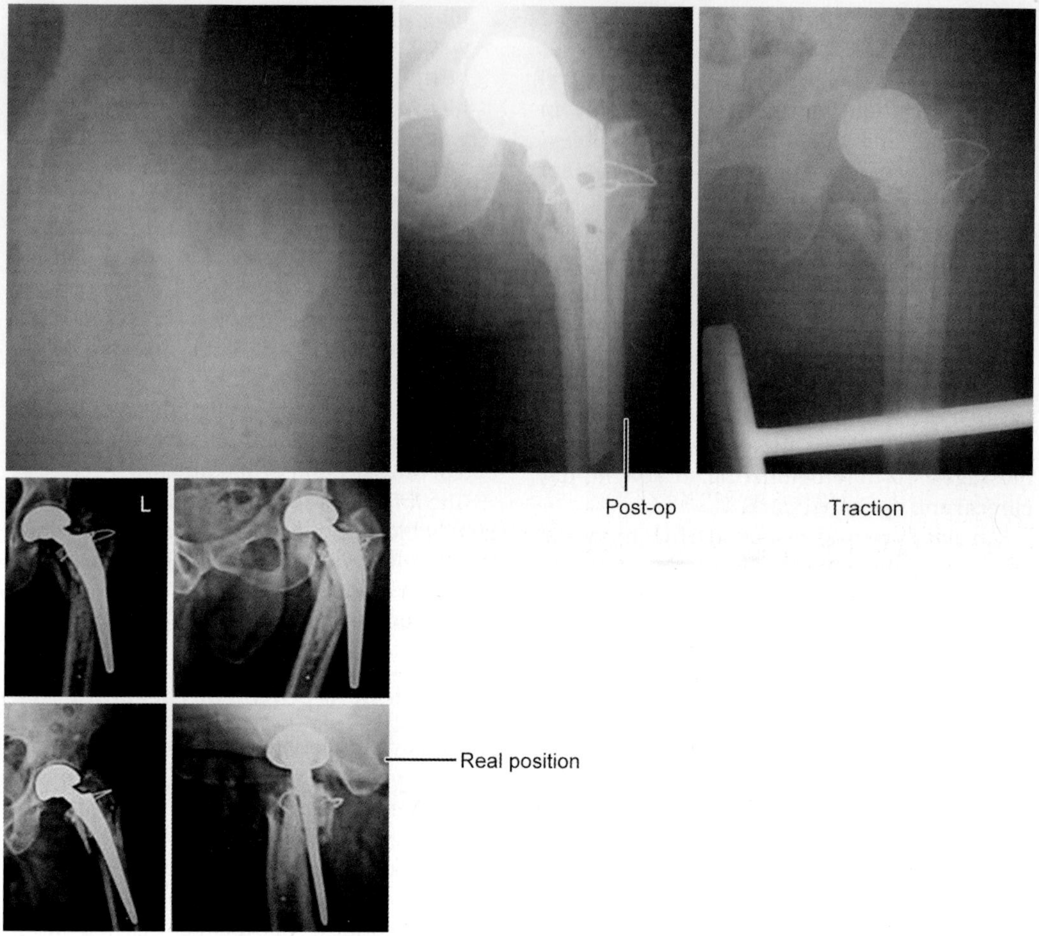

Figure 27.46 Stem extramedullary

the medullary cavity. A bipolar head cup was added. He was kept off the weight for few weeks Long-term result has been good (Fig. 27.47).

Message One Gets

- Day 1 X-ray film has to be of good quality, to know, if it is an intracapsular or an intertrochanteric fracture.
- Stem of a prosthesis needs to be well-fitting in the canal.
- In a cemented technique, backflow of cement must occur, while the stem is being inserted. This indicates that the stem is entering the medullary canal filled with a cement.

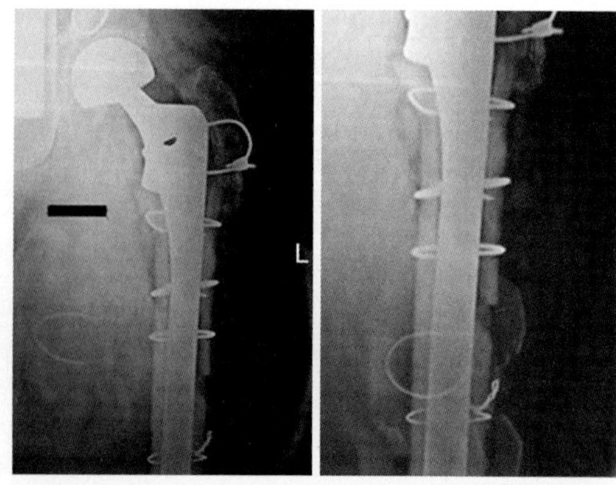

Figure 27.47 Revision of the extramedullary stem

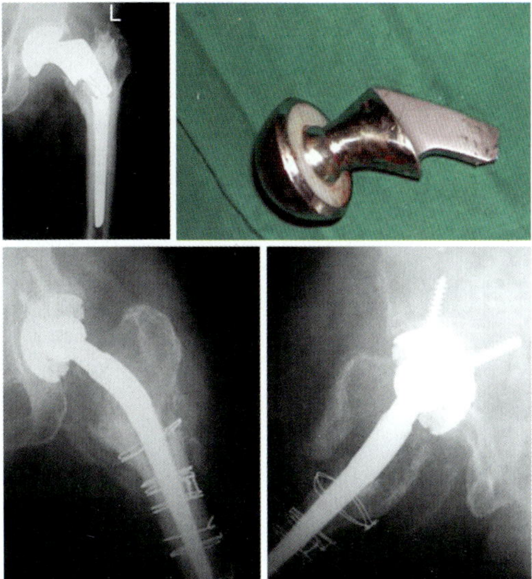

Figure 27.48 Failed prosthesis stem

- If in doubt, on the operation table, X-ray must be taken in two views. (Of course, in this case, the surgeon, perhaps did not realize, this can happen!).

Mechanical Failure of the Stem

This elderly person, more than 60 years of age, had sustained a fracture of neck of femur. A cemented non-modular prosthesis was inserted. After a few years had noted a pain and limp on the operated side and X-ray revealed a breakage of the stem in the upper/3 area. This had to be revised. The cement was removed by making a window in the shaft and the prosthesis stem was removed. An uncemented THR was done. The shaft femur was reconstructed with circlage wires. He was kept off the weight for two months, till the evidence of femur union was observed. This was followed by gradual and supervised weight bearing. Ten years, follow up is satisfactory (Fig. 27.48).

CHAPTER

28

Fracture of Trochanter

Hip fracture is a devastating injury in the elderly. It needs medical support from a team, which should include a physician, psychiatrist, rehabilitation team, social workers, besides an orthopedic surgeon. The duration of hospital stay is long and cost of the management is quite high. This is known to be more than that of a case of malignancy of breast or a cerebral vascular accident or myocardial infarction. After discharge from a hospital, home care assistance is required.

The fracture occurs in a well-vascularized area of bone and hence avascular necrosis of head of femur is rarely encountered.

In a stable fracture, postero-medial part of the trochanter is not fractured and when it is fractured, the fracture becomes unstable. Often, the fracture line extends in the subtrochanteric area.

When a hip fracture is suspected, but not apparent on a plain X-ray film, MRI examination is necessary for its diagnosis.

A stable internal fixation offers pain relief and undisturbed bone healing, permitting active mobilization in the bed at least. It thus reduces a chance of complications observed in a bed-ridden patient. A good reduction, a stable internal fixation with well-opposed fragments, offers resistance to fracture displacement. A well-reduced and internally-fixed fracture is benefitted with complementary physiological load by the muscles and enhances the stability. Some compression across the fracture is offered by the sliding screw mechanism and the compression lag screw. A stable fracture has large fragments and hence offers more resistance to the bending forces (Varus). If there is a good bone to bone contact, it resists angulatory forces. Thus in a comminuted fracture, there is less bone to bone contact and hence less stability. This leads to more stress on the implant, which may lead to angulation at the fracture site.

The Aims of Surgical Treatment

- Control of pain
- Offer stability to the fracture
- Early mobilization, in the bed at least
- Should be the only surgery for this injury
- Result should outlive the patient.

Here, a large number of cases and X-ray films are depicted. One composite picture containing few X-ray films speaks for itself. Having seen an outcome, satisfactory or otherwise, it is necessary to think and find out the possible cause of the outcome. If the outcome is not satisfactory, one should think, as to why this happened and what to avoid. One should also learn from a case with good outcome, what to do specifically, so that in future, a similar good result can be aimed at.

Historical

In the last century, internal fixation for fracture of neck and trochanter was devised. In the initial stage, it was a jointed implant, viz. The SP nail and a side plate, the Thornton plate. The assembly was held together by a top screw with a washer. In a stable fracture, where the lateral fragment is sufficiently large, the SP nail had a reasonable hold on the lateral fragment. Hence this implant usually offered stability adequate enough, to avoid a varus deformity.

The lateral end of the SP pin and the flare of the plate may not exactly match. The short end of the plate often required to be appropriately bent. A McLaughlin plate had good design, so thereby merely sliding the plate, good contact opposition between the base of the SP pin and the plate end could be achieved (Figs 28.1 and 28.2).

While operating on a fracture table, should a 'C' arm fail, it is possible to carry out the procedure, using a mobile X-ray unit. However, operating in a lateral position, if the 'C' arm fails still, after introduction of the guidewire, an X-ray can be taken with the hip rotated and take an X-ray picture and complete the procedure. This happened in a case, as illustrated (Fig. 28.3).

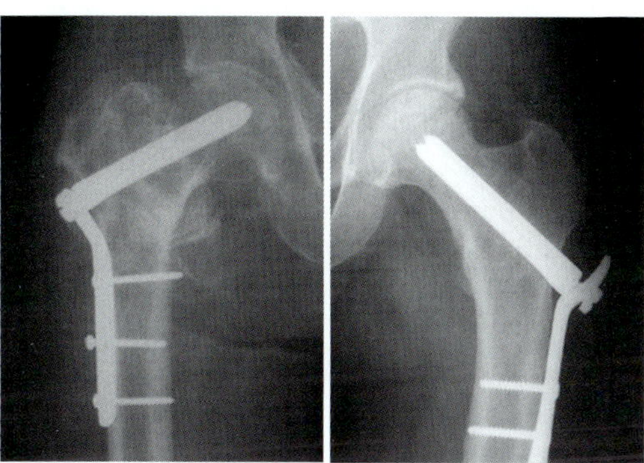

Figure 28.1 SP pin and plate

PROBLEMS OF INTERNAL FIXATION

- Pin cut out
- Pin penetration in the acetabulum
- Plate pull out from the shaft of femur
- Disengagement/breakage of top screw
- A good lateral view is desirable and necessary on arrival, to plan method of fixation.

FRACTURE MORPHOLOGY

- Fracture of greater trochanter is both avulsion and extrusion fracture:
- Fracture of lesser trochanter is an avulsion fracture and may be left as such. If the fracture anatomy permits, it is preferable to fix the fracture of lesser trochanter, anatomically. This leads to a better union, prevents fracture collapse and maintains the limb length. Often the anterior fracture line is lateral to the intertrochanteric line and hence extracapsular, while posteriorly, it is intracapsular, being medial to the intertrochanteric crest.
- Fixation of a fracture in varus subsequently increases the load on the opposite hip and this opposite hip may have a subsequent fracture.

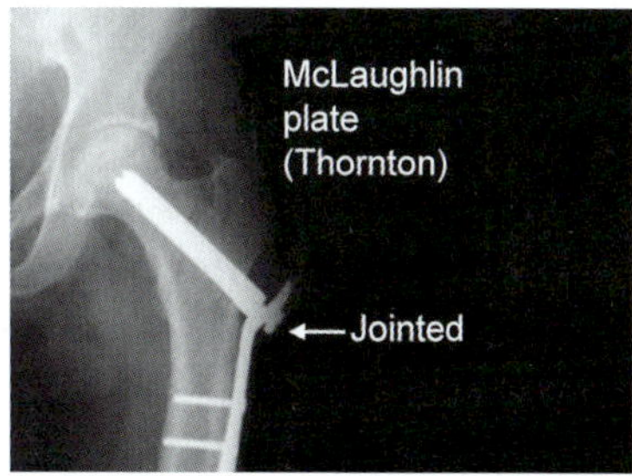

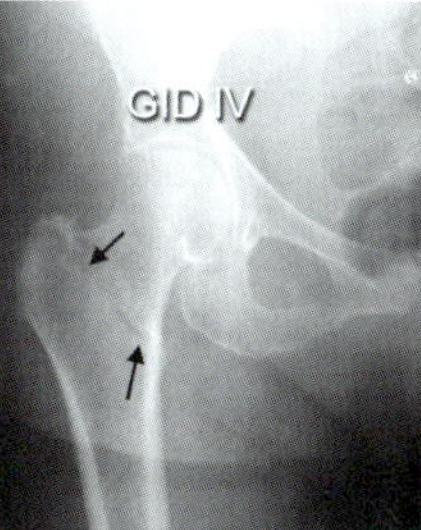

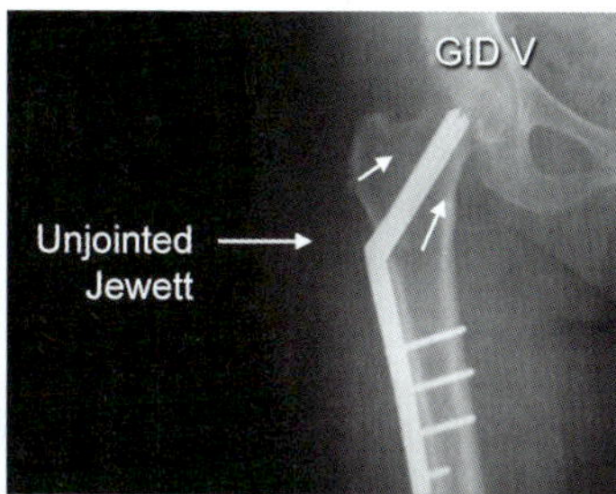

Figure 28.2 Jointed and unjointed implants

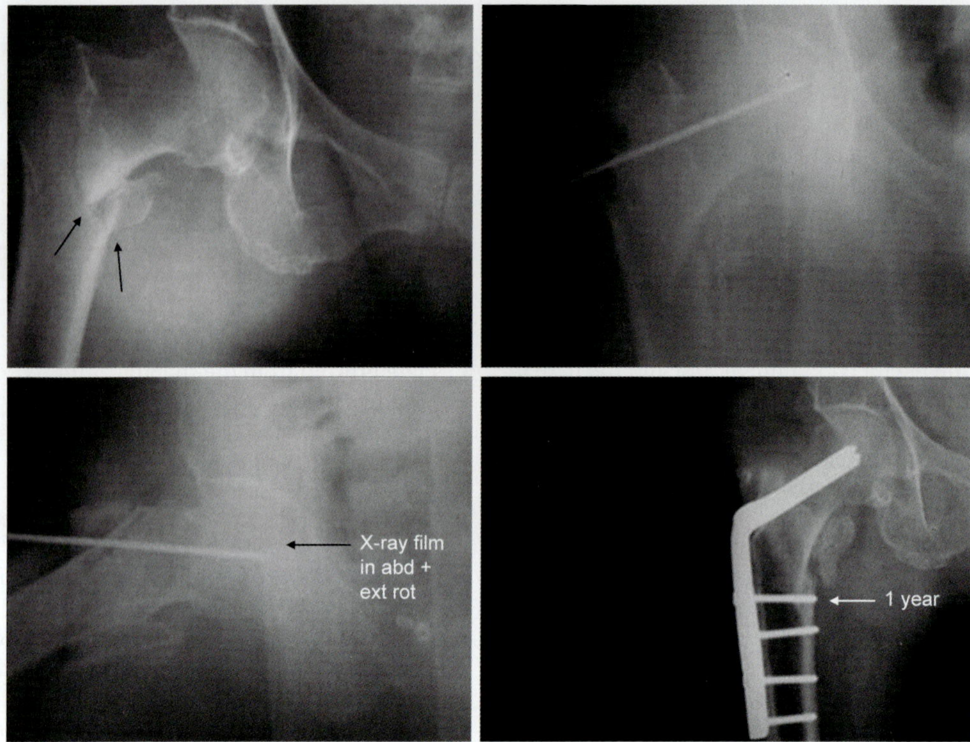

Figure 28.3 Failed 'C' arm and X-ray taken with a mobile X-ray unit

ASSESSMENT OF A FRACTURE

- Degree of osteoporosis.
- Stable or Unstable fracture.

Stable Fracture

Good contact between the medial and lateral fragments. Intact lesser trochanter.

Unstable Fracture

No contact between the medial and lateral fragment, lesser trochanter extruded.

This helps to decide the method of fixation and predict fracture collapse.

METHOD OF INTERNAL FIXATION

- Static vs dynamic implant
- Sliding vs non-sliding implant
- Sliding implant has reduced the rate of failure. However, the pin placement is the important step in fixation.

TIMING AND FACTORS FOR SURGERY

- Surgery is urgent, if not emergency
- Factors not under control of surgeon
  - Degree of osteoporosis
  - Fracture morphology
- Factors under control of surgeon
  - Quality and degree of reduction
  - Implant used and its placement.

CHOICE OF IMPLANT

- *Fixed un-jointed implants*: Jewett nail plate and condylar blade plate. However, have a danger of joint penetration
- Sliding implant—dynamic hip screw (DHS) 1981
- IM devices
- Primary replacement

PATIENT POSITION

Supine on a fracture table: in a stable fracture.

Lateral position: in a case where:
- Medialization is planned
- Multiple fragments
- When IFS to be done, esp. for lesser trochanter fixation.

FRACTURE REDUCTION

- Anatomical
- Non-anatomical
  - When medialization is planned
  - Early mobilization and perhaps weight-bearing is planned.

FRACTURE REDUCTION AND IMPLANT POSITION

- In presence of posterior comminution, slight external rotation is important to achieve a better posterior bone contact.
- A sliding implant permits the hip screw to be placed in subchondral level, reducing the TAD.
- A short barrel plate permits easy fracture collapse opposition. In a case where the screw length required is more than 85 mm, it is desirable to have a long barrel plate, for mechanical reasons.

TECHNIQUE OF DHS

I observe a stable fracture is better operated on a fracture table, when a DHS is to be used. When a 95 deg DCS is contemplated, I find a lateral position is more comfortable. In a case when it is doubtful if bone grafting would be required, it is wise to drape the iliac crest accordingly.

Prior to draping, one should confirm that both AP and lateral views are well seen in a 'C' arm image. In a lateral view (on a fracture table) often one observes posterior sagging, which should be corrected by placing a folded sheet of correct thickness, under the gluteal area. Often a good reduction is seen in the AP view, when the leg is externally rotated. The lateral view also shows an acceptable position. In such a situation, one maintains it as such. After exposure, 2 K-wires are inserted at appropriate place to stabilize the fracture and then the limb can be rotated internally and again confirmed that the reduction is maintained in both the views. This step permits one to operate, with comfort. The K-wires are so placed that the DHS/DCS guidewire and the reamer can be safely passed without any obstruction.

Insertion of a DHS/DCS Guidewire

One determines the place from where the threaded DHS guidewire needs to be inserted. A drill hole is made with a 3.5 mm drill bit. Additional drill holes are made, on all the sides in a circle. This helps:
- If one needs to change the entry point of the guidewire, these holes can be used.
- Having placed the guidewire in a correct position, when the triple reamer is used to penetrate the lateral wall, the lateral wall is already made weak by the multiple drill holes. Thus lateral wall shattering is less likely. The required length of the sliding screw is measured by a direct measuring device.
- The K-wires inserted to stabilize the fracture, hold both the fragments together and when the tap is used, the spinning of the head is less likely to occur. If the proximal part of the head cortex is too hard and offers resistance to the tap rotation, the technique of 'two half turns forward and one reverse helps to negotiate it. At this stage, while operating a right side hip, the proximal fragment is supported from the posterior surface, to prevent its excess rotation. While operating on the left side, exert pressure on the calcar from the anterior side, to prevent the calcar tilting anteriorly and the beak coming out of the shaft, so that the beak remains in the medullary canal.
- The threaded guidewire needs to be straight and easily sliding through the triple reamer and the tap. Still, while withdrawing either the reamer or the tap, another wire with both ends blunt, is placed in the butt end of the reamer/tap and gently hammered. It is kept

pressed and the outer reamer or tap is slowly withdrawn, with a T handle. This helps to maintain the initial guidewire in place. Prior to removal of the tap, the expected screw length reading is again taken on its shaft marking.

- How much depth to be tapped?
  - In a young person, with good bone stock, one needs to tap nearly 5 mm from the subchondral area. Often, one gets lot of resistance while tapping and hence, two forward and one reverse technique need to be adopted, so the tap dose not seize in the channel.
  - In elderly, with osteoporosis, the tapping is easy and as per the resistance offered, one may tap, 5 to 8 mm short of full tapping. Being soft bone, the final few turns of the screw get good grip in the bone, while it is traversing in an untapped bone. This helps to have a secure purchase of the screw in the bone.

Screw placement: In AP view, should be in the lower half of the neck and the head, while in the lateral view, preferably in the center of the neck and head.

At times, the fracture morphology is such that, on the lateral surface, one finds that the lateral edge of the large postero-medial fragment is extending nearly to the center of the lateral surface, near the proposed point of guidewire insertion.

In this situation, the entry of the guidewire has to be more anterior on the lateral femoral surface and needs to be directed more posteriorly. Then in the lateral view, the screw would appear directed more posteriorly (Fig. 28.4).

What care needs to be taken?

- The drill holes made around the hole for the guidewire need to be more in number, so that, when the triple reamer is rotated, one preserves some collar between the plate shoulder and the posterior fracture line. If unfortunately, the barrel track and the fracture line join, the fracture becomes a subtrochanteric fracture and is more unstable.

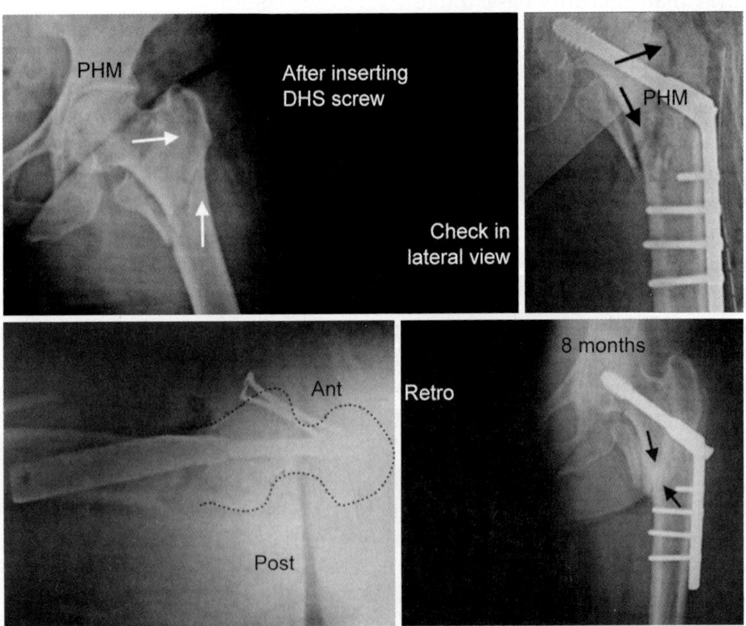

Figure 28.4 Anterior to posterior direction of hip screw

- In either situation, it is necessary to add the TSP, so that excess medialization would not occur.

The screw insertion long T handle has projections within the tube, which get purchase on the DHS screw. The final rotation and position of the T handle is so planned, that the transverse T handle tube lies parallel to the femur shaft and hence the plate would lie parallel to the femur.

Often one observes that the guidewire is inserted with a 130 degree guide and when a 130 degree plate is slided over the screw end, one realizes that that the plate required is 125 degree. This is known to occur. Similarly, one may observe that a guidewire inserted with 130 deg jig, is too vertical, while that with 125 deg is too horizontal. One may 'cheat' the procedure by using a 130 deg jig and so place that the guidewire would enter in the desired angle. After a triple trocar reaming is done, one can insert a short barrel side plate and one of the two, usually with a lesser neck shaft angle often fits well.

TRICKS IN FRACTURE REDUCTION AND PLATE FIXATION

- When the proximal fragment has a medial beak, it should be anatomically reduced. Preferably, the apex is kept slightly lateral to the medial wall of the distal fragment, i.e. inserted in the canal. This enhances the stability. Having done so, the traction on the foot should be slightly reduced, which invaginates the beak more. Thus, what is expected to occur in a few days, due to physiological forces, one has done this on table only and implant (hip screw) of correct size is inserted. When the lateral wall of the shaft is intact, this step has to be now only. Once the guidewire is inserted, triple reaming is done, further supero-inferior telescoping of the fragments would not occur. However, if there is a break in the lateral wall, either due to injury or due to osteotomy done, then after insertion of the DHS screw, it is possible to reduce the traction.
- The hip screw length be such that a short length top screw when inserted, gets adequate purchase in the screw. If this does not engage in the hip screw threads, a long top screw should be available. The hip screw length be such that, when it is inserted till the subchondral bone, it is visible a few mm deep in the lateral cortex, so, when the top screw is inserted, it would engage adequately. If the top locking screw does not engage well, it is known that the plate may get disconnected. This happens when varus forces are too much or when a patient starts premature weight-bearing against advice.
- Length of barrel: I feel, the barrel should be short. If it is a long one, often, it comes at the fracture line and then the barrel end obstructs the collapse (contact opposition)of proximal fragment and fracture opposition does not occur. However, when the screw length required is more than 85 mm, a long barrel plate is desirable.
- For a stable fracture four-hole side plate is adequate, so that 3 bicortical and one unicortical screws can be well inserted. If the plate has oval DCP holes and if the plate is not well centered on the lateral surface, then it is possible to tilt the screws and insert them, so they get a good hold on the shaft of femur in both the cortices. Besides, one can insert screws in divergent manner to have more pull out strength.
- In fixation with a 95 deg DCS in spite of insertion of the hip screw in correct direction, the side plate may not match to the shaft. In such a situation, it is necessary to change the plate angle at a point, distal to the lower of the two proximal round holes.
- In a DCS plate fixation, it is necessary to have one screw through the uppermost hole, so it holds the calcar well and increases the stability. One must be aware of the technique to insert the screw in an oblique bone surface (the calcar area). First make a drill hole in the lateral cortex by a 4.5 mm drill -> through it insert an insert sleeve → further drilling of the medial cortex of the calcar, with 3.2 mm drill, with the insert sleeve well pressed against the calcar. If this is not done

this way, the drill bit almost always breaks!

In the yester years, when medical and surgical facility was not available in remote areas, the intertrochanteric (pertrochanteric) fracture took a natural course of healing by itself. The intracapsular fracture would lead to a non-union, while trochanteric fracture would unite in varus with shortening. The basi-trochanteric fracture, even today, is rather slow to unite. In the given example, the patient gradually started walking, without any specific medical care, with some lurch, but with a pain-free hip. The basi-trochanteric area offered a support effect and the telescopic effect was minimum (Fig. 28.5).

Jewett Nail Plate

This is a fixed angle nail plate device and is non-modular, unlike a DHS. Hence, the Jewett nail inventory required is quite large.

- One needs to have different combinations in terms of the nail length, the nail plate angle and plate length, etc. Unless one has all the possible combinations, a successful fixation is not possible.
- The major fragments in a trochanteric fracture, if are adequately large with good bone density, the Jewett nail has a good hold on the bone and chances of cut out, etc. are less. The fracture has to be well reduced and co-opted and stable. Unlike a sliding hip screw contact opposition during healing process is less likely and the distraction, if any, would continue as such (Figs 28.6 to 28.11).

In a patient with osteoporosis, especially in an unstable fracture, the Jewett nail may migrate medially, penetrating the head of femur. The DHS scores over the Jewett nail plate in this aspect (Fig. 28.12).

Medialization and Use of a Jewett Nail

In some fractures, the morphology indicates a fracture in the lateral wall, below the greater trochanter area. If the nail plate is fixed *in situ*, natural medialization may or may not occur. If it occurs, it may penetrate the head of femur. If it does not occur, fracture opposition may not occur.

In a fracture with a vertical fracture line, often contact opposition is possible only when osteotomy below the greater trochanter is carried out. This level is little higher than the conventional McMurray's osteotomy, but helps

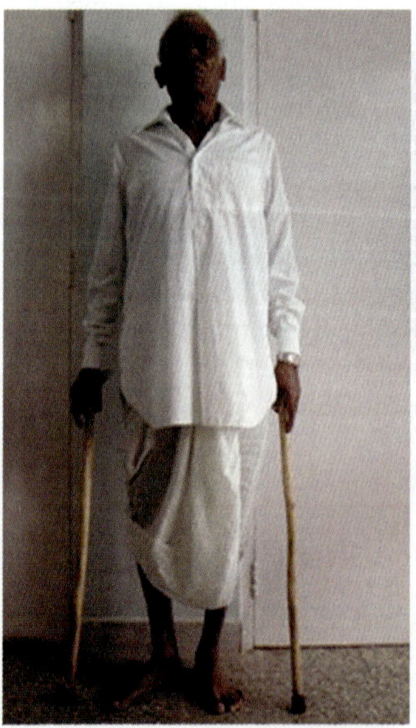

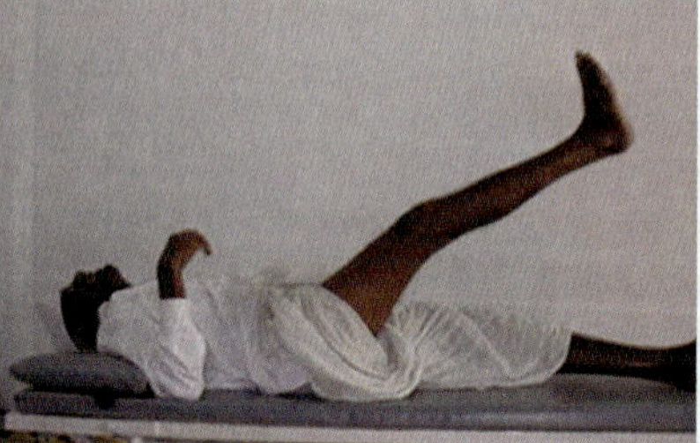

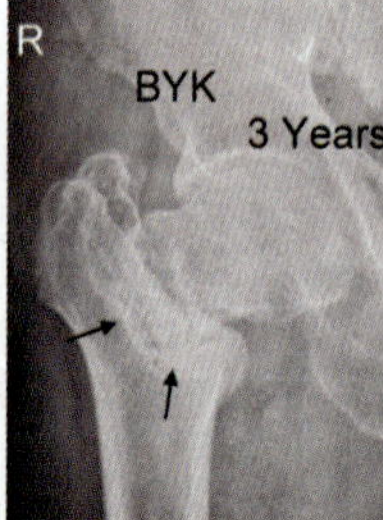

Figure 28.5 NU in a basi-trochanteric fracture

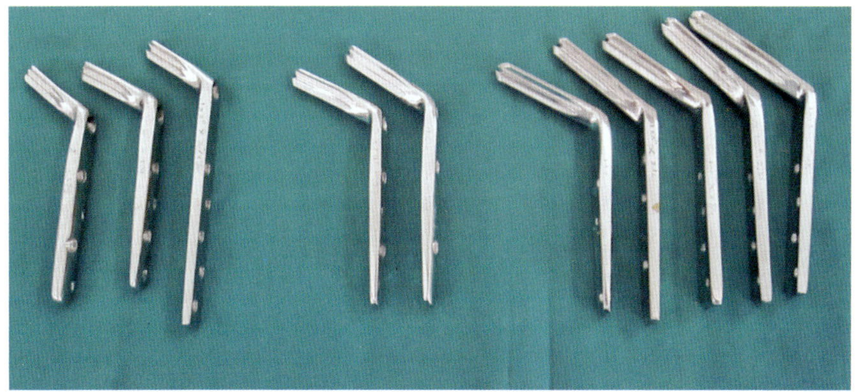

Figure 28.6 Jewett range

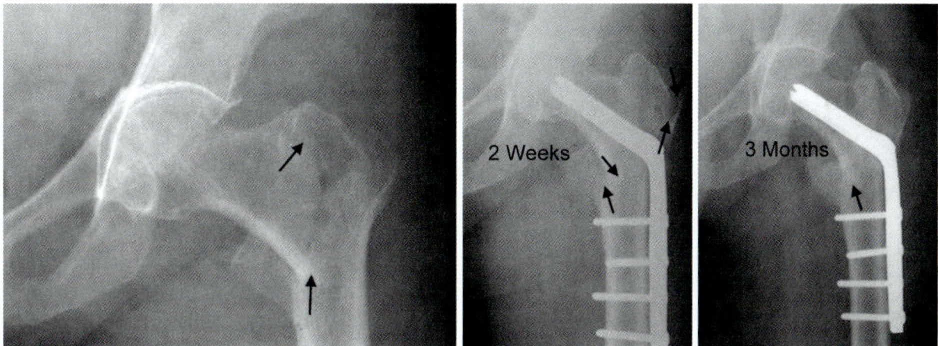

Figure 28.7 Jewett nail works well in stable fracture ii

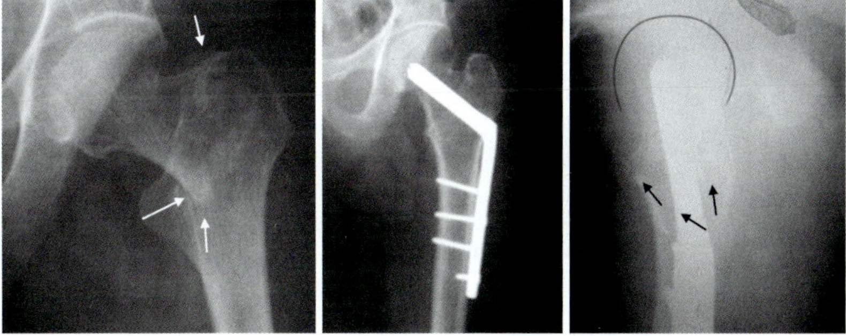

Figure 28.8 Jewett nail works well in stable fracture iv

to establish contact between the medial and lateral fragments and a good union. Any such procedure to have medialization, leads to some shortening. However, it is more acceptable, than a delayed or a nonunion (Figs 28.13 and 28.14).

Technique of Jewett Nail Plate Insertion

Which table: Fracture or conventional? Most of the surgeons operate on a fracture table, few on a conventional table in lateral position

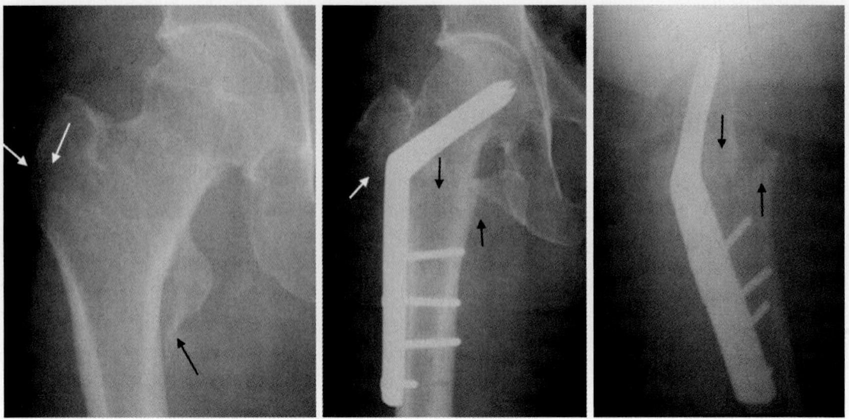

Figure 28.9 Jewett nail works well in stable fracture i

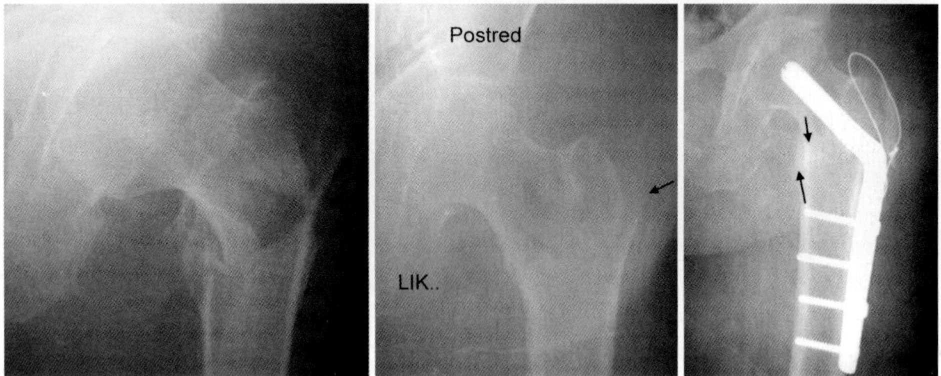

Figure 28.10 Jewett nail + TBW for fracture of gr. trochanter

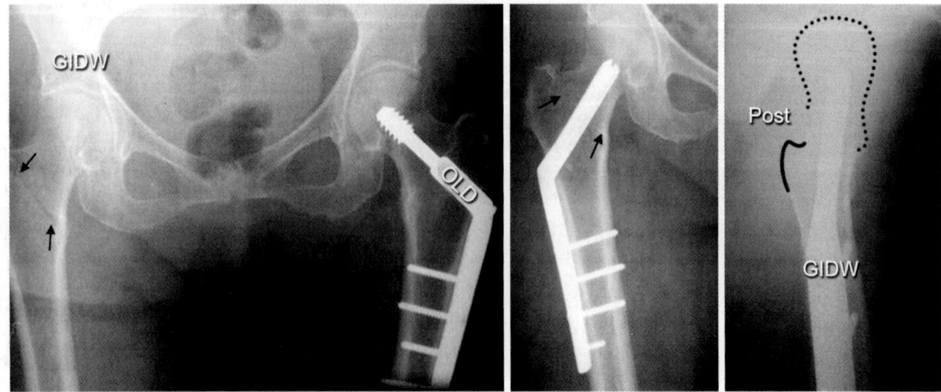

Figure 28.11 Jewett nail in stable sequential fractures

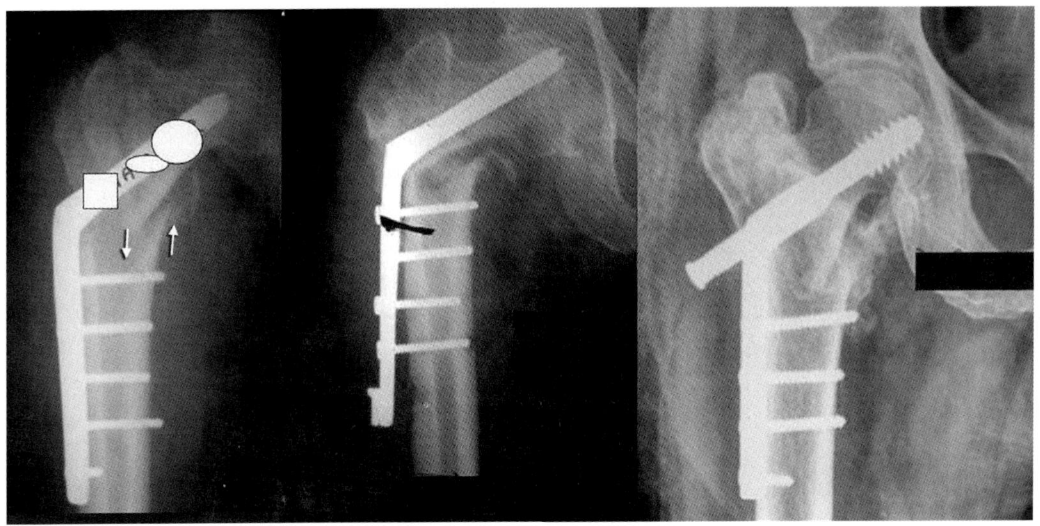

Figure 28.12 Sliding screw does not penetrate head of femur

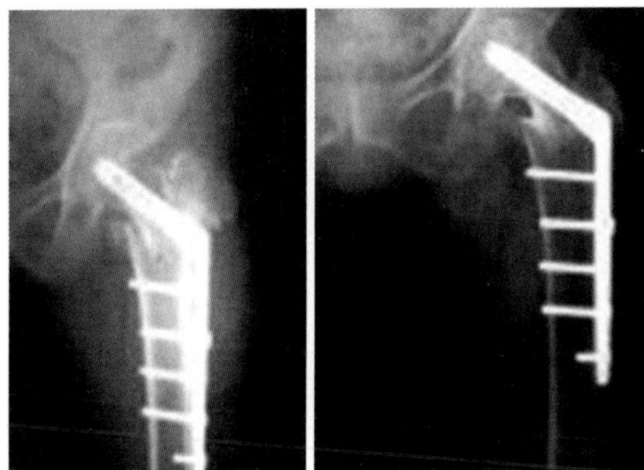

Figure 28.13 Medialization with a Jewett nail

and still less number of surgeons operate on a conventional table in supine position. I feel, it is a matter of convenience and to which one is used to. In the later two positions, a 'C' arm is nearly a must. Sliding radiolucent table top has made this possible.

Availability of a 'C' arm with an image at press of a button, has made the procedure rather too easy. Still, it is necessary to adopt a technique, 'C' arm position, to reduce the radiation and increase the life of both the X-ray tube (and the operating team!). In yester years, when a mobile X-ray unit had to be used, exposure of each film means the cost of the film and the time taken for its processing. It was possible to carry out the procedure with six to eight exposures—to know the reduction, to know the position of the K-wire and to confirm the final position of the implant. To facilitate insertion of the guidewire in a correct position, an Allis forceps was anchored to the skin, on the head of the femur. Having seen the post-reduction film and the place of the forceps tip, the guidewire would be directed accordingly. The lateral view of the post-reduction film would give idea regarding the anteversion in which the wire had to be inserted.

Having inserted the guidewire, the lateral surface of the trochanter was gently tapped with a Bohler punch to have good opposition of the stable fragments. Before the nail was finally set home, again the fracture was impacted to correct distraction, if any, has occurred. With the threaded sliding hip screw, this step is not necessary.

Today, with a 'C' arm, the number of exposures is possibly more. One wonders, if the placement of the implant has improved, with this facility (Figs 28.15 and 28.16).

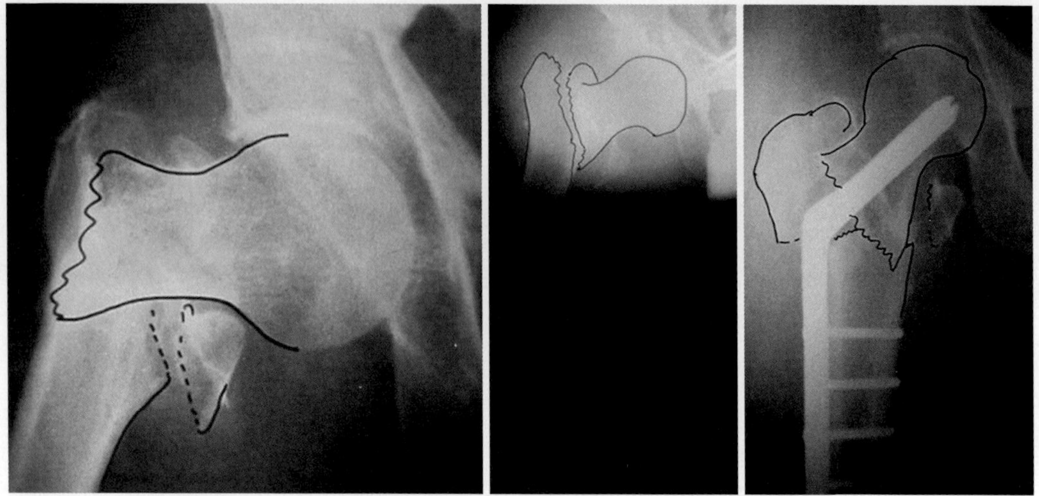

Figure 28.14 Jewett medialization II

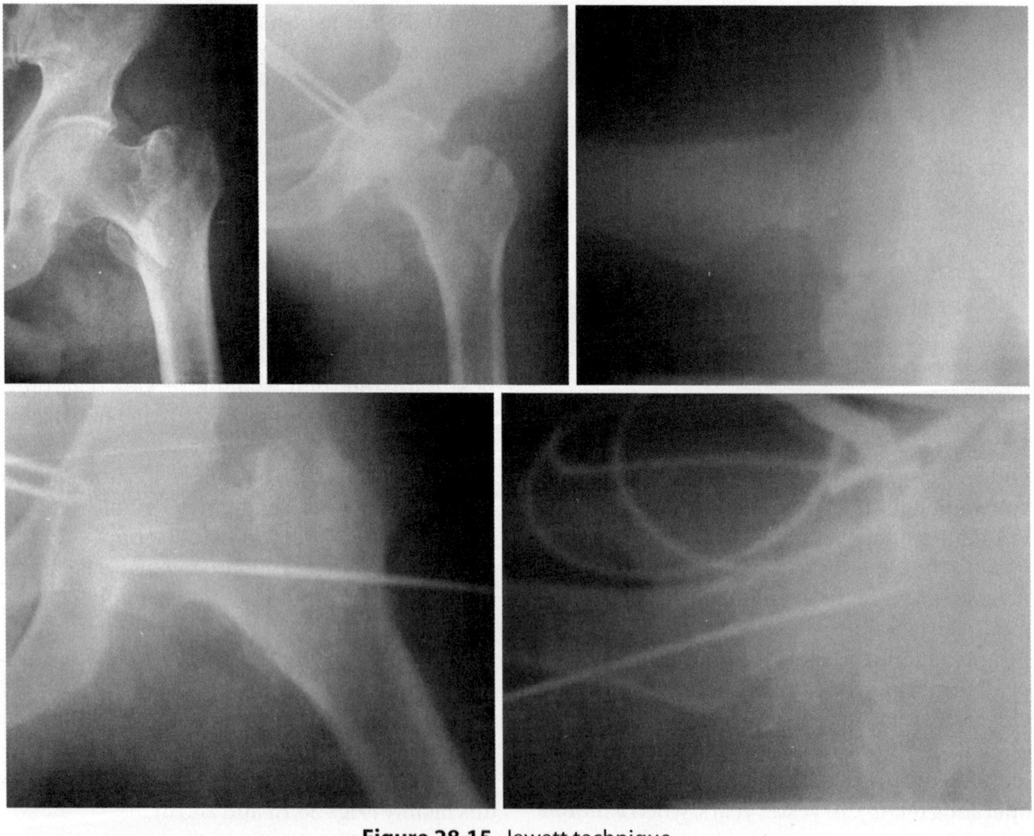

Figure 28.15 Jewett technique

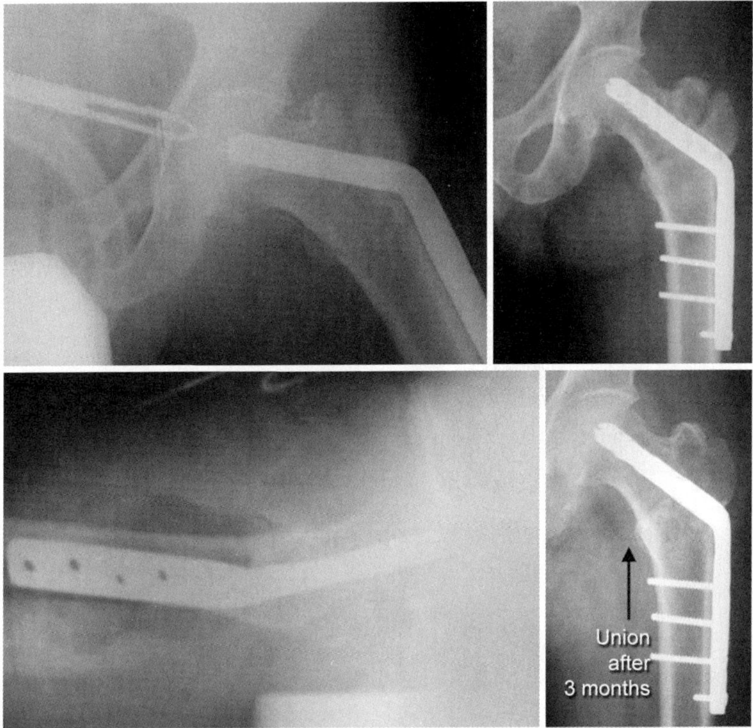

Figure 28.16 Jewett technique

In fracture in an osteoporotic bone, when a fracture is stabilized with a DHS device, collapse opposition does occur. If the screw is correctly placed, there may be limb shortening, but screw cut out is less likely. Jewett nail plate did not enjoy this advantage of sliding screw principle, and hence nail cut out was seen (Fig. 28.17).

In a case with osteoporosis, even if good fixation and medialization is carried out, the fracture collapse may be more. If the Jewett nail does not cut out, it moves medially and irritates the acetabulum (Fig. 28.18).

In a case, a Jewett nail fixation was done and the fracture was medialized. However, further medialization occurred and the nail tip was trying to penetrate the head of the femur. It did not so occur, but the plate avulsed from the shaft of femur (Fig. 28.19).

In a case done by a colleague, possibly the nail was placed more posteriorly and during follow up, it cut out posteriorly (Fig. 28.20).

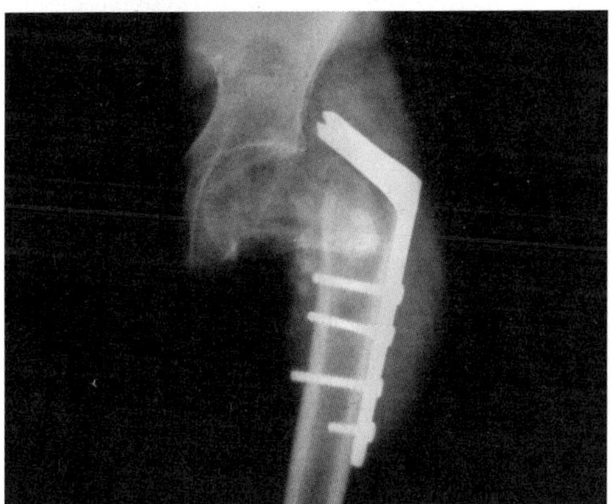

Figure 28.17 Jewett cut out

A fracture was well-fixed with a Jewett nail. However, the patient (hip being pain free) started weight bearing without permission and the nail bent. He continued to walk and the fracture consolidated (Fig. 28.21).

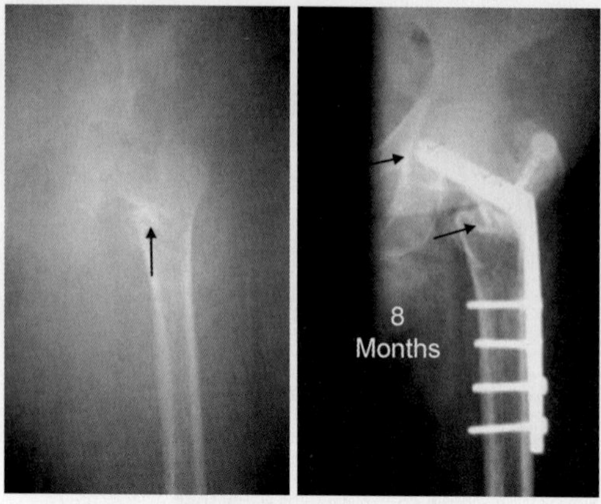

Figure 28.18 Nail irritating the acetabulum

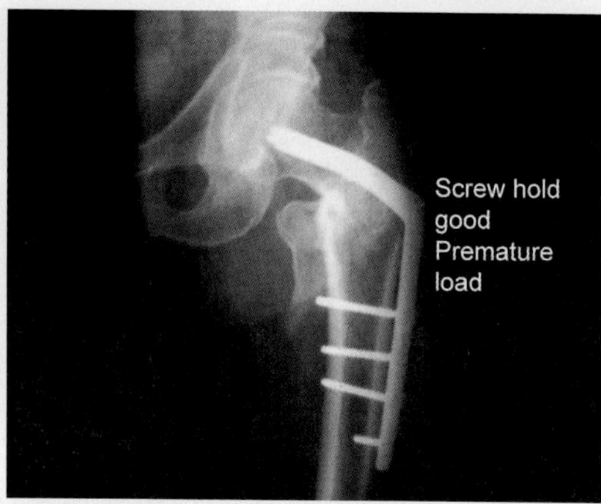

Figure 28.21 Bent Jewett nail

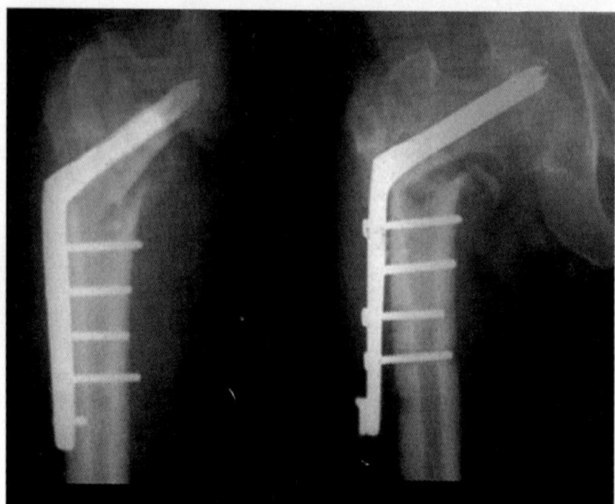

Figure 28.19 Medial migration of nail and plate pull out

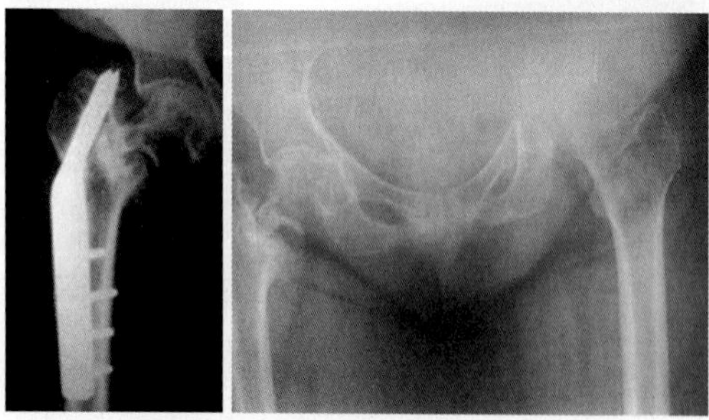

Figure 28.20 Jewett nail posterior cut out

DHS

If a fracture is two-part or three-part and stable–with good bone-to-bone contact, the stability is good. This is especially possible when the calcar medial tip is inserted—placed just lateral to the medial wall of the shaft. When operating on a fracture table, it is possible to achieve this by increasing the leg traction and maneuvering the shaft of femur. Having placed the beak in the shaft, the traction should be slightly reduced, so axial contact opposition is improved. Often, one forgets to take this step. (While the reduction maneuver is done, one should advise the assistant/theater assistant to remind the surgeon of this important step!

In presence of a postero-medial fragment, this step is relatively easier, than a case, which has a two-part fracture.

A fracture so reduced, usually unites in expected duration. The lateral view indicates the stability and contact opposition. If the AP view shows a wide bone contact and fracture area, one may add a 6.5 mm cancellous screw with a washer. This enhances the stability of fixation. Being partially threaded screw, contact opposition is possible, as the physiological load brings the fragments together.

If the TAD (Tip Apex Distance) is kept less, the fracture stability continues to be good, as the fracture collapses and shortening occurs (Figs 28.22 to 28.28).

Anatomical Reduction

In an intertrochanteric fracture, with wide fracture surfaces, contact opposition is good.

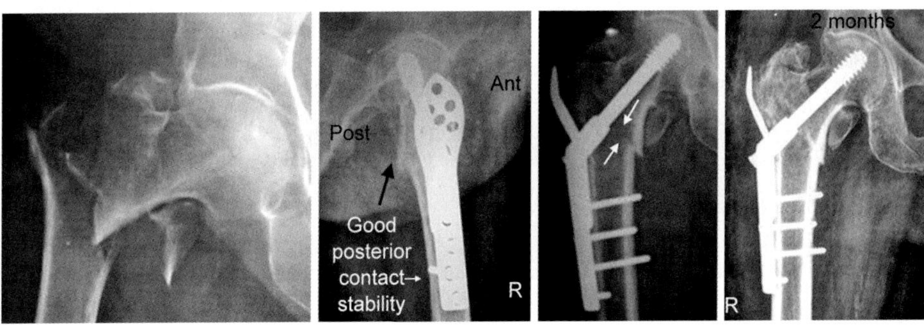

Figure 28.22 TAD less

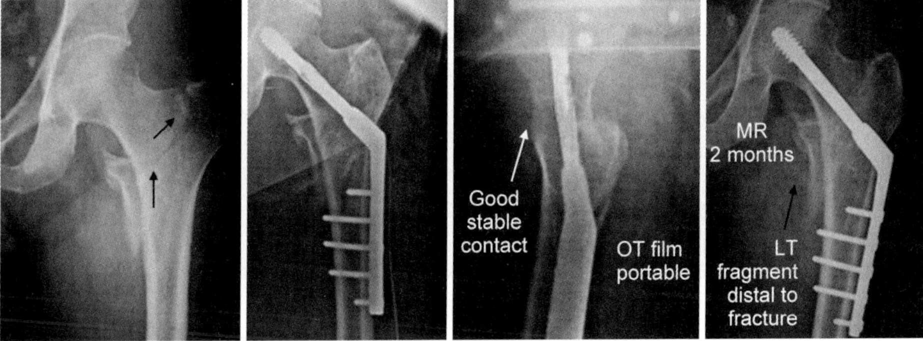

Figure 28.23 TAD less

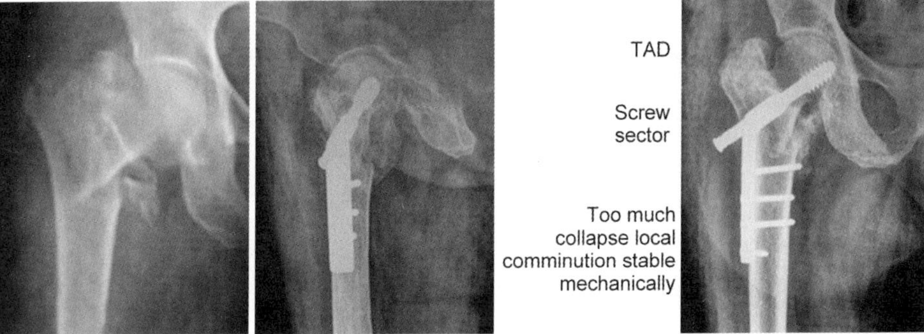

Figure 28.24 TAD less

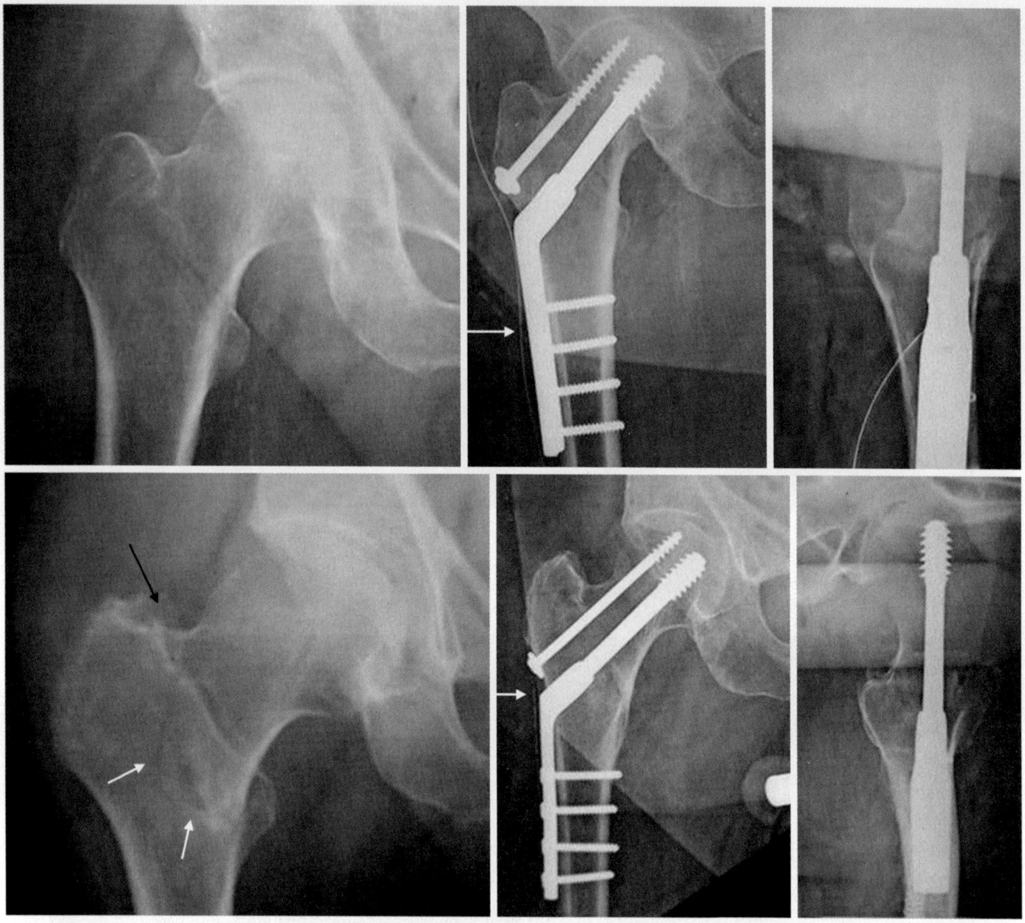

Figure 28.25 Stable fracture. No collapse

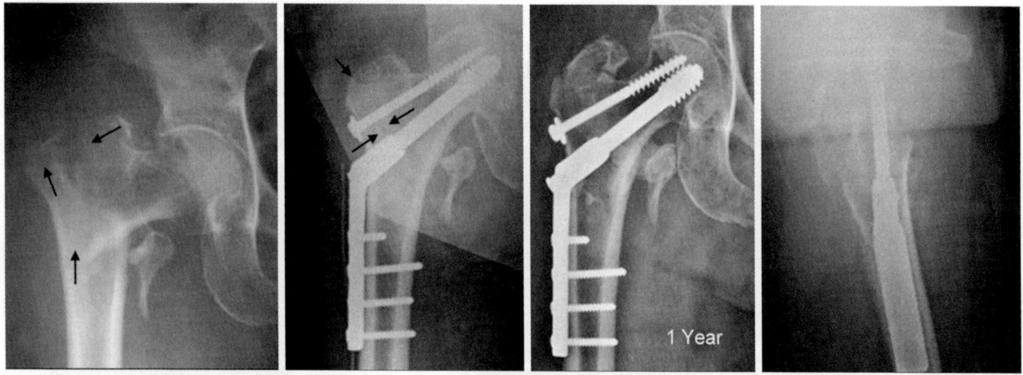

Figure 28.26 Stable fracture. No collapse

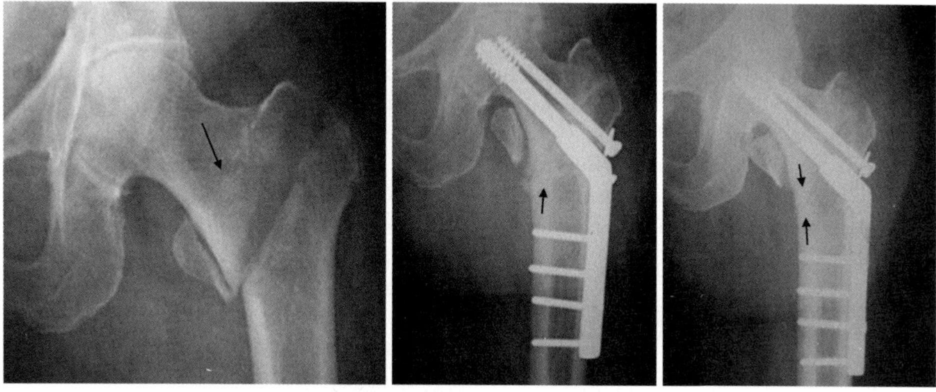

Figure 28.27 Good place for a hip screw

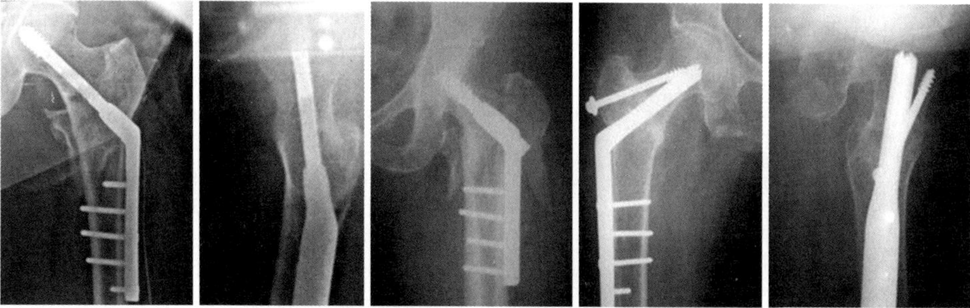

Figure 28.28 Good place for a hip screw

The small postero-medial fragment or an avulsion of the lesser trochanter, usually does not compromise the stability of fixation. If some space is available superior to the sliding hip screw, a 6.5 mm screw with 32 mm threads adds to the rotational stability. A finger tightened screw with a washer, later on, is seen to back out and migrate laterally. This is an indication of more contact opposition across the fracture.

In presence of a DHS and an additional 6.5 mm screw, follow up X-ray film may give an appearance of a varus at fracture site. One should confirm the position of the hip, in terms of rotation, when the film was exposed. Some body structures have a wide pelvis and a short stature, where in the neck shaft angle is less and this makes an appearance of fracture fixation in varus (Figs 28.29 and 28.30).

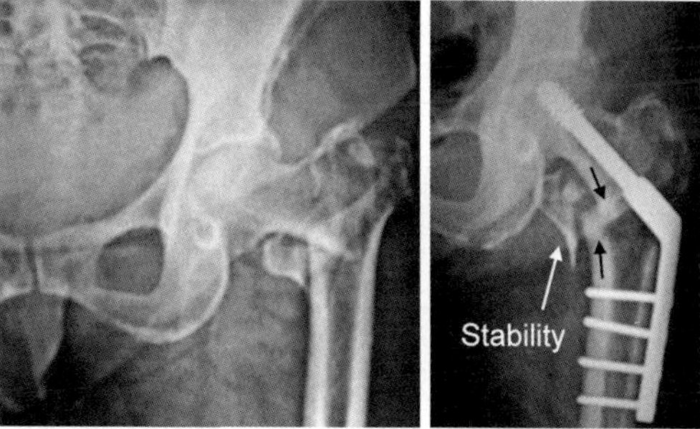

Figure 28.29 In women, wide pelvis is often associated with less neck shaft angle

A Case Example

This elderly person more than 75 years had diabetes and had old hemiplegia on the same side, that of the fracture side, with spasticity.

(Note the atherosclerotic femoral vessels). He was operated on a fracture table. It was very difficult to reduce the fracture and place the calcar beak in the femoral canal, lateral to the medial cortex. The DHS fixation with an additional 6.5 mm screw was done. The fixation was stable, but the calcar continued to be medial to the shaft. Follow up X-ray revealed, massive callus all around (Fig. 28.31).

LESSER TROCHANTER FIXATION

Lesser trochanter is an extrusion fracture. Often it has a large part of the posterior portion of trochanter. After fixation of the principal fragments, one should consider a possibility of fixation of the lesser trochanter. It is possible to pass a circlage wire, around the ilio-psoas tendon, so it does not slip and slide distally.

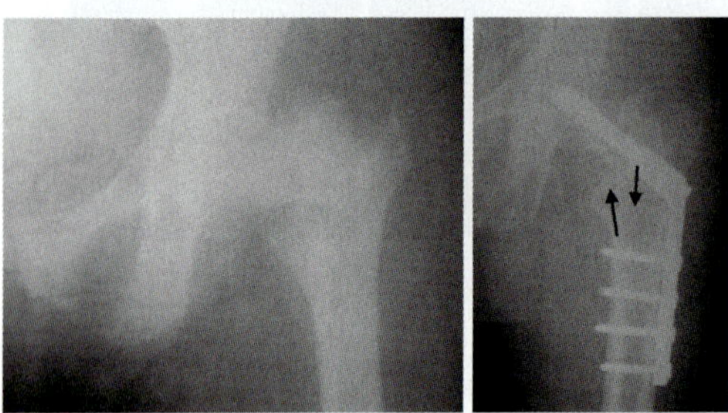

Figure 28.30 Old untreated fracture, often demands fixation in varus

(The tapering shape of the lesser trochanter permits the loop to slide distally. If semicircular cannulated wire passer is used, the tip should glide close to the bone, to avoid any important structure being caught under the wire loop.

If the fragment is large enough, it could be stabilized by IFS method.

The fragment should be reduced well. Exact anatomical reduction may not be possible, but close to it is possible. If one succeeds in doing so, medial calcar area consolidates well and prevents any possibility of late varus. Having reduced the fragment with a pointed reduction forceps, following methods are available:

Options

- If the side plate has oval holes, a malleolar screw can be passed through it, may be at an angle, which is usually needed.
- If adequate area of bone is available anterior to the plate, a screw can be inserted outside the plate. The area is sloping and hence use of a drill sleeve is mandatory, to keep it at the desired point and to prevent its breakage. A malleolar or a 4 mm shaft screw can be used.
- In some fractures there is a medial long vertical fragment. If it is possible to pass an IFS through the wider part, it at least maintains the position and does not permit to get displaced from the shaft of femur. Now, since the distance between the two fragments is reduced, with good medial

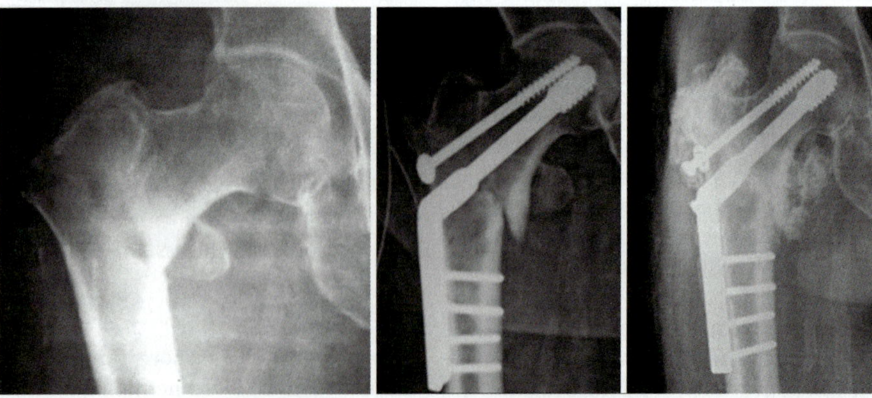

Figure 28.31 Medial beak out and union

soft tissue attachment, the union is assured (Figs 28.32 to 28.34).

If the fracture is a stable one, with wide bone to bone contact, the sliding screw should be so placed, that superior to it, a 6.5 mm screw can be inserted.

Thus when to use a 6.5 additional screw?

- Wide fracture surface in a stable fracture
- Less likely to medialize further
- Be parallel to the hip screw. (Angular placed screw gives a triangular stability)
- Adds to rotary stability
- Finger tight only, especially when lateral cortex is thin. A washer is a must.

When not to add a 6.5 mm screw?

If the proximal lateral cortex is thin, there is a danger of rupture of that area and conversion to a subtrochanteric fracture.

Prior to patient draping, one should confirm that medial calcar opposition is well maintained. At times, after the hip screw is inserted, in a stable fracture as well, the reduction appears to be a valgus one. Hence, prior to insertion of the guidewire, it is safe to insert a stabilizing 2 mm K-wire in the superior part of the neck. This helps to maintain a good reduction achieved. This is more important, in presence of a postero-medial fragment.

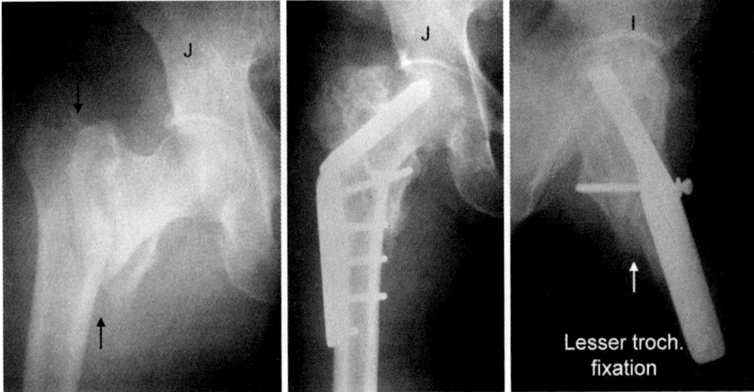

Figure 28.32 Fixation of lesser trochanter offer more stability, due to restoration of anatomy

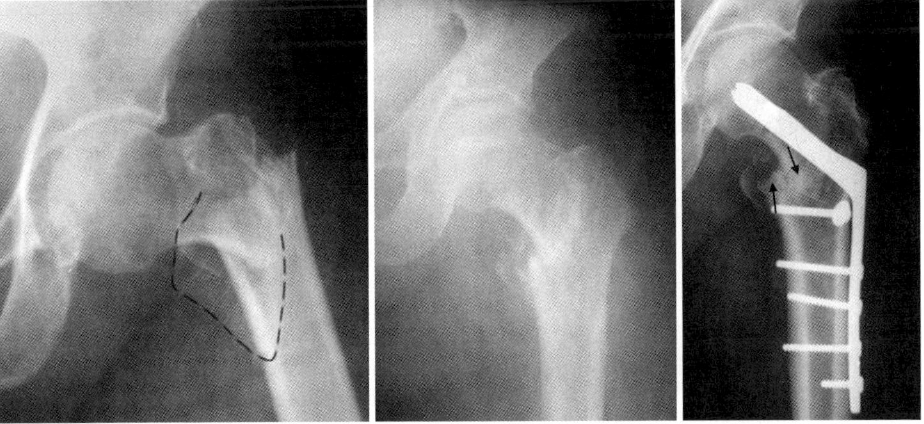

Figure 28.33 Reconstruction of postero-medial extrusion of lesser trochanter

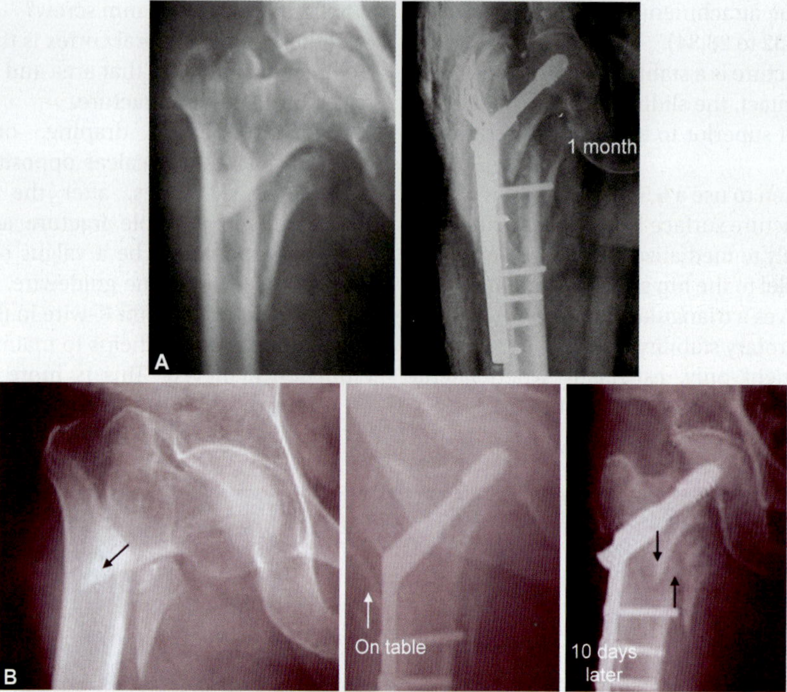

Figures 28.34A and B If medialization expected, prefer to medialize on table and offer stability on table only

However, in spite of the anatomical reduction, within few days medialization occurs, as is observed (Figs 28.34A and B).

PRIMARY BONE GRAFTING

A case of basi-trochanteric fracture on X-ray indicated comminution around the fracture area. On table, it was observed to be more than what appeared on the X-ray film. Primary bone grafting and internal fixation done. Good union.

Similarly, quite often, postero-medial comminution and bone defect is observed on table. If in doubt, it is safer to build the bone defect with autologous grafts, than a synthetic bone substitute. The former is far superior in offering good bone consolidation (Figs 28.35 and 28.36).

FRACTURE COLLAPSE AND MEDIALIZATION

In a fracture in trochanteric area, after good reduction and stabilization with a sliding screw device (DHS). Contact opposition and fracture collapse is observed during the follow up.

In a young lady under 30, anatomical reduction and fixation was done. She had to travel to a far place and expecting this outcome, a Thomas' splint too was given for three weeks. Maybe there was local comminution, which permitted gradual collapse of the fracture area, resulting in 15 mm shortening, in due course. The fracture had well-medialized and continued to be table.

Is it possible to prevent this shortening in a young person?

Options Available

- After surgery, add a minimum skeletal traction, to maintain the reduction and position, as an indoor patient for four weeks from surgery.
- In place of a sliding screw, one may use a fixed angle implant, like a Jewett nail plate.

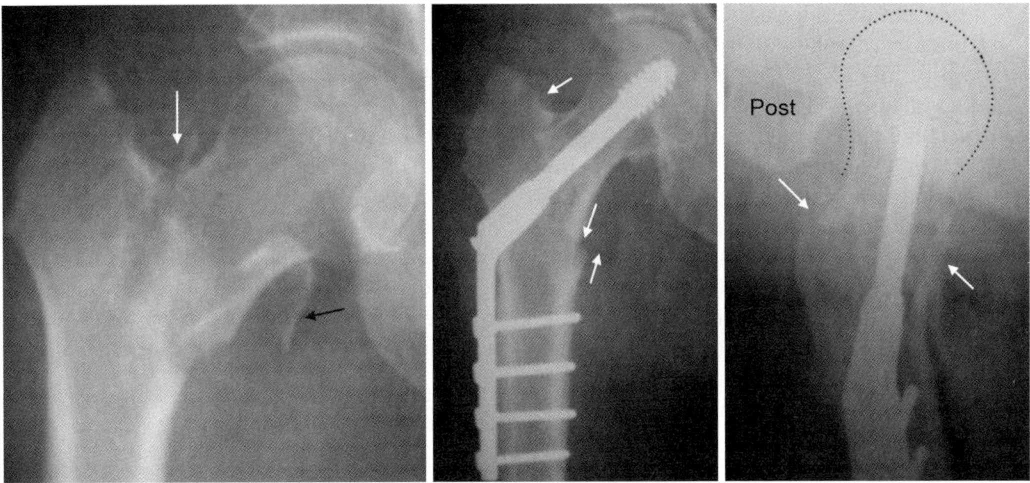

Figure 28.35 Primary bone grafting

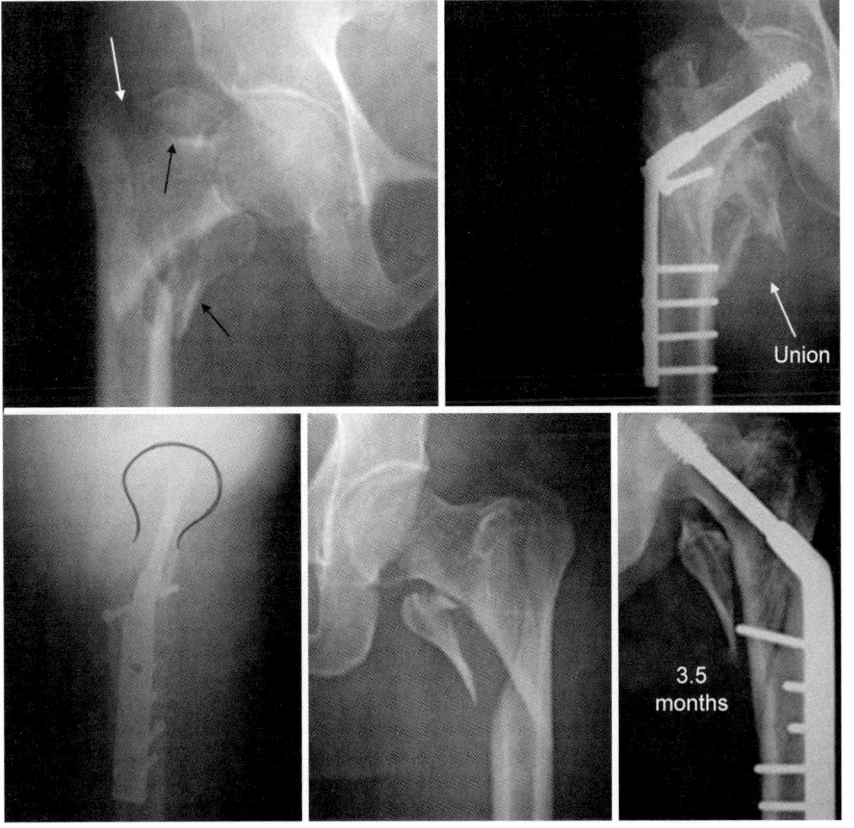

Figure 28.36 Primary bone grafting

(If one can use a locking plate for absolute stability in a diaphyseal fracture, why not use the principle also?) One has observed very little collapse and shortening after using a Jewett nail plate in such a situation.

- Above two options can be exercised in a young and middle age person, who can tolerate rest in bed and in whom the healing potential is superior compared to elderly persons. In the later, early mobilization is the concern, while in the young, restoration of anatomy and leg length is vital. The reader can imagine the patient's reaction, when such a shortening occurs.

- In such a case is there any roll of primary grafting to prevent collapse? (Fig. 28.37)

In a procedure of internal fixation with a DHS, one tries to achieve an anatomical reduction. Having achieved it, it is stabilized in the same position. The postoperative X-ray image shows anatomical reduction. However, follow up films indicate gradually increasing contact opposition. If it occurs to a small extent, the leg length discrepancy would be till 15 mm, which is functionally acceptable. Role of a trochanteric stabilization plate is discussed later (Figs 28.38 to 28.40).

MEDIALIZATION AFTER A LATERAL WALL OSTEOTOMY/FRACTURE

In a fracture, where there is a long distal beak on the proximal fragment, usually the fracture reduction is not easy, till the medialization is carried out, by an osteotomy. This is preferably done 15 mm distal to the base of the greater trochanter, which permits slight medial displacement of the lateral fragment. Often, the fact that this is possibly done, can be recognized by a trained eye only, in a postoperative film.

In a well-reduced IT fracture, the lateral fragment could be quite thin. While making a track for insertion of a guidewire or while using a triple reamer, the lateral thin cortex gives way and the fracture tends to be rather unstable.

Is it possible to keep this incidence of lateral wall fracture less?

Answer: If on the lateral surface of the shaft, one observes that the fracture line is distal to proximal and posterior to anterior, it is worth trying to have the nail entry more distally and more anteriorly. The nail entry, being more anterior, needs to be directed posteriorly in the head of femur, so it will be towards the postero-superior sector. This may possibly leave a band of bone in between the track for the barrel and the original fracture line (Fig. 28.41).

In a patient over age of 80, with osteoporosis, often comminution is observed in the trochanteric area. The fracture morphology does not permit a cemented partial hip replacement. In such a situation, one needs to stabilize the fracture, with available sliding hip screw. One should reduce the fracture, medialize as much as possible, accepting some shortening on the table. A complementary

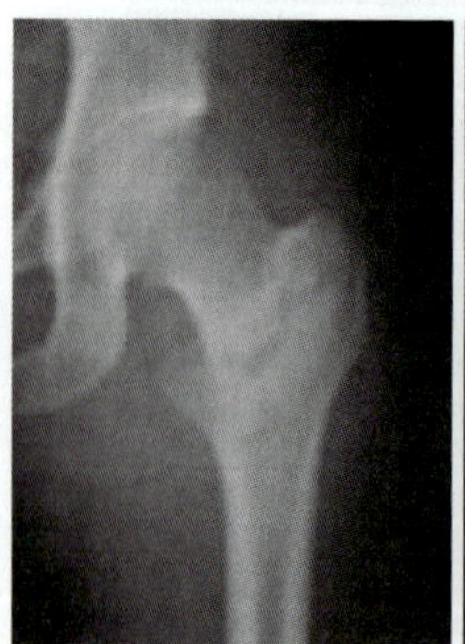
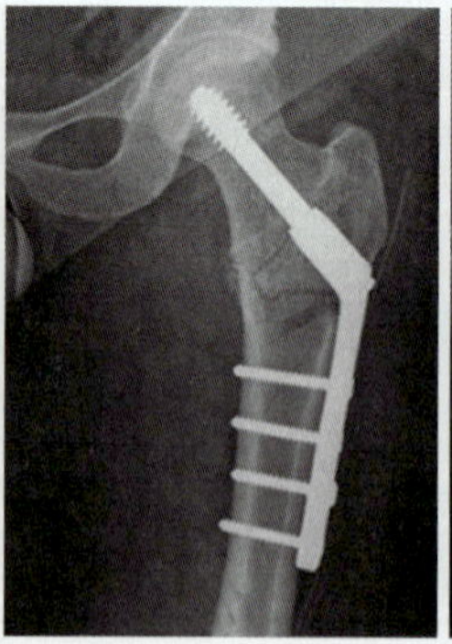
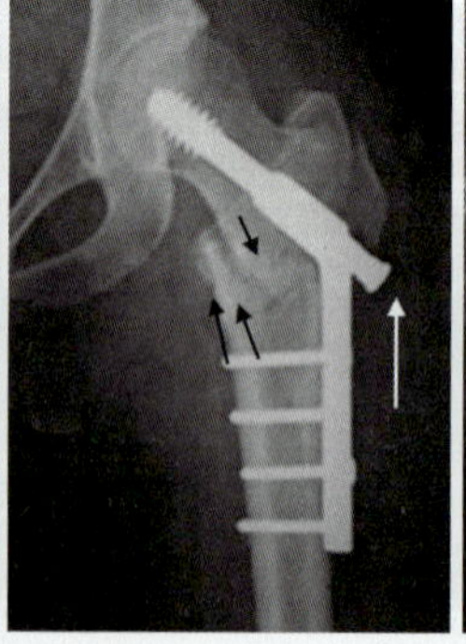
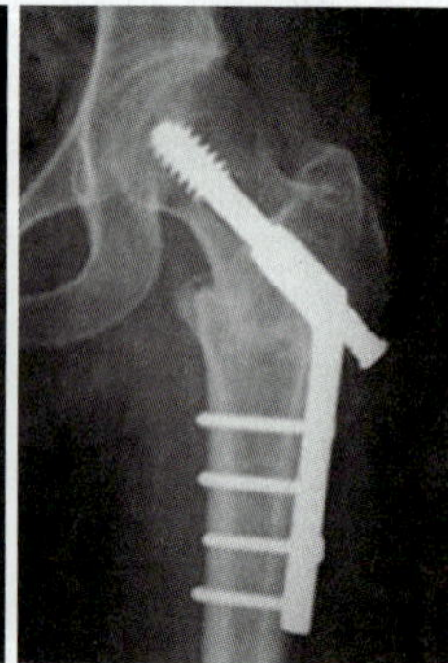

Figure 28.37 Auto-medialization in young

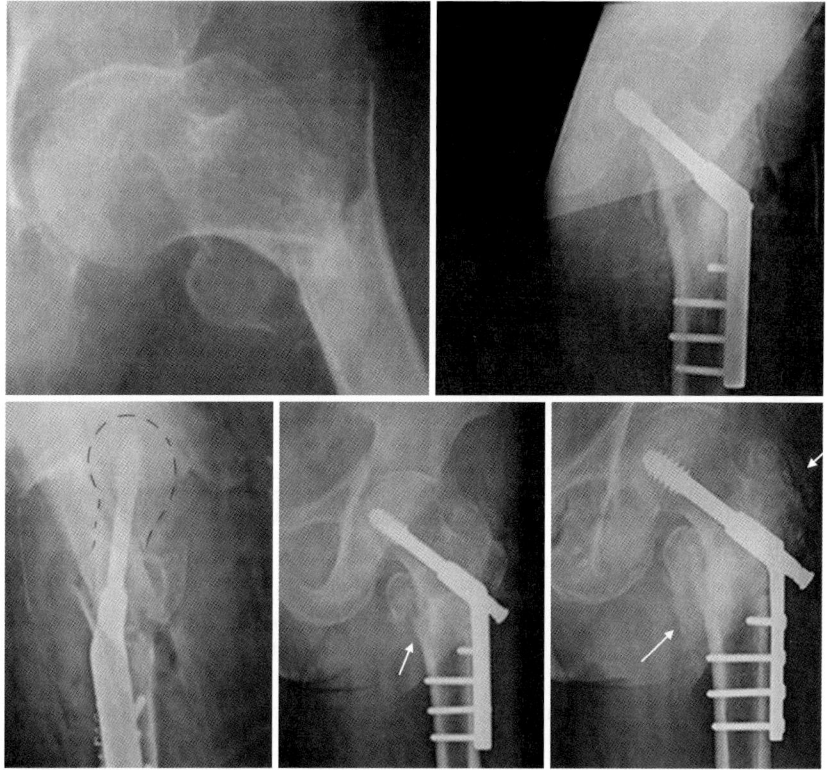

Figure 28.38 Fracture line in lateral wall necessitates making the DHS screw entry more anteriorly

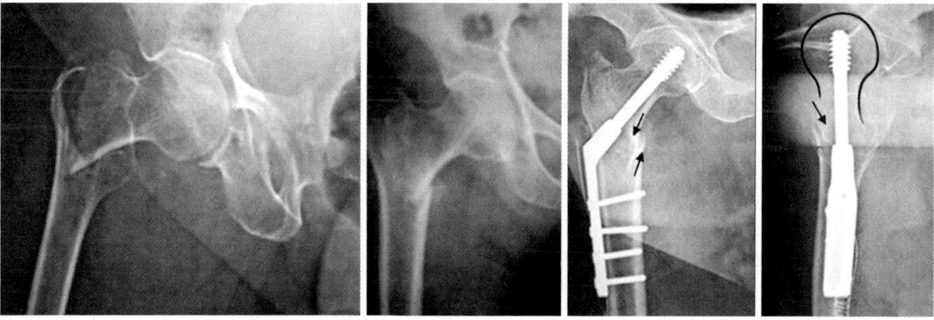

Figure 28.39 Intact lateral wall prevents late fracture collapse

trochanteric stabilization plate may be of some help, to prevent further medialization. In such a situation, it is more acceptable to have, say 2 cm shortening and a pain free, mobile hip, than a screw cut out, etc. and a revision surgery.

Remark: I did not expect so much collapse and shortening or would have used a unicortical screw, in the uppermost hole. Maybe the bicortical screw, as in this case, arrested further telescoping! (Fig. 28.42).

If not medialized:

As seen in previous cases, a stable fixation with good contact opposition in a vertical medial beak, fracture union is observed. However, before accepting a reduction, wherein the medial beak continues to be medial to the shaft, one should always consider a possibility, if it can be inserted in the medullary cavity. If this is not carried out and accepted as such, a non-union is likely to occur. One should do a procedure, which should be the only and the last procedure in a given injury, with a good end result (Fig. 28.43).

In a long vertical fracture line of an intertrochanteric fracture, often good contact opposition is not obtained on table, in spite of adjusting the adduction and abduction of the limb. In such a situation, an osteotomy of the distal fragment, just to yield the distal fragment and allow it to shift medially, is useful. Just below the base of the trochanter, multiple drill holes are made with a 3.5 mm drill bit in an antero-posterior line. After making such holes, with a 10 mm osteotome, they are joined together. The bone yields and the distal fragment is shifted medially with ease and a good contact opposition is achieved. In a postoperative X-ray film, maybe only a trained eye can notice such a procedure. The medial beak is likely to shift downwards during follow up and hence the uppermost screw is preferably a unicortical one, unlike in this case (Fig. 28.44).

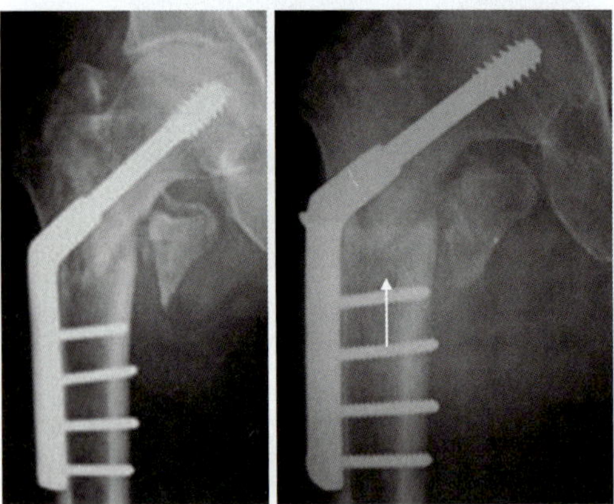

Figure 28.40 Medialization and minimal collapse offers stability, assured union and minimum leg length discrepancy

TROCHANTERIC STABILIZATION PLATE

In elderly person with osteoporosis and diabetes, comminution is commonly observed and morphology indicates an unstable fracture. A trochanteric stabilization plate (TSP) is placed under the side plate. It may need some contouring before final placement.

Its purpose is to prevent excess medialization and proximal migration of the distal fragment. To achieve this, it is necessary to insert at least one 6.5 mm screw through its proximal broad area in the neck. The screw being a shaft screw, would permit some collapse and medialization, which is accompanied by proximal migration of the distal fragment, but not too much.

It appears, the degree to which a fracture would medialize, with use of a trochanteric stabilization plate is governed by:

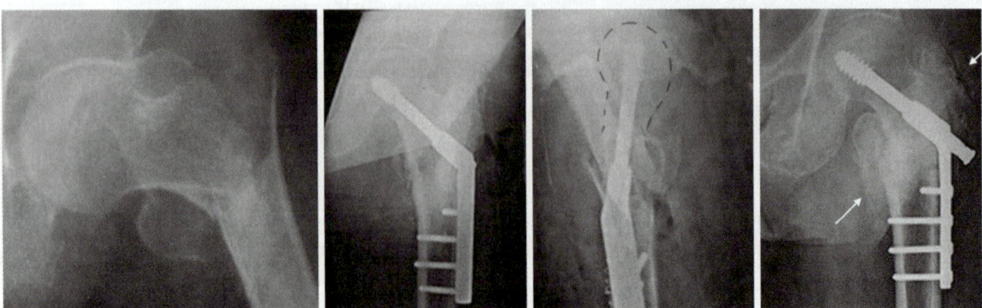

Figure 28.41 Hip screw in anterior to posterior direction

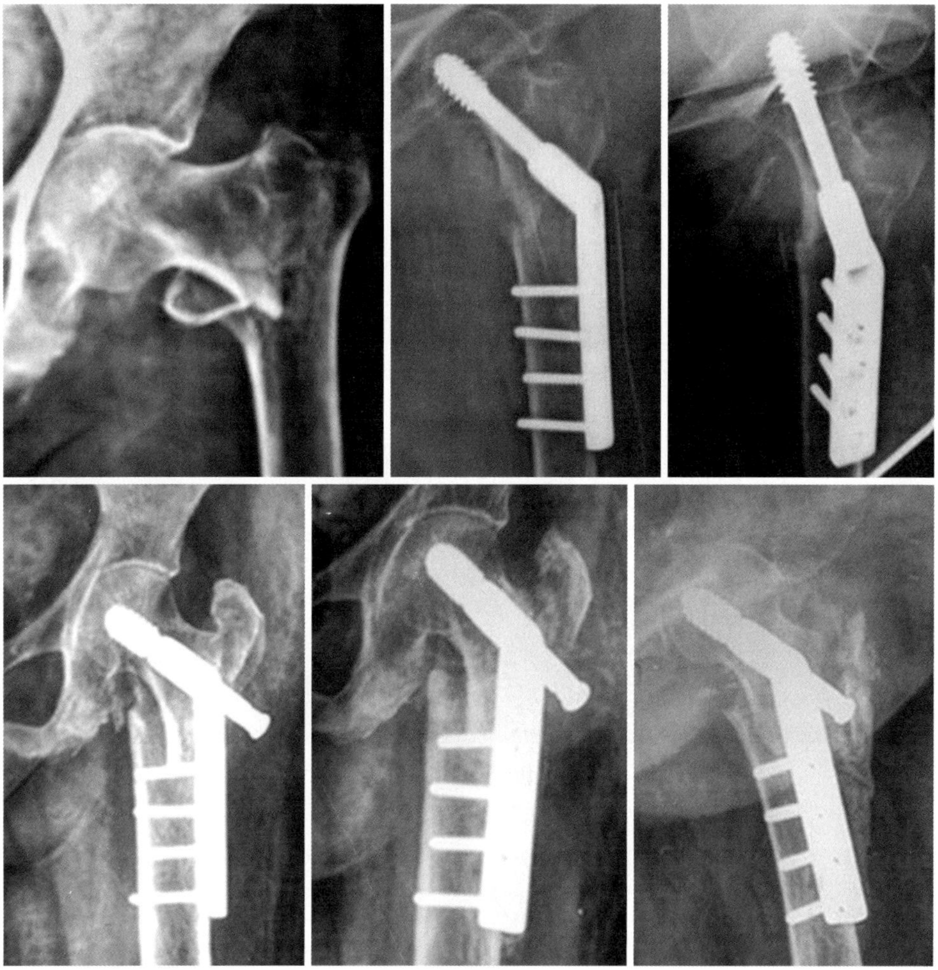

Figure 28.42 Auto-medialization after a lateral wall fracture

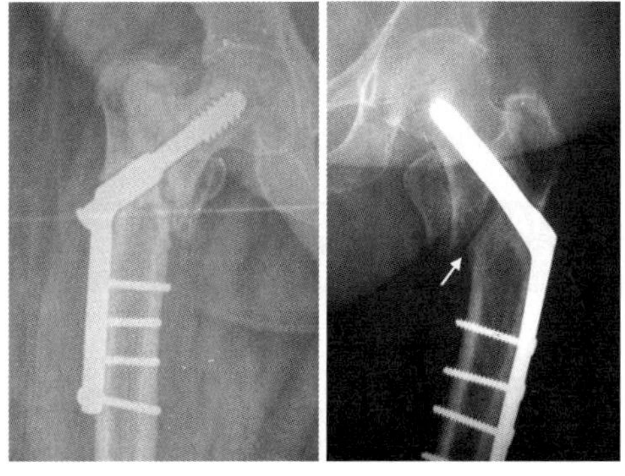

Figure 28.43 Medialize the beak

- The strength of the plate, which would resist its bending
- Contouring and good contact with the trochanter
- Presence of a screw through its proximal wide area, which would control the 'Settling' of the fracture (Figs 28.45 and 28.46).

In Figure 28.46, please note, the DHS assembly with the TSP has slightly shifted upwards, may be there was some comminution in area, where the barrel was inserted.

Today longevity of the population is increasing, especially amongst the female

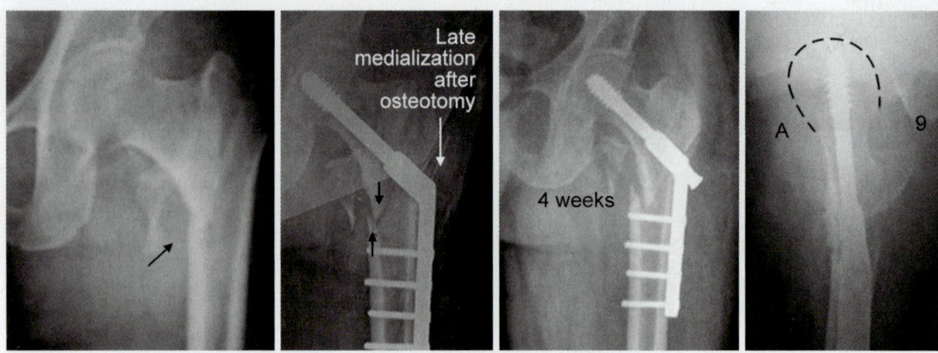

Figure 28.44 Medialization after osteotomy

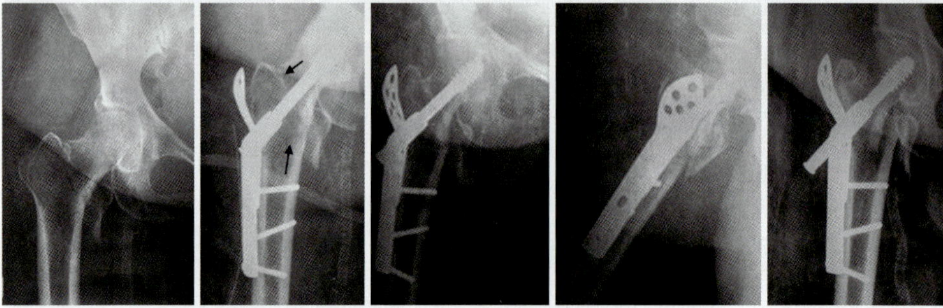

Figure 28.45 TSP

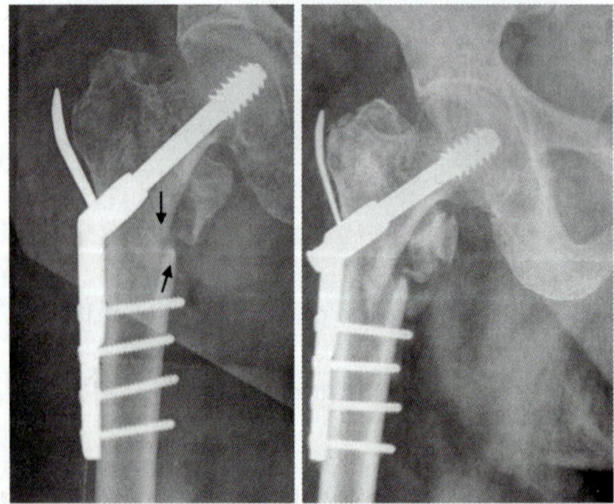

Figure 28.46 TSP

population. After a fracture in a hip, the activity level of the patient reduces.

Few factors with advancing age in a person with fracture on a hip:

- The activity level decreases.
- Due to lack of information, lack of exercises/ absence of calcium supplements/anti-resorptives, the osteoporosis would relentlessly continue.
- With advancing age, coordination of movements reduces, leading to more chances of another fall.

Hence to have a patient with a previous fracture on the opposite hip or less commonly on the same hip, is a common occurrence nowadays (Figs 28.47 to 28.49).

SPECIAL SITUATION IN INTER-TROCHANTERIC FRACTURES

Early Diagnosis

After a fall, when a person presents with pain in the hip and inability to bear weight on the affected limb, one should suspect a hip

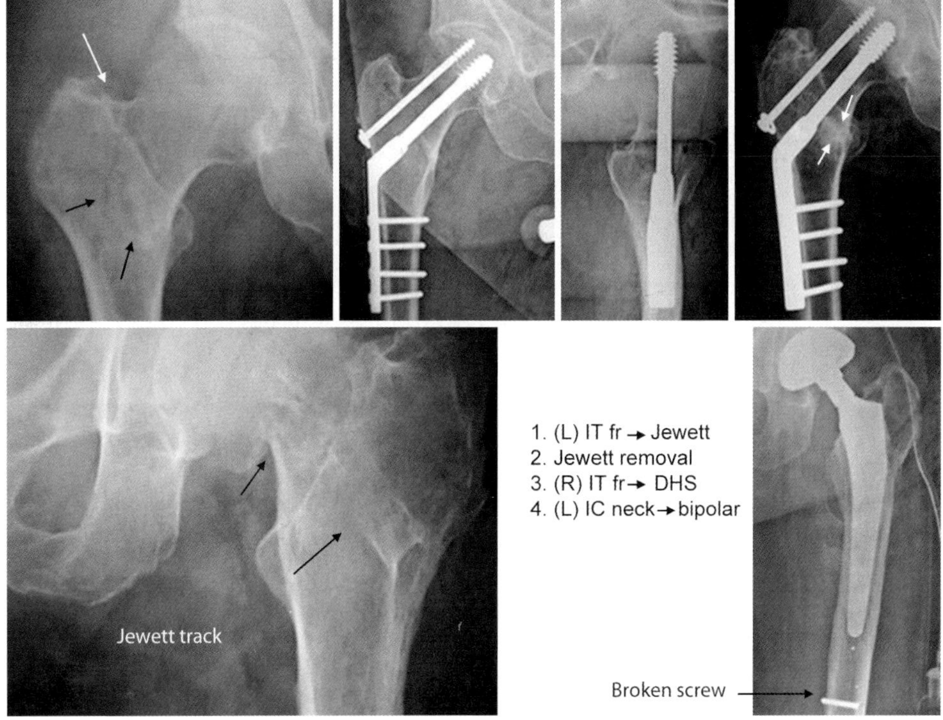

Figure 28.47 Bilateral sequential fracture in hips

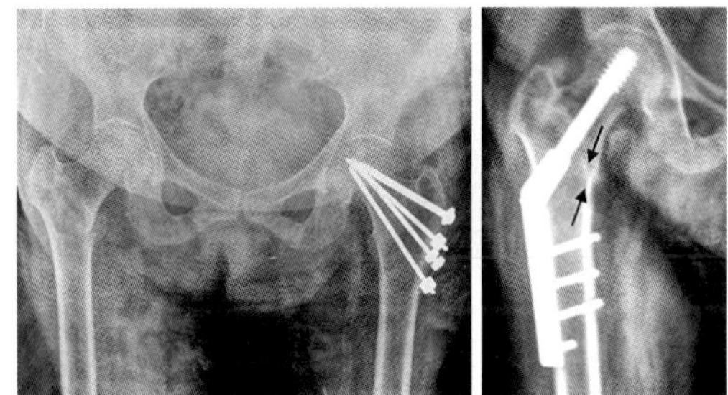

Figure 28.48 Bilateral sequential fracture in hips

fracture. X-ray of pelvis and cross table lateral view of the affected hip, may not indicate a hip injury. MRI examination is thus necessary. The MRI examination may indicate an undisplaced intertrochanteric fracture. This fracture should be immediately stabilized, so early ambulation and good end result can be achieved (Fig. 28.50).

Osteomalacia

Osteomalacia is more often seen in women. This lady (as detected in the X-ray film after a trochanter fracture) had osteomalacia with pseudo-fractures in the pelvis.

The trochanteric fracture was stabilized, with a good outcome. Necessary medical treatment helped her to restore her physical condition. Later she passed away, due to unrelated cause.

As seen in Figure 26.51, a DHS device was used. Looking at the fracture morphology again, one may also consider use of a DCS since adequate bone stock is available in the proximal fragment, wherein the transverse hip screw would have a good hold on the trochanter. A good stable contact opposition would have occurred, after the fracture was loaded with a tension device. Once a direct well-opposed reduction is obtained, there is no need for sliding the fragments, over the implant (Fig. 28.51).

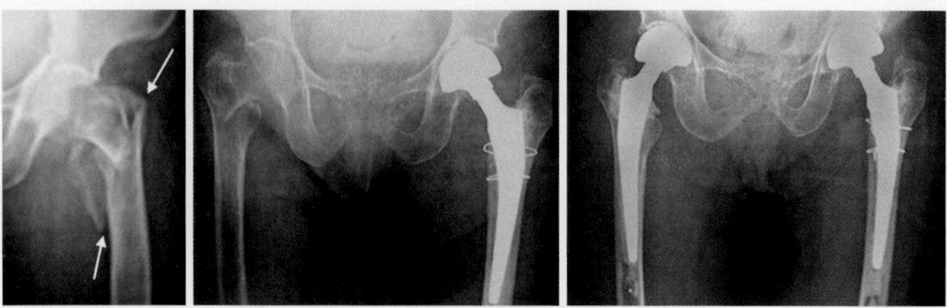

Figure 28.49 Bilateral sequential fracture in hips

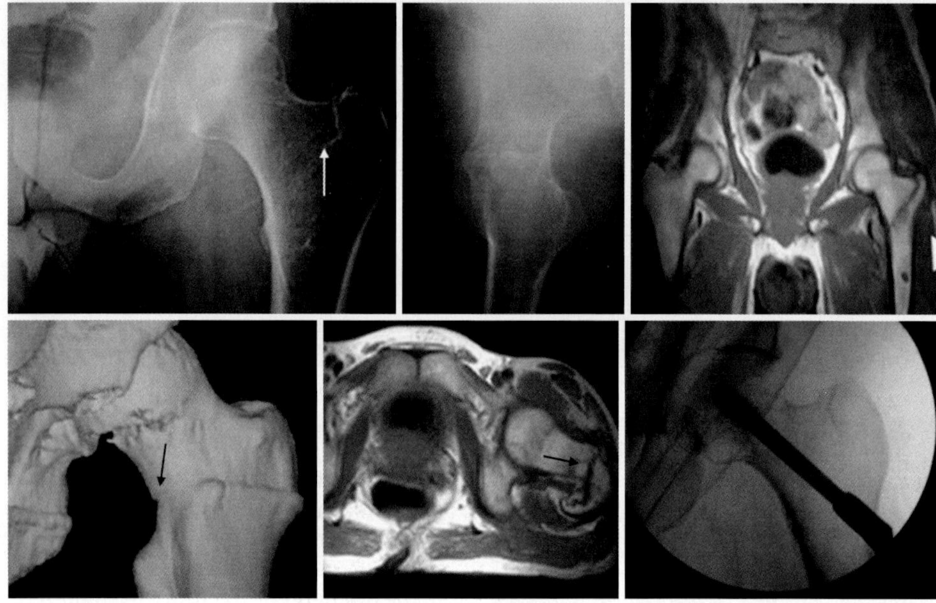

Figure 28.50 MRI diagnosis

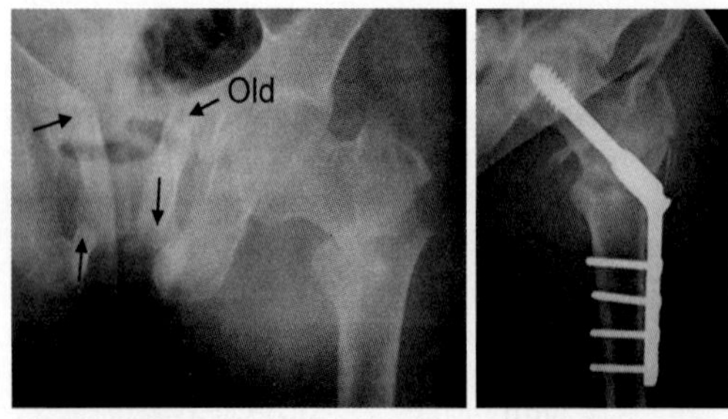

Figure 28.51 DHS in osteomalacia

Sequential Fractures in a HIP

This lady had X-ray of pelvis taken for unrelated problem few years ago, which did not reveal any injury. Then sustained a fall and being an impacted fracture (as seen in a later X-ray film), continued to walk and fortunately the fracture united. A few years later had another fall and sustained a trochanteric fracture. This was then stabilized by a Jewett nail, with good outcome (Fig. 28.52).

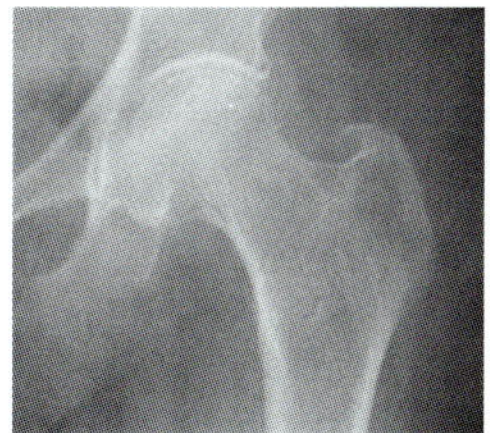

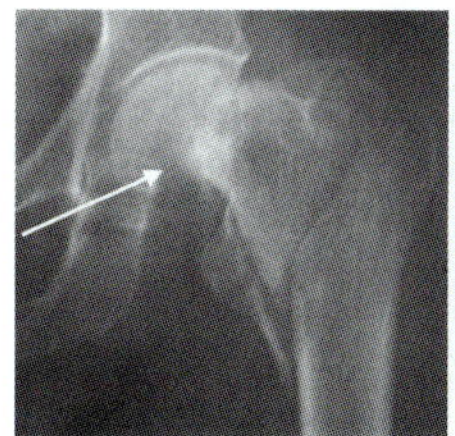

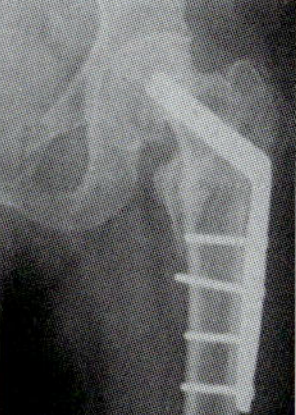

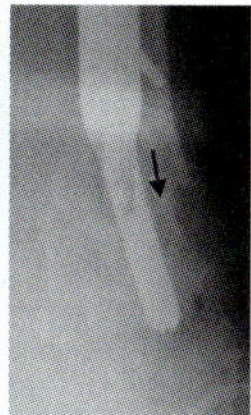

Figure 28.52 Impacted fracture and later IT fracture

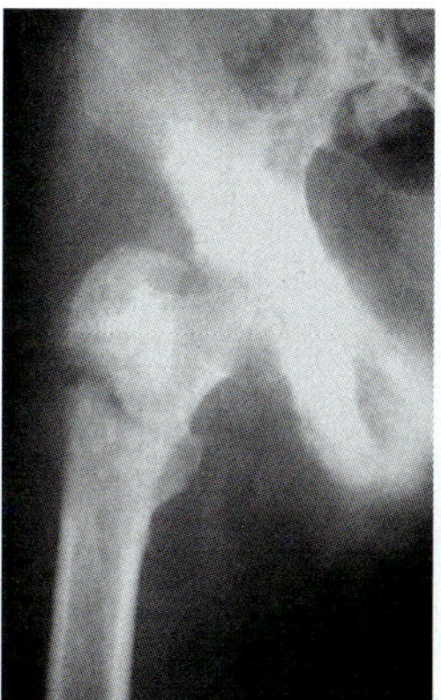

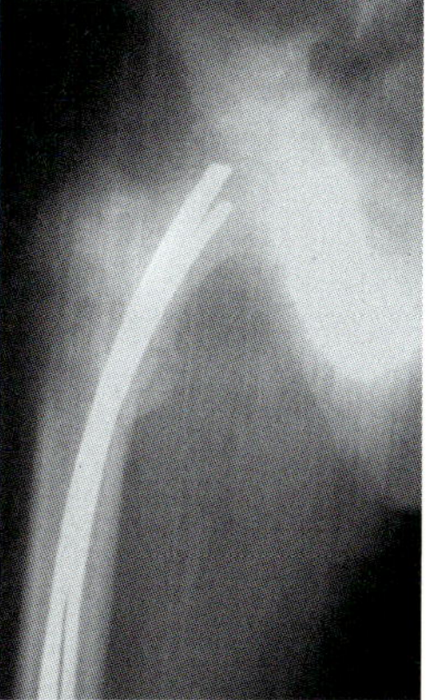

Figure 28.53 Ender nailing in pathological fracture

Ender Nail in a Pathological Fracture

This old person had sustained a fracture of the trochanter. X-ray revealed a pathological fracture, secondary to Ca prostate. The fracture was stabilized by Ender nails and the fracture gradually united well. Necessary treatment for the malignancy was carried out. Such a situation is a good indication for Ender nail (Fig. 28.53).

Untreated Fracture of Trochanter

This elderly patient reported from a peripheral area, having sustained a fall more than a month ago. On arrival, the X-ray examination revealed an inter-trochanteric fracture, with shortening and external rotation deformity. The fracture was reduced and skeletal traction was applied. After two weeks of traction, a portable X-ray with traction on, revealed that the trochanter had come down. Internal fixation was carried out, The medial beak of the proximal fragment was maintained in the medullary cavity in some degree of adduction and was stabilized as such, to achieve a good union (Fig. 28.54).

Callus in Ankylosing Spondylitis

The amount of callus seen in an inter-trochanteric fracture in a patient suffering from ankylosing spondylitis, is often much more than, what one sees in other cases (Fig. 28.55).

Another middle age person had sustained an inter-trochanteric fracture and was operated elsewhere. After 4 weeks of surgery, developed external rotation deformity and spasm in the affected left hip.

Nuclear scan with T 99, suggested a possibility of avascular changes in the hip. A Gallium scan did not indicate any infection.

With traction to the affected hip, the spasm and pain reduced and gradual mobilization was started. However, he continued to have pain on weight bearing. The range was about 30% of normal hip.

Six months later, i.e. a year after internal fixation, the hip was stiff with pain on motion. The removal of the implant was considered, with full idea that the range would not improve, but the pain may reduce (Fig. 28.56).

LONG MEDIAL BEAK

A patient suffered from tuberculosis of the left hip and was treated non-operatively about 15 years ago, with good return of function. While he was in another city, sustained a fracture on the same side. The surgeon carried out a DHS

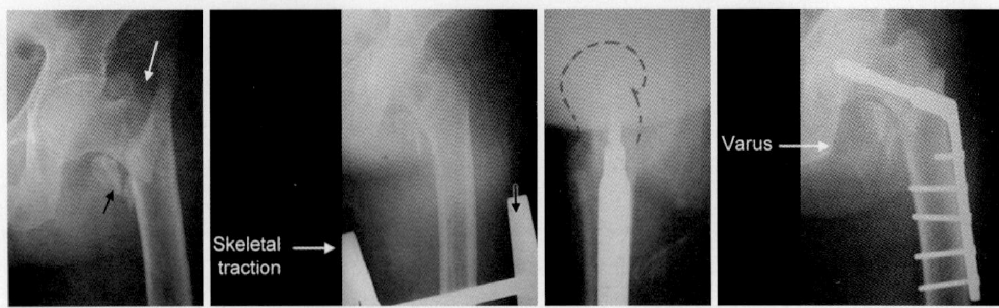

Figure 28.54 Three-week old untreated IT fracture

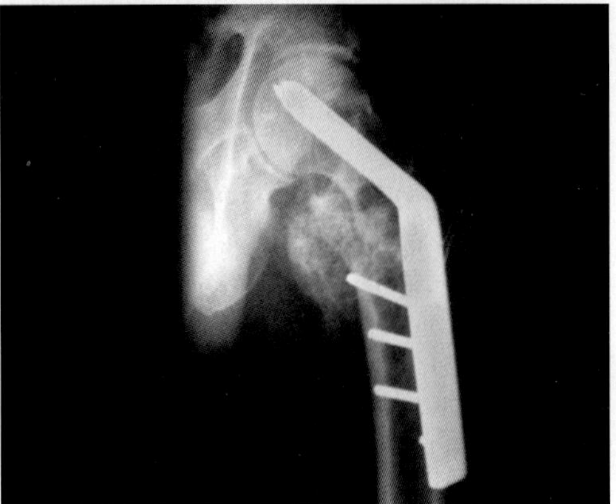

Figure 28.55 Callus in a fracture with ankylosing spondylosis

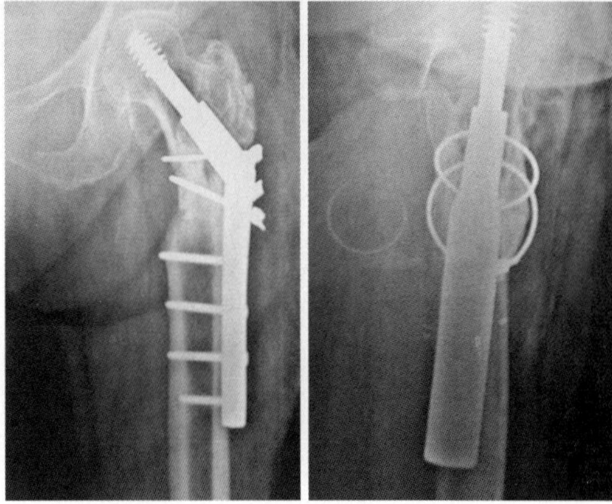

Figure 28.57 Circlage with DHS

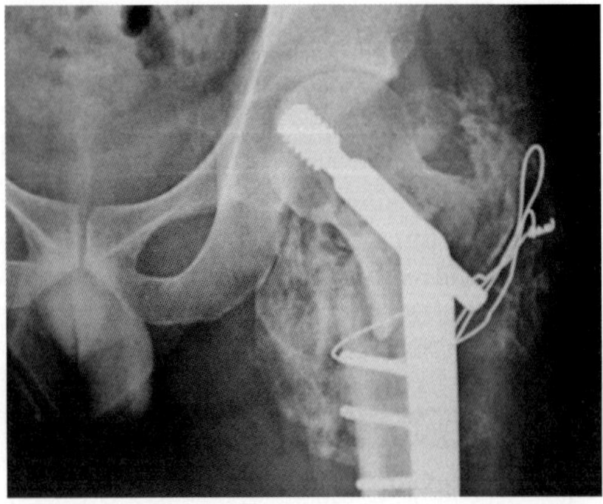

Figure 28.56 Callus in excess

fixation, with use of circlage, what appears to be cable being used. The fracture united well (Fig. 28.57).

An old gentleman of 80 had sustained a supracondylar fracture of the right humerus, intercondylar fracture of the right femur and ipsilateral fracture of the upper/3 tibia, about 20 years ago. He had multiple medical diseases and then sustained a fracture of the left hip. The proximal fragment had a long beak. It was stabilized with a circlage and a DHS. The fixation was well-maintained and could stand with support. He became progressively more ill due to unrelated ailments (Fig. 28.58).

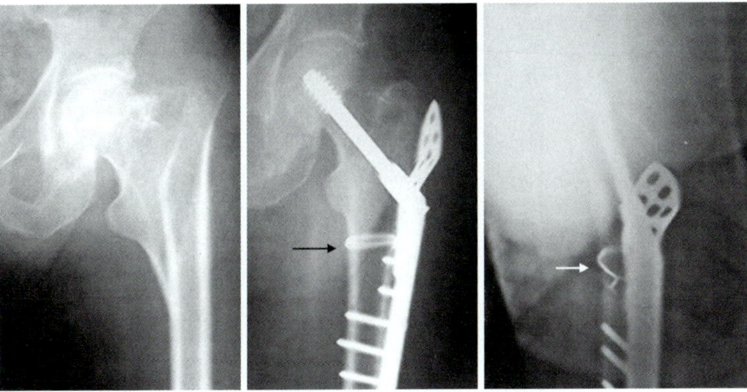

Figure 28.58 Circlage, DHS and TSP

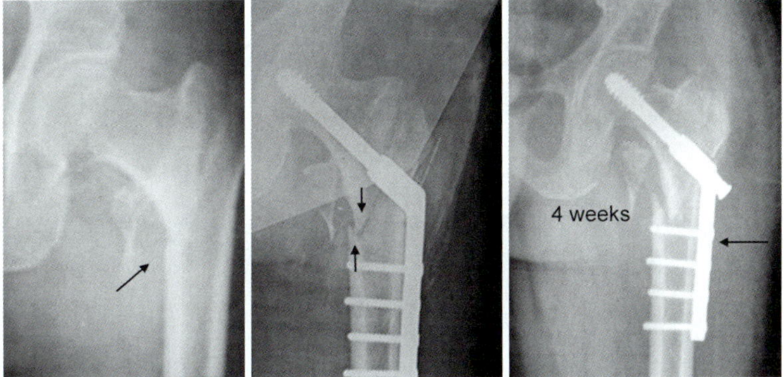

Figure 28.59 Need of uppermost screw to be short

WHEN FURTHER MEDIALIZATION AND TELESCOPING IS EXPECTED

In a fracture, where the proximal fragment has a long medial beak, one may achieve anatomical reduction. However, in presence of posterior comminution, one should expect medialization and more telescoping of the vertical beak. In such a situation, the screw in uppermost hole of the plate, should be a unicortical, permitting telescoping of the beak and increasing the fracture stability. If the screw is bicortical, the beak may not slide downwards (FIgs 28.59 to 28.61).

In spite of this care of inserting a short screw, at times, the shaft medializes, so much that the unicortical screw may be pushed laterally!. In the given example, may be the screw was inserted through a thin cortex, had a poor hold and hence it was shifted laterally (Fig. 28.62).

In an intertrochanteric fracture, if both the fracture surfaces are wide and without comminution, it remains stable. In a fracture at a slightly proximal area, as in a basi-trochanteric fracture, and with some comminution the distal narrow part of the neck easily invaginates in the wider lateral trochanteric area, leading to fracture collapse to some extent. Fortunately, the stability continued to be good and hence the fracture united well (Fig. 28.63).

Often the bone is very osteoporotic and one is concerned about the hold of the screws

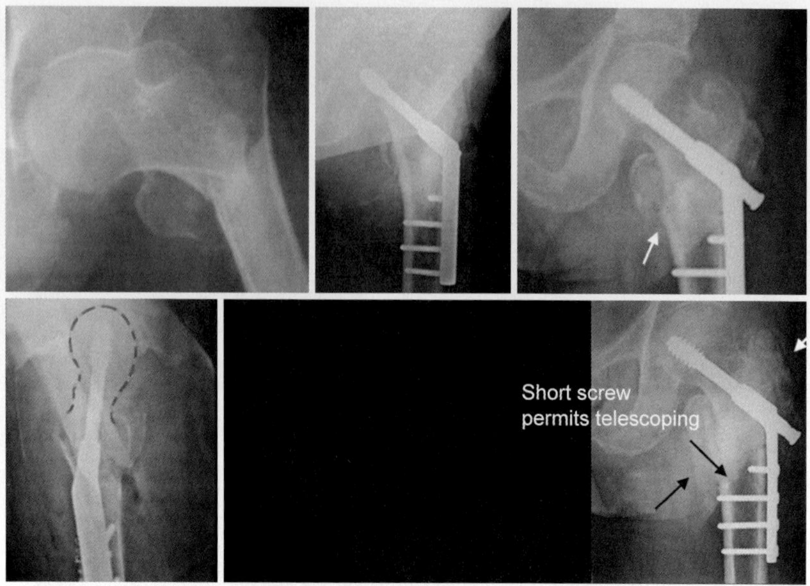

Figure 28.60 Need of uppermost screw to be short

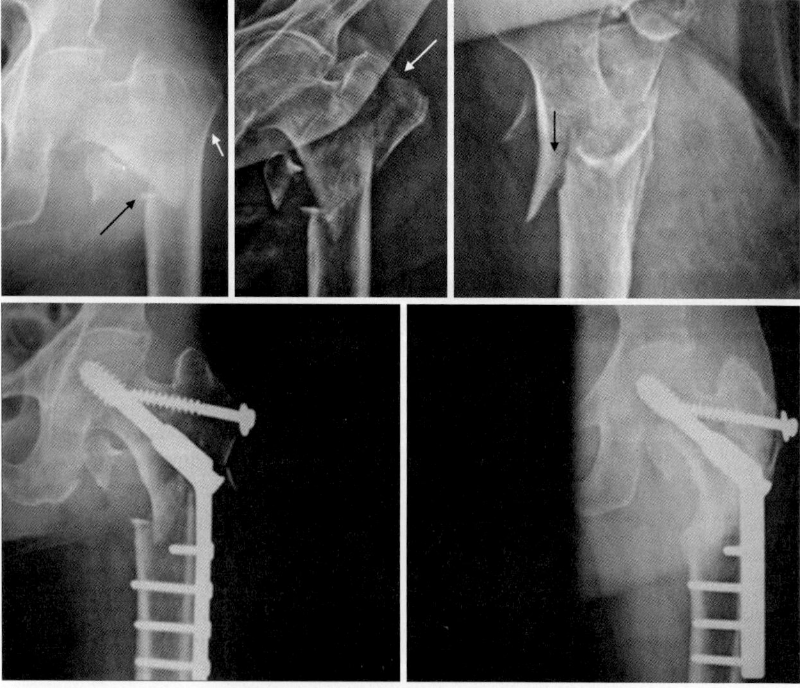

Figure 28.61 Need of uppermost screw to be short

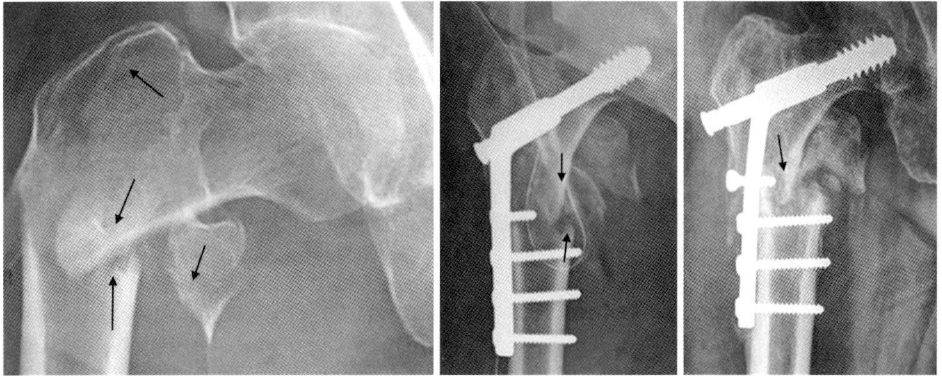

Figure 28.62 Upper short screw migration

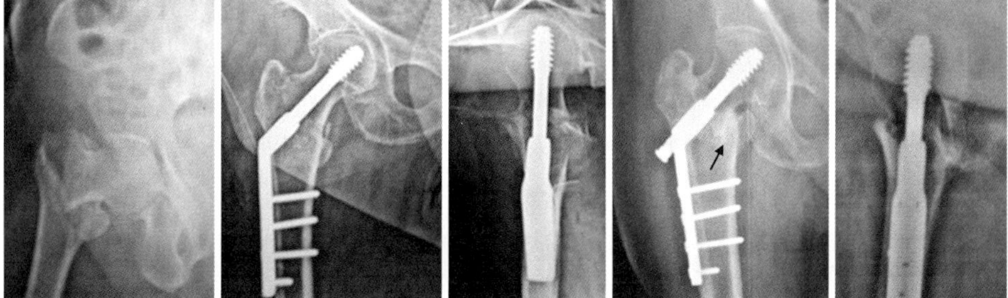

Figure 28.63 Wide lateral fragment and narrow medial fragment

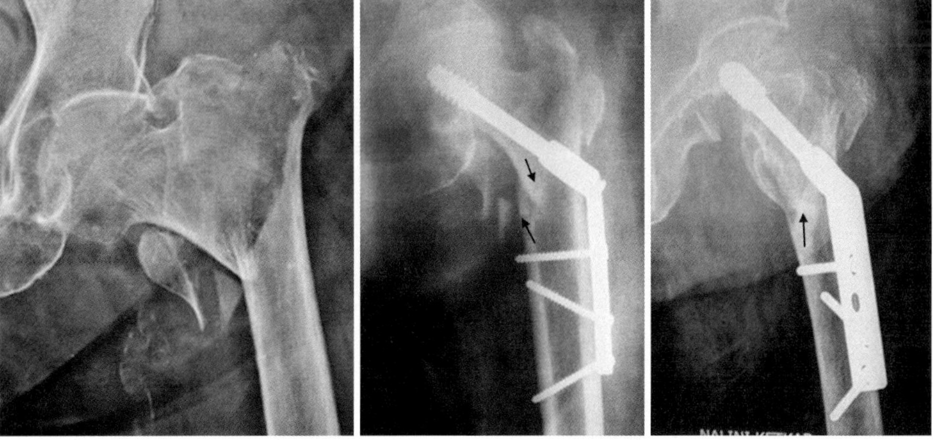

Figure 28.64 Divergent screws in plate

inserted in the side plate and a possibility of screw pull out. In such a situation, one can consider insertion of the distal two screws in an oblique direction, so they offer more resistance to pull out. Naturally, the side plate should have oval holes, to be able to insert the screw in oblique direction. The oblique screw would come in the way of adjacent screw path and which has to be a unicortical. The screw tracks being quite close to each other, it is safer to leave that plate hole unused. In such a situation, it is worthwhile to use a five-hole plate, instead of a four-hole plate.

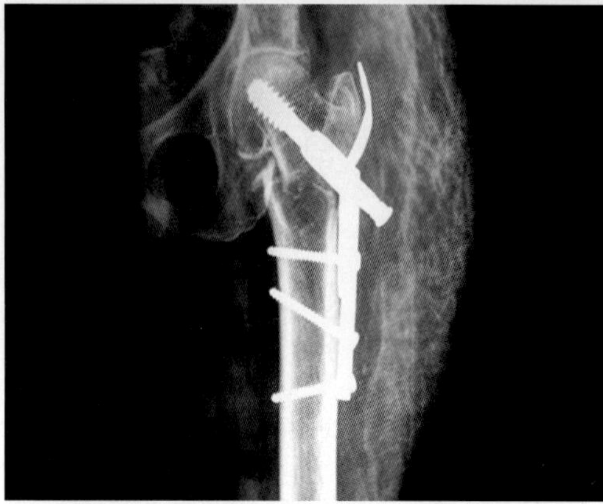

Figure 28.65 Divergent screws in plate

Order of screw insertion. The uppermost screw should be inserted first. The distal most two screws be inserted in divergent directions. Now, one can plan, if the hole above the divergent screws should have a unicortical screw or may be left unused (Figs 28.64 and 28.65).

Due to a direct impact on the greater trochanter, a fracture of the greater trochanter may occur. Often, the fracture may not be clearly visible and the fracture line plane cannot be defined. A CT scan defines the fracture and indicates the direction of the fracture line. If the fragment is small, it is stabilized with two

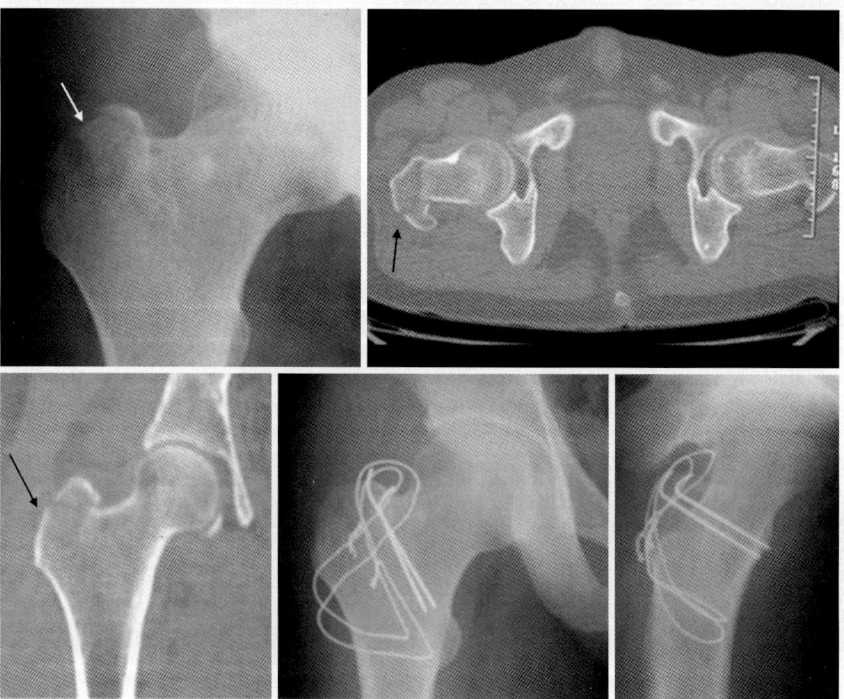

Figure 28.66 Fracture of greater trochanter

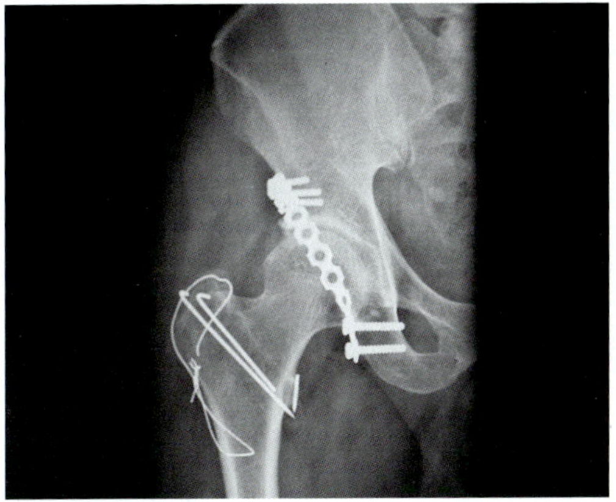

Figure 28.67 Wire fragmentation

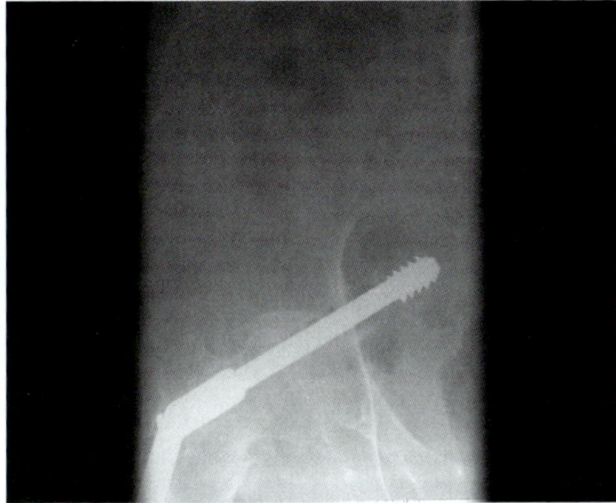

Figure 28.70 Screw penetrating acetabulum

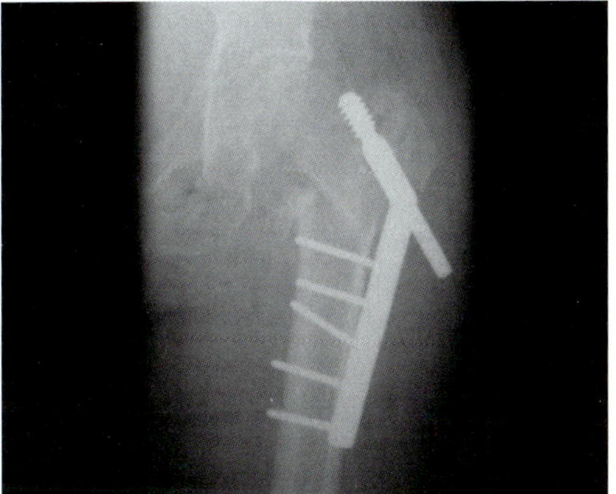

Figure 28.68 DHS screw cut out

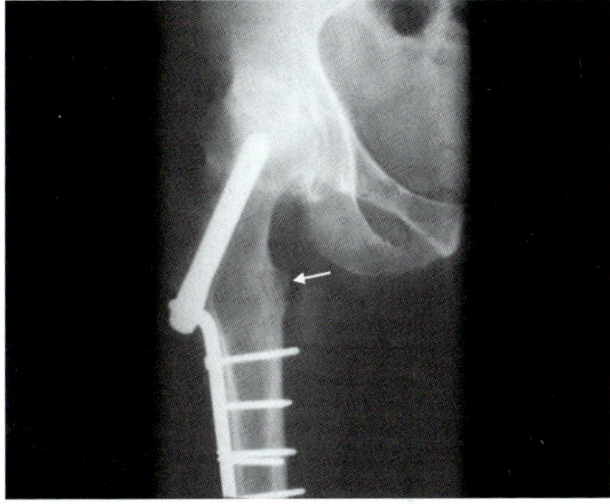

Figure 28.71 Note, it is SP nail and plate, machine screws and a broken drill bit

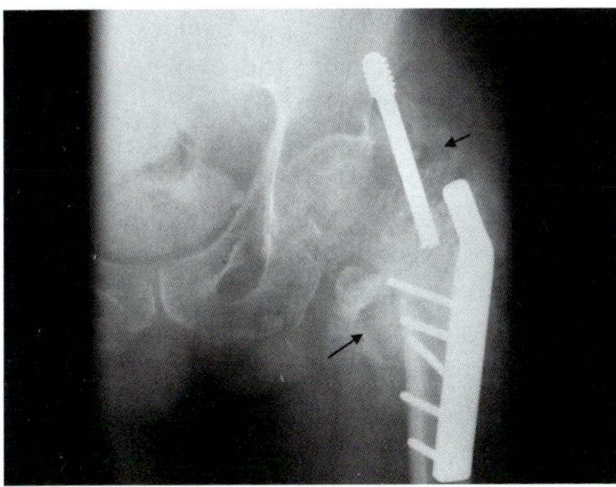

Figure 28.69 Cut out screw migration, in the absence of a compression screw

K-wires and figure of eight wire loops.

It is necessary to advise the patient to come for removal of the implants at the end of a year, before the wire fragments and/or migrates (Figs 28.66 and 28.67).

MECHANICAL COMPLICATIONS

Often, one may come across a case, treated elsewhere. This old person was operated elsewhere and came with pain in the left hip on the trochanter. X-ray revealed a screw cut-out and a possibility of deep infection. He went away and reported after three months, with pain on the lateral side of the iliac wing with a

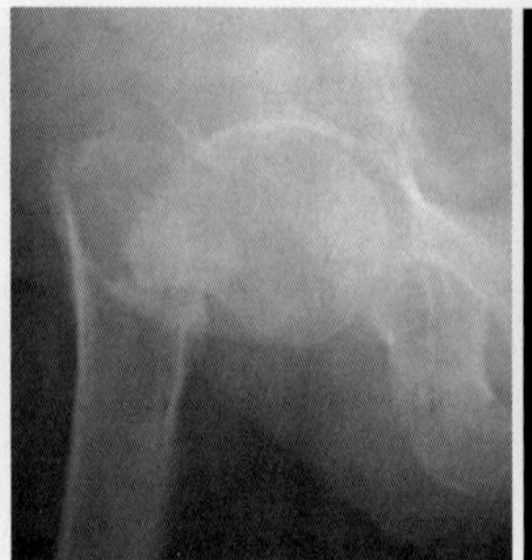
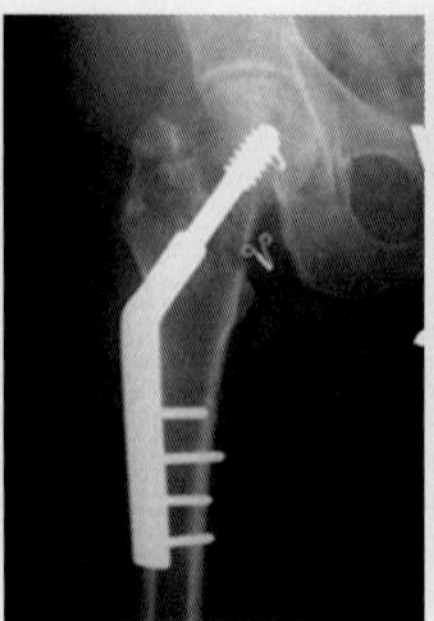
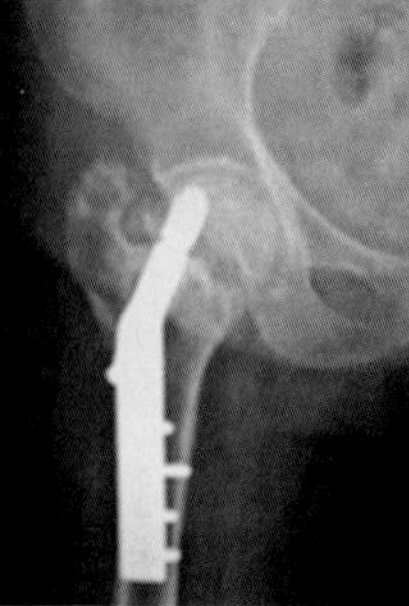
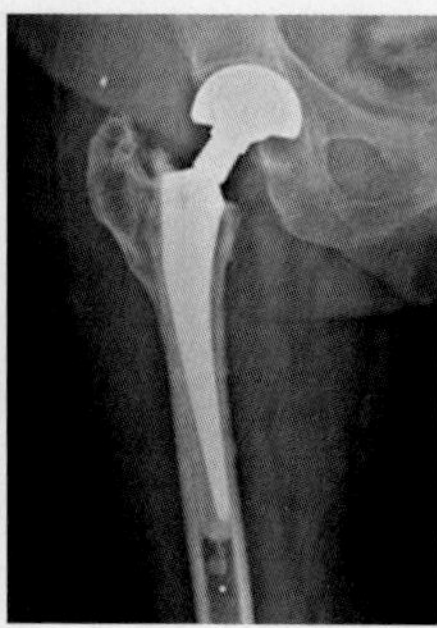

Figure 28.72 Avoid excess valgus

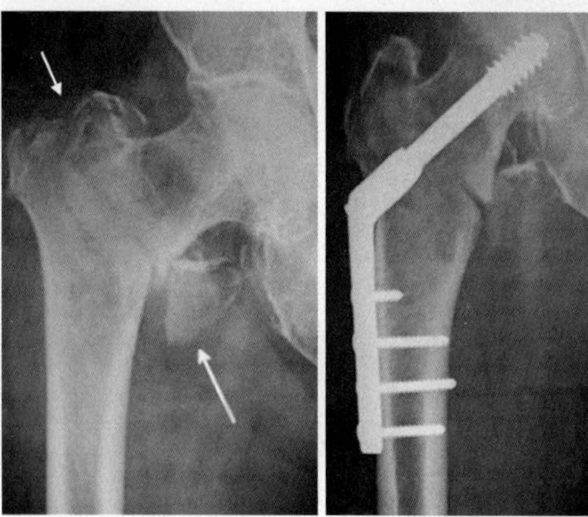

Figure 28.73 Avoid excess valgus

bursa. X-ray examination revealed a migrated sliding screw, towards the iliac wing (Figs 28.68 and 28.69).

An X-ray film was brought for opinion. The lady had a hip fracture and was operated elsewhere. Detailed history was not available, but at present, had pain in the hip with restriction of movements. The X-ray showed a long hip screw, penetrating the floor of the acetabulum and some medial migration of the DHS assembly.

How and what may have happened?

Possibly the triple reaming was done through the floor of acetabulum and a long screw was inserted.

Message, during triple reaming, one should stop in between and take the reading on the shaft, as to how deep the reaming has occurred! (Fig. 28.70)

The fracture reduction be such that, there is no excess valgus angulation at the fracture site. Too much valgus is not safe, as it increases the leg length and there is a chance of AVN of the head of the femur (Fig. 28.71).

If the fracture is reduced in excessive valgus, often changes of painful arthritis develop. This lady of 80 years, following internal fixation of an intertrochanteric fracture had a persistent painful hip. She reported at this stage and a cemented bipolar partial hip replacement relieved her pain (Figs 28.72 and 28.73).

Decision: Whether to fix a fracture and preserve the head of femur, Or Carry out a bipolar replacement?

In elderly patient with osteoporosis and a comminuted fracture of trochanter, after internal fixation with a DHS there is a possibility of delayed weight bearing, due to fracture morphology. The complications of prolonged rest in bed are likely to occur. Besides, there is a danger of implant cut out and/or plate avulsion. Hence, there is a trend to carry out a bipolar hip replacement in such a situation.

Even if the fracture morphology is suitable for internal fixation, the patient's health may require early mobilization and perhaps early ambulation. In fact, the demand of such a patient is also quite less and usually is already leading an assisted living. Hence a partial hip replacement is considered.

At times, the X-ray film taken on arrival may not be able to offer the exact anatomical appearance. Hence the hip needs to be examined under anesthesia and a 'C' arm, to

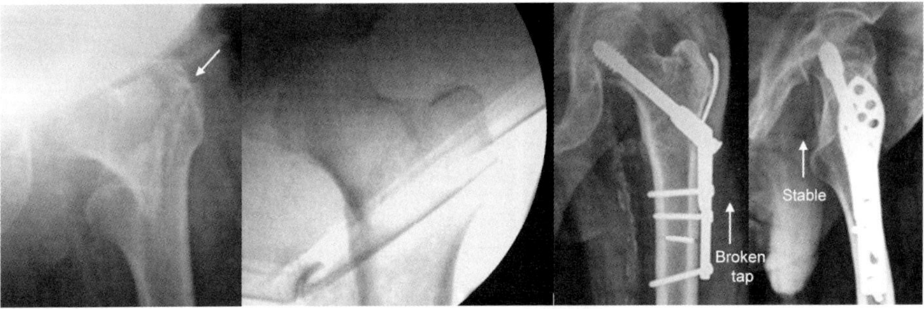

Figure 28.74 Assess under anesthesia and decide

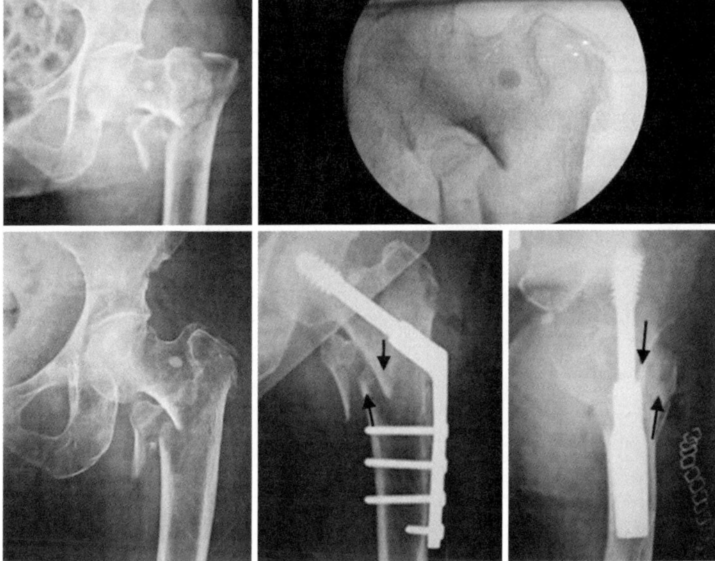

Figure 28.75 Assess under anesthesia and decide

study the same. An X-ray film should be taken for documentation.

In such a case, one has to make a decision, as to which procedure is to be done. Both the options should be explained to the family. Necessary equipment for both the procedures, internal fixation and bipolar replacement should be kept ready.

Under anesthesia, the fracture is reduced and post-reduction image taken with a 'C' arm is studied. Then, as per the fracture geometry, bone stock available to hold the prosthesis is studied. If one feels, internal fixation is possible, it is carried out accordingly. In this case, we thought, it would be prudent to fix the fracture and was carried out accordingly. As the decision is taken, it is necessary to take an X-ray film of the fracture after traction and reduction under anesthesia, to document the reasons for carrying out a given procedure and to plan the procedure. In the given case, the fracture morphology was such that internal fixation was thought to be a correct decision and was carried out.

In the X-ray photo, please note the broken tap. One can appreciate that the axis of the tap did not match that of the drill and hence, while it was against the endosteum, it gave way (Figs 28.74 and 28.75).

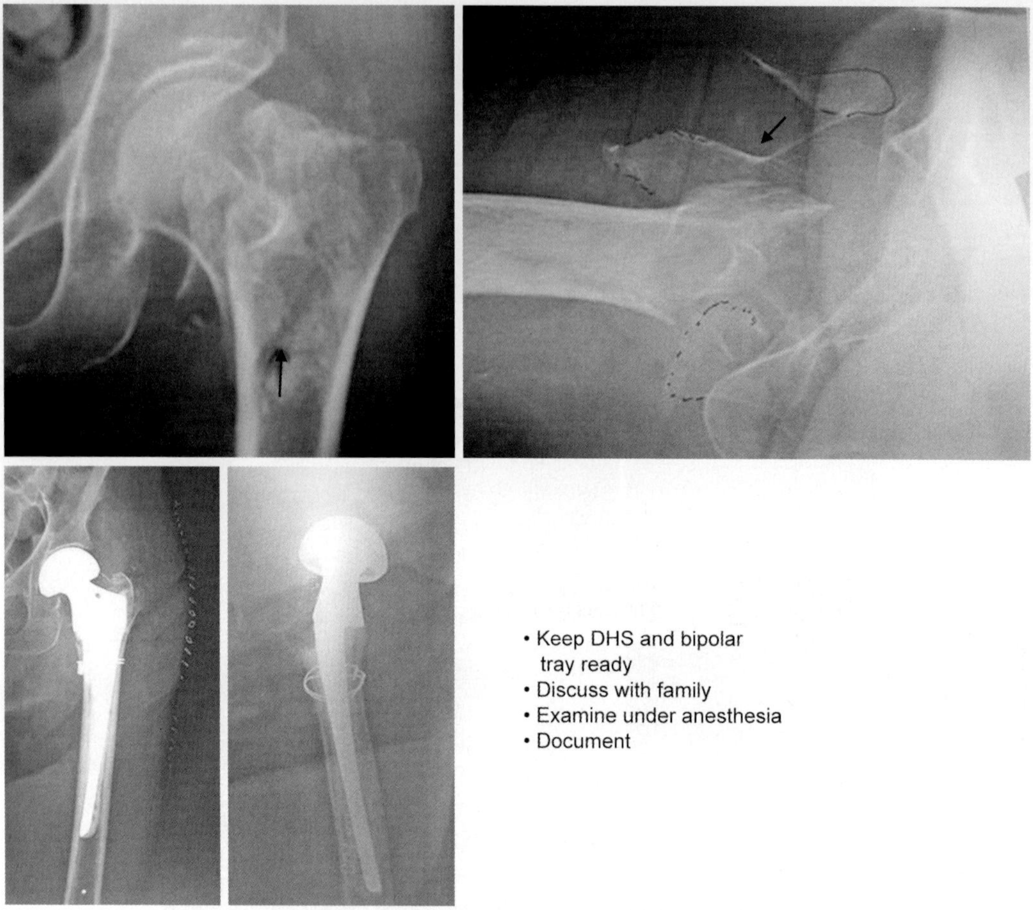

- Keep DHS and bipolar tray ready
- Discuss with family
- Examine under anesthesia
- Document

Figure 28.76 Bipolar replacement in a trochanteric fracture

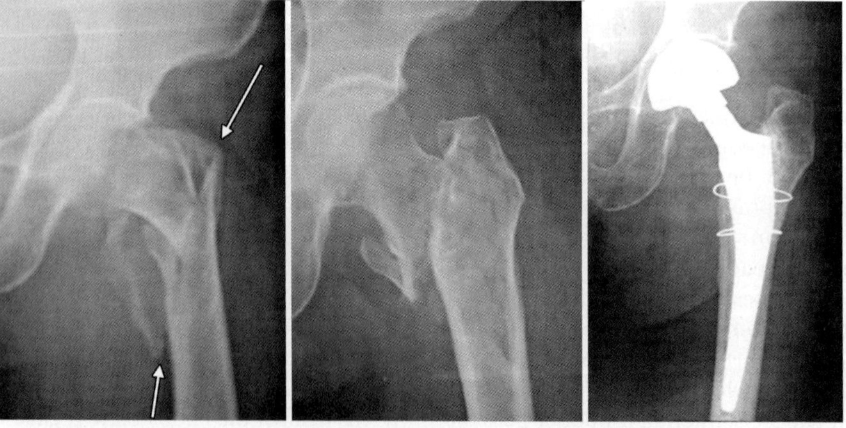

Figure 28.77 Bipolar replacement in a four-part fracture of trochanter

If the local area is comminuted and one expects too much fracture collapse, shortening and perhaps a possibility of implant cut out, it is preferable to carry out a partial hip replacement. In yester years, we were using a monoblock prosthesis and now prefer a cemented bipolar modular prosthesis for a better outcome. This procedure of replacement permits early and a safe mobilization in the bed, bedside sitting and ambulation, The complications of rest in bed are also reduced (Fig. 28.76).

Technical Details in Bipolar Replacement

In a four-part fracture of trochanter in a lady of 94, there was a large fragment on the posterior side, which we desired to preserve. In lateral position, after the fracture was exposed and the head extracted, the posterior fragment was studied and the soft tissues were well preserved. If one passes a circlage wire over it and take around the proximal shaft, while tightening the wire, it often slips downwards, due to the tapering shape of the shaft. Hence two holes were made through the fragment, one below the other on the medial side. A 1 mm soft bone wire was threaded through each of them and the ends were kept apart. The canal was prepared and a trial prosthesis was inserted. While the trial prosthesis was in the femur, over the shaft of femur, the wire was taken around and manually loaded, without the use of a wire tensioner (Tractor bow) and the ends were cut off. Then the trial stem was removed, cement restrictor was inserted and bone cement inserted with a cement gun. Final stem was inserted in the shaft and further procedure carried out. This technique helps to keep the circlage wires in desired position and maintain the shape and structure of the proximal femur, close to prefracture status (Fig. 28.77).

In a short stature person, especially in Asian ladies,, in presence of local comminution, it is necessary to keep a 55 and 60 mm hip screw ready in the implant tray. In its absence, one has to use a longer screw and then the locking top screw cannot be used (Fig. 28.78).

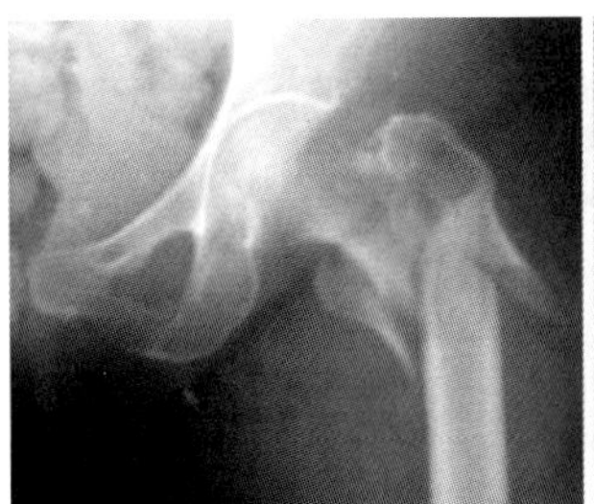

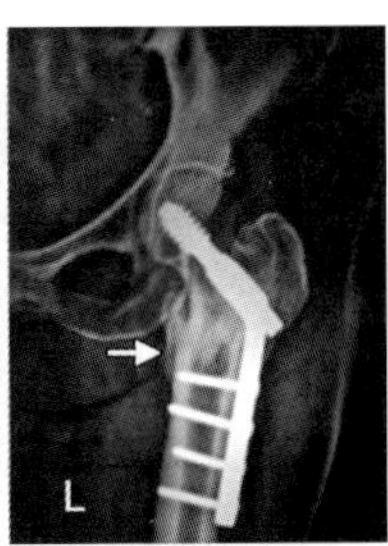

Figure 28.78 Short hip screw be available

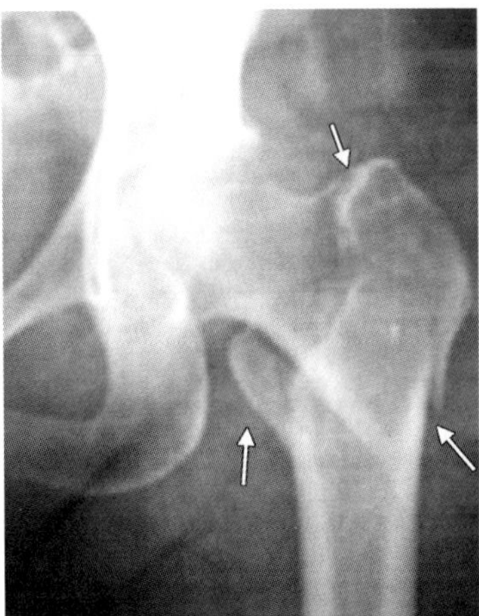

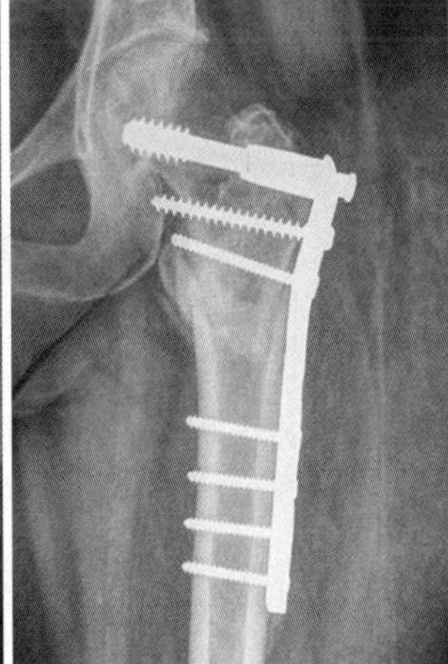

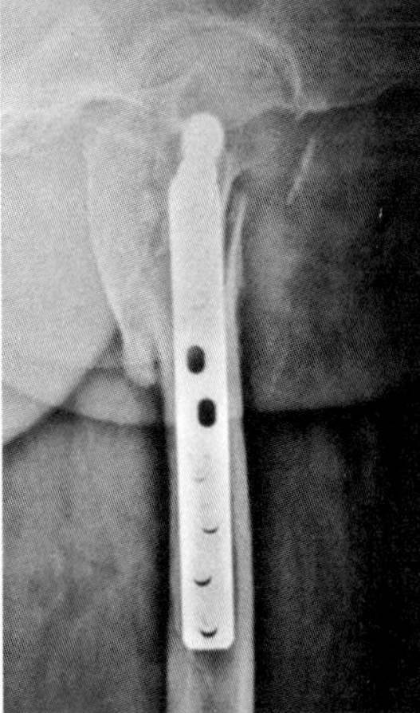

Figure 28.79 DCS fixation in a trochanteric fracture

95 DEGREE DCS IN TROCHANTERIC FRACTURE

In an intertrochanteric fracture with subtrochanteric extension, use of a 95 degree DCS is a good alternative.

- My preference is to operate such a case in a lateral position.
- The position of the guidewire needs to be more precise than that in a DHS screw, in terms of its position with respect to the calcar. The inferior part of the head has more dense bone and offers a good hold of the screw.
- The physiological load in the subtrochanteric area being very high, complementary bone grafting should be carried out, prior to application of the plate. It is possible to place few grafts in the fracture area and few in the medullary cavity and should be done, so that the fracture consolidates well in expected duration and mechanical failure of the assembly is forestalled.
- At times, when the plate is inserted over the screw, it may not lie flush with the shaft. In such a case, the 95 degree DCS plate needs to be gently contoured, so that it is flush with the shaft. (Plate bending tools be ready)
- At least one, preferably two, screws should be able to take a good purchase in the calcar for better stability (Figs 28.79 to 28.81).

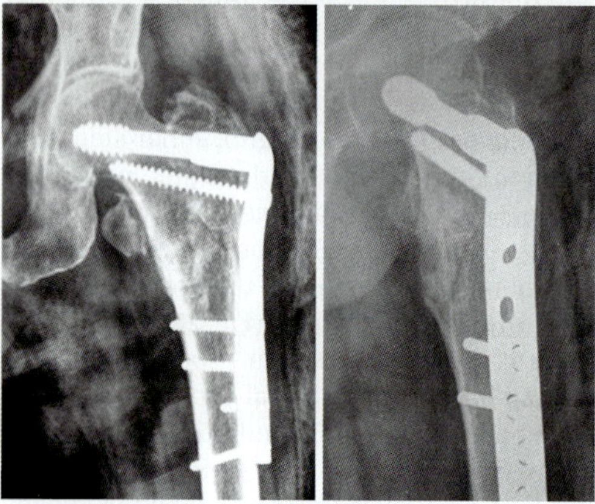

Figure 28.80 DCS fixation in a trochanteric fracture

INTRACAPSULAR AND EXTRACAPSULAR FRACTURE

This old lady had osteoporosis and sustained a fracture in the hip. The injury was: intracapsular fracture, associated with a subtrochanteric fracture. Any form of internal fixation would be associated with a possibility of cut out. Besides, early mobilization was necessary to reduce

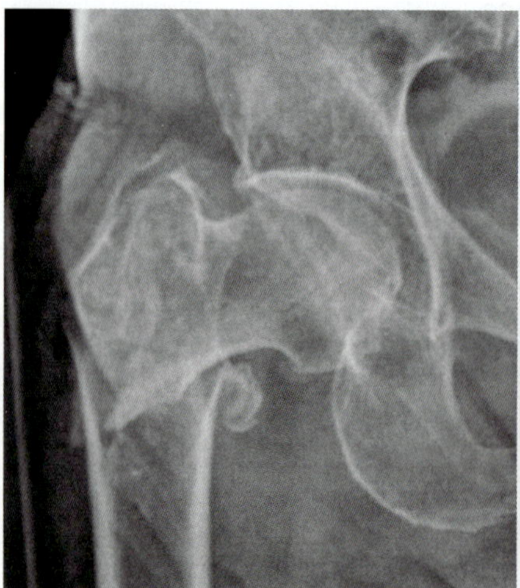

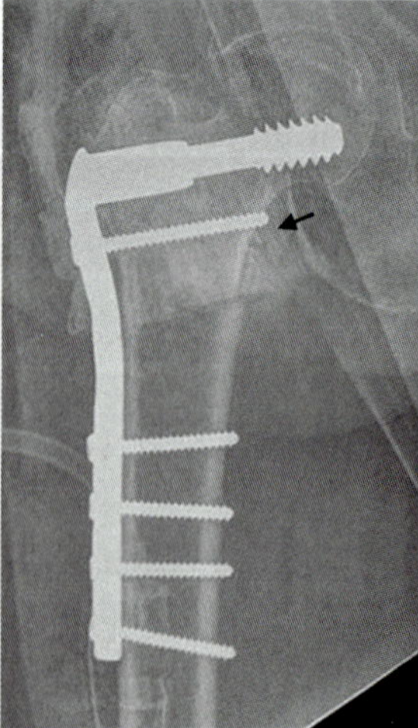

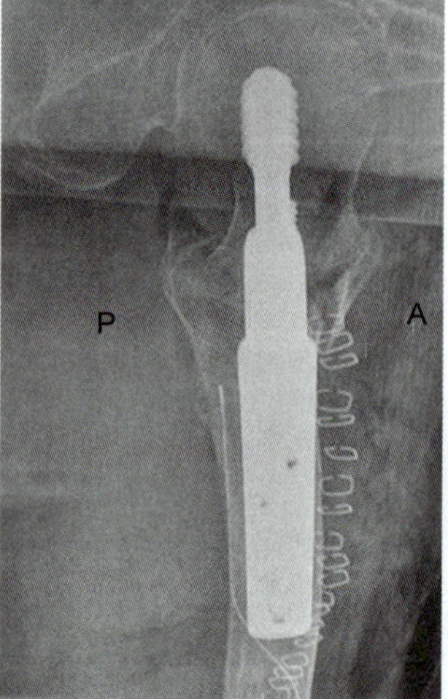

Figure 28.81 DCS fixation in a trochanteric fracture

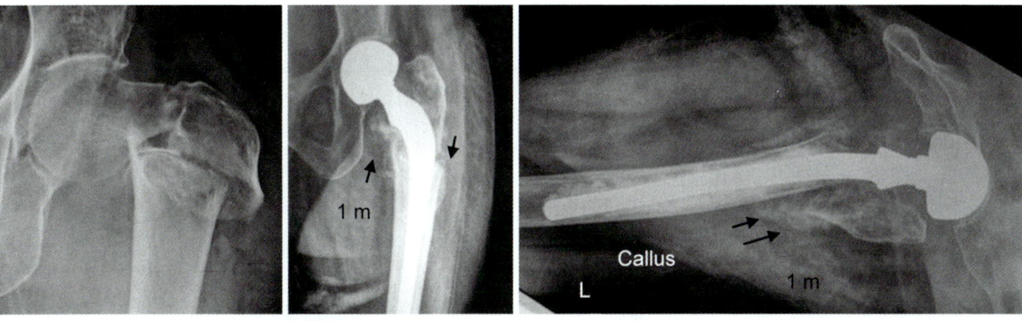

Figure 28.82 Intracapsular fracture with a subtrochanteric fracture

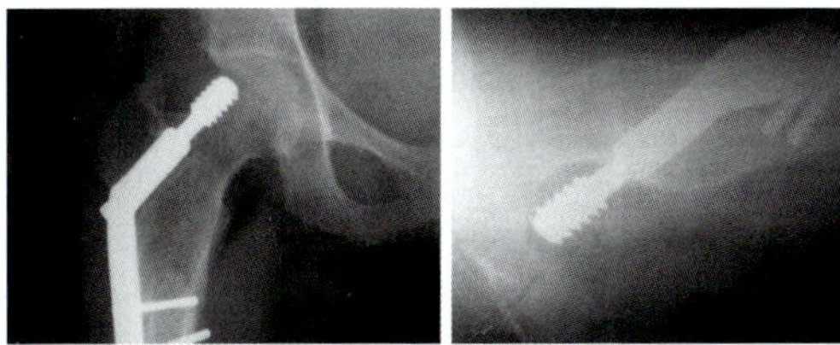

Figure 28.83 Screw penetrating the neck

complications of prolonged rest in bed. Hence a cemented bipolar replacement was done. An X-ray taken after a month shows presence of callus formation around the subtrochanteric area (Fig. 28.82).

FEW UNFORTUNATE SITUATIONS

- A patient came with ache in the right hip. Had good range of motion and had sustained a fracture of the same hip, few months ago. The X-ray film revealed, the hip screw was placed in the superior sector as seen in AP view. The lateral view showed, it had penetrated the neck and was directed posteriorly. The assembly must have been stable and hence the fracture united well. I wonder why this happened?
  - The 'C' arm may have failed during the surgery
  - The 'C' arm image may be poor
  - The procedure was done with a mobile X-ray unit and quality of film may be poor

  Fortunately, the nail had pierced posteriorly and was irritating the posterior capsule in flexion of the hip. If it had penetrated the anterior area, then flexion would be restricted (Fig. 28.83).
- This case reported with pain and inability to bear weight on the operated limb. X-ray of the hip revealed postero-superior cut out of the hip screw. The screw must have been placed too posteriorly, resulting in cut out. Had good relief after replacing the hip. The specimen of the excised head shows the position of the screw in the head (Fig. 28.84).
- X-ray film was shown for a second opinion. The postoperative film indicates that the reduction was not correct and there was a distraction at the fracture site. The nature had done its best to achieve as much collapse as possible, but eventually the plate avulsed.

Message

- The reduction on table has to be good with as much contact opposition as possible.
- The drill bit needs to be sharp and drill should not have high RPM, which may generate excess heat, leading to bone necrosis.
- The tap too needs to be sharp (changed as and when necessary) (Fig. 28.85).

TECHNIQUE AND OBSERVATIONS IN A BIPOLAR REPLACEMENT IN A FAILED DHS

- During a revision surgery in a hip, the tissues are often not supple and hence, exposure is rather tedious. The bleeding also could be more.

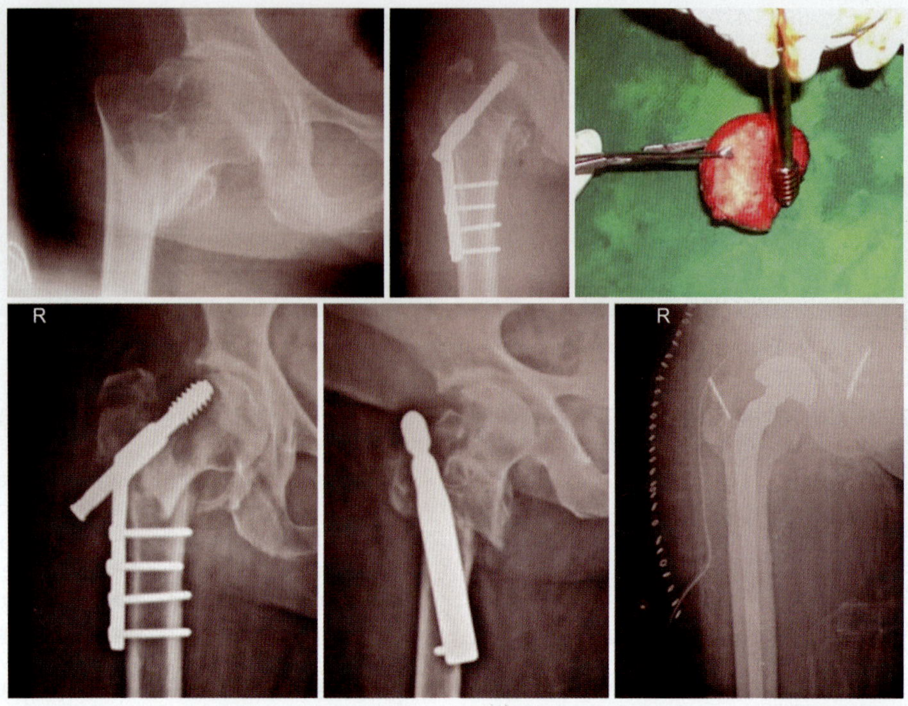

Figure 28.84 Screw cut out

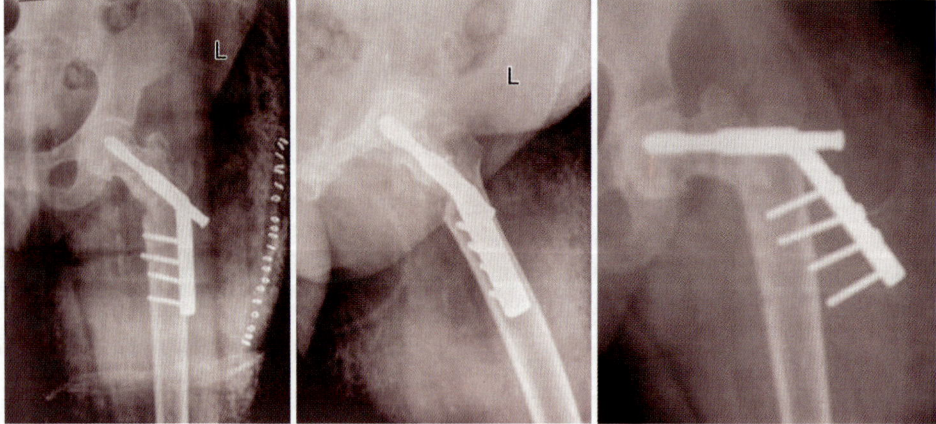

Figure 28.85 Plate avulsion after fixation in distraction

- If the greater trochanter was fractured in earlier injury, often some abnormal mobility is observed, due to a fibrous union. One needs to be careful, while rotating the hip internally, so that the greater trochanter union does not get disturbed. Usually the soft tissue and muscle continuity is observed along the glutei and the vastus lateralis, which should be preserved.
- On the tip of the DHS screw, often a bursa forms and some fluid comes out, during the exposure, which should be sent for Gram stain and culture.

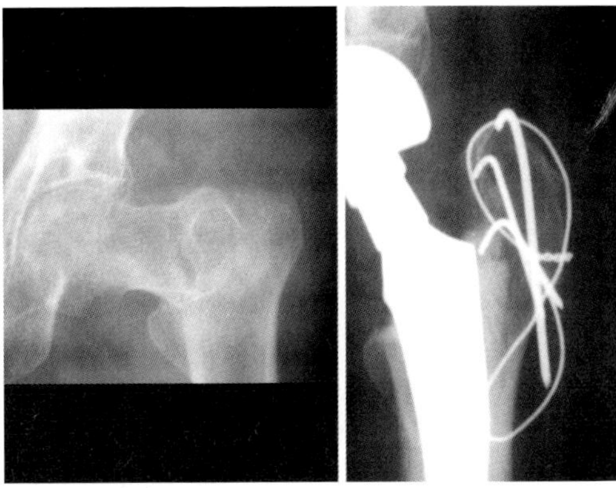

Figure 28.86 TBW for greater trochanter

- During the exposure of the side plate of DHS, the vastus lateralis should be erased, just necessary.
- Later on, one has to have a posterior approach and access for inserting the stem and hence this care.
- One should study the status of external rotators and identify them. Prior to their erasing from the inter-trochanteric crest, they are tagged with vicryl. It serves as a mark for them and then attaching them to the bone is relatively easy. Even if one cannot bring them close to the bone, it is worthwhile to anchor them to the bone, with a hope, that tissues would grow along the sutures.
- On the X-ray film, taken prior to the revision surgery, one may find that the tip of the trochanter has shifted proximally and associated soft tissue contracture may have occurred. In such a situation, it is worthwhile considering preoperative skeletal traction, to bring the proximal end down and to have an ease in exposure and reduction of the head in the acetabulum.
- *Removal of the hip screw*: In the first place while stabilizing a fracture, one should select a hip screw, which has reverse cutting threads also, so while its removal, it is easy. Still, while removing, one should adopt a technique of two reverse and one forward technique, so the threads do not get jammed in the neck. (Remember the technique of bone tapping, prior to insertion of a screw) One should keep an extra T wrench for screw removal, preferably made of stainless steel. (Often the T wrench is of aluminum and while a force is applied, to rotate it to withdraw the hip screw, the barrel key lock gives way, i.e. the ridge present on the inner wall of the wrench yields). Barrel key lock is a raised part within the barrel of the side plate and the screw wrench, which locks the screw in the barrel.
- After a successful removal of the DHS screw assembly and after extraction of the head and neck portion, one needs to locate the femoral canal. Often it is found to be blocked by fibro-osseous tissue. One should study the local anatomy, to avoid creating a false passage. To confirm and create a canal, one should serially use a cobbler awl, a diamond awl and a taper pin canal finder and reamer. At times, while preparing the femoral canal, the endosteal tissue growth is firm to hard and to remove it is difficult. Hence, one should keep rigid straight femur reamers ready. Keeping 6 and 7 mm reamers (needed in a shoulder replacement) and of more diameter along with necessary power reamer tools is a great help. If the direction and place of the femoral canal is in doubt, one may insert a Steinmann pin mounted on a T handle, for some length and confirm in 'C' arm.
- During reduction of the replaced head in the acetabulum, some difficulty may be encountered, which could be due to contracture of the anterior capsule. If so, it should be carefully released—remember the anterior important structures!
- If the DHS side plate is longer than 5 or 6 holes, one needs to keep long stem for bipolar procedure also ready and sterile.

Stem Insertion

After insertion of a trial stem in correct anteversion, one should do a trial reduction. At this stage, one needs to be extra careful, to avoid

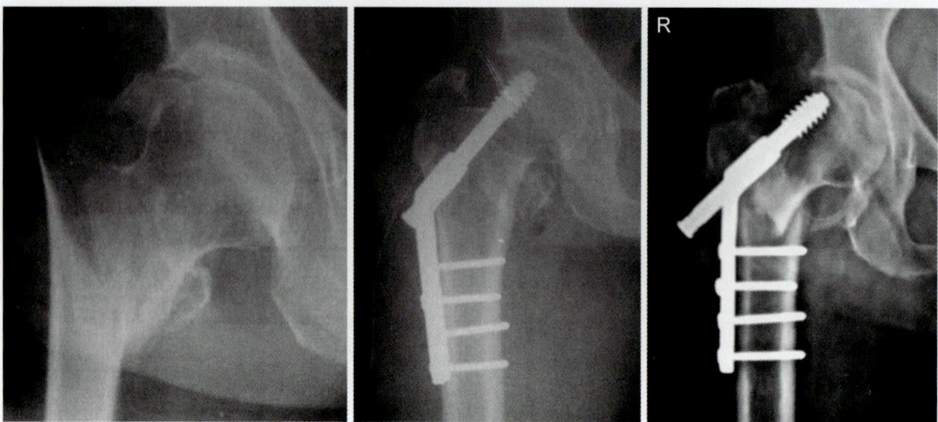

Figure 28.87 Use of ethibond to anchor greater trochanter

separation of greater trochanter. Thereafter, the trial stem is removed and cement restrictor inserted till correct length and the trial stem is inserted again, to confirm the restrictor has reached the correct level.

RE-ATTACHMENT OF GREATER TROCHANTER

Use of a TBW Method

If the bone stock in the trochanter is adequate, one can use a TBW technique, using a bone wire circlage. While the trial stem is in, a drill hole is made in the lateral cortex, 2 to 3 fingers distal to base of trochanter and a 1 mm soft wire is threaded through it.

The greater trochanter is reduced and through it 2, 1.8 mm, K-wires are driven distally in the anterior and posterior cortices of the femur. The circlage wire is taken around the K-wire tips, proximal to the greater trochanter and TBW completed. The tension may be given by hand or may be a tractor bow, with minimal tension. Thus the trochanter is built over the trial stem.

The screw holes in the lateral cortex can be plugged with short 12 or 14 mm screws, so cement does not leak through them. Those holes on the medial side have to be accepted as such. Cement insertion with a cement gun, pressurization, insertion of final stem in anteversion is carried out as usual. Once the cement has set in, ideally one should do a trial reduction with the final stem in place. However, if the trochanter stabilization is not that strong and one envisages a possibility of its displacement, one may skip the step and insert the final head and neck assembly (Fig. 28.86).

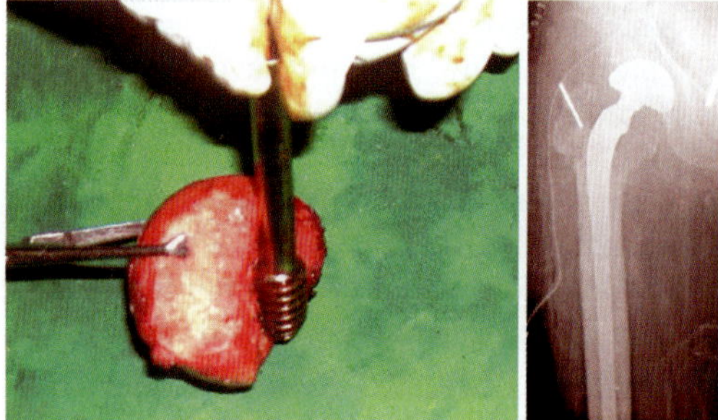

Figure 28.88 Use of ethibond to anchor greater trochanter

Use of Ethibond Material

If the greater trochanter has two or more parts and is soft, not adequately strong enough, to offer a hold for K-wires, one should prefer to use no: 2 ethibond to reattach the greater trochanter.

After a trial reduction with a stem, it is removed. In the upper margin of the shaft, three holes are made with a 2.5 mm drill at a distance of 5 to 6 mm and no. 2 ethibond is passed in each, keeping the needle attached to each thread. Restrictor insertion, checking its level with a trial stem again, is done and cement is inserted with a gun. Final stem in correct anteversion is inserted and kept pressed down, to prevent its proximal migration, as the cement expands. At this stage the assistant should move the ethibond threads to and fro, so a track is created for each and the threads do not get anchored in the cement and can freely slide.

After the head neck component is inserted and the hip is reduced, one by one thread is taken around the trochanter/muscle attachment, etc. and tied, so the trochanter is stabilized well. The needle is quite strong enough to penetrate the trochanter, which is usually osteoporotic and hence soft (Figs 28.87 and 28.88).

CHAPTER 29

Fracture of Subtrochanteric Area

INTRODUCTION

In the young, a subtrochanteric fracture is a high energy injury, while in the elderly, this fracture can occur with a domestic fall. Various methods of internal fixation have been practised and there is an evolution in the methods. In the early era of internal fixation, SP pin and a plate fixation was practised. If, at least, one screw could be inserted in the proximal fragment, the stability and the result achieved was reasonably satisfactory.

An intramedullary nail did not offer a stable fixation, due to wide medullary cavity in the proximal fragment. However, with a possibility of a derotation plate, the result improved remarkably.

It was then realized that, this is an area with high stresses and hence a complementary bone grafting was advocated, so the fracture union occurred, before the implant failure.

With advent of interfragmentory screw fixation, the stability was further improved and thus, a Jewett nail-plate or a DHS plate fixation also offered a good outcome. In the last two decades, the proximal femoral nail is invented and has improved the outcome immensely.

In this chapter, various historical methods are shown, with a purpose, to demonstrate benefit of various methods and one can adopt some of the principles, while using various methods.

DHS is modular device and hence needs less inventory, compared to a fixed angle implant, as a Jewett nail.

SUBTROCHANTERIC FRACTURE AND JEWETT NAIL PLATE

In the years gone by, SP pin and plate fixation helped to mobilize the patient early and reduced the complications due to prolonged rest in bed. In a stable inter-trochanteric fracture, it worked well. However, when used in a subtrochanteric fracture, often the top screw could not resist the angular load and often gave way, leading to a varus deformity. The screw would usually pull out from the nail or cut out. This gave to the idea of a fixed nail plate device, without any joint. This non-jointed implant offered more resistance to the varus stresses and thus the Jewett came in the armamentarium.

The device in not a collapsible or a sliding one, as is a Dynamic Hip Screw. Hence in situations, where a collapse of fracture occurred, due to physiological stresses or due to local comminution, Jewett plate had problems, such as: persistent distraction at the fracture site or medial migration of the entire assembly and penetration in the hip joint.

Surgeon's judgment, measurement of the nail plate angle and precision are important factors in a successful internal fixation with a Jewett nail plate. In a DHS after the screw is inserted in the neck, one can assess the angle again and select the specific plate with a matching angle, so it would fit flush with the lateral cortex of the femur. However, this facility is not possible with Jewett nail plate. Since the device has gone out of vogue, one would not discuss the tricks here.

In the last decade, increasing use of a PFN in a fracture of the proximal femur is observed. It needs a minimal exposure, the blood loss is less and recovery is relatively faster. Perhaps, weight bearing may be safe and earlier than that after a DHS or DCS plate.

A subtrochanteric fracture takes little more time to unite than an intertrochanteric fracture and due to mechanical reasons, weight bearing is advised later than that in an IT fracture. It is necessary for a fracture to unite and consolidate, before mechanical failure of any implant. Hence it is always recommended to do the fixation, with a complementary bone graft. In situations, where there is local comminution, which would leave a defect in the medial and postero-medial area, it is prudent to think of bone grafting in the preoperative planning. In fact, this needs to be explained to the patient's family and accordingly the draping needs to be done. After a DHS or a DCS device is fixed, the bone void area may not be accessible, to fill it with bone grafts. Hence, it is essential to take the grafts and deposit in the voids, prior to fracture reduction and fixation of the device chosen. At the end of surgery, few slivers are also laid on the medial side, along the calcar. This helps to assuredly consolidate the fracture, in expected duration and build the calcar area.

LIMB LENGTH

In a transverse fracture, the leg length is usually restored well. In a spiral or a short oblique fracture, some shortening is expected, due to mechanical reasons. In comminuted fracture, it may be difficult to exactly reduce a fracture, to have a good contact opposition, yet maintaining the leg length. A fracture union in expected duration is more important.

FEW CASE STUDIES

Case 1

A few decades earlier, SP pin and plate fixation was order of the time. If the patient was young, at times, even a hip spica was advocated after internal fixation, and was accepted by the patient and the treating community. If the physiological load was not realized and the limb was left unsupported, at times, the top screw gave way, leading to a varus deformity. The fracture would unite with varus and shortening. Raised shoe would not reduce the limp, as the hip mechanics was altered, due to a raised trochanter (Fig. 29.1).

Case 2

This reverse oblique fracture was stabilized with a Jewett nail and a circlage took care of the fracture of the greater trochanter. After a few years, the implant was removed. A 13-year follow up is shown, when he presented with ache in the hip, due to OA hip (Fig. 29.2).

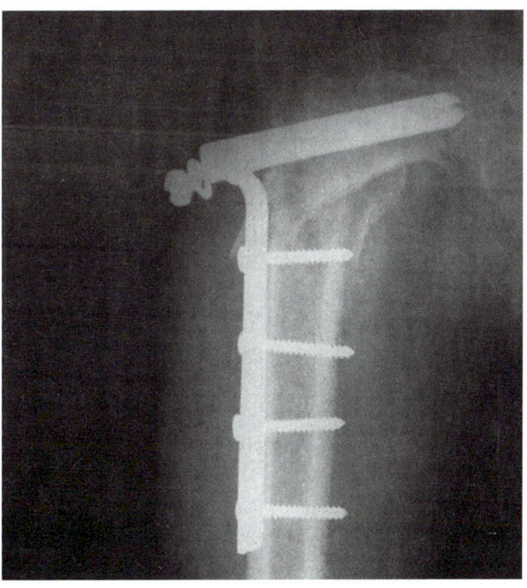

Figure 29.1 Top screw pull-out

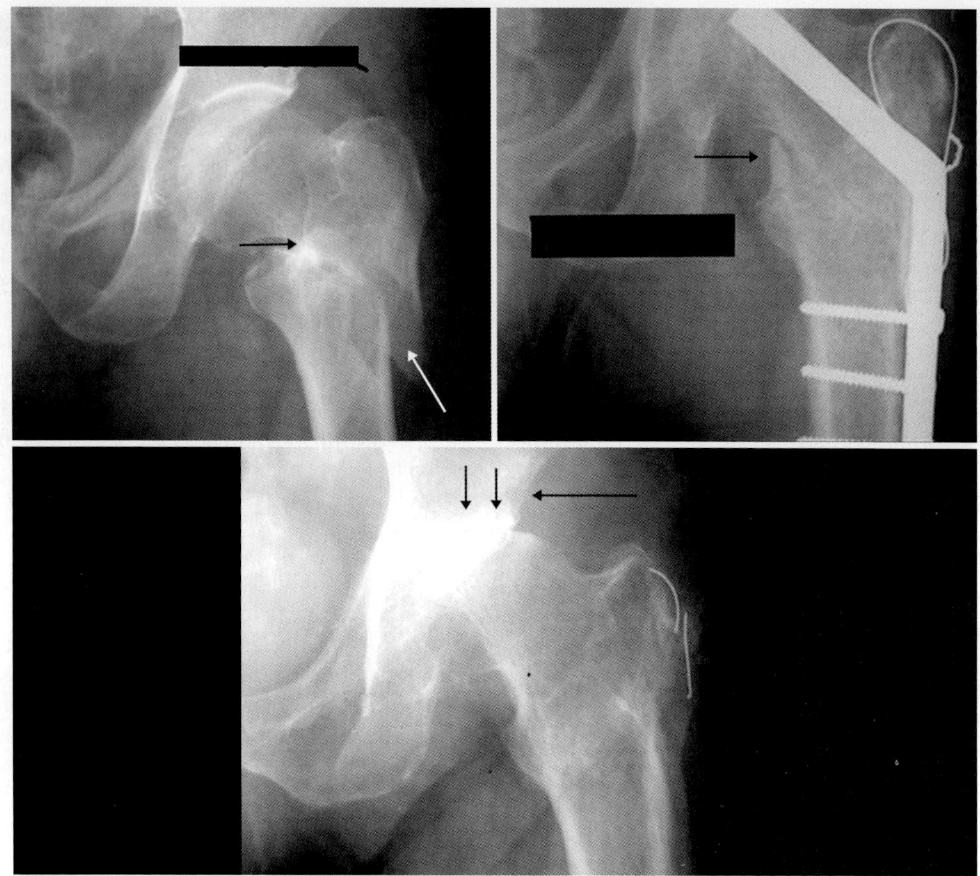

Figure 29.2 Jewett in reverse oblique fracture

Case 3

A subtrochanteric fracture in a lady more than 60 yrs of age, had a five-part fracture, with huge hematoma. The limb was reduced and the limb kept in a skeletal traction. Once a limb is on a Bohler frame with skeletal traction the fragments fall in their place. In due course, internal fixation with a Jewett nail and bone grafting was done and a good union was observed (Fig. 29.3).

Case 4

This young person had a subtrochanteric fracture with multiple fragments. He was operated in a lateral position. Internal fixation with a Jewett nail and bone grafting was done. In spite of all the care, he had 10 deg of external rotation deformity. However, function was good. In Indian community, one needs to sit cross-legged, which was possible for him (Fig. 29.4).

Case 5

This young man had an IT fracture with a subtrochanteric fracture. It was fixed with a Jewett nail, with good outcome (Fig. 29.5).

Case 6

This old man had a spiral fracture and the fracture surface was rotated. The fracture was

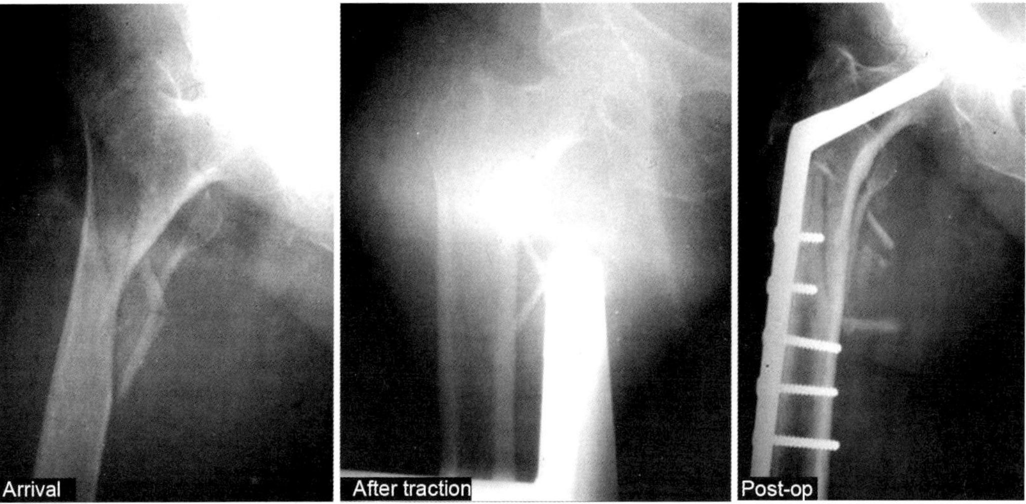

Figure 29.3 Preoperative traction

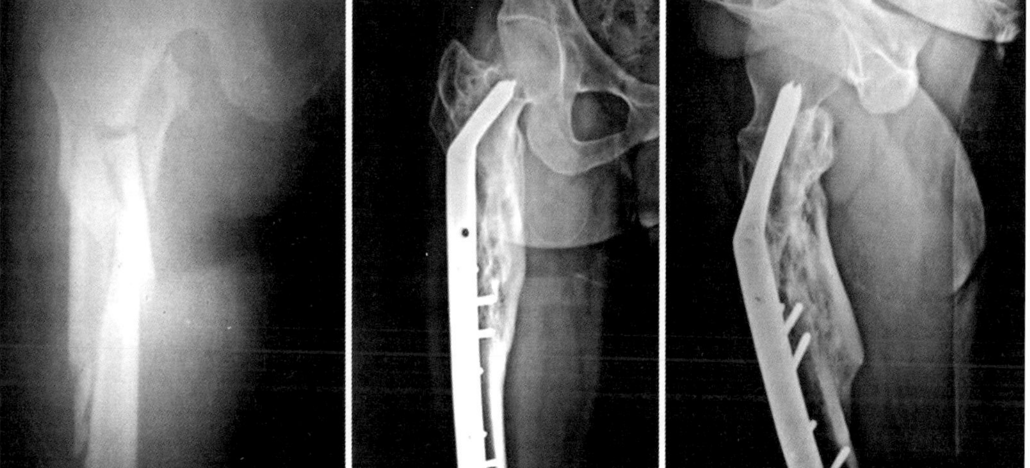

Figure 29.4 Jewett nail in comminuted fracture

stabilized with a Jewett nail and bone grafting: The fixation stability improved with IFS. Good union and function (Fig. 29.6).

Case 7

This another old man had a spiral fracture and was fixed with Jewett nail plate. United well (Fig. 29.7).

These examples reveal internal fixation with a fixed angle device, like a Jewett nail plate, is also useful in managing a subtrochanteric fracture with a good outcome. Application of the principles of fixation is more important than which implant is used.

The Jewett device has a cannulated nail component and hence passing the nail over a guidewire permits one to pass the nail in the

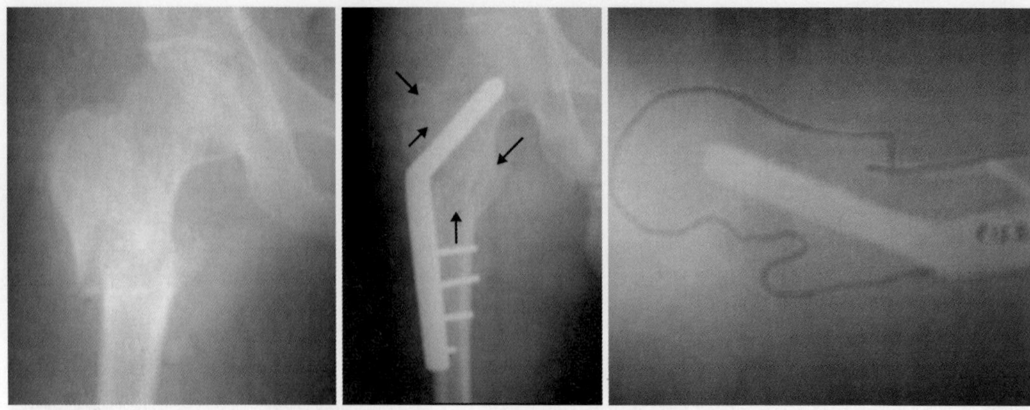

Figure 29.5 Subtrochanteric fracture with IT extension

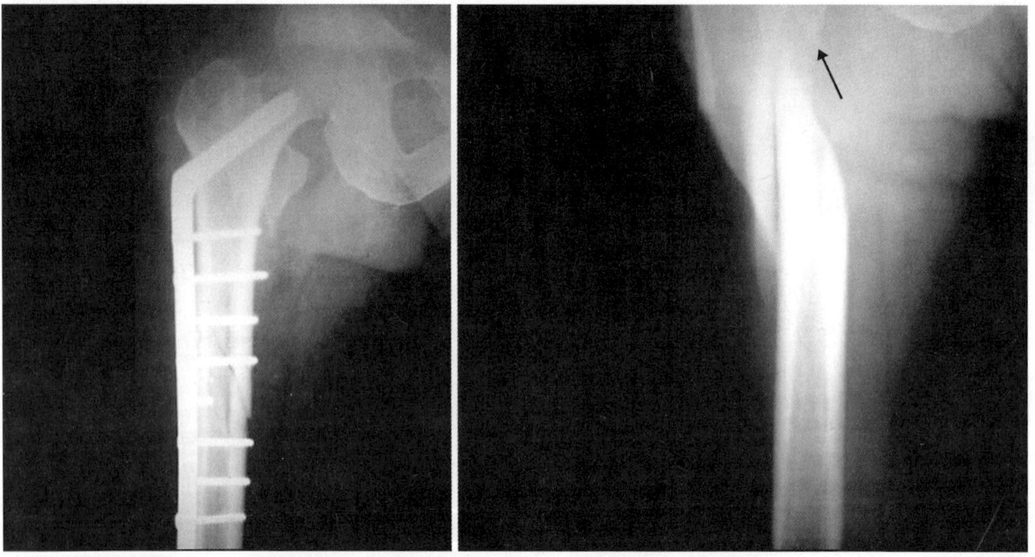

Figure 29.6 Spiral fracture with extrusion of LT

desired direction. In fact, I desired to have 95 degree one piece Jewett nail, with a notch at the distal most hole. This would make it possible to load a transverse fracture with either a Charnley compression device or articulated tension device. The holes also could be oval, with a facility to have a sliding hole geometry. Unfortunately, no manufacturer was willing to make an implant of this type. The proximal nail being cannulated would have an advantage over a 95 degree blade plate, to pass it over a guidewire.

SUBTROCHANTERIC FRACTURE: DHS FIXATION

In the given examples, the lateral and medial walls of the fragments did not have comminution. In the given cases, it was possible

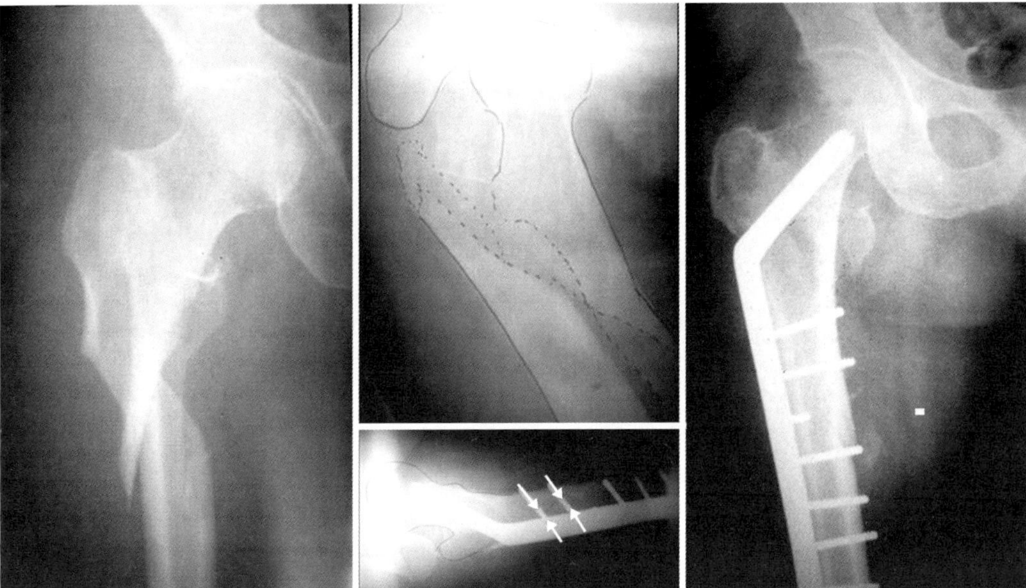

Figure 29.7 Spiral fracture II

to insert an IFS across the two fragments which enhanced the stability of fixation and led to good union in an expected duration.

Case 1

This patient over 70 years of age, presented with a fall and severe deformity in the hip and great discomfort. After X-ray examination, soon it was reduced under anesthesia and upper tibial skeletal traction was applied. The traction helped to align the distal fragment with the proximal one and offered good pain relief. The fracture was operated on a fracture table. Iliac crest grafts were taken as step 1. A guide-wire was placed and confirmed the position. Prior to final reduction and cooption of the fragments, few cancellous grafts were inserted in the medullary cavity (and later on few grafts medial to the reduced fracture). After the plate was passed over the hip guidewire, the fracture reduction was done. The reduction and the plate was held with a self-centering forceps.

Few screws were inserted distal to the fracture. The fracture line was such that, a screw could be passed through the plate hole as an IFS by a sliding hole and threaded hole principle.

Hence, the IFS through the plate was inserted. The fixation was completed. Few grafts were laid medial to the fracture area. Since the skeletal traction was already in situ, it was continued with a Bohler frame. This offers good elevation of the limb and could maintain the neutral position of the limb. At times, when the limb lies in external rotation on a Bohler frame, foot drop is known to occur, due to pressure on the common peroneal nerve. Tissue reaction was minimum, due to elevation. Water bed prevented bed sores. After five days, the skeletal traction was removed and patient was mobilized in the bed.

The patient was old and asthenic and unable to walk with a non-weight bearing technique. At the end of 10 weeks, the fracture showed evidence of good union and then he was permitted to start partial weight bearing, using a walker (Fig. 29.8).

Case 2

This patient in mid-fifties had a road accident and suffered a 3-part intertrochanteric fracture with subtrochanteric extension. The thigh hematoma was quite large with extensive tissue

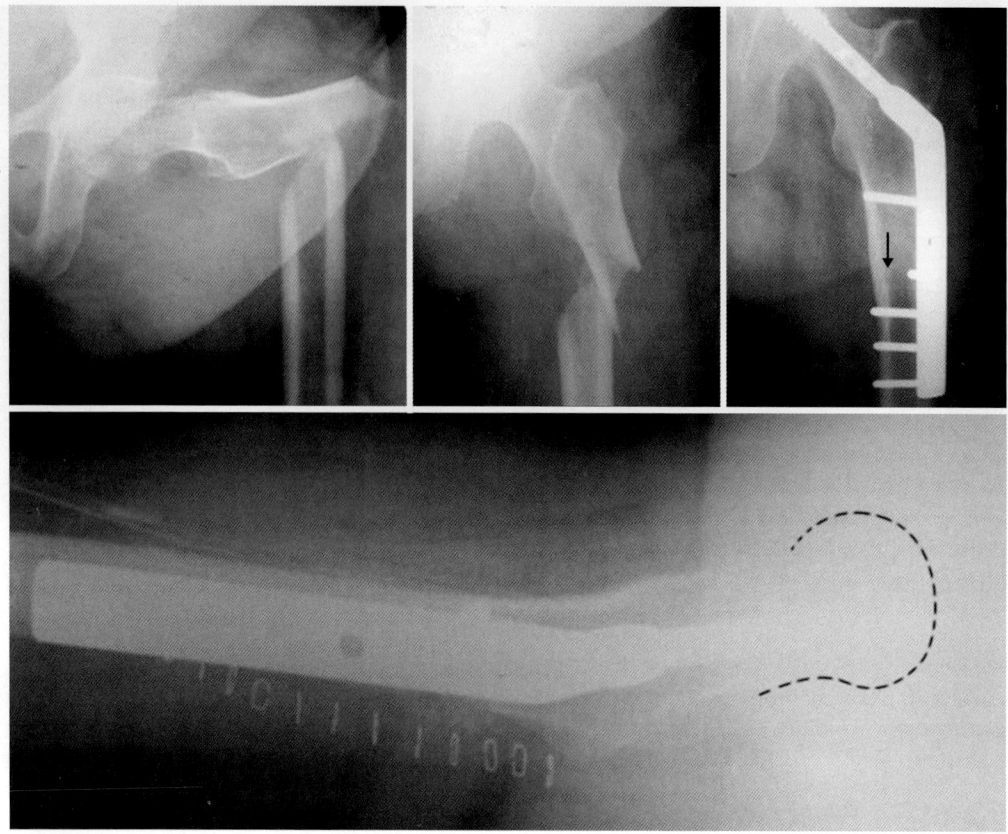

Figure 29.8 Spiral subtrochanteric fracture

swelling. Hence, closed reduction and upper tibial skeletal traction was applied. In a week, the tissue reaction settled down and internal fixation with a DHS was done. As in prior case, cancellous grafts were laid in the fracture area and medial to it. The IFS very well stabilized the fracture.

The Steps

- The fracture site was exposed and studied. Ipsilateral iliac grafts were taken and laid in the fracture area.
- After the hip screw insertion, the appropriate angled side plate was slid over the screw. Before the plate was fully inserted, the fracture was well-reduced, with a combination of manipulation, adjustment of traction and angulation. The distal end of the proximal fragment was well-aligned in both the planes. The plate and the reduced fracture together was gently held with a self-centering forceps and the traction was slightly reduced for fine adjustment.
- Distal to the fracture, a bicortical screw was inserted. Screws above it were unicortical, as were near the fracture line. Then the IFS was inserted, with a little tilt, to be at right angles to the fracture area and then the rest screws were inserted. The fixation of lesser trochanter fragment was thought of. However, the required place of the screw was too close to the important IFS and hence was left as such. Total stability achieved was good and hence a circlage was not done.

- Continued the traction for a few days and then he was mobilized. Being able to walk non-weight bearing, was ambulated in two weeks. Good union and range of motion (Fig. 29.9).

Case 3

This person of 75 years, had a four-part IT fracture with subtrochanteric extension and a medial beak. The fracture was operated on a fracture table and a DHS fixation was carried out. As in the earlier case, grafts were laid in the fracture area and medial to it. After achieving good reduction, it was maintained with 2 × 1.8 mm K-wires. The reduction was also held with a pointed reduction forceps, especially when a triple reamer and tap for the femur head was used. All these steps prevented rotation of the proximal fragment during the steps carried out. On the lateral fragment, adequate bone was available, to insert an IFS to fix the lateral fragment with the calcar. This was done and enhanced the stability. Fracture consolidated in due course. Extensive callus was seen between the fracture area and the lesser trochanter (Fig. 29.10).

OBSERVATIONS AND SUGGESTIONS

Supine position on a fracture table:

- A stable two-part IT fracture is well-aligned after reduction on a fracture table. Having reduced and adjusted the traction, it can be fixed with ease.
- In a fracture, with a medial beak on the proximal fragment, it is necessary to insert it in the medullary canal, to lock it. This offers more stability. However, it leads to some shortening as well, which needs to be accepted. To achieve assured stability and mobility is more important than having an anatomical reduction. (Often an anatomical reduction, in due course, is known to lead to medialization and hence preferable to carry out so, primarily on the table).

Lateral position on a conventional or a wooden table, which offers a lateral view in a 'C' arm:

- The exposure is easy and the blood loss is less. Assistant can stand on the opposite side and there is ease of exposure, tissue retraction, etc. One can have a good view of both anterior and posterior surfaces of the fracture area.

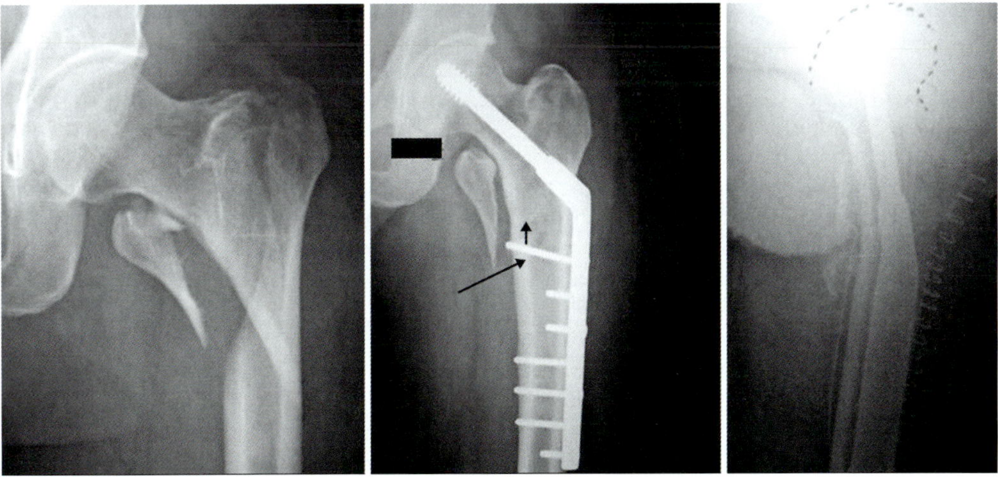

Figure 29.9 Subtrochanteric fracture: DHS and IFS fixation

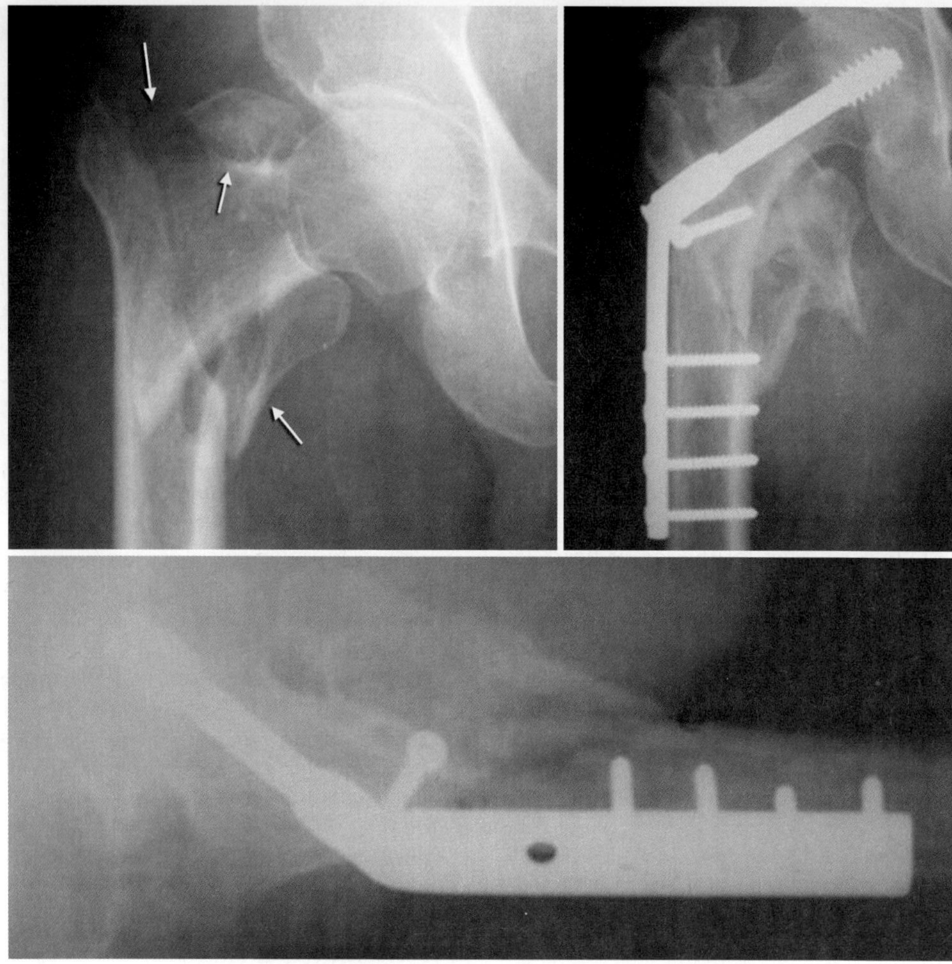

Figure 29.10 Subtrochanteric fracture: DHS and IFS fixation II

- With hip flexed, one can palpate the calcar area well and can medialise it well. Usually, having achieved this medialization, the fracture remains well reduced, especially with a pillow below the knee, etc.
- If an IFS is to be inserted, one can do it as well, perhaps with more ease.
- Disadvantage: In the lateral view in 'C' arm, both the hips are overlapping. One may have to keep the patient slightly tilted OR tilt the X-ray tube, with exact lateral position of the patient. If the opposite hip has some implant or prosthesis, following an earlier fracture, it comes in the way of lateral view.

It is a matter of training and individual preference for the patient position. Most of the surgeons feel, a stable fracture is better operated on a fracture table, while an unstable one, in a lateral position.

SUBTROCHANTERIC FRACTURE: DCS

In a certain morphological type of a subtrochanteric fracture, DCS offers more stability, as a surface implant. The screw is a sliding hip screw, and is so inserted, that the threaded tip is in the lower quadrant of the head of the femur. This area has relatively good bone stock. Mediolateral sliding is possible and does occur, with a better contact opposition in the fracture area, during the fracture union. Often the fracture line is at a place where the DHS screw entry should start. Hence use of a DCS is a better option for stabilization. The limb length achieved on the table remains as such and no further shortening occurs. Often the medial bone defect needs to be filled with bone grafts. This leads to fracture union and consolidation in an expected period, prevents a varus deformity and thus, a mechanical failure of the plate.

Few typical examples are shown. In some cases, the patient is from a different city and follow up may not be complete. An attempt is made to make a complete follow up in the cases, demonstrated.

Technical Tips

- The guidewire needs to be inserted, using a 95 degree jig. However, I find it easier to insert the guidewire, with a drill sleeve, in the desired direction and depth, so the hip screw threads anchor in the good subchondral area in the inferior part of the head.

  The point of guidewire entry is important, so that, a 95 degree DCS will be so placed, that the plate component will lie flush against the lateral femoral cortex. However, in every case, this may not be exact and at times, some change in the plate angle is required. This is better done below the proximal two rounded holes, where the plate span between the two holes is more. Use of a plate press is a safer method. However, it is observed that a good plate bending press is not available in each OR which one should have for a gentle contouring of the plate. In addition to it, plate bending irons and a three-point plate bender are of great help (Fig. 29.11).

  A well-contoured and fitting plate is threaded over the hip screw. It is preferable to have a plate with oval holes, so that should

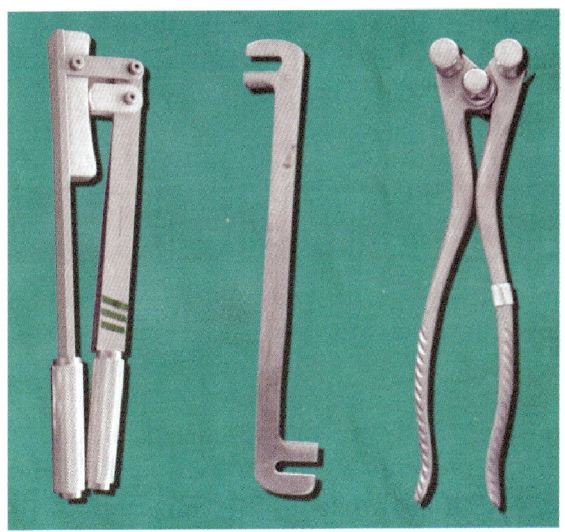

Figure 29.11 Plate bending press

  tilting of screw if required, to get a hold on a 3rd fragment, it is possible. In a few cases, there is a medial comminution and bone loss, due to crushing. This loss needs to be made up by autologous bone grafts.
- Having prepared a suitable plate of correct angle and length, grafts are placed in the fracture area, with few slivers in the intramedullary area as well. Grafts placed at this area are more helpful for fracture consolidation, while those placed on the bone surface, also help to maintain the bone width and hence, the strength.
- After inserting of the grafts, the plate is slid over the screw and aligned with the shaft of femur. It may be necessary to remove the plate and turn the screw by few degrees, so the plate is exactly aligned with the lateral surface of the shaft. Thus, the distal-most screw in the plate is well-centered on the shaft and has a good hold.
- The plate is held against the shaft with a self-centering forceps, without tightening its speed lock. Having studied the reduction, it is confirmed under in a 'C' arm image. The distal fragment is manually pressed proximally, by pushing the knee superiorly. This would close any voids in the fracture area and offer a good opposition. Thus, if the fracture area is well-opposed manually,

further screw placement in the area distal to the fracture in the oval holes, in eccentric mode, will enhance the stability and help the union.

TECHNIQUE OF THE SCREW INSERTION IN THE CALCAR

In a DCS implant, the proximal two-round holes are at the level of the calcar. Every effort should be made to insert a 4.5 mm screw through these two holes. This gives a good hold on the proximal fragment and prevents displacement of the fracture reduction, in flexion and extension movement of the limb.

Through the round hole, a 3.2 mm drill bit is inserted thro' a round hole drill sleeve. Having pierced the near cortex, it abuts against the far cortex, the calcar, at an angle, without any protection of a drill sleeve. The drill bit is making a hole in the oblique calcar, with respect to the drill bit and the drill bit usually breaks at this stage. Hence, the following steps are followed:

- Drill the lateral cortex with a 4.5 mm drill bit. Remove the drill bit.
- Insert in the hole, an insert sleeve, till it touches the calcar.
- Through it, insert a 3.2 mm drill bit and make a drill hole in the calcar. Now, the insert sleeve protects the drill bit, which makes a hole in the calcar safely.
- With a depth gauge, measure the screw length required → tap and insert the screw.

Having inserted one screw in the proximal fragment, the rest of the screws are inserted in the distal fragment. The bicortical screws are inserted through the distal holes of the plate. In the fracture area at places, where a medial fragment is present opposite the plate, insert an IFS through the plate hole. The fixation is completed with a second screw in the proximal fragment. If there are at least 3 (preferably 4) bicortical screws in the distal fragment, the last screw can be unicortical, to distribute the load.

The length of the plate: If there is a medial comminution or a medial 3rd fragment, the distal fragment should have at least 3 bicortical screws and a few unicortical screws. Thus at least eight cortices must be held. It is safe to have a plate with an extra screw hole, so that should a hole cannot be utilized, due to a fracture line below a hole, an additional screw hole is available (Fig. 29.12).

If one finds that the calcar is so fractured that the width is rather less, in place of a 4.5 mm screw, one may insert a malleolar screw. Though the thread diameter is the same, one finds this screw safer than a 4.5 mm screw (Fig. 29.13).

The fracture morphology may be such that the proximal fragment would accept only one screw engaging the calcar and the second screw

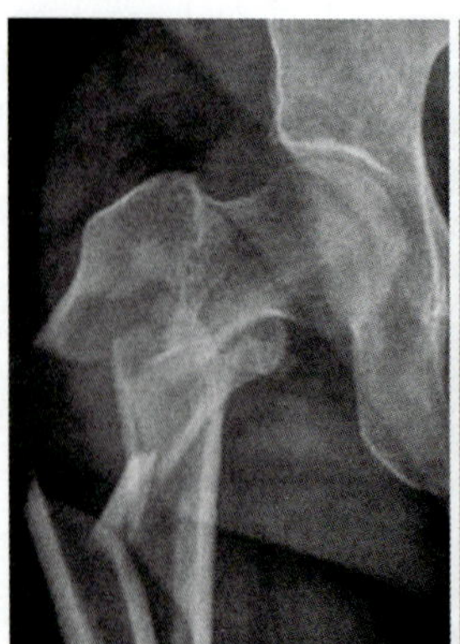

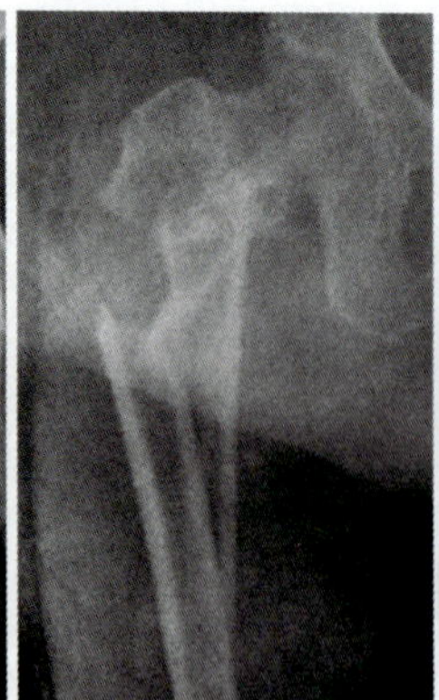

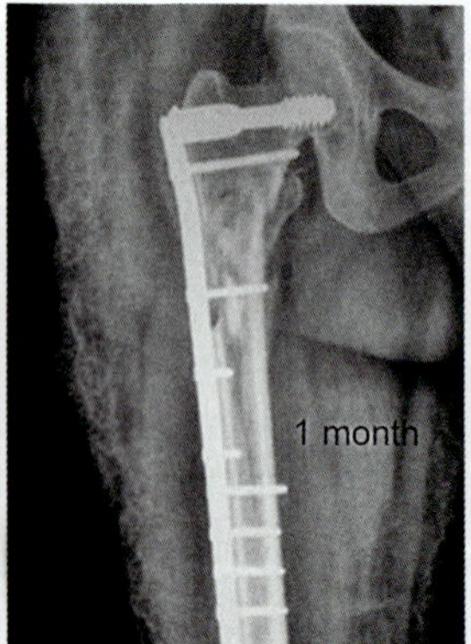

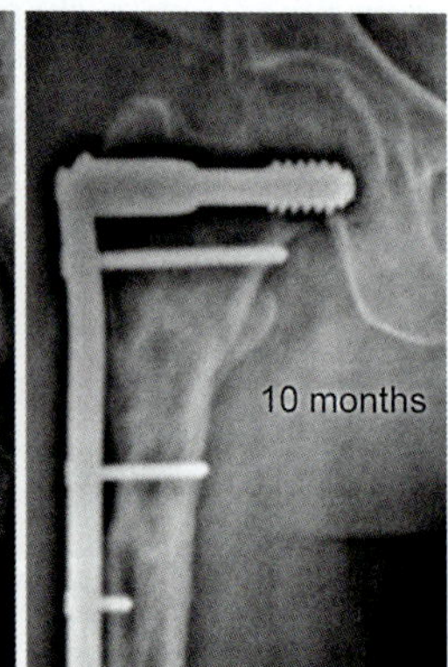

Figure 29.12 Fracture with multiple long fragments: I FS

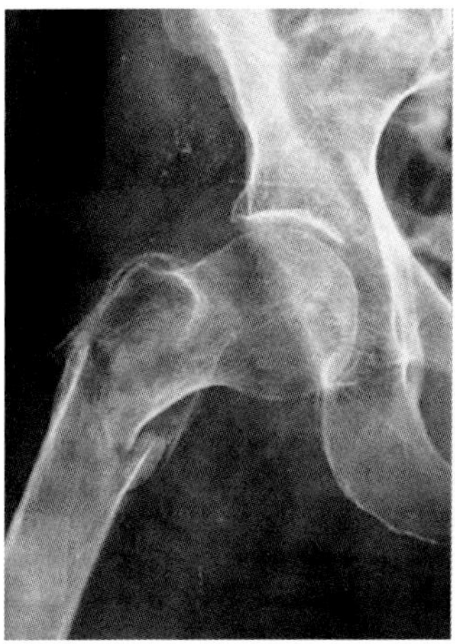
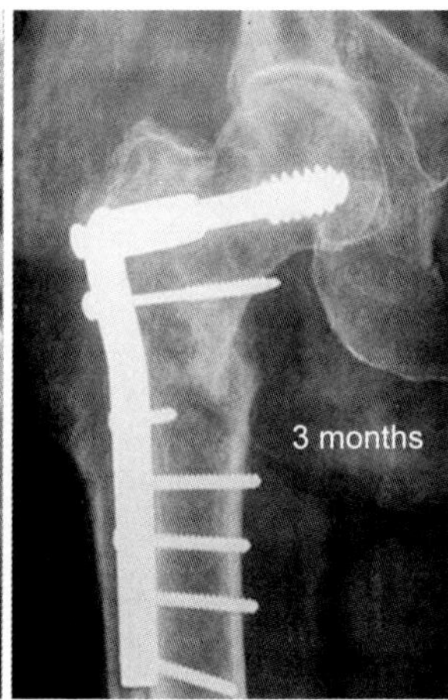

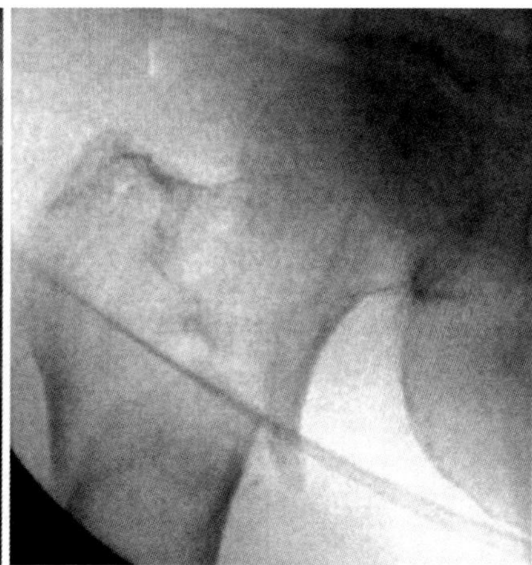

Figure 29.13 Malleolar screw

needs to be unicortical in the lateral cortex alone (Figs 29.14A to C).

In a reverse oblique fracture, a screw cannot have a purchase in the calcar. However, a unicortical screw through the lateral cortex is possible (Fig. 29.15).

In a short proximal fragment, may be only one screw has a place in the proximal fragment (Figs 29.16 and 29.17).

In an oblique fracture, if possible, one should insert an oblique screw in an IFS mode for better stability (Figs 29.18 and 29.19).

Less often one may come across a transverse fracture in the subtrochanteric area. It is a good morphology to do PFN. However, a surgeon, who prefers a surface fixation with a DCS, this is a situation, where, compression across the fracture is possible with an articulated tension device for absolute stability (Fig. 29.20).

In a subtrochanteric fracture with intertrochanteric extension, a DCS was used. The bone comminution was substituted with synthetic substitute and some bone grafts. The initial progress was satisfactory. However, at the end of the six months, she developed progressive limb shortening. A follow up X-ray revealed a mechanical failure in the plate and was revised. The plate was changed. Prior to application of another plate, the area was grafted with autologous bone grafts. At the end of four months, good consolidation was observed.`

Technical information: In this case, a screw was broken, during the removal. Fortunately, the screw holes of the revised plate did not match the earlier ones. The plate was taken longer, to overcome mechanical problems (Figs 29.21 and 29.22).

This lady over 80 years and rather malnourished had this subtrochanteric fracture. As the proximal fragment was being prepared for insertion of the hip screw, very little resistance was observed during triple reaming. Hence gentle tapping in the head part was done, short of full length. This helps to have a good purchase of the final screw threads, without tapping. As it is, we had planned to carry out bone grafting at the fracture site. Hence at this stage only, iliac grafts were taken and few long slivers were inserted in the screw track and final screw was driven in. This increased the screw hold on the bone, as some resistance was encountered now. We preferred bone graft to bone cement.

Prior to application of the 95 degree plate, a 0.8 mm circlage wire was carefully added, with minimum soft tissue erasing, for undisplaced flake of the distal fragment.

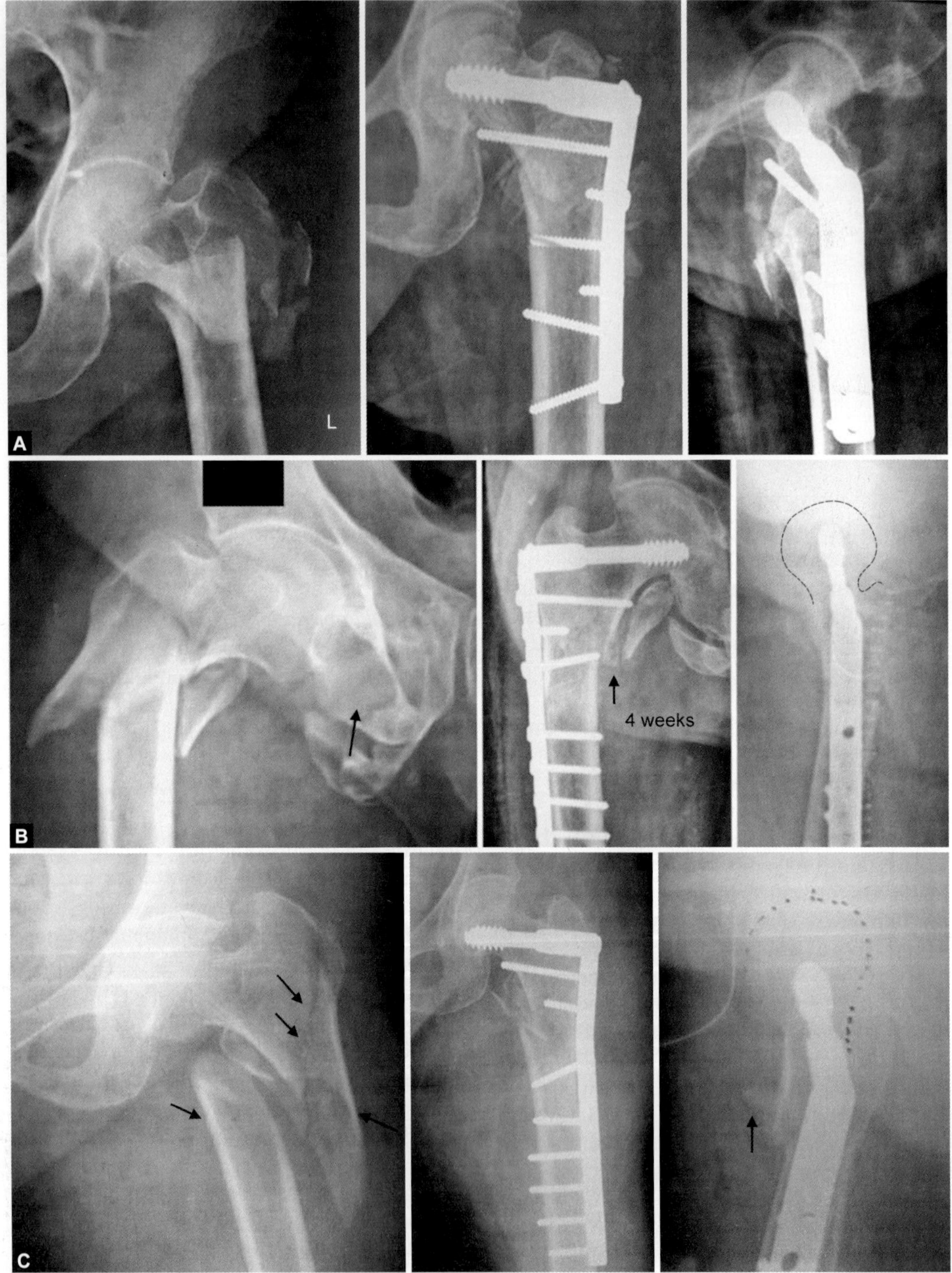

Figures 29.14A to C DCS in subtrochanteric fracture: Second round hole screw be unicortical

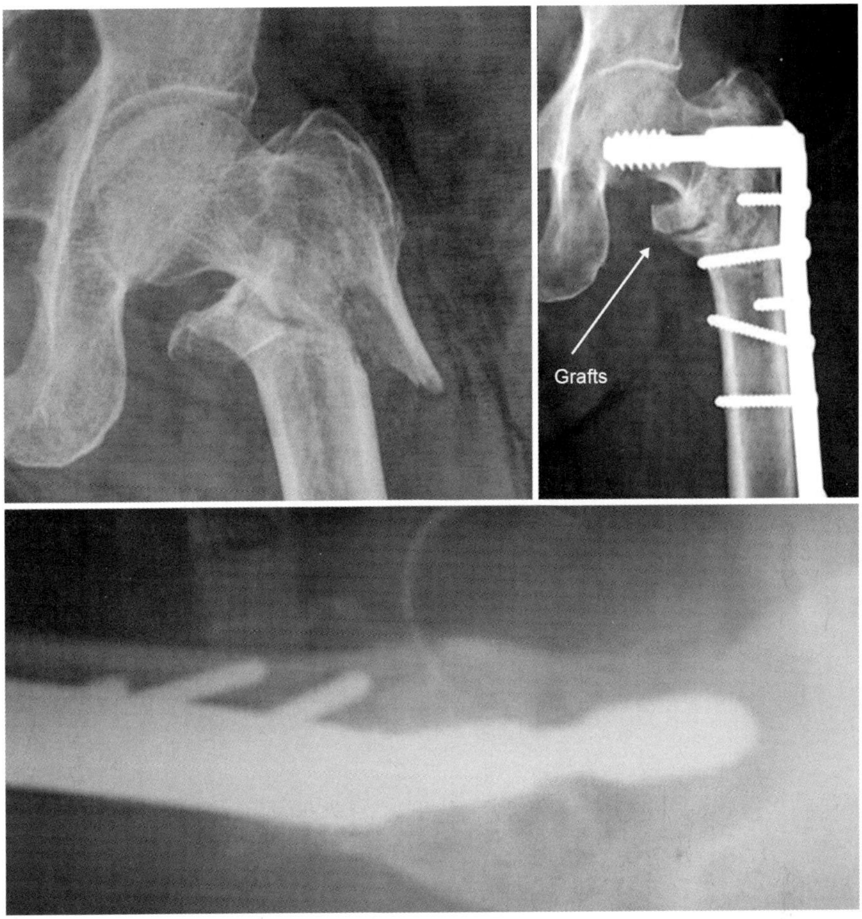

Figure 29.15 Reverse oblique fracture

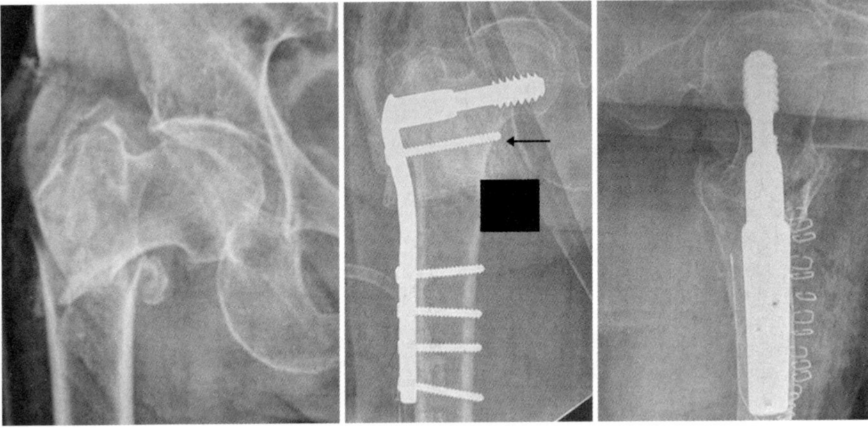

Figure 29.16 DCS in subtrochanteric fracture only 1 screw in calcar i

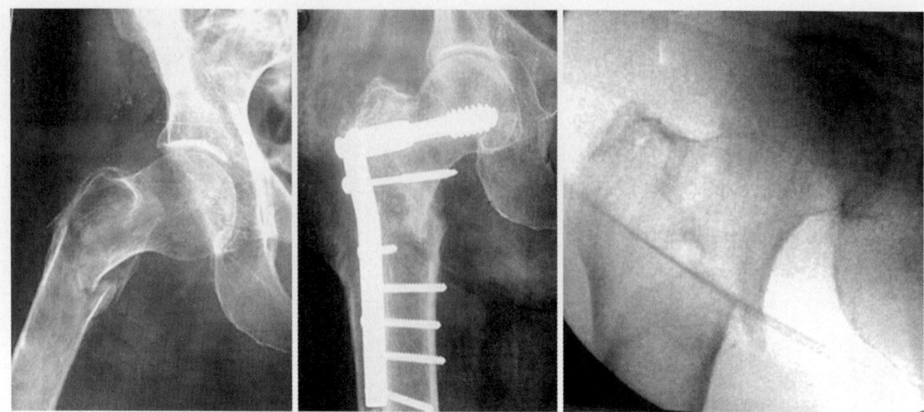

Figure 29.17 DCS in subtrochanteric fracture. Only 1 screw in calcar ii

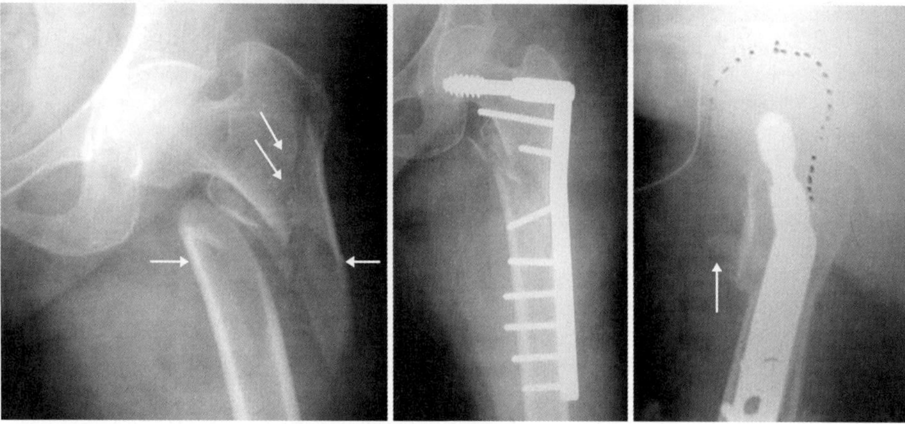

Figure 29.18 IFS

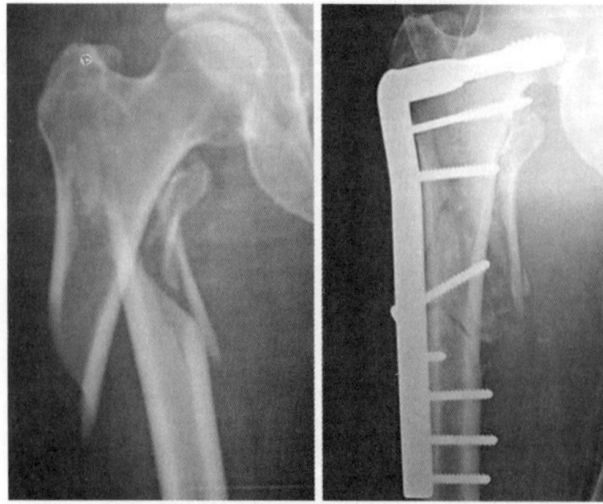

Figure 29.19 IFS

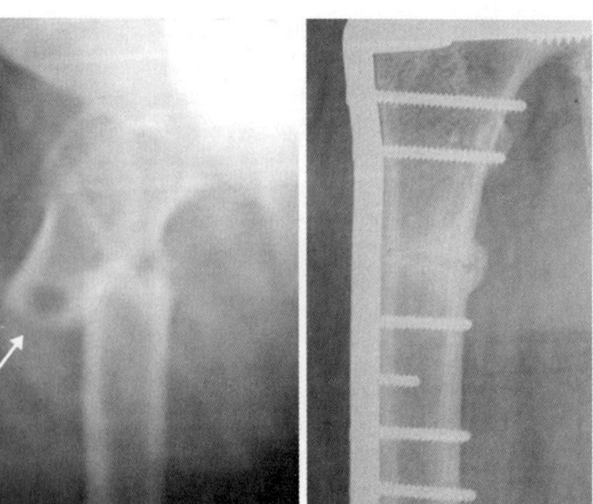

Figure 29.20 A transverse fracture loaded with oval hole geometry or an articulated tension device

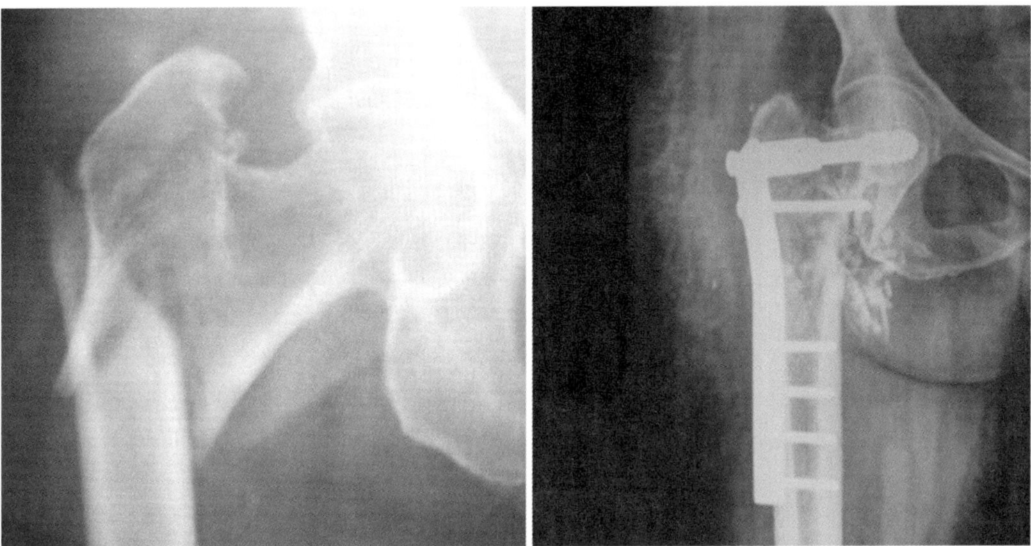

Figure 29.21 Machanical failure of a DCS

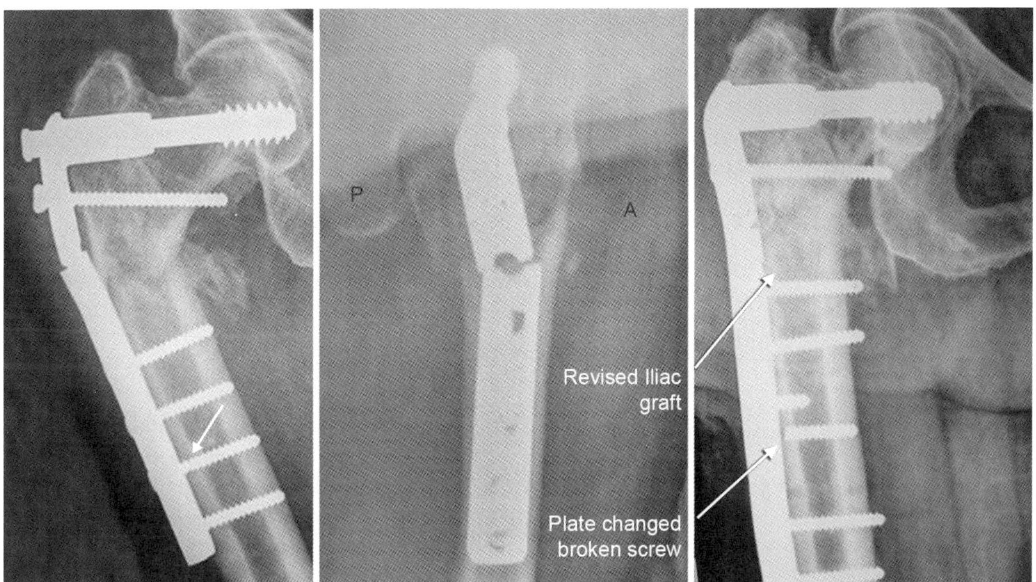

Figure 29.22 Revised with another plate and revision bone grafting

In cases, where the bone is observed to be osteoporotic (as per the resistance encountered during drilling, the distal screws were inserted in divergent mode, to improve the pull out strength of the implant. Follow up films not available, as patient did not turn up (Fig. 29.23).

INTRAMEDULLARY DEVICE IN SUBTROCHANTERIC FRACTURE

Intramedullary nail is a mechanically sound device. Due to the length of the device, good stability is offered. However, it is essential to

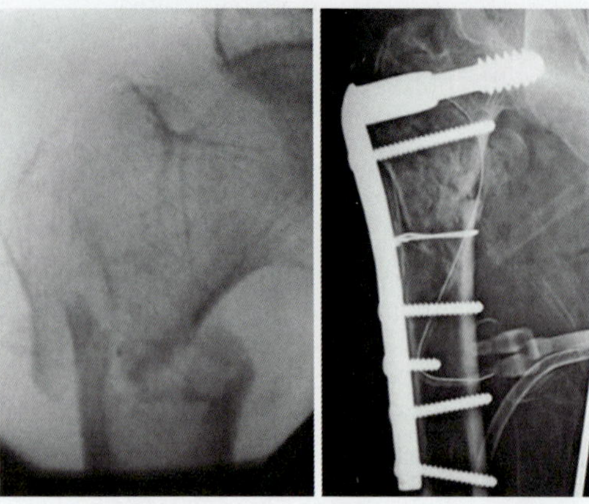

Figure 29.23 Assess in 'C' arm

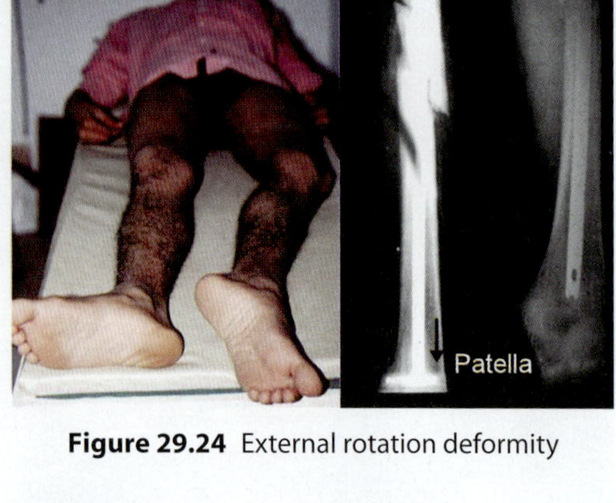

Figure 29.24 External rotation deformity

observe few technical and biological principles, to achieve a successful outcome. Deviation from any one of them would lead to a poor outcome. Few cases of failure of IM internal fixation would highlight the importance of necessary steps to be observed.

Reduction with good rotational alignment is important. In a closed interlock nailing or open method of a K nailing, rotational alignment is important. If this is not carefully done, the deformity is often very troublesome for the patient.

Case 1

The patient presented for opinion to know, if the leg could be made straight. Here one clinically observes the external rotation deformity of the leg. The X-ray shows a part of the lesser trochanter. The distal end of the femur in external rotation (Fig. 29.24).

Case 2

In a closed interlock method, how one can achieve an exact rotational reduction?

After a guidewire insertion, reaming, when the nail is advanced, following technique needs to be adopted. I assume, one is doing the procedure on a radiolucent table, with the patient in the lateral position. When the tip of the nail is at the fracture site, one should keep the leg on a sterile wrapped pillow and keep the

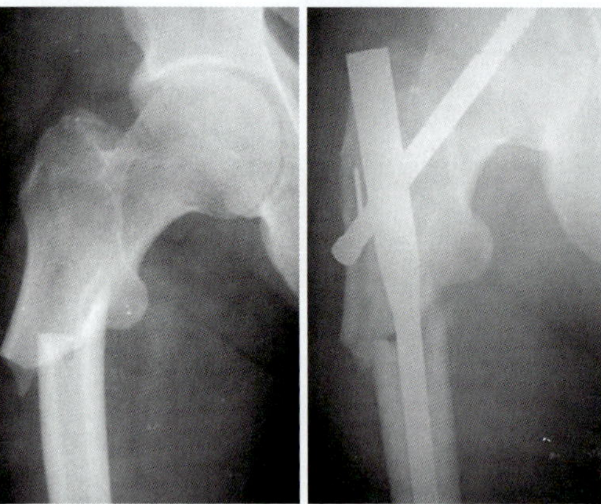

Figure 29.25 Malrotation of femur in a closed IM nail with a non-union

distal fragment such that the femur condyles are exactly overlapping. Now, the 'C' arm is moved towards the hip joint and a lateral view of the hip is taken, in 'C' arm. Now when the lateral view of the hip shows approximately 15 deg. of neck anteversion, while the femoral condyles are exactly overlapping, it indicates the femur shaft fragments are exactly aligned. Having achieved this, the nail is advanced and one can be sure, the rotational alignment is perfect.

If this method is not practised, often, it leads to an appearance, as in the case, who presented with pain on weight bearing (Fig. 29.25). (Dr Rahul Damle).

Case 3

A subtrochanteric fracture with a medial segment was well stabilized with a reconstruction nail. However, the fracture line was persistent. Decortication, medial bone grafting and application of a derotation plate lead to union.

Message

In this highly stressed area, a good reduction must be achieved and complementary bone grafting be done. In spite of the locking bolts, absolute stability may not be always achieved. If fracture does not show evidence of union in expected period, early bone grafting and a derotation plate fixation is necessary (Fig. 29.26).

Case 4

In a comminuted intertrochanteric fracture with extension in the subtrochanteric area, a closed PFN was successfully carried out elsewhere. The patient was ambulated in a few days. As we all are aware, even though, patient is advised not to put weight on the limb, some weight does pass through the limb, while rising from a chair, on the steps, etc. Patient noticed gradual shortening of the limb and pain in the left hip and attended the clinic for a second opinion. X-ray examination at this occasion revealed a broken nail.

One should understand the subtrochanteric area is a highly stressed area (perhaps the highest stressed area in the body). Every implant is known to fail, if the union does not occur in an expected period. If the nail breaks, the magnitude of revision surgery, to remove the broken nail, to revise the fixation and to do bone grafting is much higher than the primary procedure with a staged grafting.

Therefore, I feel all such fractures should have a complementary bone grafting in addition to a successful closed nailing. The grafts when laid medially, help to build the calcar area, which transfer the weight (Fig. 29.27).
What I practise?

Case 5: A Typical Case Study

This elderly person sustained a five-part subtrochanteric area. A CT scan of the hip was done, especially for a suspected fracture at the tear drop area. It revealed an undisplaced fracture of posterior lip of the acetabulum, which was treated nonoperatively. A Thomas' splint was applied as a first aid.

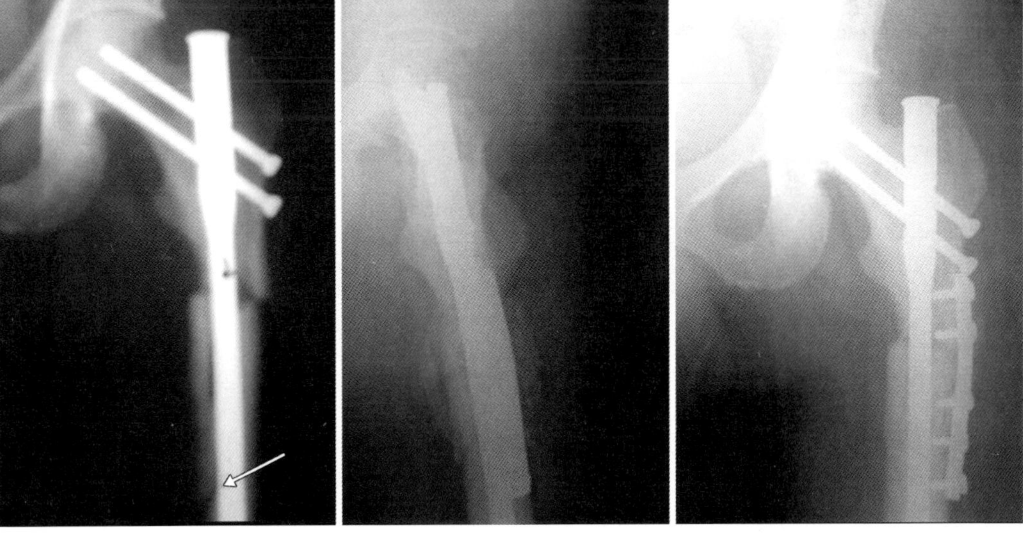

Figure 29.26 Union after a derotation plate and bone grafting

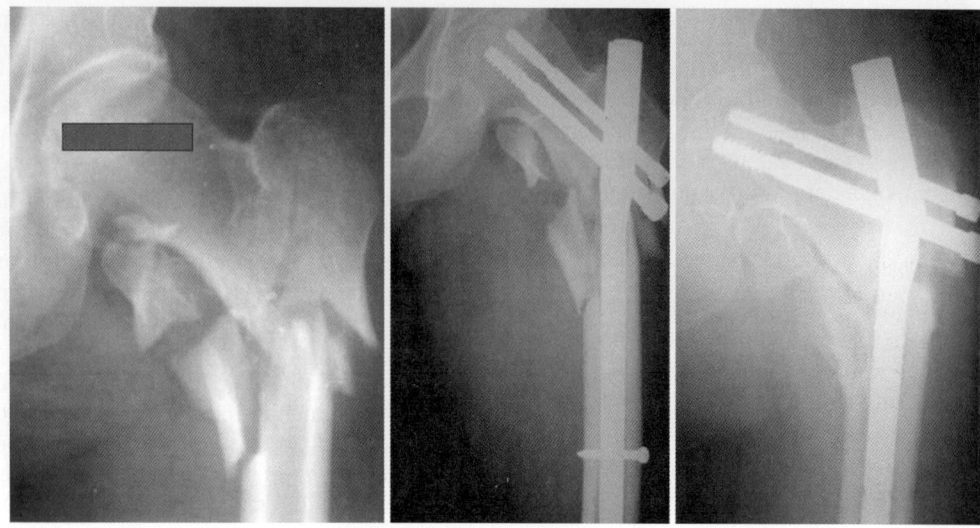

Figure 29.27 A nail failure after a successful closed nailing (No grafting done)

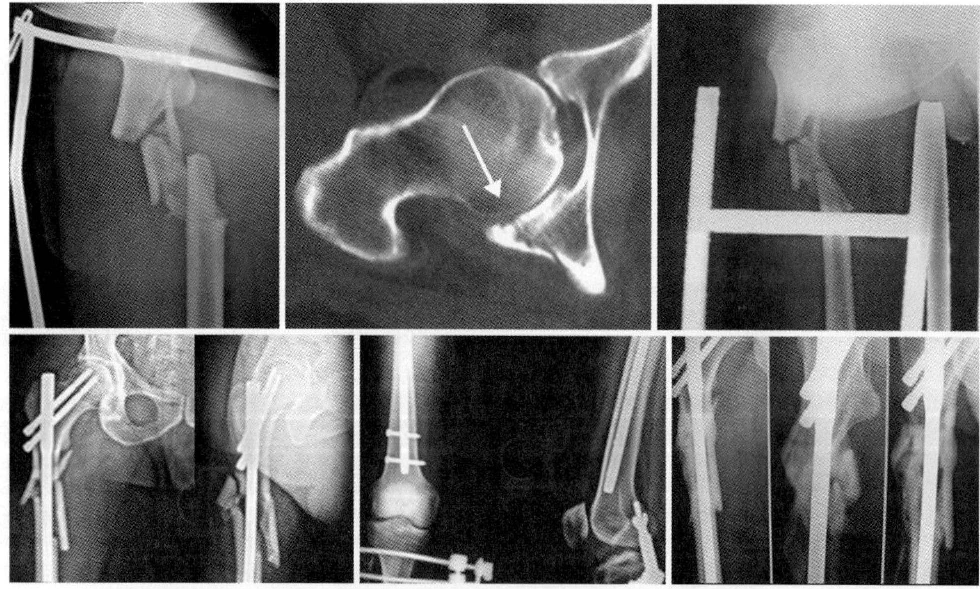

Figure 29.28 Important steps in management of a subtrochanteric fracture

The thigh had a large hematoma and to reduce the tissue reaction, it was necessary to wait till it settled down. A skeletal traction was applied through the proximal tibia and we waited for ten days or so. Then a successful closed PFN was carried out and the traction was continued. The traction weight was naturally, just to maintain the position. This postoperative elevation on a Bohler frame, helps to keep the reactionary swelling to a minimum. After two weeks, the skeletal traction was removed and the mobilization in the bed was permitted.

A week later, when the thigh swelling settled, cancellous bone grafting was carried out and patient was kept in the bed. At the end of six weeks from the internal fixation, he was permitted to use a walker, with non-weight bearing mobilization. At the end of four months from the internal fixation, the fracture united and the consolidation continued (Fig. 29.28).

Message

- In this high-energy injury, it is necessary to wait till the initial tissue reaction settles, for a definitive surgery.
- If a closed nailing is successful, a staged bone grafting must be done.
- Mobilization in the bed is safe and ambulation should be started at appropriate time, after bone grafting is done.

CHAPTER 30

Fracture of Femur Shaft

Fracture of shaft of femur is a major injury, because the femur is the longest and the strongest bone in the body. Let us assume that this fracture was the only injury with which a patient has come to the emergency room.

Immediately after arrival, a clinical examination, especially the pedal pulses and toe movements must be recorded. IV fluids, analgesic must be administered and the limb immobilized in a Thomas' splint. This should be done prior to X-ray examination. Later on, if necessary, on the X-ray table, the splint may be temporarily shifted downwards, for a clear X-ray of the hip area. Hemodynamic stability is taken care of.

One should be able to boast of a well-equipped splint room, next to the emergency room, containing splints of all sizes. It requires the spirit of good first aid by the treating surgeon and the hospital administrator and does not cost much. Mere thigh brace or only a skin traction without a splint is insufficient method of immobilization. A well-applied splint of correct size relieves pain and prevents further tissue damage (Figs 30.1A and B).

Clinically, a fracture in the middle/3 of the thigh can be diagnosed. The X-ray examination must cover an area from the hip to the upper/3 of tibia. Time and again, one comes across missed injuries in the hip area (including undisplaced fracture of posterior lip of acetabulum), and around the knee, associated with fracture of femur, especially in high energy injuries. Hence, importance of the extent of X-ray examination. The hip must be at least in neutral rotation, if not in internal rotation, to exclude a hip fracture. If the proximal fragment is in external rotation, one can angulate the X-ray tube accordingly and try to take a film, which would exclude associated such an injury. Now-a-days, many institutes do take 'Trauma X-ray set' X-ray of chest/cervical spine and pelvis as a routine in road traffic injuries, and deserve praise.

Here is an example how a fracture can be missed. I had an opportunity to see few X-ray films of a case. I am predicting, as to what may have had happened in the given case.

Clinically, a fracture in lower/3 femur was observed and was confirmed by an X-ray. As per the teaching, X-ray of the hip was taken, to exclude any associated fracture of the neck of femur. It revealed a fracture of neck of the femur. The surgeon did fixation of the neck of femur fracture with cancellous screws. The distal femur fracture was fixed with a DFN. A short DFN nail was used and the proximal bolts could be fixed with a jig and perhaps X-ray or a 'C' arm image may not have been taken and a Thomas' splint was applied. X-ray taken later on through the splint showed another fracture at the upper/3 area! This was later fixed with a plate.

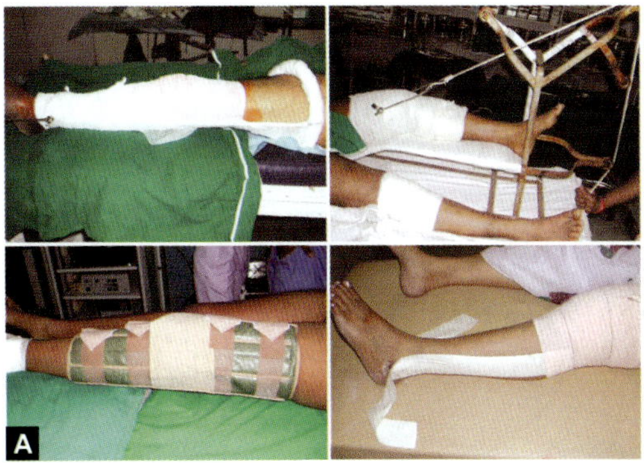

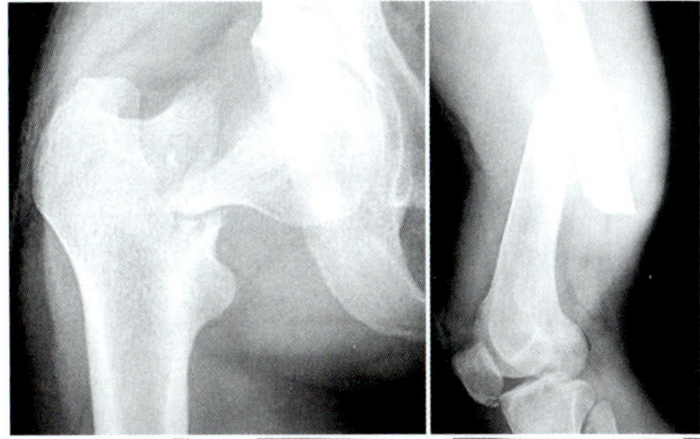

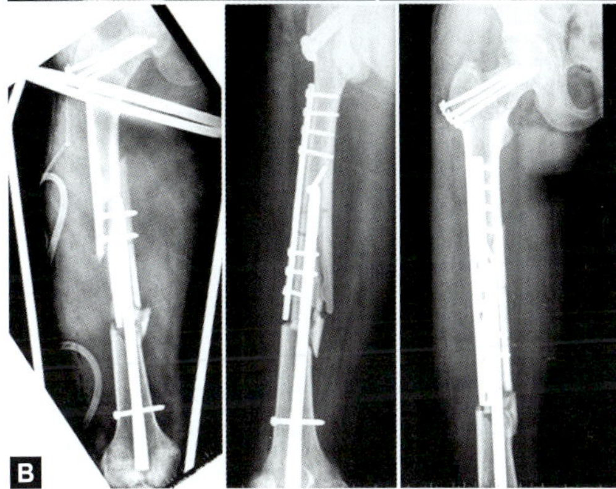

Figures 30.1A and B (A) First aid and splint; (B) Missed fracture of neck of femur

Message: In a fracture of femur, the entire femur must be examined in continuity, to avoid such a situation (Fig. 30.2).

There is an increasing trend to stabilize such an injury, soon after arrival. It is safe to do so only, if a trained clinician assesses the case personally, necessary tests, including USG of abdomen if necessary, are properly done and results available. Assessment of cardiovascular status by a physician is equally important too.

THE OPERATION ROOM AT ANY TIME

It is important to have the necessary equipment ready and available, with infrastructure beyond the routine working hours. Sterile supply of necessary instrumentation and implants is very necessary. Operation room assistants, nursing services including recovery area, etc. need to be available. These services are necessary part of the entire exercise of operating at any time of a day or night.

Sterile instrumentation and implants is of prime importance, as everyone knows.

At times, the patient has severe pain and is unable to co-operate to apply the splint correctly. In such a situation, even the X-ray of pelvis/ipsilateral knee may also not be possible. Hence, once the patient is stabilized, it is a good idea to carry out a procedure *under general anesthesia*, in an emergency theater.

What Needs to be Done?

- X-ray examination of the pelvis and the entire thigh till the upper/3 tibia.
- Attending associated injuries, which may need wound lavage/suturing/dermabrasion etc. is done. In fact, shaving of the area to be operated is also done with comfort, now only, rather than to do this in a theater, where a planned procedure is to be done later on.
- Application of skin traction and Thomas' splint can be done more efficiently.
- If the thigh swelling and hematoma is too much or the blood sugar is too high or other conditions, which may need to wait for a few days for a definitive surgery, my preference is to add an upper tibial skeletal traction, which is maintained on a Bohler frame later on. A skeletal traction can efficiently reduce the pain and spasm. The limb is automatically elevated, on the Bohler frame and due to the head low position, the hematoma and edema is taken care of. Due to adequate skeletal traction, the limb and

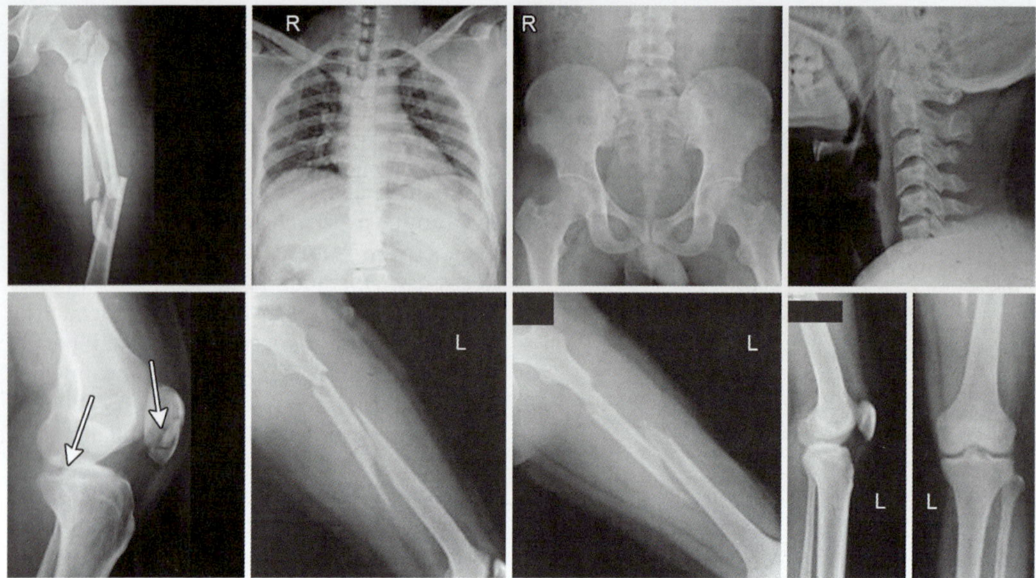

Figure 30.2 Trauma X-ray films

muscle length is maintained well, which would increase a chance of a successful closed IM procedure. In an oblique or a spiral fracture, a bone spike may have penetrated adjacent muscle, making a closed procedure difficult or perhaps unsuccessful. A skeletal traction aligns the bone ends and the bone spikes, which have pierced adjacent muscle, may come out, and are well-aligned with adjacent bone ends.

- In a closed interlock nailing, presence of a Steinmann pin helps to give a traction to the distal fragment and can be of help to achieve a correct rotational alignment.

NON-OPERATIVE METHODS

In earlier years, for many reasons, non-operative method of treatment was given to the patient. If managed well, a fracture of femur usually responds well to such a treatment.

Case shown, had a head injury, fracture of shaft of femur with a puncture wound and an ipsilateral fracture of tibia. This was in an era when CT scan and external fixators were not yet invented. The patient had cerebral contusion and fever, which could not be explained. Hence, a non-operative method for both the fracture had to be used. In due course, both the fractures united well and for the next 35 years, he could actively continue his profession, including driving a scooter (Fig. 30.3).

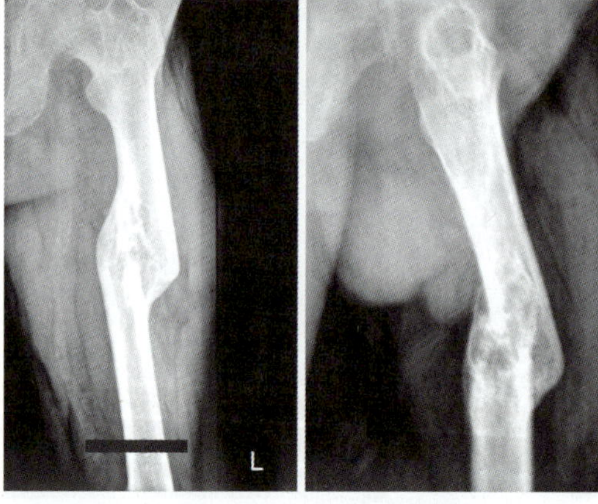

Figure 30.3 Non-operative method for fracture mid/3 femur: 30-year follow up

In a lower third fracture, quadriceps exercises help to prevent muscle adhesions and restore good knee range of motion (Fig. 30.4).

FRACTURE OF FEMUR SHAFT IN INFANTS AND ADOLESCENCE

A two-year old baby, sustained a fracture at the subtrochanteric area and was an incomplete fracture. Any movement, carrying her in arm was painful. Application of a Thomas' splint for two weeks made her comfortable. Another five-year-old child had a spiral fracture in the mid/3 area. A Thomas' splint aligned it well and in three weeks, adequate callus formed, to be able to keep her free (Fig. 30.5).

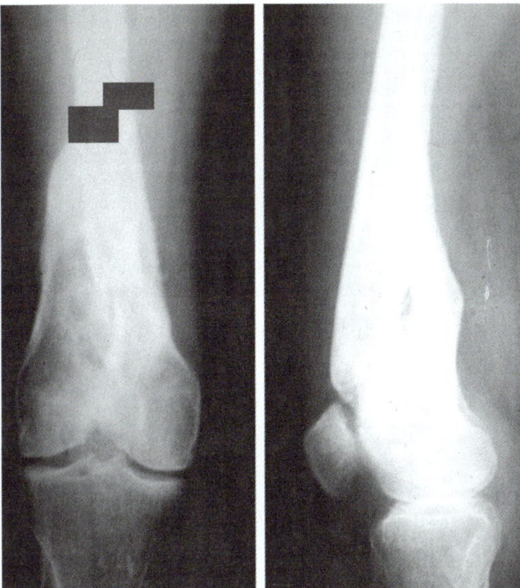

Figure 30.4 Non-operative method for fracture of L/3 femur

In a girl of 11 years, a closed reduction was successful and a Thomas' splint was applied. Follow up X-ray every week arranged. At the end of two weeks, the fracture was noticed to be getting displaced and hence a plate fixation was done, with a good outcome. (This was in a pre-TEN nails era) (Figs 30.6 and 30.7).

A young sportsman of 15 years had a transverse fracture in mid/3 femur. He was well-built and being a sportsman had to be offered a precise reduction and result. A plate fixation was carried out. Please note the precontoured plate. At such an age, the implant needs to be removed, once the remodeling has occurred. This would prevent another fracture adjacent to the plate end. Besides, in the second growth spurt, the stress shielding would also get corrected rapidly (Fig. 30.8).

Today, with advent of elastic nails and a 'C' arm, a closed method of nailing, using an elastic nail, is possible. The nail, as an implant, being a load sharing one, the stress shielding is much less, compared to a plate (Fig. 30.9).

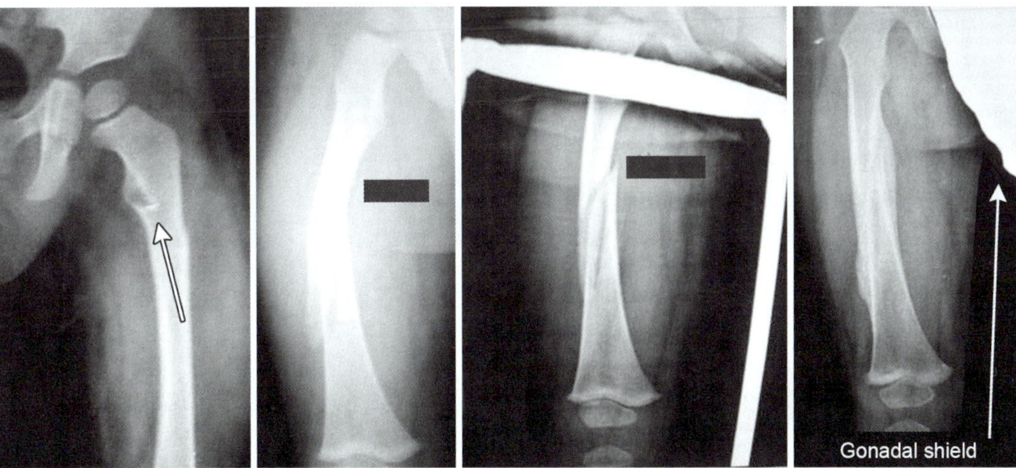

Figure 30.5 Fracture of femur in infancy and childhood

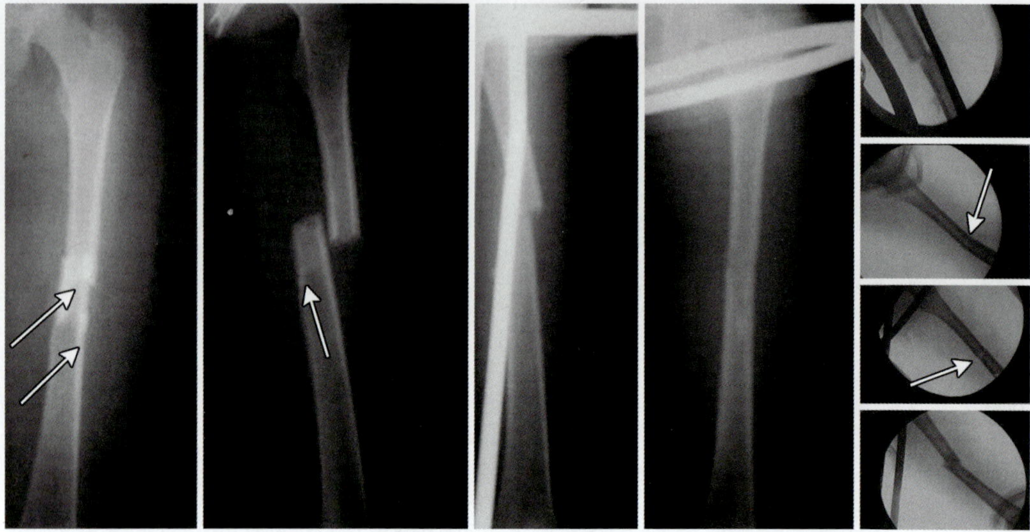

Figure 30.6 Fracture of femur in adolescent; plate

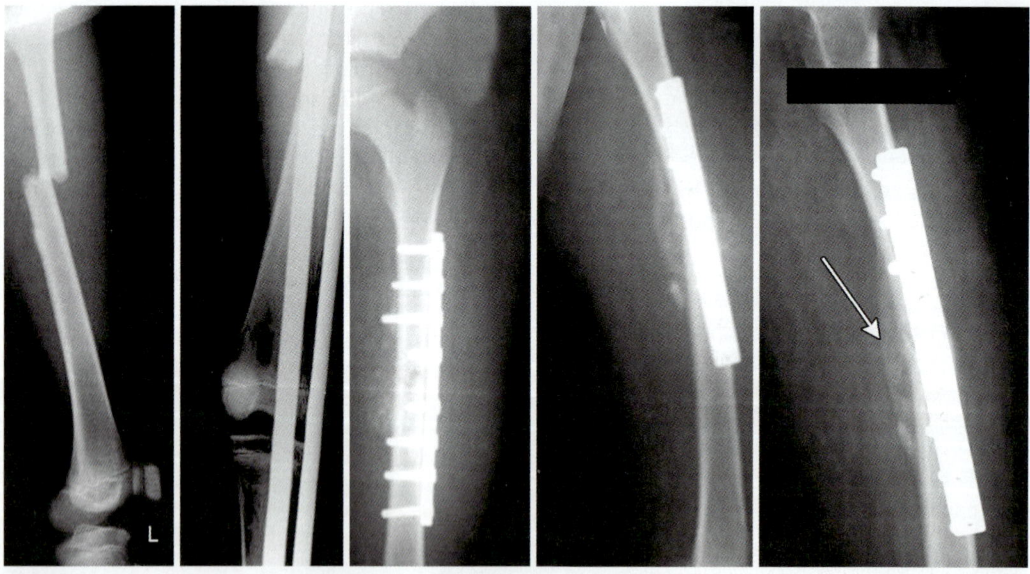

Figure 30.7 Fracture of femur in adolescent; plate

TECHNIQUE TO ASSESS ROTARY ALIGNMENT IN A SHAFT FRACTURE

A young man came with a deformity in the leg. He had undergone open reduction and internal fixation of a femur fracture by a K-nail. He had an external rotation deformity. The X-ray depicts slight presence of lesser trochanter at the proximal femur, while the lower end shows an appearance of complete lateral view of

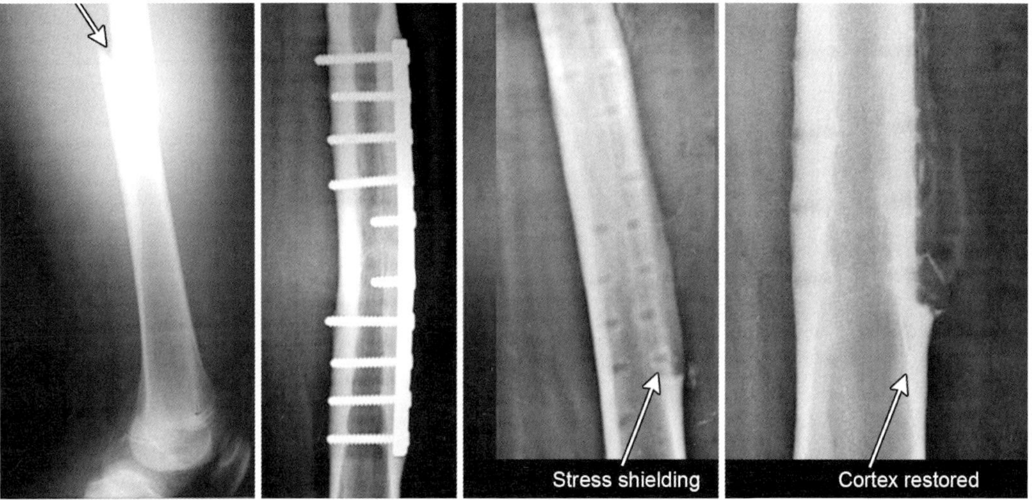

Figure 30.8 Stress shielding

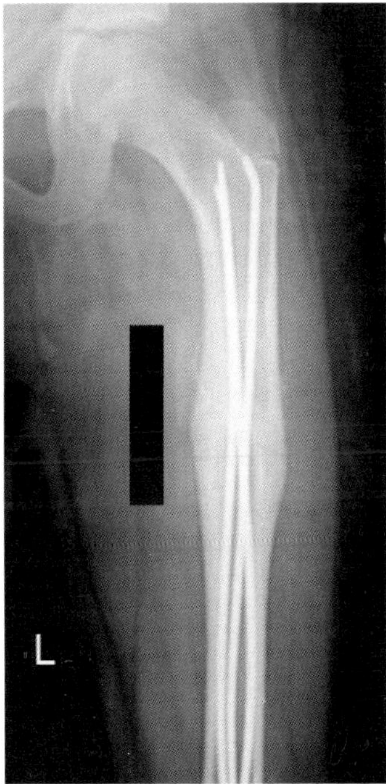

Figure 30.9 Elastic nails

femoral condyles, superimposed on each other. This indicates at least 70 degree of external rotation deformity in the femur.

How to Obtain a Correct Rotational Alignment while doing by a closed IM Nailing?

I prefer to carry out a femur interlock nailing in a lateral position. After adequate reaming is done, one inserts a nail mounted on a jig. As the nail tip reaches the fracture area, one takes a lateral view of the hip. The position of the patient, if is in exact lateral position, one sees the neck of femur, springing out from the shaft at an angle of anterversion. Now, the 'C' arm is moved towards the knee and a lateral view of the lower end of femur is taken. Now, if the femur condyles are seen exactly superimposed, it indicates that the distal femur is in neutral rotation and the neck is in correct anteversion. In each case, this should be followed to confirm the rotational alignment and then the nail is advanced in the distal fragment. (This case shown was in pre 'C' arm era. Still, having done quite a few open K-nail fixation, in yester years, I feel, this is an exceptional case with extreme external rotation deformity).

In addition to this, one should compare the thickness of the cortex adjacent to the fracture area in a 'C' arm image. If it is the same on either side of the fracture, the rotational alignment is correct (Fig. 30.10).

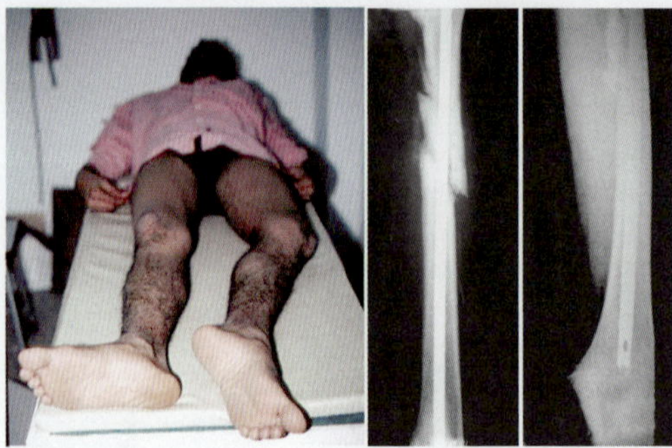

Figure 30.10 External rotation deformity

Achievement of a Successful Closed Nailing in a Segmental Fracture

The technical details are available in various books of surgical technique of interlocking nailing procedure. Usually the beaded guide wire negotiates the proximal fracture. At this stage, a narrow diameter nail (narrow because, it easily enters the medullary cavity) is advanced over the guide-wire, till the distal fracture. It is then used as a joystick so, the beaded guidewire can negotiate the second fracture. However, in presence of soft tissue interposition, it is worthwhile to carry out an open reduction of the distal fracture, through an incision of necessary length. In such a situation, the proximal and the middle fragments have a nail within and the distal most fragment can be controlled by the knee. To align and reduce both the fragments, a Kuncher diamond awl is inserted in the fracture site and the bone ends can be aligned well, so the guidewire can be advanced further in the distal most fragment. It is necessary to learn this technique of reduction using an awl and levering the fragments in place, so that use of Hey Groves or self-centering forceps can be avoided and soft tissue attachment to bone ends is well maintained.

In such a 3 segment fracture, usually the upper segment out of the three is in flexion and passage of guidewire in the middle segment could be painstaking and difficult. Hence one may have to do open reduction of this fracture. Having passed the guidewire further, crossing the distal fracture, to enter the 3rd (and the distal most) fragment by a closed method is usually successful. During reaming of the fragments, often the middle segment rotates along with the rotating reamer and especially when an open reduction of this fracture is done, one should hold it with a self-centering forceps, to prevent its spinning and losing the soft tissue attachments. The reamed material draining out through the fracture area, is carefully allowed to remain there only and should not be mopped or sucked away. This has a good capacity to promote union.

How to Assess Rotatory Alignment of the Proximal with the Distal Fragment in a Segmental Fracture and Keep the Nail in the Desired Position?

In a lateral position: After a successful reaming, a nail is advanced till the distal fracture site. The greater trochanter and the femoral condyles are palpated. The jig attached to the upper end of the interlocking nail, should be in plumb line (at right angles to the nail).

- With a 'C' arm, an AP projection of the hip, in neutral position should show, just a small amount of lesser trochanter. The limb is kept stable in this position and the 'C' arm turned, to have a lateral view of the hip.
- In the hip, correct lateral view should show anteversion of the neck as the neck springs from the shaft.
- The 'C' arm is moved to the knee to show the femoral condyles. If the femoral condyles are overlapping exactly and the distal holes of the nails are full moon shape, it means the fragment alignment is correct. Often at this stage, the holes appear biconvex, indicating the nail is lying in external rotation. The nail may be slightly withdrawn and advanced again in correct rotational position, so that the proximal jig is exactly lateral and the distal holes are in full moon shape.
- *An Important Step:* Let us imagine, both the fragments are well-aligned, as per above criteria. Now, one must consider placement of the IM nail with respect to the bone.

- If the lateral view of the distal fragment shows, exact overlapping of the condyles and the nail holes appear oval, it indicates that the nail is in external rotation in the medullary cavity and then the distal bolts need to be passed from a posterolateral to anteromedial direction, which is a painstaking exercise (Fig. 30.11).

Bent K-Nail

Few years ago, when flexible reamers and 'C' arm was not available in every hospital, ORIF and K nailing was usually practised. One had to take a judgment, as to which diameter K-nail has to be used. Since the nail is a pressfit one and passed by tapping, without any reaming, it had to be of a diameter of the narrowest part of the medullary cavity. Hence often, it would not be able to resist the physiological forces on the limb. At times, may be the patient had tripped or did some premature weight bearing, some leg deformity is noted and patient reports to the clinician.

Hence, after any internal fixation, if a patient had a fall, it is necessary to examine and take an X-ray of the area, to confirm that the implant has not given way or bent.

Technique: Under anesthesia, the fracture is manipulated. Note the radiopaque fulcrum. The K-nail is gently straightened and removed. Usually adequate fibrosis and soft tissue healing has occurred around the fracture area, so the fracture does not get displaced. A guidewire is passed and progressive reaming is done and the reamed material created thus penetrates around the fracture area and union occurs in due course of time (Fig. 30.12).

Slow Healing After a Plate Fixation

In a three-part fracture of upper third area, a surgeon did a plate fixation. In a plate fixation the plate has to be prebent adequately, to bring the opposite cortex under compression. In addition to this, the teaching has been, whenever a plate fixation is done for fracture of femur, a complementary bone grafting must be done. In this case looks like both the principles were violated. There was some local swelling and pain in the area. Hence, removal of the plate and an interlocking nailing was planned. In such a case, the medullary cavity is usually obliterated and the procedure to open the medullary canal and to pass the guidewire may not be easy.

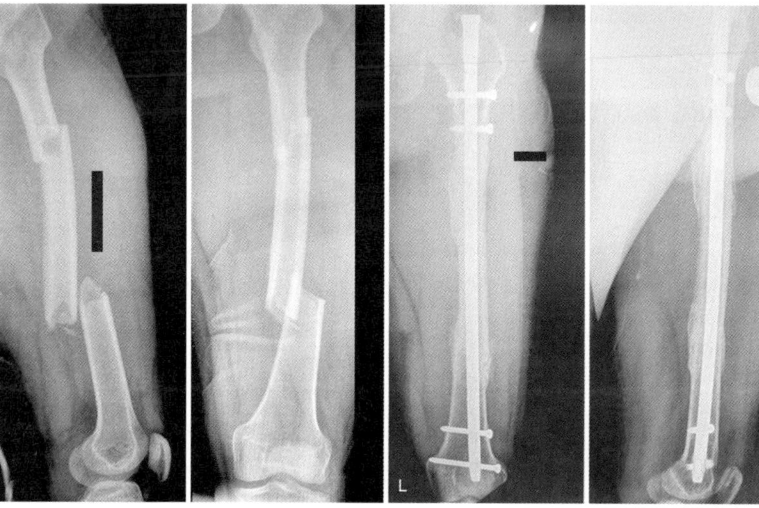

Figure 30.11 Segmental fracture closed IM nailing

On exposure, local tissue did not appear healthy and may have had a lingering infection. The fluid was sent for culture. The decision to consider IM nailing was rather difficult to take. Mild abnormal mobility was noted. The wound was closed over a drain and upper tibial skeletal traction was applied. The skeletal traction was maintained for three weeks, followed by three weeks of Thomas' splint. The patient accepted this well. Serial X-ray films indicated evidence of union on the medial side first, as is always seen.

The limb became gradually pain free. At the end of six weeks, the limb was gradually mobilized and patient ambulated. The fracture consolidated at the end of three months and he returned to his profession. He has full range of hip and knee movements, without any limp. X-ray at the end of 12 years shows good remodeling and restoration of medullary canal.

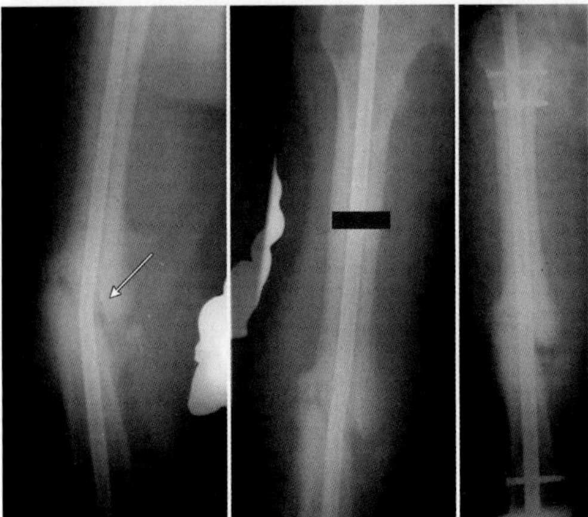

Figure 30.12 Bent K-nail

Thus, even after an operative procedure, at certain stage, it is worthwhile to change to a time-honored nonoperative method (Fig. 30.13).

A case of fracture of the upper/3 femur had medial two fragments and the distal end of the proximal fragment was oblique, above downwards, medial to laterally.

- A retrograde nailing was performed. Being an oblique fracture, the nail almost always takes a course that it penetrates the tip of the greater trochanter and the alignment of femur is disturbed.
- The two fragments were opposed to the shaft with circlage wires. Almost in each case, where a circlage is done, the surgeon, first completes the nail fixation procedure and then observes that the fragments are not well-opposed to the host shaft area. Thereafter, with a curved hemostat or a wire passer, the wires are passed around the 3rd fragment and the femur. This strips the soft tissue attachment to the 3rd and the 4th fragments and the fracture fails to unite. May be if the fragments were left as such, without

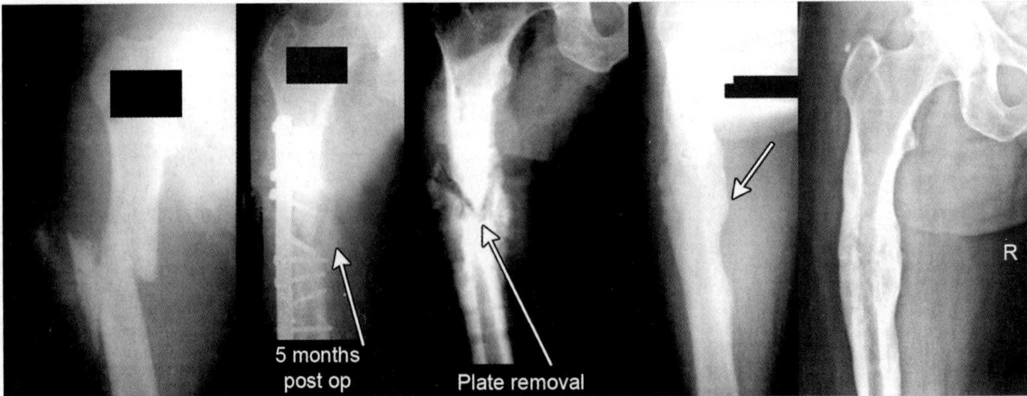

Figure 30.13 Plate removal

a circlage wire, they all may have united. Alternatively, it is a good practice to lay a few cancellous grafts between the fragments and the host shaft, in the fracture area.

- *Recommendation:* In such a situation of an open nailing, in any long bone, the procedure can be done in this way. As the fracture is opened, retrograde nail is passed. Before the fracture is reduced, the 3rd fragment is easily accessible. With a circular wire passer, gently a wire is passed, close to the bone, with a minimal stripping and the ends are held with hemostats and laid apart on either side. After the procedure of nailing is complete, then the wire is tied around the femur.
- In such a case my preference would be to add a derotation plate on the lateral surface. When a derotation plate is to be used, it should be a 12 mm narrow plate.
- In the given case of ununited fracture, the fracture was exposed. The 3rd and the 4th fragments were found to be united to each other, but the host principal fragments were ununited. The circlage wires were removed, decortication was done and bone grafts added. The fracture consolidated well (Figs 30.14 and 30.15).

In a fracture at the junction of mid/3 and the lower/3 area, the distal fragment is quite wide and the nail may not have adequate hold on it. Abnormal mobility was seen on table. Hence a derotation plate was added for rotational stability. Cancellous grafts were added on the medial side of the fracture. These steps make the procedure complete and lead to assured union.

It is a teaching that whenever a plate fixation is done for femur, complementary bone grafting is necessary, including when a plate is used as a tension band plate or as a derotation plate with a nail. Unfortunately, not all surgeons follow this principle and advice and it leads to an ununited fracture (Fig. 30.16)

A man in late 40s had a fracture of lower/3 femur and was treated with a K-nail fixation elsewhere. He was permitted to be ambulated with a pair of crutches. In a few weeks, patient noted gradual bowing in the thigh and prominence in the gluteal area, due to backing out of the K-nail. At this stage, he reported to us. By then, the interlock system was available and a revision surgery was planned. In spite of two locking bolts in the distal end of femur, one cannot get absolute stability in the fracture area and hence, additional derotation plate and bone grafting was planned.

Area of decortication: On the lateral surface of femur shaft, the 12 mm plate is to be applied. The decortication is done medially, till anterior and posterior to the area, where the plate would be fixed. The screw hold is better in an intact

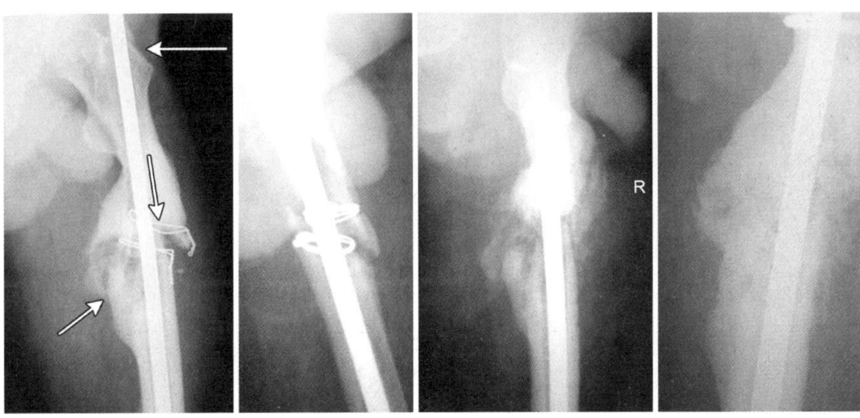

Figure 30.14 Circlage wires and nonunion. Only grafts added

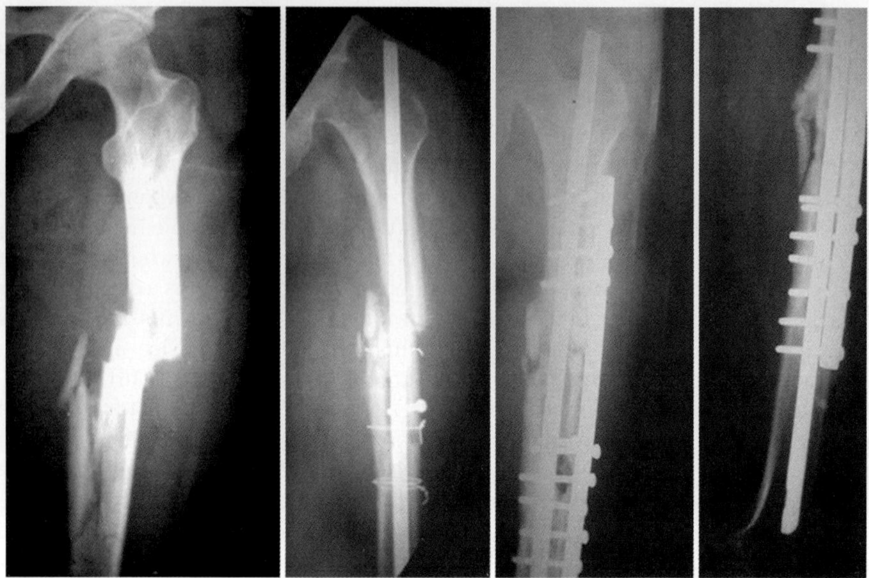

Figure 30.15 Long medial fragments: Grafts and derotation plate added

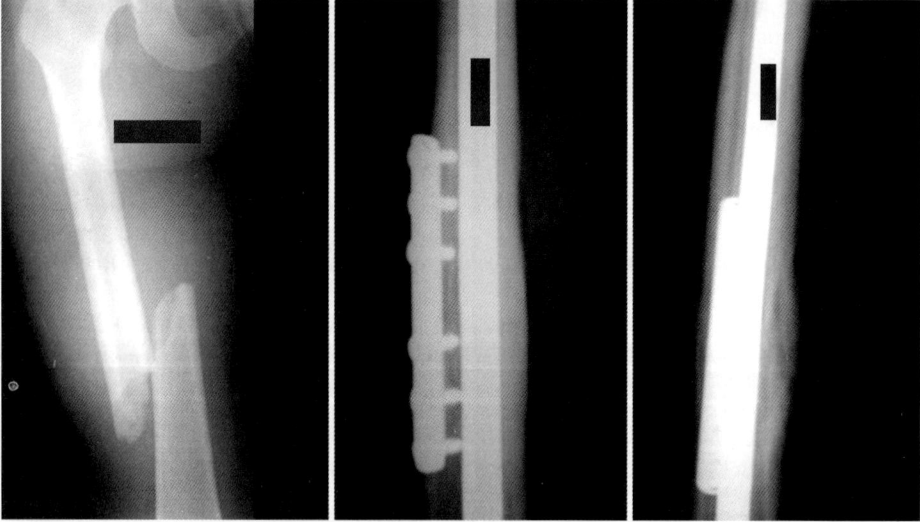

Figure 30.16 Derotation plate

cortex, than in an area, where the decortication is done. Due to presence of the nail within the marrow cavity, the screw length needs to be short. Today, if such a need arises to add a derotation plate, a locking plate and screws will be a good option than conventional screws.

Interestingly enough, the place of the second screw hole in the plate was just over the upper locking bolt. Hence, it was passed through the plate (Fig. 30.17)!

An old man had an oblique fracture in the lower/3 femur and the surgeon carried out an

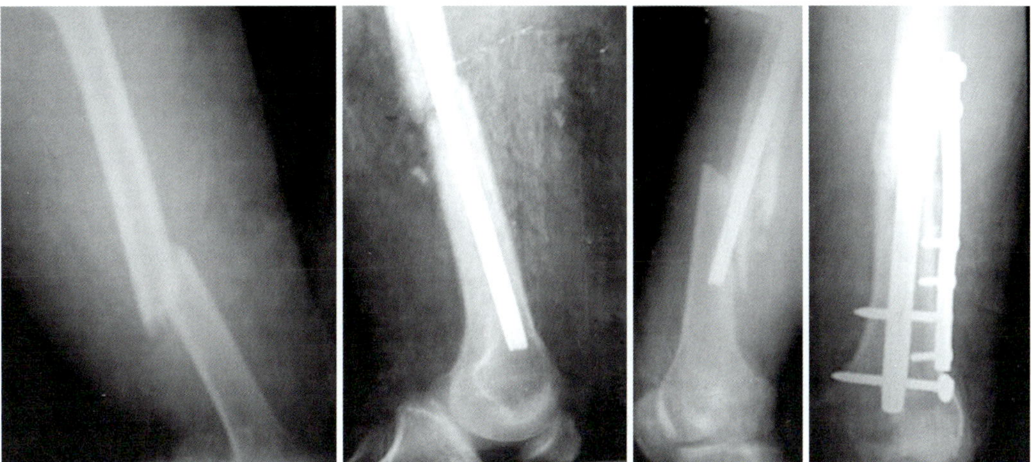

Figure 30.17 Derotation plate II

interlocking nail, in another hospital. In due course, the limb was mobilized. Later on the family noticed progressive limb shortening and external rotation deformity and was brought for further treatment.

The X-ray taken on operation table, during the previous surgery was studied. As is clear in the picture, the film did not cover the entire distal end of the femur and the nail end. *The fact that both the distal bolts did not pass through the distal holes in the nail was overlooked.* The distal end of the nail, therefore, was free to move and had migrated and penetrating the articular surface of the femur.

How was this Managed after this?

- *Step I*: Upper tibial traction was applied on a Bohler frame. In few days, the distal fragment came down and was confirmed by an X-ray taken with traction on.
- *Step II*: During the revision surgery, the fracture was exposed. A femoral distractor was applied, to achieve further distraction. One distal locking bolt was inserted, While there was an already broken drill bit in another hole area. Derotation plate and bone grafting completed the procedure and the fracture united.

Lesson Learnt

On table final 'C' arm image has to be clear. When an X-ray film is exposed, two views must be taken and they should cover the distal end of the nail, beyond doubt. If for some reason, on table X-ray film cannot be taken, it should be done so, at the earliest, in the postoperative period, prior to mobilization of the patient (Figs 30.18 and 30.19).

Fracture of Femur at Lower/4 Area

At this level, the distal fragment has a wide medullary cavity and even if two bolts are passed at the distal end of the nail, still the stability achieved is not adequate enough for a primary union.

In yester years, I would fix it with a condylar blade plate or a DCS. Today other options like, a DFN and locking plate are available and the reader may make his choice of the method to be used (Figs 30.20 to 30.22).

TYPICAL CASES

Case 1

An elderly person sustained a fracture of femur at the junction of mid and lower/3 area

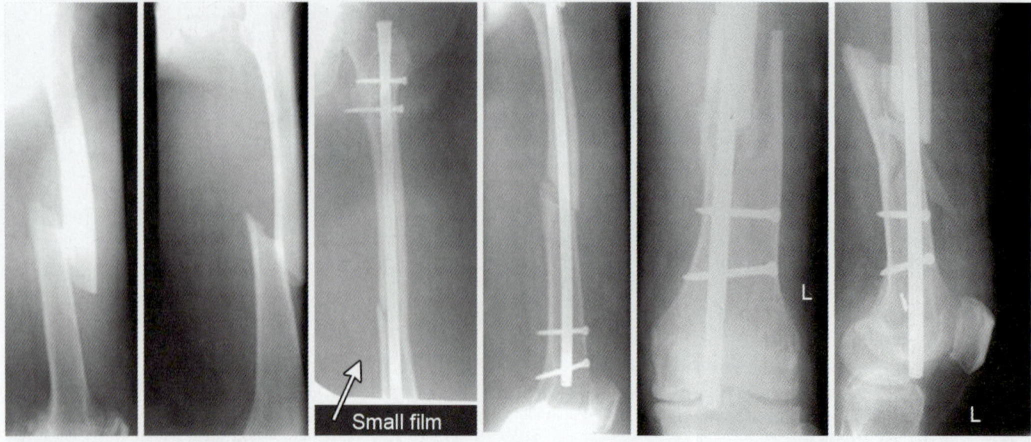

Figure 30.18 Derotation plate iii

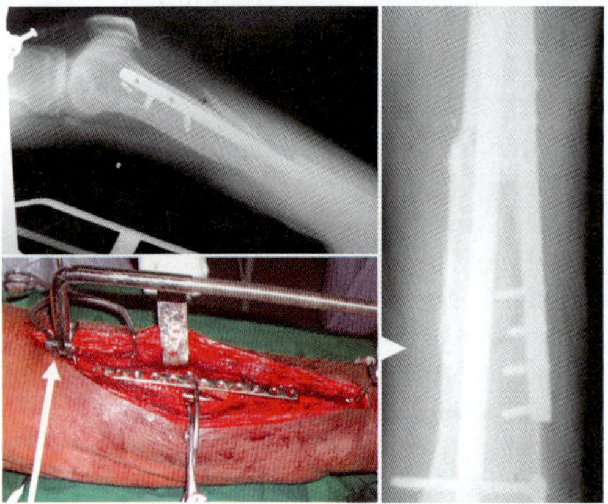

Figure 30.19 Derotation plate iv

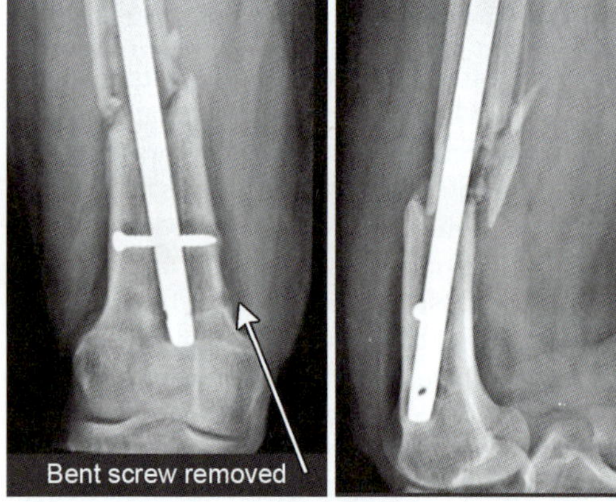

Figure 30.20 Wide medullary cavity

in another state. Open interlocking nailing was done, elsewhere. The fracture did not unite. Hence a surgeon in his home town did dynamization by removing both upper and the lower bolts! The preoperative, postoperative films were not available. He was on non-weight bearing ambulation for two years. The X-ray revealed that the proximal end of the nail had sunk below the pyriform fossa and the distal nail tip was about to penetrate the distal end of the femur and enter the knee joint.

Why this occurred? Possibly the initial nail was too long and had created a track in the femur condyle. Then it may have been changed to a

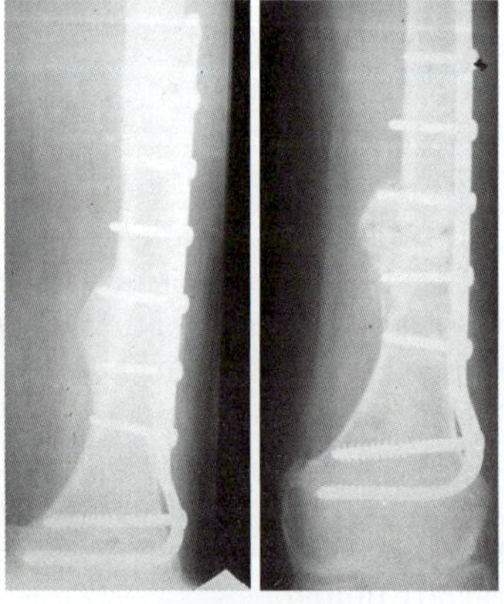

Figure 30.21 Blade plate

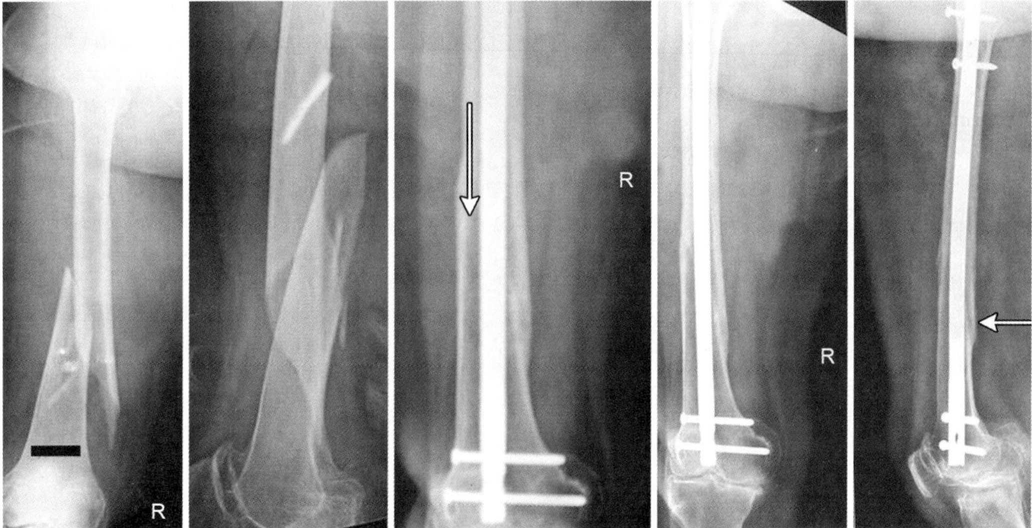

Figure 30.22 DFN by a closed method

nail of lesser length and locking was done, After removal of all screws, the nail slowly migrated in the femur condyle, to come to the subchondral area, because a track was created on day 1 of surgery, being a longer nail then.

He reported for further care to us.

How it was Further Managed when Came for Further Treatment

- The nail had to be exchanged.
- Decortication and bone grafting was necessary.

Steps of the Procedure

- In a lateral position, the area of nail entry was exposed. The nail had sunk below the bone surface. With the help of a 5 mm osteotome and a 15 mm straight gouge, a canal was created at the expected position of the nail end. Shining metal end guided its place. The end of the nail had a flare, which resisted its bringing out. Hence the canal was further made wide and with an extractor, it could be retrieved.
- There must be fibrosis around the fracture site, which held the fracture ends together. A beaded guidewire was inserted and the length of the nail removed measured. Another nail short by 2 cm was selected.
- The fracture site was exposed and area was decorticated as much as possible. Iliac crest grafts were laid around the area. A 12 size drain was inserted and the muscle layer was sutured back. Thus the muscle layer was sutured back, prior to the reaming to be done. *This step is important.*
- Then progressive reaming was done. At this stage, whatever reaming material is generated, it flows through the fracture area and remains in that area, because the muscle layer is sutured back. The local area has bone grafts and reaming material in addition, which thus has a good healing potential. It thus remains localized and does not flow out, because the muscle layer is sutured back.
- Patient was ambulated. At the end of four months, dynamization was carried out, by removing the round hole screw from the proximal end. Gradually weight-bearing was increased and in a few more months, the fracture consolidated well. Please note the nail track seen in the intercondylar area (Figs 30.23 to 30.25).

Case 2

A middle age lady sustained a 4-part fracture in the mid/3 area. The surgeon did a plate fixation and no bone grafts were added. After a few weeks, the plate avulsed from the distal end and the surgeon revised the procedure by changing the 4.5 screws to 6.5 mm screws. One can notice, that the screw tips did not engage the opposite cortex, which may have been the cause of avulsion. Again no bone grafts were added.

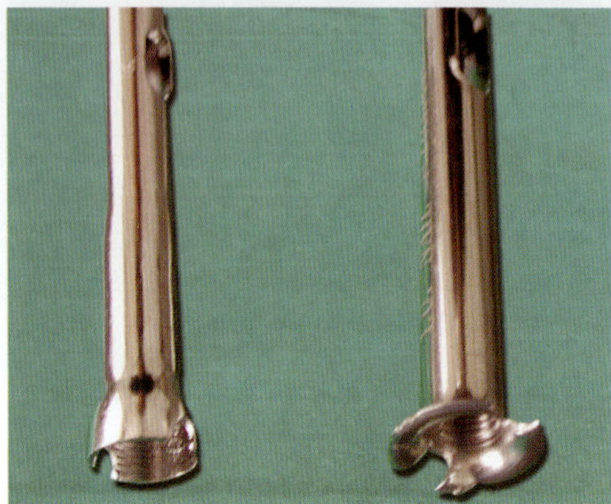

Figure 30.23 Nail-end design

The fracture united in due course and for reasons not known, the surgeon removed the plate (As can be seen, the medullary cavity in the opposite femur is very narrow). Though, the bone had united, stress shielding took its toll and the lady had a refracture in the same area.

Hence, the surgeon did an interlocking nailing. There was one screw at the proximal end through the oval hole in the proximal end and only one screw in the distal end. A broken drill bit is also seen in the distal end, which happens at times. The fracture did not unite and at this time, I came in the picture. Due to repeated procedures, a possibility of latent infection was kept in mind. Options and equipment kept ready:

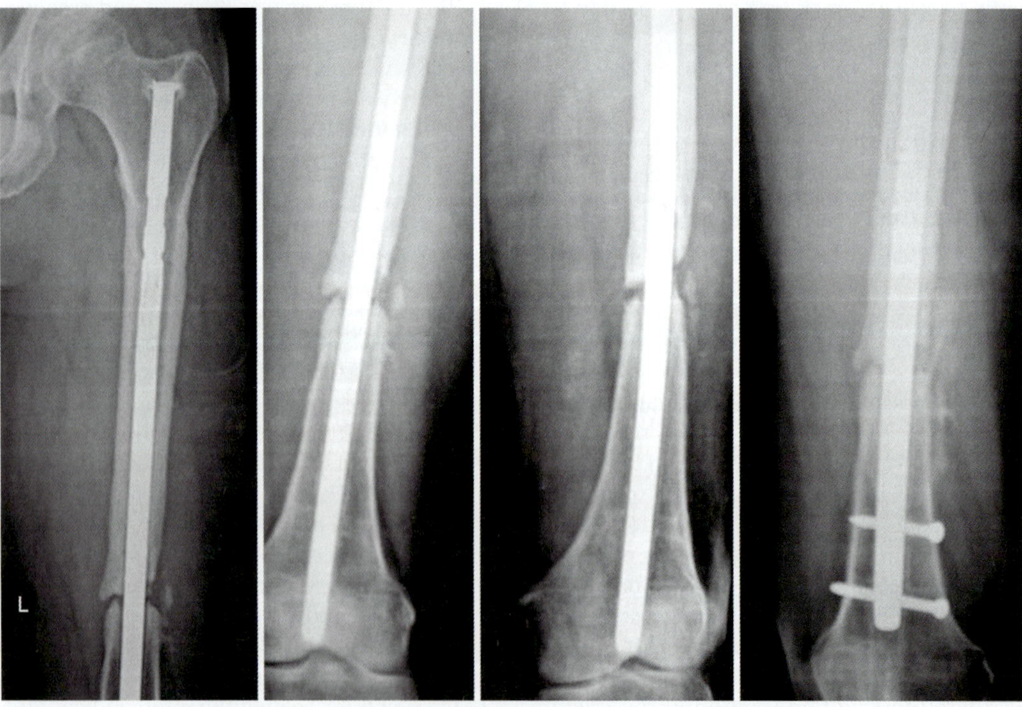

Figure 30.24 Revised interlock nailing and bone grafting

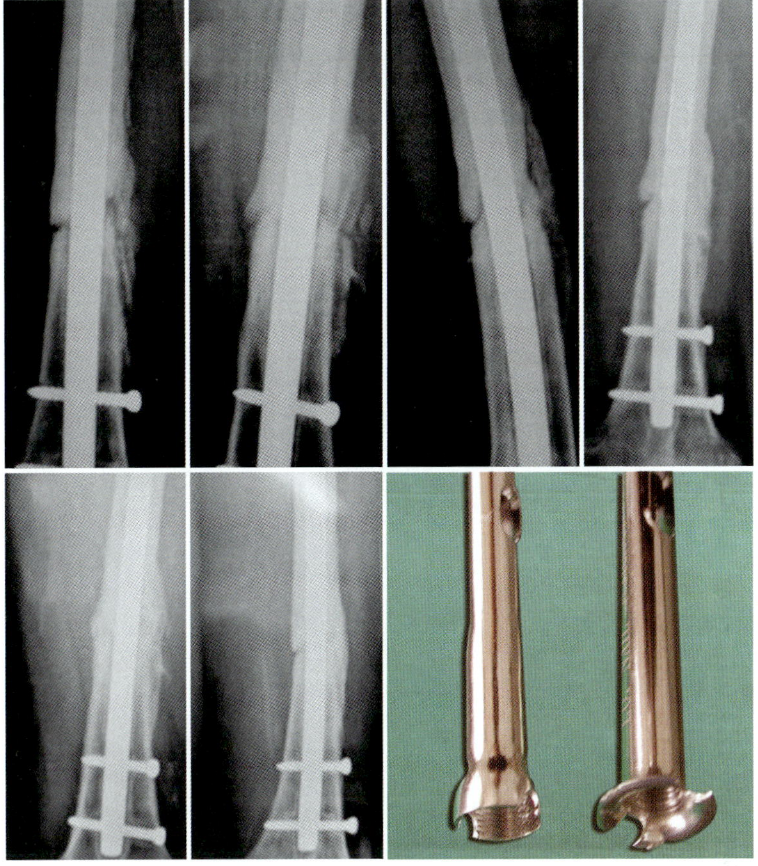

Figure 30.25 Post-dynamization

Options

- Revision nailing
- Retaining the present nail and decortication, bone grafting, derotation of plate and addition of locking bolts
- Should local area is indicated infection, removal of the nail and stabilization with a tubular external fixator.

On exposure of the fracture area, there was no evidence of any infection. Hence, decortication and bone grafting was done. In the distal end, a second locking bolt over a washer was inserted. The limb was well elevated and gradually mobilized. The wound healed kindly and knee range returned. Progressive union occurred (Figs 30.26 to 30.28).

Lesson Learnt

- The plate must adequately span the fracture. Plates of necessary lengths must be available. For both the femur and humerus, 16 mm broad plate is necessary.
- With sharp drill bit and tap, good screw fixation should be achieved.
- The screw lengths should be adequate, must cross the opposite cortex, may be 2 mm more. At least eight cortices must have a good purchase on either side of the fracture. In a plate fixation a complementary bone grafting is necessary.
- After a union after a plate fixation, one needs to wait for adequate duration to remove the plate. After plate removal the patient must

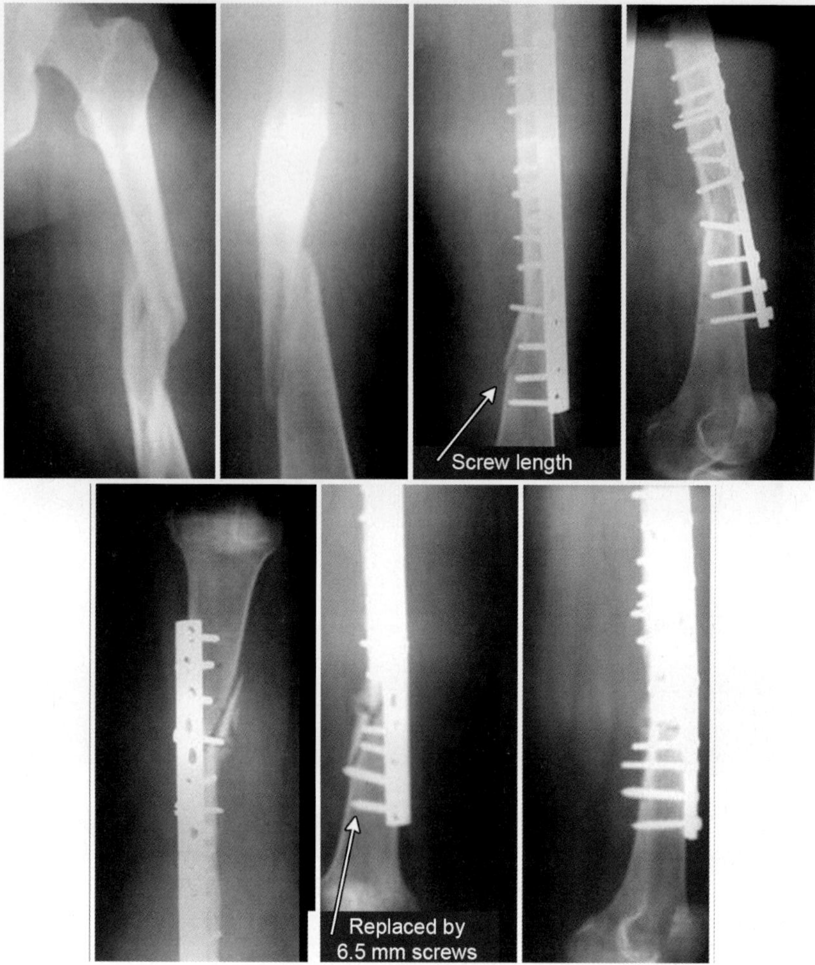

Figure 30.26 Plate to nail

be off the weight for few weeks, as per the radiological appearance.

- In a procedure of interlocking nail fixation, two locking bolts at either ends are necessary. When a secondary procedure of nailing is done (after removal of the plate) addition of bone grafts may have led to a union.
- In such a case of 4-part fracture in mid/3 area of a femur, IM nailing is mechanically far superior. If the medullary cavity appears to be too narrow, one should arrange for a good quality of flexible reamer set, power reamer, etc.

Case 3

A young well-built man, in early twenties, was on a bike and sustained a high speed and a high energy accident. Sustained fracture of right radius and ulna, fracture of lower/3 of right femur and an ipsilateral fracture of tibia. Necessary first aid was given.

In stage I: Radius and ulna nailing and closed interlocking nailing of femur was carried out. After a few days tibial interlocking nailing was done. (May be if DFN was launched and available), then a DFN for femur and

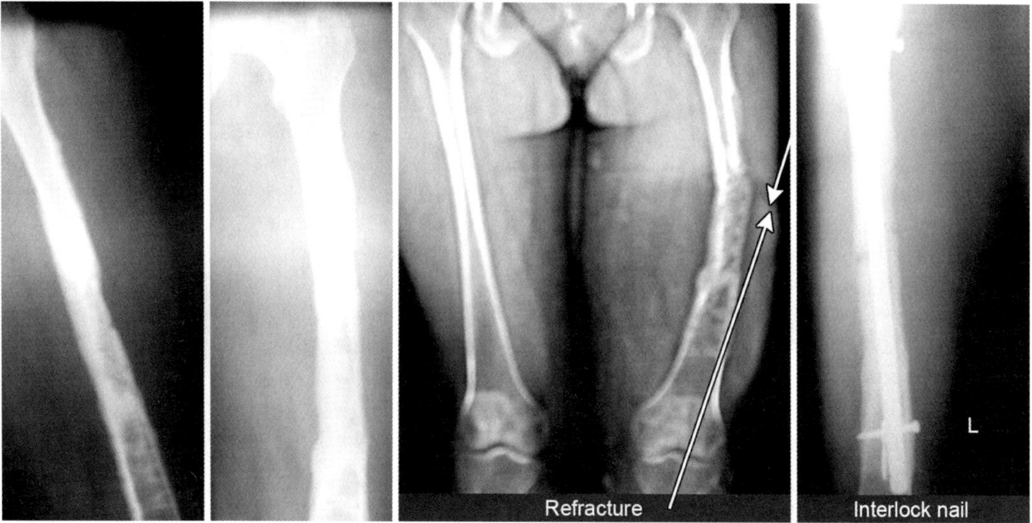

Figure 30.27 Plate to nail

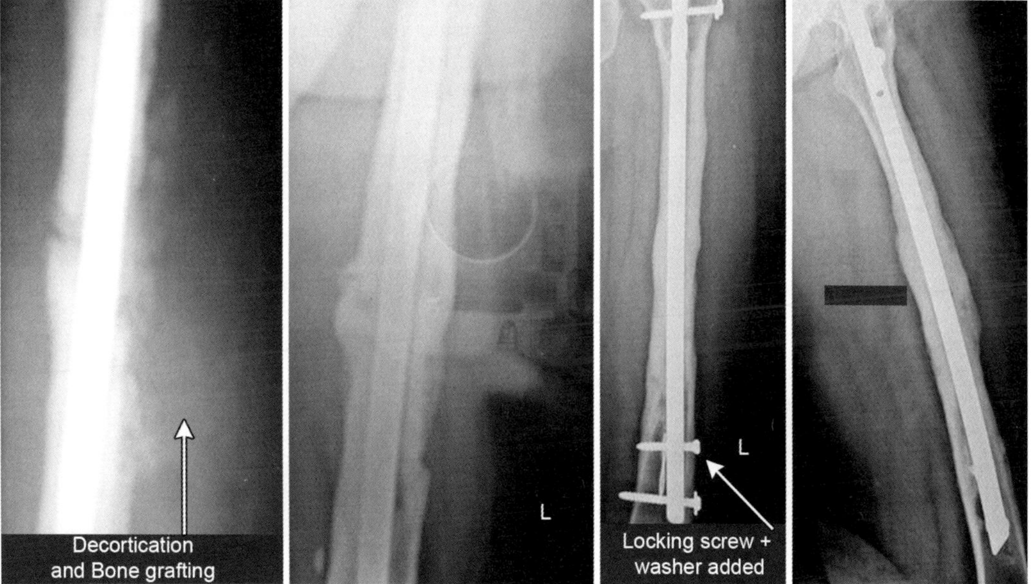

Figure 30.28 Plate to nail

interlocking nail for tibia could have done in one stage).

At the end of four months, the femur showed no signs of union and hence, a derotation plate and bone grafting was carried out.

Still at the end of further 3 months, in the femur, no bridging callus was noted. However, the fracture ends of the femur fracture showed some thickening and an attempt of union. Hence, a revision nailing was planned, as at this stage there was a likelihood of fatigue fracture of the nail. (This decision is important and must be taken timely. If one has to do an exchange nailing/removal of a plate/bone grafting, etc. one needs not open the medullary cavity of the femur. The soft tissue cover and the soft tissue sleeve continuity is well maintained. If one has to do the same procedure, for a broken nail, then one needs to angulate the fracture area to retrieve the distal segment of the broken nail. During this procedure, whatever fibro-osseous union has taken place, one has to disturb it. The former procedure will always lead to an earlier and assured union than the second one).

Hence, procedure carried out as per steps described:

- Fracture exposure
- Plate removal and decortication
- Laying of bone grafts from iliac crest
- Closed suction drain tube laying in and closure of muscle layers
- Exchange nailing. The reaming material did collect at the fracture site, because the wound muscle layer was sutured and the material remained localized around the fracture area. The screw holes came exactly at the same area and hence a 13 mm washer was added on the distal bolts.

Final outcome was satisfactory. All the fractures consolidated well. At the end of five years from the accident, all the implants have been removed in stages.

Looking back, I am unable to find a reason, why the first procedure of closed interlock nailing of femur, did not work, while the next one worked. May be with time, the local bone circulation had improved and the second surgery reaming stimulated union (Figs 30.29 and 30.30).

Case 4

This elderly person had a fracture in the upper/3 femur and a closed interlocking nailing was carried out. During follow up, shortening of the leg and a prominence in the upper thigh

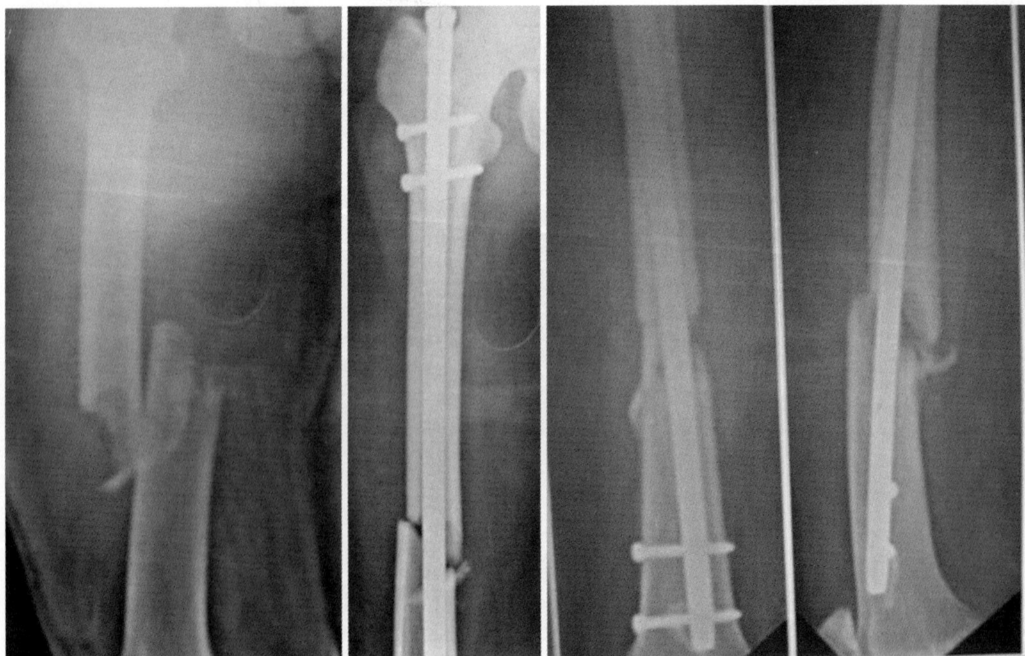

Figure 30.29 Lower/3 femur fracture interlock nailing

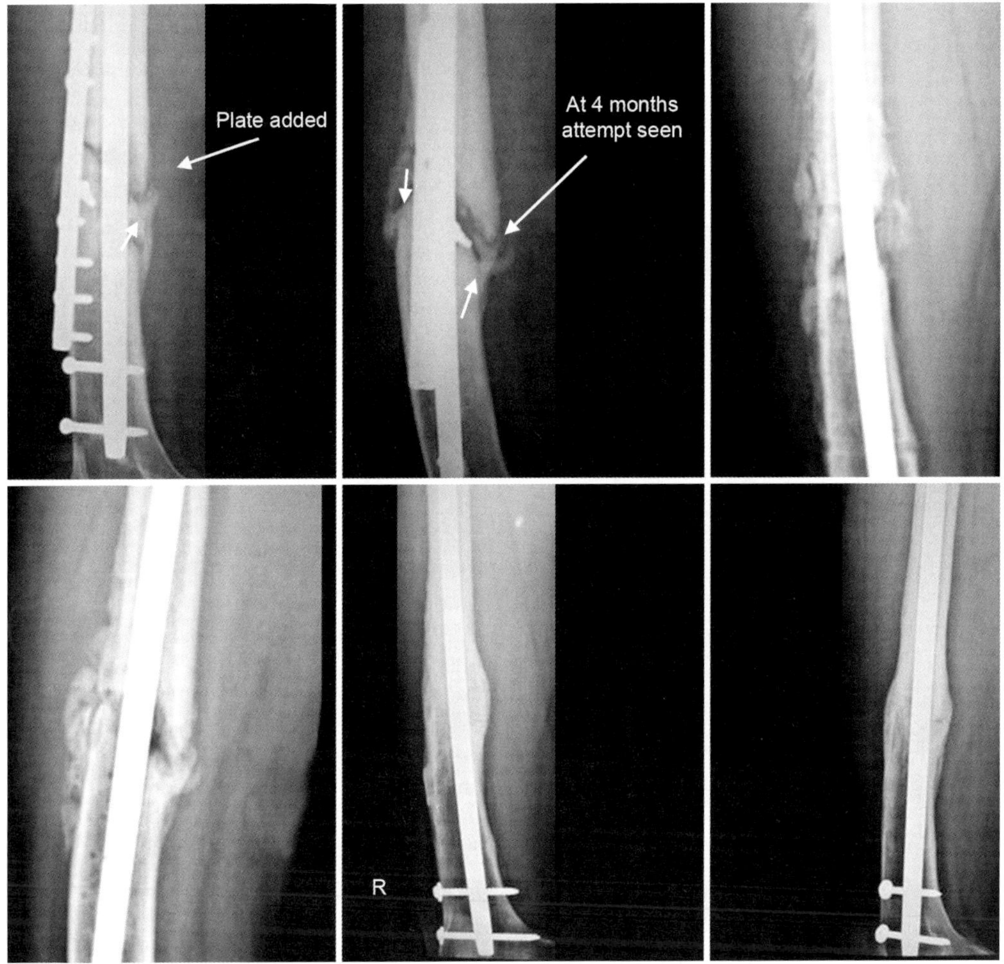

Figure 30.30 Failed derotation plate: Revision nailing succeeded

was observed. He denied any history of fall. Obviously, the nail had to be changed. The X-ray film revealed that the fracture was about 6 cm distal to the second screw hole.

To exchange the bent nail, one needs to straighten the nail first and then remove it. The femur was first straightened and then the nail removed. The nail extractor was attached to the proximal end and the locking bolts were removed. Only the short proximal segment of the nail came out, indicating that the nail had broken. The fracture was exposed and the distal segment of the nail was removed.

Comments

- On the X-ray it is difficult to know, if the nail is broken either complete or incomplete or otherwise.
- As seen, the nail was bent at the fracture site, while it was broken through the second screw hole.
- May be the nail breakage was complete, when the X-ray was taken, but not visible in the X-ray film or it was incomplete and during the manipulation it became complete

- If the nail breakage had not occurred, one could have done exchange of nailing, without opening the fracture site (FIg. 30.31).

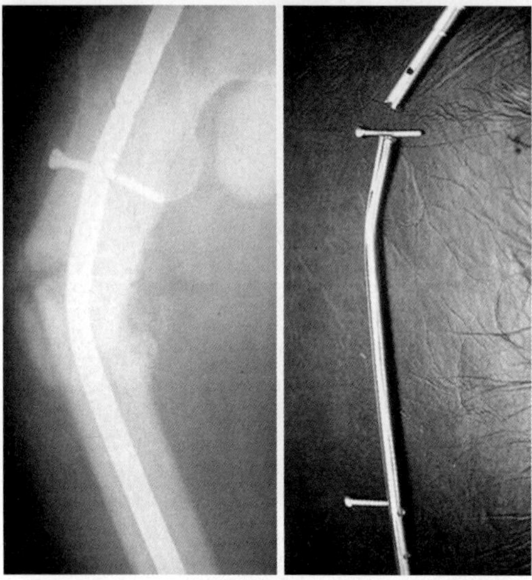

Figure 30.31 Bent and broken nail

Case 5

Twenty years ago, a young man had sustained fracture in lower/3 femur and a K-nail fixation was done. The limb was mobilized and gradually partial weight bearing was permitted. As seen in the X-ray, the nail was rather short and the tip was against the anterior cortex. During follow up X-ray, it was found that the distal end of the nail was broken, possibly, because it was against the anterior cortex of the bone and due to load, it gave way. I was consulted at this stage. This was prior to interlocking nails were available. Hence, it was changed to a blade plate implant with bone grafting and the fracture united well (Fig. 30.32).

Case 6

For a fracture in lower/3 area, an internal fixation with an interlocking nail was done elsewhere. However, the nail length was less than the desired one. Follow up X-ray showed, the fracture was getting angulated, having only one bolt in the distal end of the femur and hence the same surgeon changed the nail to another nail of a correct length, indeed a wise decision.

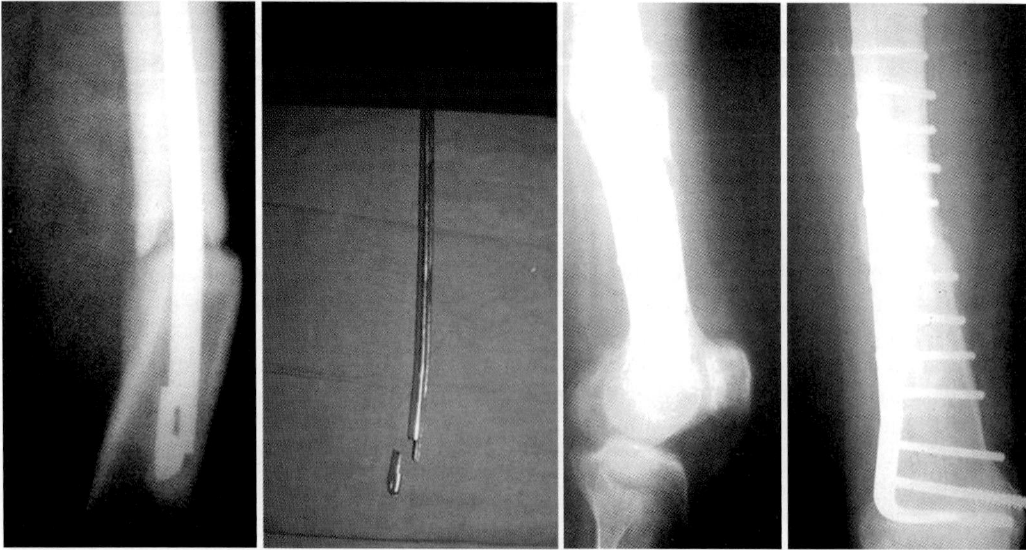

Figure 30.32 Broken nail tip

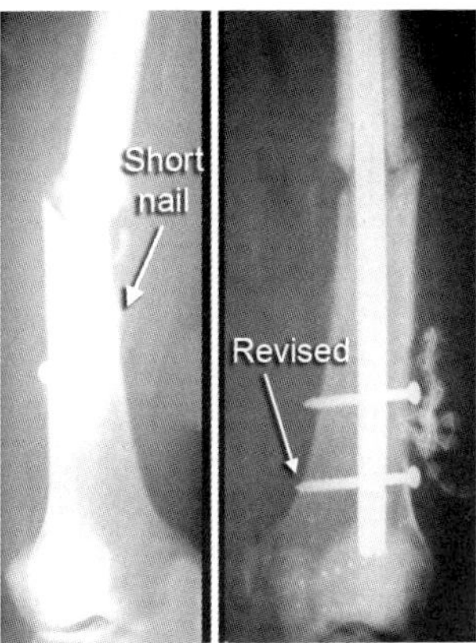

Figure 30.33 Short interlocking nail and sinogram

Unfortunately, there was local infection in the lower wound, after the second procedure and hence a sinogram was done, as seen in the film. I was consulted with X-ray films only for another opinion. The patient was from a distant place and did not report back (Fig. 30.33).

Cases 7 and 8

Both the cases had a fracture in lower/3 of femur. In the first case, a blade plate was used, which was bent and the fracture did not unite. He reported to us. Hence, the removal of the blade plate, bone grafting and interlocking nail was done.

In the second case, the distal fragment was not excessively wide and hence, the stability was maintained, The fracture united after the primary procedure. In a few cases shown previously, the fractures in distal/3 had to be re-operated. Looking at the X-ray films, I feel, the cause may be too wide distal fragment. In spite of adequate reaming, a nail of adequate thickness and the two bolts could not offer good rotational stability and hence the fractures did not unite (Fig. 30.34).

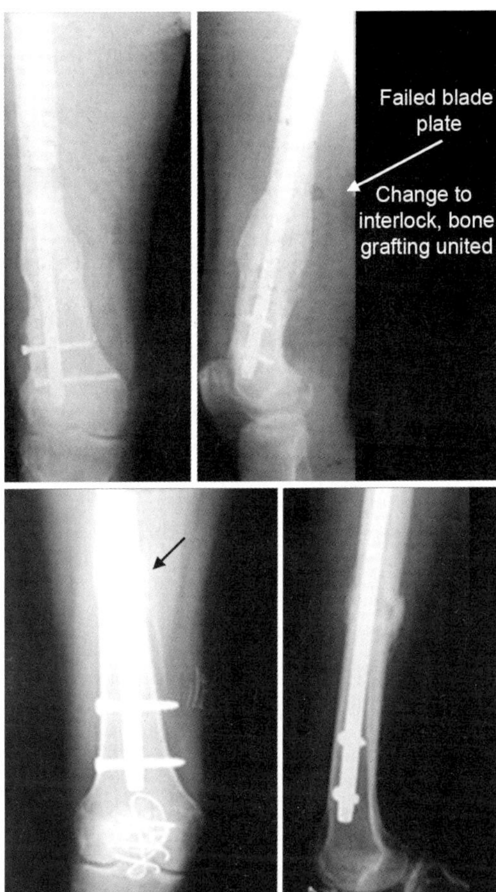

Figure 30.34 Fracture in lower/3 femur

Case 9

Patient had a four-part fracture in the middle/3 area. Previous surgeon did a duel plate fixation and no bone grafting was done. The fracture was slow to unite. When reported for a second opinion to me, bone grafting was recommended. However, he was lost to follow up.

Comments

- Is a duel plate fixation biologically a correct option? Quite a large area of bone surface must have been deprived of blood supply.
- How one would fix another such a fracture? This was prior to interlocking nail era. Even then, I would prefer to carry out a K-nail fixation. If the fracture was not well-opposed, primary bone grafting would

be the preferred option. Complementary derotation plate can be thought of, if there was rotary instability on table. The area for the plate should be such that the blood supply to the lateral fragment should be preserved, as much as possible (Fig. 30.35).

Case 10

In a case of ipsilateral fracture in the basi-trochanteric area and a shaft, K-nail fixation and multiple AM. Pin fixation leads to a good outcome. With advent of DHS and precisely made plates and screws, DHS for the basi-trochanter area and plate fixation for the shaft was carried out.

Later on antegrade femoral nails were available and both the procedures could be carried out by a close method (Fig. 30.36).

Case 11

In a four-part fracture in lower/3 femur, today one has locking plate as an implant. This can be done with MIPO technique. However, if a good reduction is not obtained, one should carry out an open reduction, to align and reduce the fracture well. If the reduction obtained is not acceptable, only because, it is an MIPO technique, fracture would not unite. This is amply demonstrated in fractures in lower tibia chapter. Addition of bone grafts in the medullary cavity and in between the fragments assures a union in expected duration (Fig. 30.37).

Case 12

An old lady had sequential fractures of femora in the pre-interlocking nail era.

On the right side, a K-nail with derotation plate was done, while on the left side, a K-nail was used. Both the fractures united well.

After a few years, she had a fall again and sustained a fracture of the left femur, distal to the previous one, while the K-nail was in situ. The nail was bent. This was treated by a closed method of exchange nailing. The bent nail was

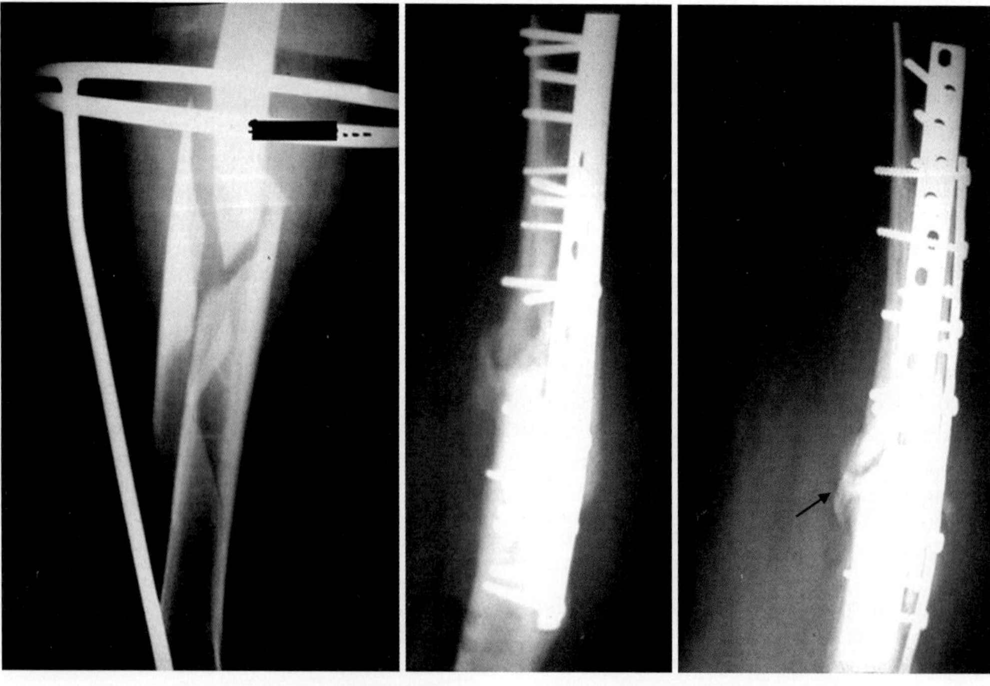

Figure 30.35 Dual plate fixation

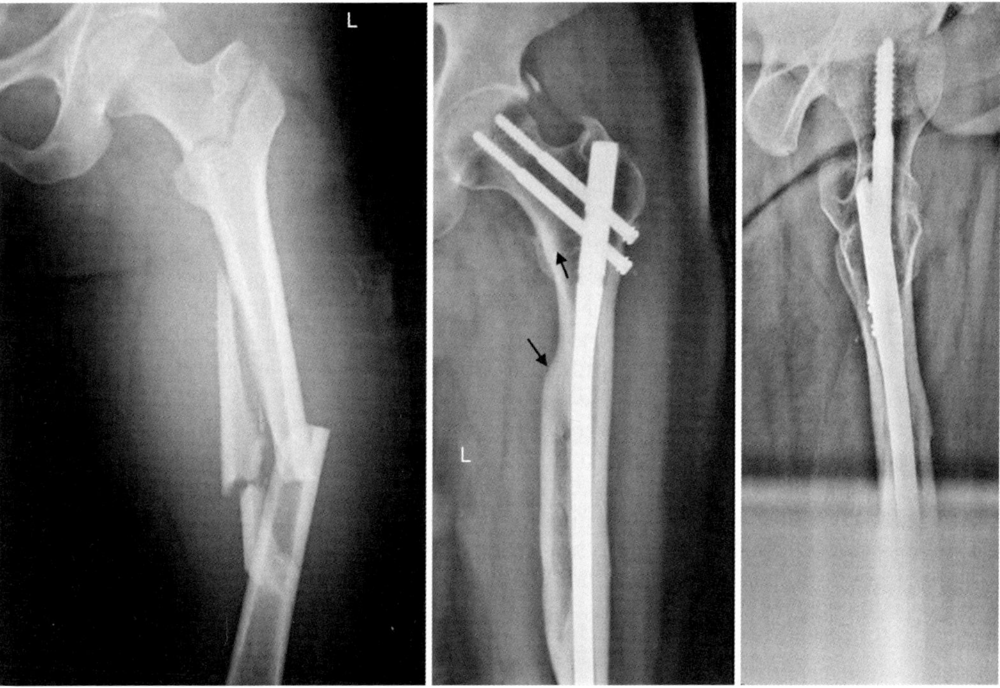

Figure 30.36 AFN for ipsilateral neck and shaft of femur fractures

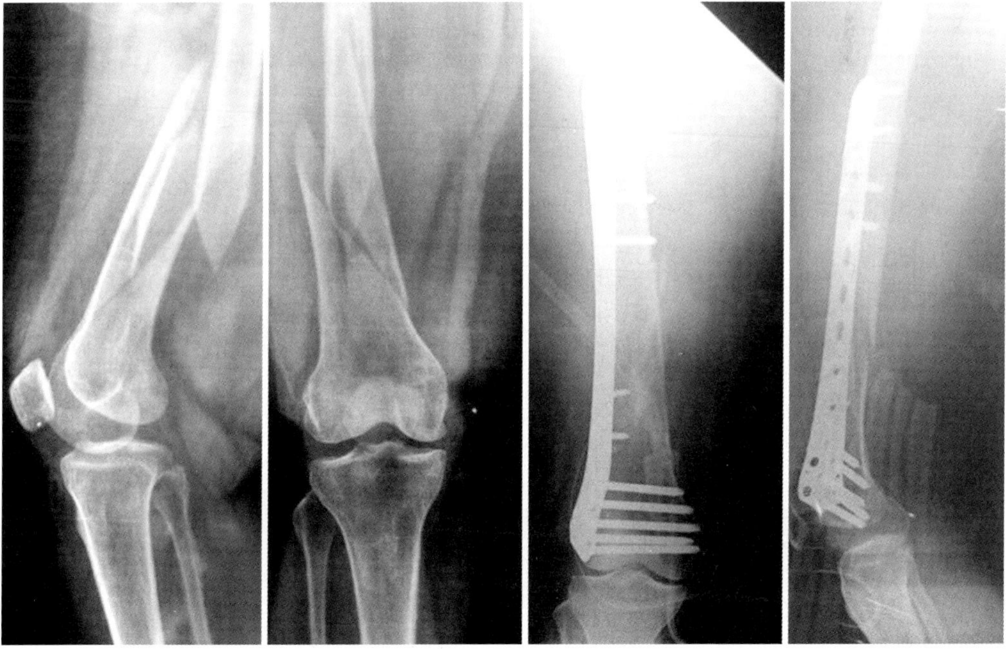

Figure 30.37 Locking plate in 4-part fracture of lower/3 femur

gently straightened and removed. Reaming was done. In due course, the fracture was dynamised and proceeded to union (Fig. 30.38).

Case 13

A patient had a fracture shaft femur at junction of mid and lower/3, 20 years ago. Open K nailing, derotation plate and bone grafting was done. As a routine, AP X-ray of the operated hip and fracture area was taken. The hip X-ray is taken to know, as to how much length of the K-nail is outside the bone. The hip X-ray revealed a fracture at the basi-trochanteric area. The proximal end of the fracture looked to be stabilized by the nail. It was conserved and ambulation was delayed by a month. Both the fractures united in due course.

The preoperative X-ray films of the hip in two angles were studied again, but did not reveal nay fracture.

Message

It is absolutely necessary to take an X-ray of pelvis after an accident, especially with a fracture of femur, to exclude associated fracture of neck of the femur.

After every case of femur nailing, at the end of surgery, it is necessary to take an AP X-ray of the hip area. Since the fracture looked to be crossed by the nail, it was taken to be stable and hence mobilization was delayed, with a satisfactory outcome (Fig. 30.39).

Case 14

A young boy had sustained a 3-part fracture of the upper/3 femur shaft. The X-ray of the hip was included on day 1 X-ray, which did not reveal any associated fracture in the neck of femur. At this time, interlocking nail was available and hence a closed nailing was carried out. After inserting all the four locking bolts, final 'C' arm examination was carried out. The nail design was such that the two proximal bolts were transverse, adjacent to the lesser trochanter. It revealed an undisplaced fracture at the base of the neck. It required to be stabilized. AM pin fixation, passing adjacent to the nail, across the fracture was necessary. However, the pins were not sterile. Hence, we did not close the wound and waited, till the sterile pins were available. Pins were inserted adjacent to the nail. The mobilization of the patient was permitted in bed only. Both the hip and the shaft fractures consolidated in due course (Fig. 30.40).

Case 15

A middle age person sustained a fracture in the upper/3 femur shaft. A closed interlock nailing under 'C' arm control was planned and carried out. (Having experienced, that at times, one

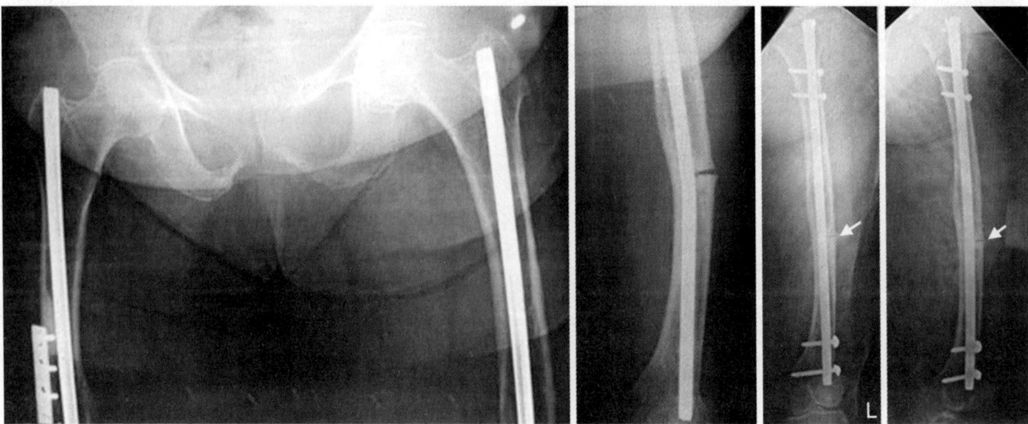

Figure 30.38 Bilateral fracture of femur: refracture

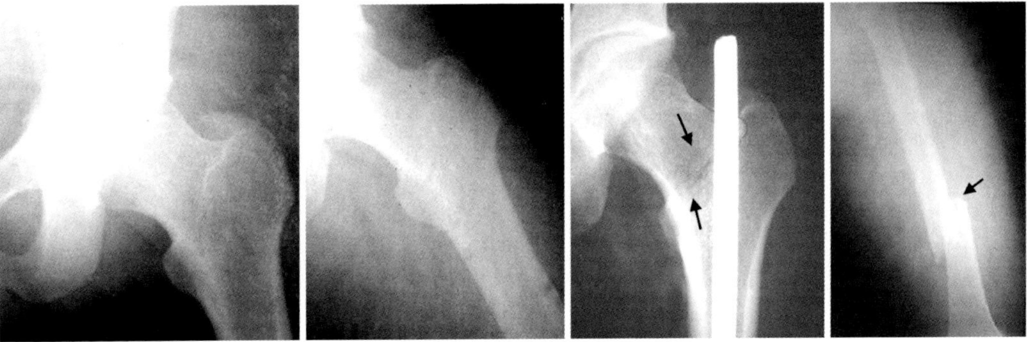

Figure 30.39 Fracture of neck of femur noted after K-nail insertion

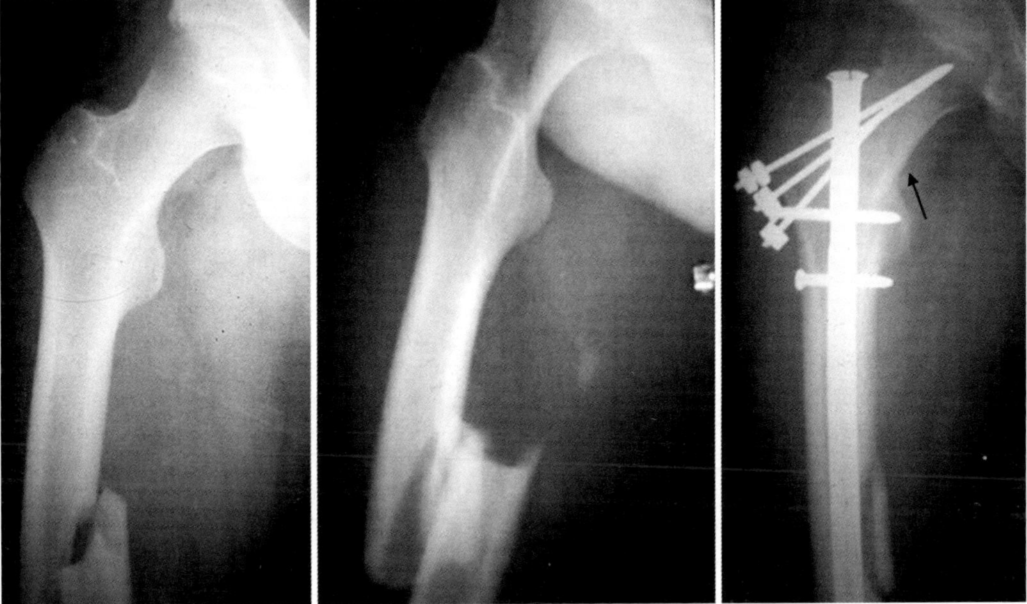

Figure 30.40 Fracture of neck of femur noted after interlock nailing i

observes appearance of a basilar fracture at the end of surgery, I always kept necessary implants and instrumentation for AM pin insertion, in each case).

A few cases after the case no. 14 above, were successfully done. However, in this case, at the end of the procedure of nailing, a fracture line was visible at the base of the neck. The AM pins were already kept ready and were passed across the neck (Fig. 30.41).

Looking back the above two cases:

1. During prograde nailing and making a canal at the pyriform fossa, one has no problem, The track created by a diamond awl should be exactly in alignment with the medullary cavity. If it is initially directed anteriorly, we had some reason to doubt, if the fracture occurred at that stage.
2. In this second case, the nailing system had only one proximal locking oblique screw,

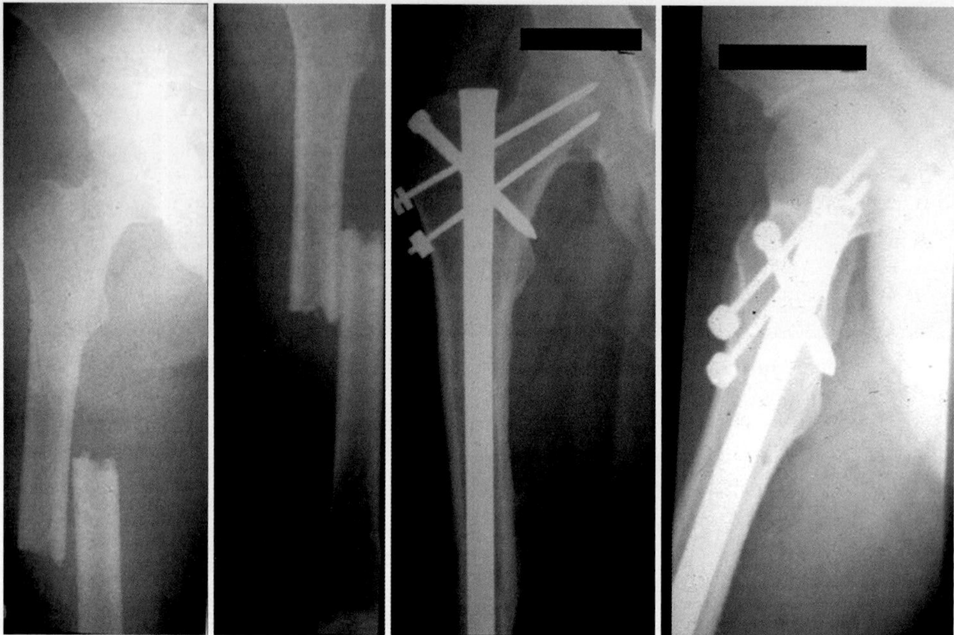

Figure 30.41 Fracture of neck after interlock nailing ii

while in the earlier case, they were transverse two bolts, much distal to the basilar area.

3. A possibility exists that there was an undisplaced invisible fracture, at the time of injury, which became visible, after some impact of canal opening/reaming and may be final setting of the nail.

Message

In each case of interlocking nailing procedure, AM pins and related instrumentation must be ready:

- AM pins of various lengths
- Appropriate 2 mm long drill bit
- Pin cutter to cut the excess length
- 0.8 mm soft bone wire, to take around the nuts, to keep them in place, or else, often, they unwind and get separated from the pins. (The wire was not used in theses cases, which should have been).

A Thought

While removing a shaft screw (partially threaded 4 mm or 6.5 mm screws), often the screw is known to break at the junction of the shaft with the threaded portion. Now the screw threads are so made that, there is a reverse cutting edge, where it joins the shaft. While removing such a screw, at the initial stage, one should slightly tighten it further and then move anticlockwise. If one does this motion, two half turns anticlockwise and one half turn clockwise, the screw keeps on moving and less likely to give way and break.

While carrying out a closed interlocking nail in a femur, the teaching is to keep reaming the shaft, with a moderate speed, using a low speed, high torque reamer. It is a good practice to keep the drill motor running, continuously, while reaming is done, in forward direction. While reamer is to be withdrawn, it should be first kept running in forward direction and while it is rotating, it should be withdrawn.

In a four-part fracture of femur, while the reamer was running in a clockwise direction, it was being withdrawn. (Trying to remove it in opposite direction (anticlockwise) at times unwinds the flexible reamer shaft). It could no more be withdrawn. The proximal end of the reamer head had slightly moved medially (in the comminuted area) and was hitched against medial wall of the proximal fragment. With the reamer running, moving it to and fro, could not negotiate it. With a few attempts, it could be withdrawn, without a need of opening the fracture area. This makes me feel, it is desirable to have cutting edge at the proximal end of the reamer head as well. This will help, to make a track for itself, should it get locked, as happened in this case.

PERIPROSTHETIC FRACTURE

After a procedure of AM replacement, another fall often leads to a periprosthetic fracture. The patient has grown more old, having pulled through a major surgery. Traction with a Thomas' splint application, usually leads to fracture union. However, complications of prolonged rest in bed, like pressure sores, DVT, chest congestion etc. need to be taken care of. To reduce the duration of the splint, one may use a long 12 mm span plate in such a case. Bicortical screws are passed distal to the stem tip. On the proximal end, one needs to pass oblique screws in the trochanter area, to have some purchase. To make this possible, one has to use a DCP, which has oval holes, permitting insertion of screws at an angle. If it is possible to pass a circlage, with minimal soft tissue erasing, it may be added (Fig. 30.42).

Fracture distal to the prosthesis or a short PFN can be stabilized better, if some bone segment is available for screw fixation in the proximal fragment. Today, with availability of locking plate, short screws can be used, in bone, over the stem. In a given case, there was a fracture 4 cm distal to the tip of the stem. A locking plate was applied. Today, one has an additional device, a transverse malleable plate, which can be mounted on the proximal end of a locking plate. On sides, it has few screw holes, which are directed in an oblique direction, so they pass along the side of the stem in the shaft cortices, adding to the stability of the plate. Having few such short screws, enhances the stability and indeed is a boon for such a case (Fig. 30.43).

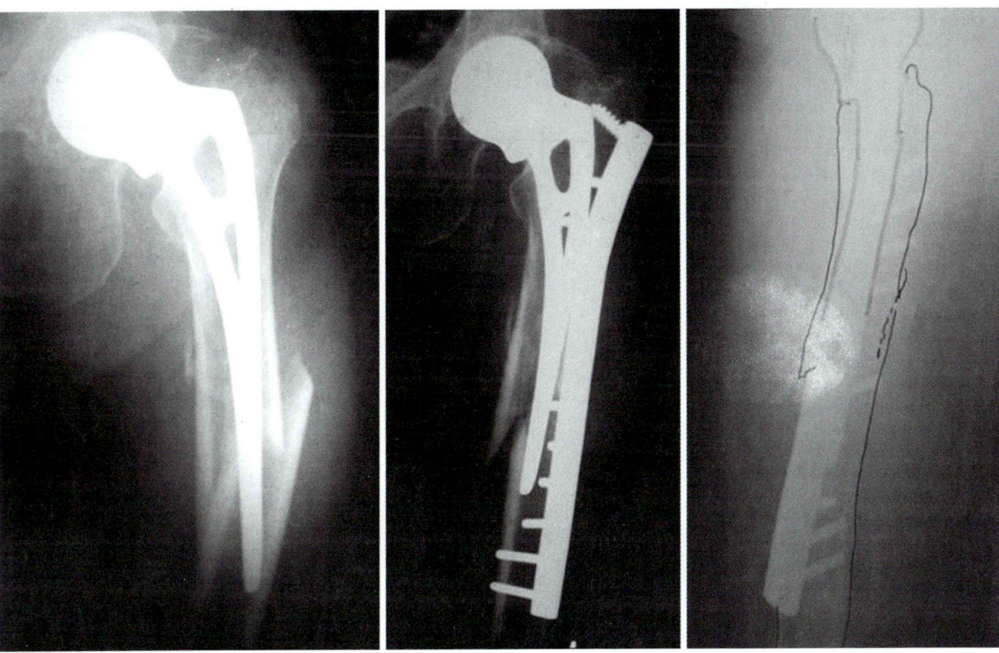

Figure 30.42 Periprosthetic fracture

Fracture just distal to a short PFN occurred in an old person. Today availability of locking plate made the procedure relatively easy and assured. Removal of the PFN makes the plate fixation easy and more stable (Fig. 30.44).

A middle age person had a fracture of femur, which was treated with internal fixation. There was infection and the knee became stiff and he was used to that way of life. Unfortunately, following a fall, 17 years ago,

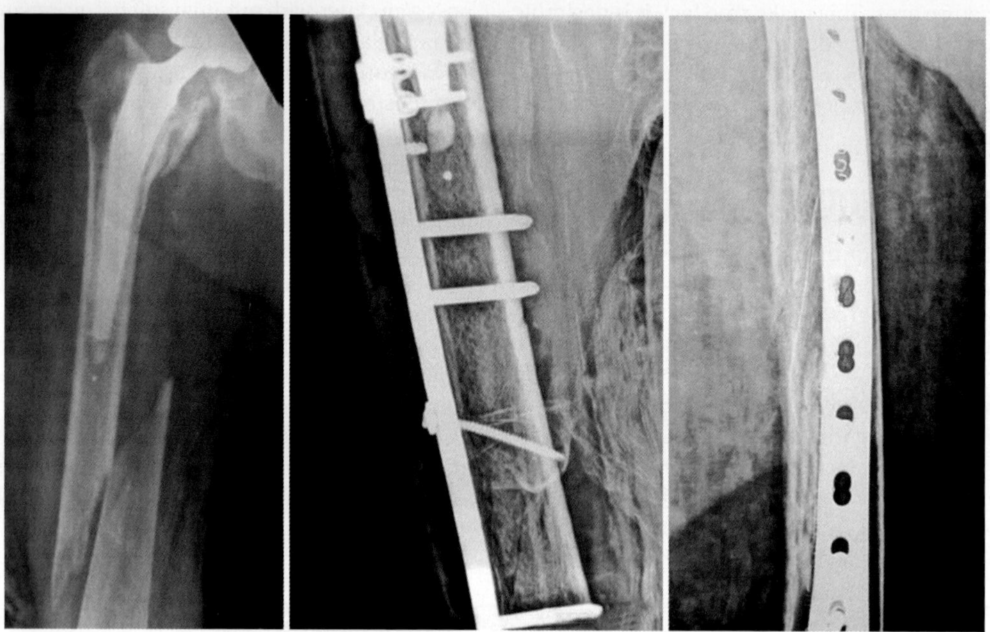

Figure 30.43 Periprosthetic locking plate I

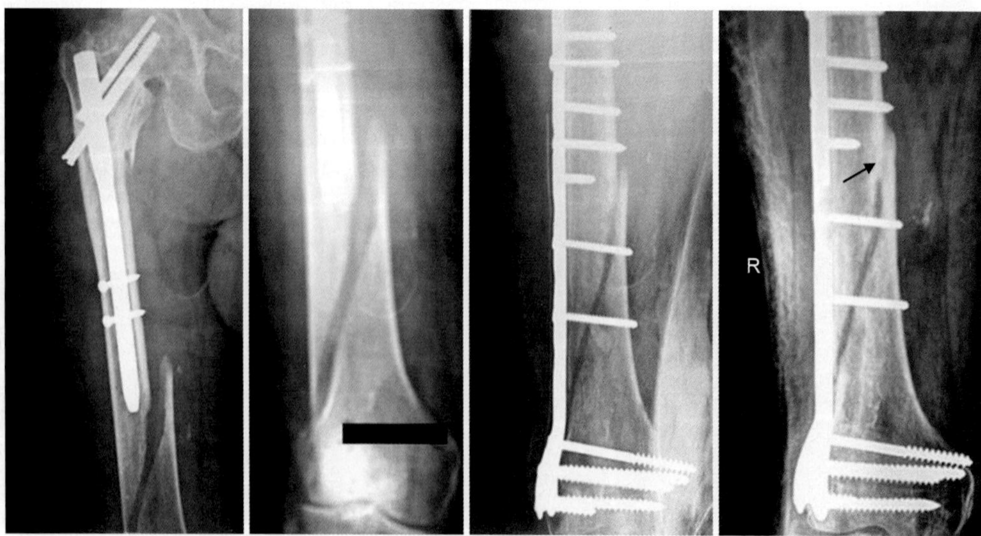

Figure 30.44 Periprosthetic locking plate II

he had a supracondylar fracture. There was a sinus around the knee and lingering infection, as seen in the sinogram. In view of the deep infection, the surgeon, perhaps opted for a non-operative method and a long leg cast was applied. However, the fracture failed to unite and he is managing with a knee brace (Fig. 30.45).

Few Useful Instruments for Femur Interlocking Nail

For a free hand locking of the distal hole in either a femur or a tibia, a 2 mm K-wire is usually used. A wonderful device is available for this purpose. This device is strong and rigid, with a pointed end, which should be protected with a rubber tube cap, when not in use. It has a butt end with a radiolucent handle, which takes blow of a hammer. It is very useful instead of a K-wire. The butt end being translucent, one can easily confirm the location of the tip with respect to the hole in the nail. I am sure, anyone who uses this device, will be pleased to use it forever (Fig. 30.46).

- While using an AFN, the available drill bits and the depth gauge are very long, as they are to be used over long sleeves. For the

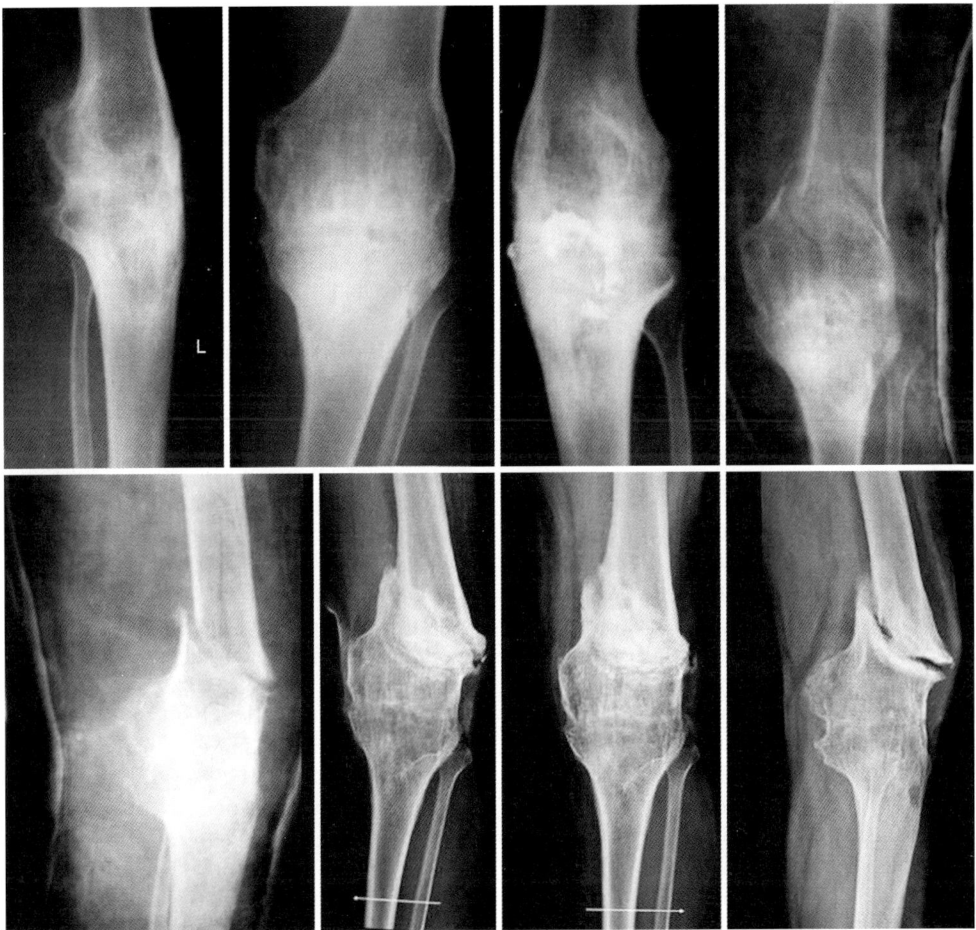

Figure 30.45 Post-knee stiffness fracture of femur

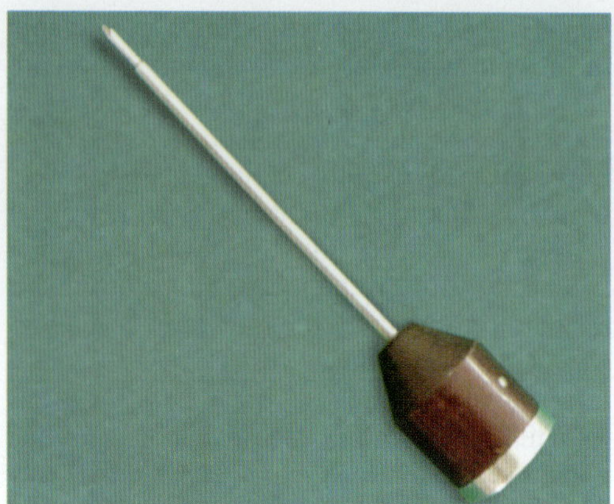

Figure 30.46 Distal aiming device

distal locking, one needs a short drill bit of Jacob or quick coupling type, a standard depth gauge, a screw driver of standard length is required and should be available in the set.

- Often, for a procedure, loaner instruments and implants are provided by the manufacturer. The commonly used screws are needed to be replaced. This is more important for the hip DH screws, which need to be of exact length and the inventory MUST be checked by a knowledgeable person, prior to sterilization.

Removal of Femur Interlocking Nail: Few Steps

Express consent must be obtained, to make it clear that the nail may not come out and one may have to carry out a vertical osteotomy of femur to remove it and then weight-bearing will have to be delayed. At times, even after carrying out a vertical osteotomy, the nail extraction may fail. An open discussion prior to the surgery with the patient and the family is necessary.

An X-ray film taken even a day prior to the procedure, may not indicate, if the interlocking nail is broken or otherwise. While the nail is being removed, if the nail is broken, either partially or completely, only proximal segment would come out, and the other part remains in the medullary cavity. Removal of the remaining part could be quite difficult and demanding too.

Preoperative Planning

X-ray examination in three views of the entire femur is necessary. The area of the distal hole in the proximal end should be carefully examined, since this is the common site of nail breakage. Even if the X-ray film may not indicate so, one should keep the possibility and an informed consent obtained prior to the surgery.

- The proximal end of the nail is exposed and the threaded part of the nail is cleared of the fibrous tissue in growth and the extraction bolt is attached to it and tightened.
- The proximal bolt/bolts are exposed and removed, followed by removal of the distal bolts. The extraction rod is attached to the bolt and with backward blows of the ram, the nail is removed. It is necessary to thread the extraction bolt in the nail first and then remove the locking bolts. (If the bolts are removed first and then one tries to thread the extraction bolt, the nail may rotate in the medullary cavity. If at the time of insertion of the nail, if a longer nail was first inserted and then exchanged to a shorter one, a track is already created in the femur condyle and while attaching the extraction bolt, the nail may slide distally).
- Whenever, an interlocking nail is to be removed, one should always assume that nail is broken somewhere and one will have to remove the distal segment as well. Even if X-ray film shows no evidence of any mechanical failure of the nail, often during extraction, only a part of the nail comes out! Hence, every instrument needs to be kept ready.
- Preferably, one should know from earlier record, as to the make and size of the nail, so its corresponding extractor can be kept ready. It is also necessary to keep extractors for other brands of nails, as a precaution.
- Some design of an interlocking nails, have large bolts, which need wider hex drivers. The common 3.5 mm wide hex driver used for 4.9 mm bolt is smaller for such a screw head.

- If during extraction, one finds that the nail is broken and only a segment of the nail comes out:
  - There a chance that the distal segment of the nail has not moved at all. Quickly, one should insert the distal aiming device or a 2 mm K-wire through the distal holes each, so the nail is locked again and will not rotate, while a threaded extractor is inserted in the broken distal segment.
  - Take a broken nail extractor, with conical threaded end and see which one of the two fits in the distal end of the removed segment of the nail.
  - Insert this extractor in the medullary canal and gently progressively tighten the nail. At this time, since the 2 mm K-wires are in the distal locking holes, anchoring the nail, the nail will not rotate in the medullary canal and the extractor can be well tightened. The nail in all probabilities will come out (Fig. 30.47).

Broken Femur Nail

- There is a hook extractor also available. The long rigid shaft with a hook at the other end is inserted through the nail. However, as it reaches the distal end, one may have to remove the temporary inserted K-wires in the distal holes, to allow the hook to travel further. The hook has to exit from the distal end of the nail. It is then rotated and try to take a grip on the nail wall. An extraction rod is attached to the butt end and nail extracted. During these steps, the tension on the bar is maintained, or else, it slips from the engaed area, at the distal tip of the nail. The ram is tapped backwards and the nail segment is extracted. Common problem is that the distal segment of the nail may be tightly gripped by the bone and the hook may straighten out. The material from which the hook is made, needs to be quite hard and is not easily available.
- *An observation*: Usually in the distal locking holes of a nail, bone growth occurs, which anchors the nail to the bone. This is especially seen, in an empty hole, rather than in hole occupied by a locking bolt (Fig. 30.48).

Pushing the nail proximally from the distal end:

- Having done a procedure of DFN nail, one is acquainted with exposure of the distal end of femur. The area is exposed and a canal is made to enter the distal femur. Through it a nail pusher is introduced.
- The narrow shaft of the extractor should enter the nail cavity at the distal end and the distal knob abuts against the nail. The pusher is gently hammered to push the nail proximally. In some cases, especially when there is excess anterior bowing of bone, the distal end of the nail may lie against the anterior endosteum. In such a case, this extractor may not reach to the distal nail

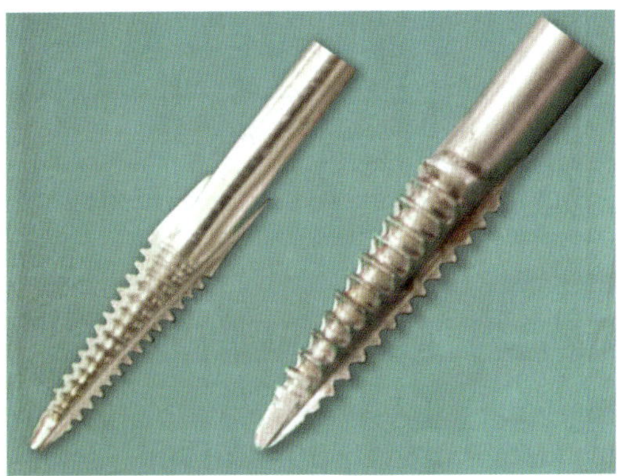

Figure 30.47 Broken nail extractor

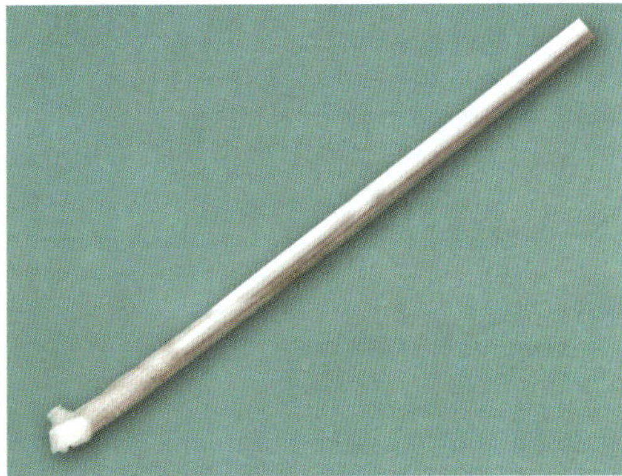

Figure 30.48 Hook extractor. My preference is for the conical extractor to the hook extractor

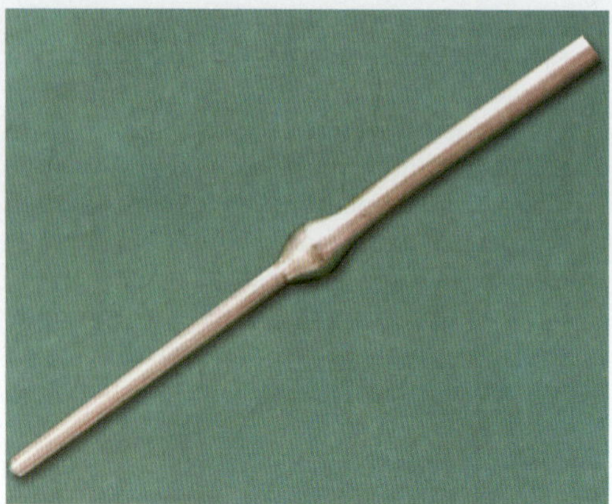

Figure 30.49 Broken nail pusher

tip. Pre-operative study of a good lateral view of distal femur X-ray can indicate this possibility (Fig. 30.49).

- In general, if the initial reaming is done 1.5 mm more than the diameter of the nail used, the nail should come out well. So also, if during introduction of the nail, if one had to tap the nail a little more, it means, the nail was closely fitting inside the medullary cavity or the patient being young, the endosteal bone growth was too much. Bone growth can be in and around the nail and may be it has grown in the screw hole also. This is especially true, if one of the holes was left unused, wherein the bone grows in it.

Case Study

This young man had ipsilateral fracture of neck and shaft of femur. Approx 15 years ago, *another surgeon* had carried out interlocking nail and then patient reported to me for further treatment. X-ray examination from hip to knee was carried out.

Unfortunately all the previous analogue X-ray films were not available.

Findings

- The fracture of neck of femur was missed and there was shortening.
- Both the bolts in the distal end of femur were not in the holes of the nail.

What was Done?

- The distal screws were revised and upper tibial skeletal traction was applied, to bring down the trochanter, which had migrated proximally because of untreated fracture of neck of femur. This is possible, only when distal locking bolts are correctly inserted, so the traction force can be transferred to the entire shaft of femur.
- The neck was stabilized by miss a nail technique, with 6.5 mm screws and AM pin.
- In due course, the femur was dynamised and both the fractures united well. 4-year follow up of X-ray reveals the nail continuity.

Further, after 6 years thereafter, he developed pain in the hip, due to OA changes. X-ray taken at this time revealed a break in the nail at the level of distal of the proximal two holes.

May be the mechanical failure of the nail had occurred some time, but was not visible in earlier X-ray film. Later on, as he continued to walk, as the fractures had united, the break in continuity was visible. The proximal nail end may have been caught in some muscle fibers and due to the muscle movements, it displaced proximally.

Note: X-ray Appearance

The length of proximal part of the interlocking nail above the trochanter looks to be more. The tip has been irritating the ilium and caused erosion there.

He was advised to get all the implants removed, so the bone and soft tissue reconditioning would occur. This would help the possible next surgery of THR, which he is very likely to need for the OA changes. The advice is not yet followed by him (Fig. 30.50).

SPECIAL SITUATIONS IN REMOVAL OF FEMUR NAIL AND/OR A PLATE

Removal of Interlock Femur or Tibia Nail in a Patient in 20s and 30s

The nail is a load sharing device. After removal of a K-nail, one can gradually resume physical

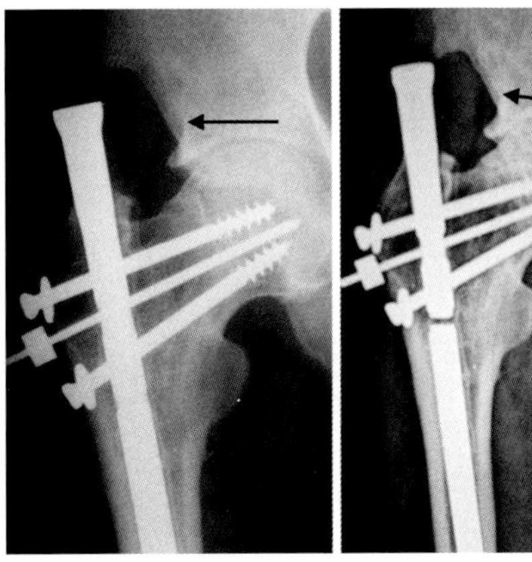

Figure 30.50 Broken femur nail

activities and if the remodeling has occurred well, no refracture is observed.

However, after removal of the nail and all the screws, cases have been reported to have developed a fracture through the screw hole, which is a possibility. This can occur, if contact sports have started prior to consolidation of the screw tracks or if there was another major injury. It is recommended that, first all the locking bolts only are removed and the patient continues to walk with a stick. No contact sports are permitted. After about six months, when one expects that the screw tracks have healed well, the nail is removed. I feel, this is a safe staged option and of less magnitude than facing a refracture.

Removal of a Kuntscher or an Interlocking Nail and the Complementary Derotation Plate

I have come across a case of an elderly lady with diabetes. A colleague had carried out a K-nail fixation with a 16 mm derotation plate. (In fact a 12 mm wide derotation plate is recommended and is adequate to serve its purpose).

The nail and the plate were removed in one stage and was given a walker to gradually load the leg. Still, unfortunately, she had perhaps a little jerk and a refracture occurred. (One cannot say for sure if the fracture occurred first and then she had a fall or vice versa).

Interlocking nailing was done, which was available by then, with a closed method. However, the fracture went in a delayed union.

Thought

May be it is worth considering a two stage removal of the implant assembly:

- *Stage 1*: Remove the plate only and permit partial weight bearing.
- *Stage 2*: May be after few months to a year, as per restoration of the stress shielding of the cortex, the removal of the nail be considered.

A Thought on Removal of a Plate on Femur Shaft from a Middle 2/3 of Shaft

Prior to advent of interlocking nailing, plate fixation was in vogue. A person, who has undergone a plate fixation, about 25 years ago, would be of 50 years of age now. If the procedure of removal of plate is planned, how one should proceed?

- During personal discussion with those who have wide experience in the field suggested, one should remove the plate and may insert an IM nail as a protection device, for a year or so, till stress shielding recovers.
- I have no experience to carry out this logical procedure. However, it is observed that bone trabeculi form along the screws in the medullary canal. They form an obstacle in insertion of a nail. I do not know, if one will be able to pass a guidewire through them or if one can attempt to pass a flexible reamer with a fixed taper head reamer, without a guidewire, to make a canal, in such a situation.

CHAPTER

31

Ipsilateral Femur and Tibia Fractures

In a RTA, one comes across ipsilateral fracture of femur and tibia. Let us assume, both are closed fractures and patient is unconscious with head injury. The head injury may not need surgery and on arrival needs only observation.

To maintain a splint, etc. is rather difficult in an uncooperative and restless patient. Often the patient is aggressive and abusive. Usually an air mattress is given, to prevent pressure sores. Often, due to his condition, a skin traction, keeping the leg over a pillow is given. It is observed, if one tries to keep the leg on a Bohler frame, sores develop near the adductor area.

At the end of say 8 to 10 days, the condition may be the same and then one plans to carry out internal fixation for both femur and the tibia. Due to the spasticity and overriding of fragments, a closed femur nailing is difficult and one has to do an open reduction. Hence, I observed, following tips useful:

ON ARRIVAL

- A below knee padded POP slab + skin traction for fracture of femur. One should discuss the situation with the anesthesiologist and the physician, and
- At the earliest, carry out femur nailing. At this stage, there is more chance for a successful closed femur nailing. If the general condition and time taken permits, tibia also may be fixed at the same time.
- If the femur fracture is in the mid/3 area many surgeons choose to use a DFN for femur and interlock nail for the tibia. This is because, the exposure for the nail entry for both the femur DFN and the tibia is anterior on the knee.
- If the neurological condition indicates that the patient may settle in, say, a week or so and is not much aggressive and manageable, an upper tibial skeletal traction maintains the femur length well, to help a successful closed femur nailing. This pin insertion is possible under LA. If for some reason, the patient has to be given GA, then at the same time, the tibia is reduced, especially in a transverse fracture, which maintains the muscles length well. At the same time, associated soft tissue injuries/wounds can be better managed under anesthesia.
- When a definitive surgery of femur nailing is planned. the Steinmann pin is cleaned and is taken in the sterile field, but again covered with a sterile sheet. This is helpful to give traction to the distal fragment of femur. It

is removed after a successful femur nailing. If the track is healthy, one can proceed with tibia IM nailing at the same time. In exceptional situation, if one is not so happy with the pin track, tibia plate fixation can be considered.

Once both the segments, the femur and the tibia are stabilized, patient nursing and care becomes much easy. However, above decision needs to be taken in conjunction with the intensivist and the anesthesiologist. Often an anesthesiologist finds it easy to manage such a patient on day 2 or 3, rather than on day 7 or 8, when a possibility of a closed nailing is less.

CHAPTER

32

Fracture of Patella

Tension band wiring for management of fracture of olecranon and patella is one of the important inventions in fracture management. The engineering principle of a Derrick Crane is very well applied. The tension band is at right angle to the distracting forces and hence the distracting forces are converted into compressive forces. Early mobilization and restoration of function is possible. The plaster cast application is no more required and there is patient satisfaction.

However, if good reduction, axial alignment, stabilization with K-wires and appropriate load application using correct mechanical principles, is not carried out, the outcome is less than satisfactory. Besides, if unfortunately infection occurs, the knee stiffness is difficult to overcome. This is especially true, in a case with diabetes.

INCISION AND EXPOSURE

Earlier a *transverse* incision was commonly used, when patellectomy was a commonly done procedure. One could easily reach the medial and lateral ends of the retinaculi, which need good approximation. The fracture hematoma usually creates some tissue plane, which makes the dissection and raising thick skin flaps easy. During wound closure, exact subcutaneous opposition of tissues helps to reduce tension on the skin, during mobilization. The incision being in skin fold, the healing is satisfactory and often the scar inconspicuous.

Now, with advent of tension band wiring, which needs more cephalo-caudal exposure, a vertical incision is preferred. This also facilitates insertion of the K-wires from the superior pole of the patella. To gain access to the extreme medial and lateral part of the retinaculi, often the length of the incision needs to be more. The incision being at right angle to the skin folds, often keloid formation is noted.

TIMING OF SURGERY

If fracture of patella is the only injury in a case and the patient is fit to undergo surgery, one can operate within six to twelve hours of the injury. However, if for some reasons, such as uncontrolled diabetes or associated injuries, delay is necessary, it is preferable to aspirate the hematoma and apply a Robert Jone pressure bandage. This makes the patient comfortable. A posterior plaster slab or even a knee brace is adequate. Elevation of the limb helps to keep the reactionary swelling to a minimum.

ANESTHESIA

Regional anesthesia, like a spinal anesthesia, is adequate. Additional epidural anesthesia with a catheter and continuous monitoring or with a pump, offers good pain relief and one can start early mobilization or addition of a CPM which helps to restore good range of motion.

INSTRUMENTATION

Following instruments are necessary and make the procedure easy:

- Curved wire passer
- Cobbler awl with an eye
- Front and a side wire cutter/narrow nose pliers to handle the wire/K-wire bender, which makes an acute bend in the K-wire
- Tractor bow: either a Kirschner wire tractor or a rocket design
- Flat Bohler frame, with various heights, as per patient height. This is an important gadget to have necessary and stable elevation of the knee and the leg.
- A wooden quadriceps board, which offers gravity assisted knee bending and at the same time, permits knee extension exercises against gravity. Both the above two gadgets are economical, long lasting and offer a good return of range of motion.
- A continuous passive motion unit. Out of the above three devices, which one to use, is the surgeon's choice (Figs 32.1 to 32.7).

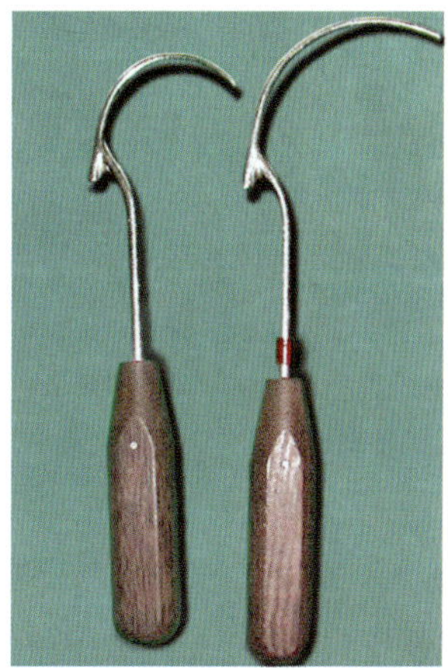

Figure 32.1 Curved wire passer

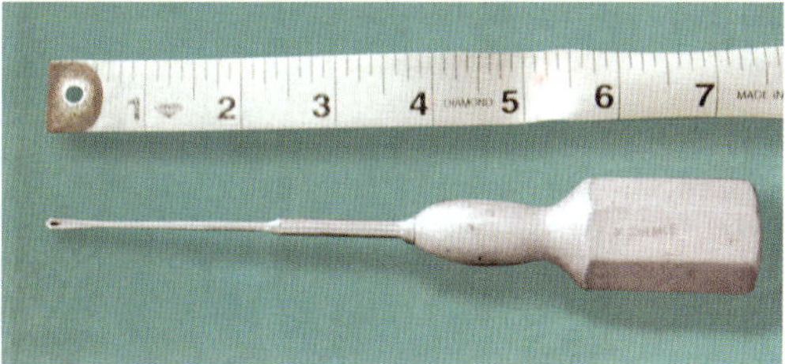

Figure 32.2 Cobbler awl

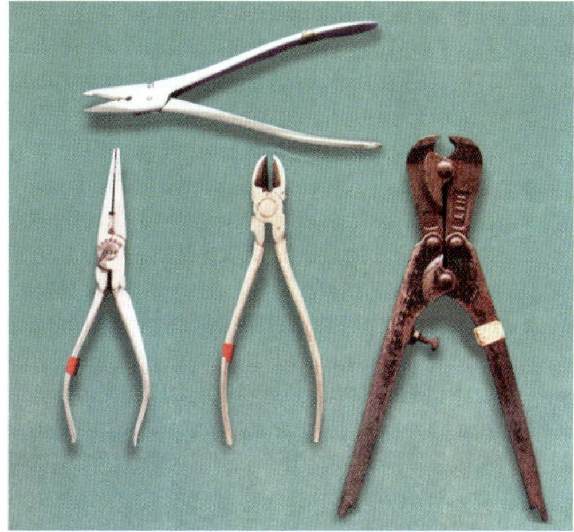

Figure 32.3 Cutting and bending tools

IMPLANTS

- 1.8 and 1.6 mm double ended 150 mm K-wires. Additional 1.4 mm K-wires in a case of multiple small fragments.
- 1 mm cold drawn soft wire, for the figure of eight circlage. In a fresh fracture, where the knee was mobile prior to the injury, the 1 mm circlage wire is adequate. It may be tempting to use a 1.2 mm wire. However, it offers more resistance to bending and sliding, when loaded and thus, may not sit close to the bone surface. If it does not lie close to all edges of the patella, during mobilization, the fracture may get distracted. If the patient has a heavy built, one may consider addition of another figure of eight loop with a 1 mm wire. Mechanically, this is far superior to having a single 1.2 mm wire for the loop.

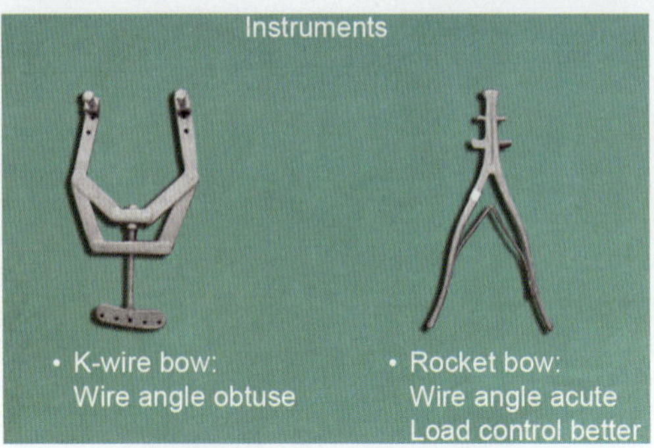

Figure 32.4 Wire tensioner types

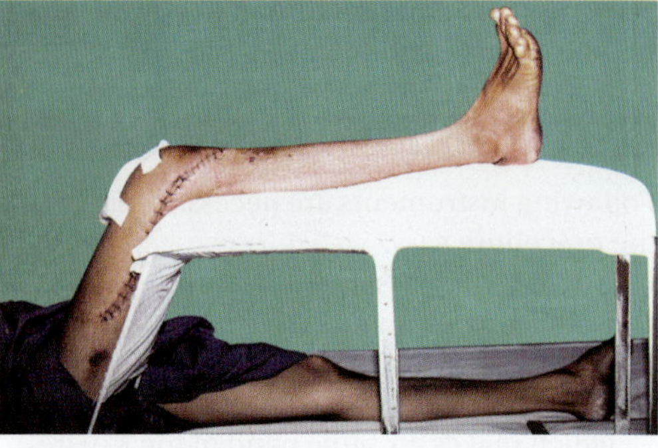

Figure 32.5 High Bohler frame

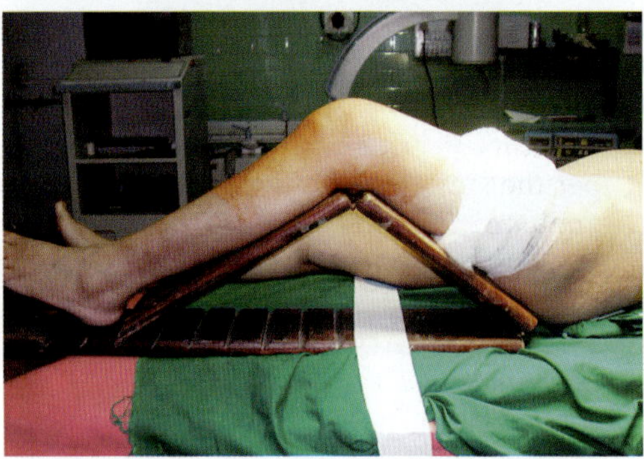

Figure 32.6 Quadriceps board

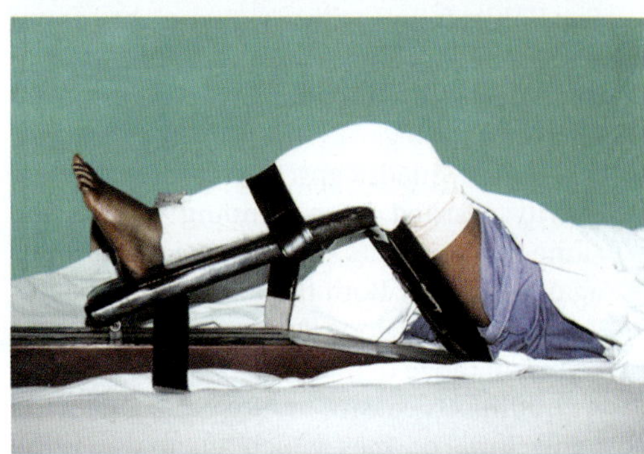

Figure 32.7 Continuous passive motion machine

PRINCIPLES

- In a transverse fracture in the middle/3 area, the axial K-wires stabilize the bone fragments. The K-wires should be parallel to each other, so, during active mobilization of the knee, the fragments would slightly slide along them and help to compress the fragments, during knee flexion. In a three- or four-part fracture, one needs to pass the K-wires at right angle to all the fracture line, to keep the assembly stable. The K-wires are passed close to the articular surface, where the subchondral bone is strong and offers a good hold. During the loading of the figure of eight loop anteriorly, such posteriorly placed K-wires also help to prevent distraction of the fracture surface in the articular surface. Even if such a distraction is observed, during active knee flexion, it gets adjusted.
- The circlage wire has to be in a figure of eight configuration, anterior to the patella, so it prevents anterior fracture distraction and holds the fragments well opposed.
- A circumferential wire may keep the fragments together, but, would not prevent their opening anteriorly. It thus may keep the fragments together, but cannot resist distraction forces.
- *Combination*: In a comminuted fracture, especially when the displacement is not too much, a circlage is placed first, to keep all the fragments together. Additional anterior figure of eight loop would load the assembly and prevent their distraction.
- Tension band wiring works well, when the articular surface of patella is not comminuted and has a good contact opposition. If so, then only it resists distraction forces well and undisturbed fracture union occurs.

TECHNIQUE

- A pneumatic tourniquet makes the surgery easy and tissue planes are better developed. Just prior to inflating the tourniquet, manually the proximal fragment should be kneaded to bring it as distally as possible, so the quadriceps muscle is brought down. This helps ease of reduction of the fragments. If it is not done, the quadriceps muscle is locked under the tourniquet cuff and then bringing down the proximal fragment is not so easy.
- A quadriceps board (wooden angled frame) helps to keep the knee stable, at an angle as per the stage of surgery. It is usually kept at an angle of 30 deg. After the exposure of the fracture, the fracture hematoma is cleared and a wound lavage makes the fracture surface well exposed and clear.
- With a pointed forceps (or a large Blackhaus towel clip) the proximal fragment is brought down and the assistant holds it as such. With a medial and a lateral pointed reduction forceps, the surgeon reduces the fracture and with necessary movements of the fragments, the anterior surface is well aligned. The serrated edges of the fracture line should be well interdigited for accurate reduction. This is a trial reduction. The reduction is undone and the fracture surface of the proximal fragment exposed again. Through this surface a retrograde 1.8 mm K-wire is drilled towards the superior pole and is brought out proximally. At a distance of 15 to 17 mm distance another wire is drilled similarly. The fracture is reduced as before and both the wires are sequentially advanced towards the distal fragment. The first wire is drilled till the tip penetrates 3 mm beyond the distal pole and is then gently withdrawn by 3 mm or so. The second wire too is driven this way. This makes a track for each wire. The assistant continues to hold the medial and the lateral reduction forceps, may be with less pressure, as the K-wires stabilize the fragments well. At this stage, one may take a 'C' arm image in the lateral view to confirm the alignment of articular surface and depth at which the K-wires are placed. The level up to which the distal end of the K-wires lie, is also checked and some adjustment is made, if needed. The assembly can be slightly tilted on either side to confirm reduction of the articular surfaces, under vision.
- A stab incision is made 5 mm on lateral side of either K-wires at the superior pole. A cobbler awl with an eye is passed through one incision, very close and deep to the posterior part of both K-wires and the quadriceps, towards the opposite side and is brought out. A 1 mm soft wire is threaded through it and is bent acutely. The cobbler awl is withdrawn, with the wire. The path of the wire so passed, should be *deep to both the K-wires and the quadriceps tendon.* Use of a curved wire passer is also possible, as per the surgeon's choice. The circlage wire ends are kept 2/3 on one side and 1/3 on the other side. At this stage, if fascia anterior to the patella is present, the wire ends are taken deep to it with a cobbler awl.
- A cobbler awl is passed just deep to the ligament patellae from the side of the long end and brought out on the other side, very close to the distal end of patella. Wire is drawn by the awl, to the opposite side. By holding and pulling apart the wire ends with two pliers, the wire slack is taken away. This long end of the wire is taken across the anterior surface of patella and crossed against the other end. The ends of the wires are threaded through the eyes of the wire tensioner. While threading the wires in the tensioner, about 3 cm of free wire be available between the tensioner and the expected site of the crossing and the knot. (At this stage, the knee should be in extension, so the fracture is well stabilised in an extended knee). The handles of the tensioner are pressed together, to stretch the wires, so adequate load is created across the fracture area. One often observes that the patella tends to have slight posterior angulation, indicating adequate load is applied. The wires are rotated/twisted by 180 degrees and little more. This makes a knot,

which would not loosen. Now, the tension in the handle is slightly reduced and further twist is added. If the tension is not reduced and one continues to twist it further, often the wire breaks at this stage! At this stage one observes, that the quadriceps tendon has narrowed slightly, indicating good tension in the wire. The tractor/tensioner is removed. One moves the knee through 10 to 50 degrees, to assess maintenance of stability of the implant and reduction. Then the circlage wire ends are cut 3 mm beyond the knot. With a nose pliers, the knot is bent and buried, so that it will not irritate the subcutaneous tissue.

- The quadriceps tendon around the K-wire is slightly slit and with a K-wire bending pliers, using the slot in the jaws, the wire is bent more than 90 deg. Surgeon may choose to bend it with a nose pliers or a metal small suction cannula. The excess length is cut off. The wire ends are rotated, so they point posteriorly and gently tapped, so they travel distally in the predrilled track already prepared in the distal fragment.
- The tourniquet is deflated and as the quadriceps is freed, range of knee motion and the stability of fixation confirmed again. Finally the reconstruction is checked under a 'C' arm and an X-ray film exposed. I have observed that, at times, some problem is noted in an X-ray film, which was not visible on 'C' arm image. Hence, exposing an X-ray film and seeing it personally, prior to wound closure is a safe and makes a documentation also.
- Medial and lateral extensor retinaculi are sutured with vicryl. It is preferable to start the repair from extreme medial and lateral ends and come centripetally. This assures good closure. They transfer substantial part of the force, during the knee extension and hence the importance of good opposition. The prepatellar bursa is also sutured well.
- Postoperative leg elevation is important. As the effect of spinal anesthesia wears off, leg elevation on a high Bohler frame is done. In presence of continuous epidural anesthesia, the knee position of flexion is well tolerated by the patient. Early active knee extension is recommended. Such an elevation keeps the knee at 40 to 50 deg of flexion and returns of further flexion is relative easy and comfortable. Besides, due to the elevation, the reactionary tissue edema and hence the pain is less.
- At the end of three days, one may use a quadriceps board. It has an arrangement for changing the angle, at which it is kept. One can keep the angle of 30 deg flexion, which is usually comfortable for the patient. From this angle, the patient is encouraged to carry out knee extension. Having gained confidence in himself, he can do carry out the exercises well. One should progressively increase the knee flexion. The knee extension also improves well and the extensor lag is kept to a minimum.
- Having achieved this, non weight bearing ambulation with toe touch is possible.

Note: In a fracture of patella with multiple fractures, it may not be possible to have a look at the articular surface after stabilization of every fragment. Often all the fragments cannot be anchored, well-aligned and held by K-wires. In spite of this, the outcome is more often satisfactory. It is observed that one has come across very few, cases, if at all, of osteoarthrosis of a patello-femoral joint after a comminuted fracture of patella!

LATE PRESENTATION OF FRACTURE OF PATELLA

Undisplaced Fracture, Patient Came Walking

Was able to slowly walk. Was able to lift the leg up, with knee at 20 deg flexion. 80 to 20 deg extension was possible.

Options

- Apply a padded crepe for support and allow non-weight bearing mobilization. Gradually advise active knee extension.

Danger: If unfortunately has another fall, the uninjured foot slips, before the fracture has united, the fracture may get displaced.

- In situ fixation with axial K-wires and figure of eight tension band. This offers safety and the knee can be mobilized early.

However, the patient was reluctant for surgery, but was prepared for a cast application (Fig. 32.8).

Technique of a Cylinder Cast

A cylinder cast extends from two fingers above the ankle till the upper thigh. It prevents knee flexion and permits toe touch weight bearing. As the thigh disuse atrophy sets in and the knee swelling reduces, the cylinder cast tends to slide down the leg and hurts the ankle. Hence it needs to be kept *suspended* on the leg.

5 cm wide adhesive tape is applied on either side of the calf and the ends are kept 6 long, distally. The knee is kept at 10 degree flexion and a cylinder cast is applied. Just before the final plaster roll, the adhesive tape is turned up and kept pulled upwards by an assistant and is kept close on the partially applied cast. A roll of plaster is taken over it and thus the tape is incorporated in the cast. Thus the cast is suspended from the calf by the adhesive tape and does not slide down.

During follow up, one must supervise static quad exercises and permit assisted and later free straight leg raise with the cast on. This maintains the tone and strength of quadriceps (Fig. 32.9).

Displaced Untreated Fracture of Patella

This young man had an untreated displaced fracture of patella. He had lost active knee extension, as expected. On clinical examination, one could bring down the proximal fragment fairly distally. Prior to inflating the tourniquet, the knee was flexed and the proximal fragment was pushed distally, as much as possible. The fracture surfaces were cleared of fibrous tissue and internal fixation with tension band wiring was carried out.

Postoperative recovery was satisfactory. However, X-ray taken a few months later shows a united patella with a good flexion of the knee and a broken wire at the superior end (Fig. 32.10).

FRACTURE OF PATELLA OF DIFFERENT PATTERNS

Vertical Fracture of Patella

After a fall, the patient had pain, limp and was able to walk unaided. Knee had hemarthrosis. A skyline X-ray view was also taken, which revealed a vertical fracture. The extensor expansion continuity was present and was able to raise the leg straight. Hence was treated with a crepe support only. This is not a bipartite patella (Fig. 32.11).

Undisplaced Fracture of the Inferior Pole of Patella

The lady had a fall on road on both the knees: On one side contusion, while on the other side small hemarthrosis with tender distal patella

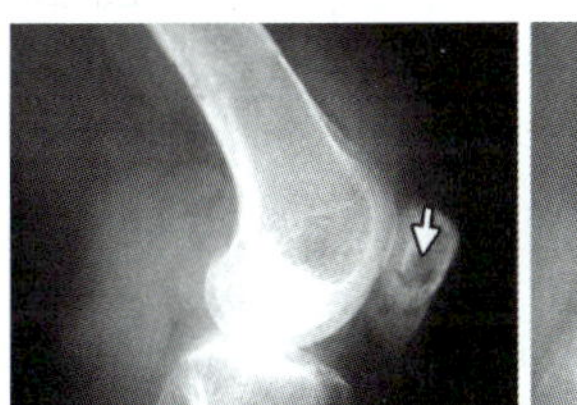
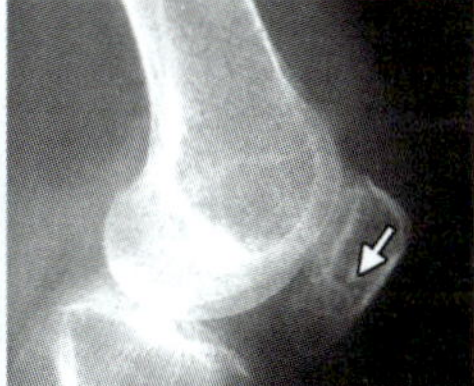

Figure 32.8 Undisplaced fracture

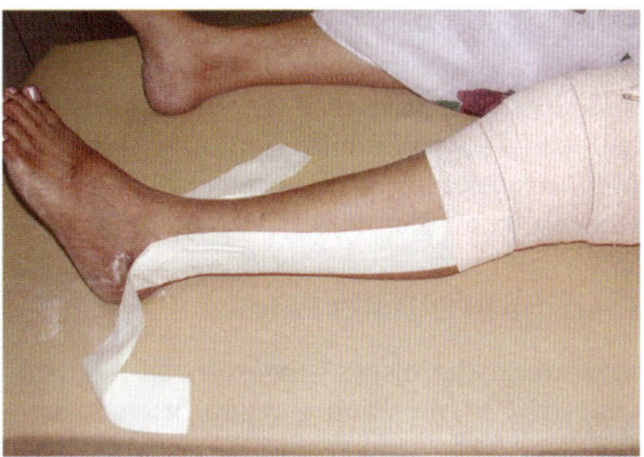

Figure 32.9 Cylinder cast

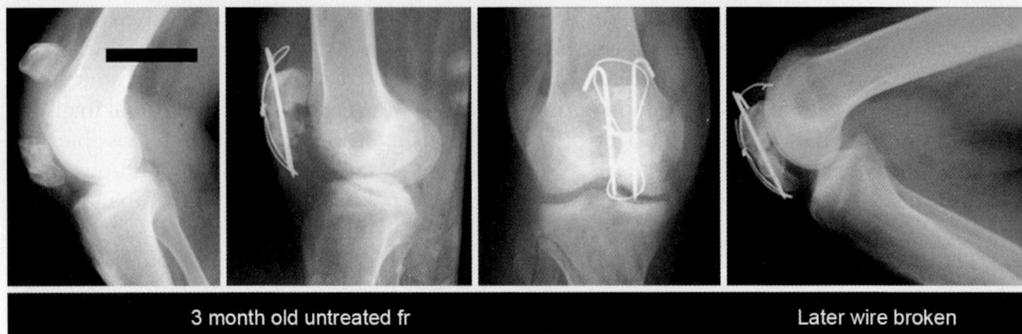

Figure 32.10 3-month old untreated fracture of patella

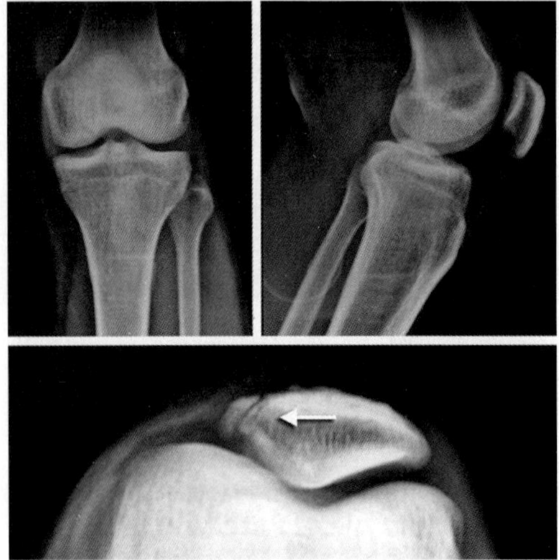

Figure 32.11 Vertical fracture of patella

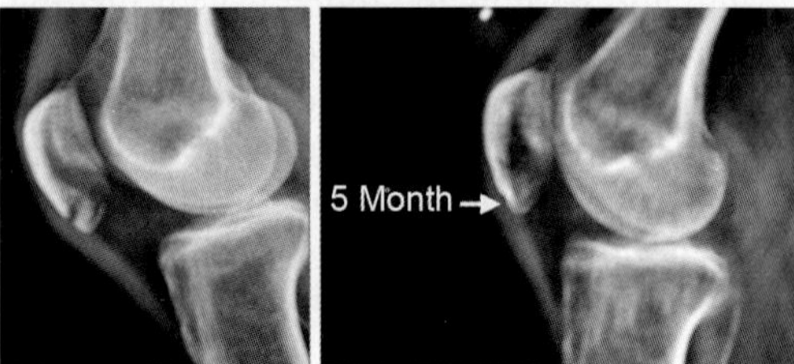

Figure 32.12 Undisplaced fracture of inferior pole of patella

was noted. She was able to stand and walk with support. Active straight leg raising was possible. The X-ray revealed an undisplaced fracture of the distal end of patella. It was treated with padded crepe, advised to keep off the weight and early active mobilization. The continuity of the extensor expansion protects the fracture. Good outcome (Fig. 32.12).

Fracture in Distal/3 Patella

Fracture at the distal/3 area can be managed with axial K-wires and a figure of eight loop. However, the K-wires are inserted from the distal pole proximally, for better stability (Fig. 32.13).

Fracture of Distal Pole

The distal fragment, if too small, when the circlage loop is loaded, tends to tilt posteriorly. Hence to gain more axial stability and prevent such a tilting, a 4 mm shaft screw with a washer is used. The fracture is reduced and the screw with a 7 mm washer is inserted from the distal pole towards the proximal pole and is finger tightened. Being a shaft screw, during the axial loading, fracture opposition does occur. The figure of loop is added from above the upper surface of patella and distally is deep to the ligament patellae, as usual. The rigidity of the screw prevents any angulation of the fracture, while the wire is being loaded (Fig. 32.14).

Four-Part Fracture of Patella

As seen in the film, all the fragments could be well assembled with K-wires and a TBW (Fig. 32.15).

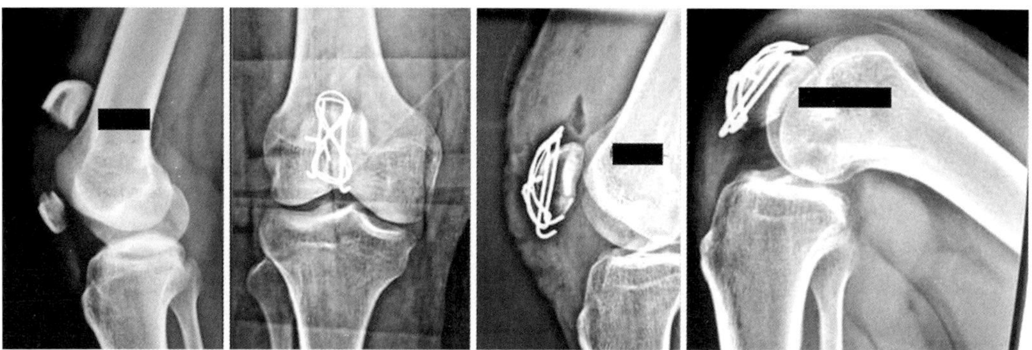

Figure 32.13 Distal to proximal K wires

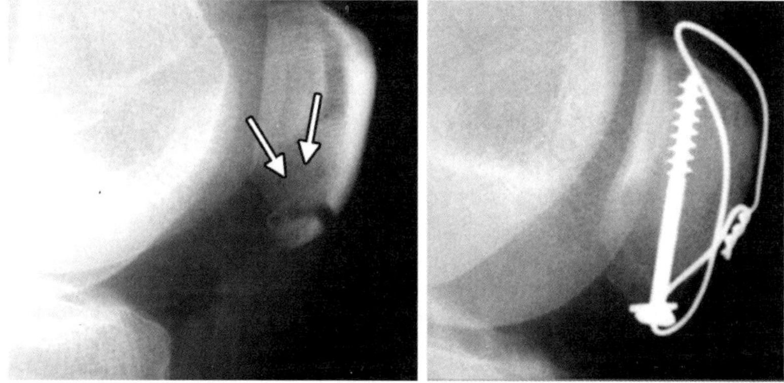

Figure 32.14 Distal to proximal screw

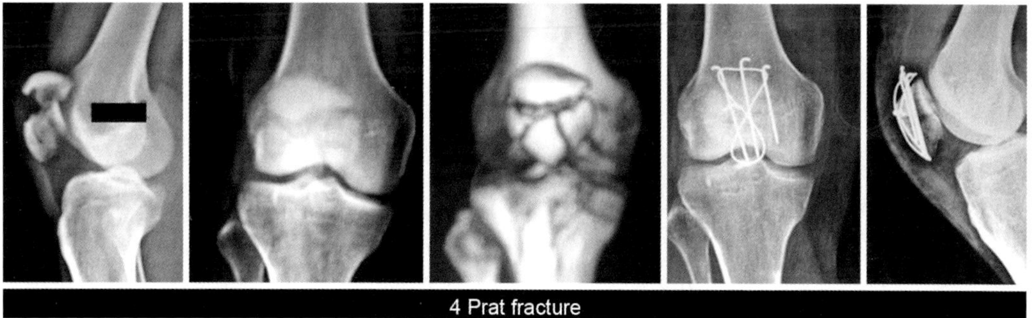

Figure 32.15 4-part fracture: TBW

Broken Circlage Wire

Follow up of a case treated with tension band wiring is important. The fracture unites well and an X-ray taken later on reveals that the wire is broken at a place. This is observed to occur even after the fracture has well consolidated. Case shown was operated elsewhere and came for follow up after few years. X-ray revealed the breakage of wire. The wire was removed. It

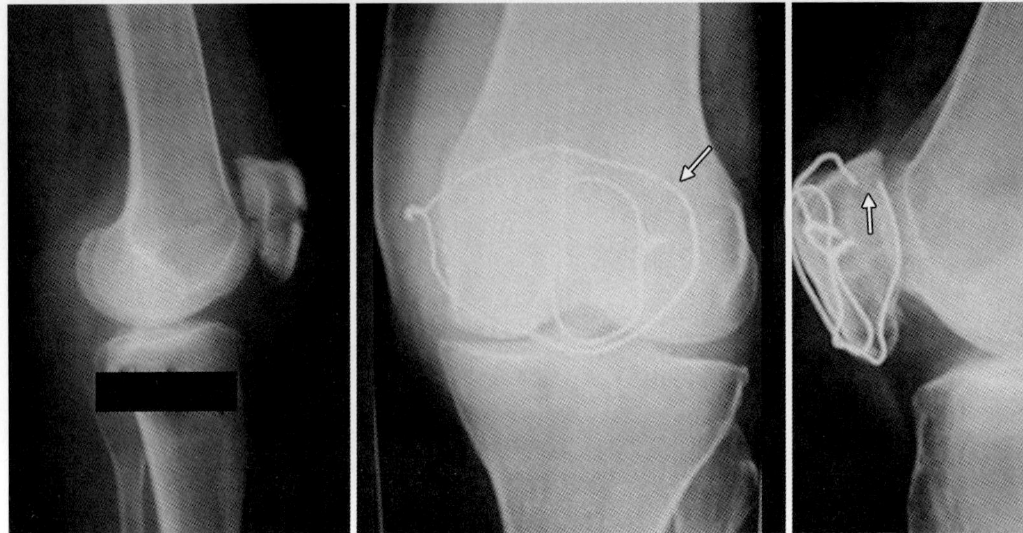

Figure 32.16 Broken wire

is observed that, if the figure of 8 wire ends are crossed, twisted and thus tightened by a pliers, such a breakage is not observed. Maybe with the use of a tensioner, the wire strength at some place is reduced, due to some elongation and hence later on gives way at that place (Fig. 32.16).

The case was operated by me and after a few years the wire was found to be broken. He was advised to remove the wire, which he did not follow up (Fig. 32.17).

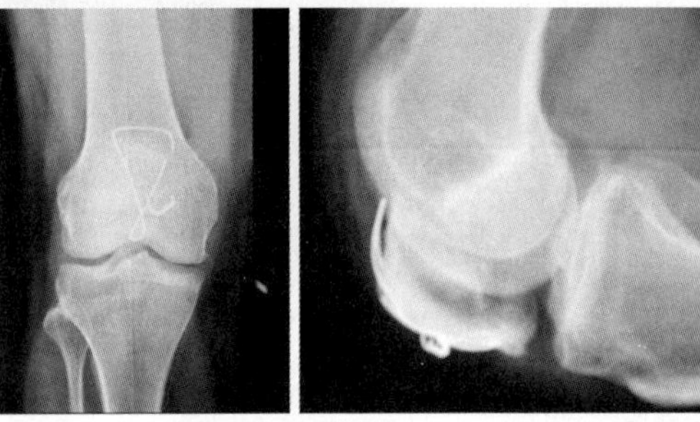

Figure 32.17 Broken wire

Broken and Migrated Wire

In another case, the patient came for follow up, rather late. X-ray revealed that the wire had broken at two places and the segment had migrated posteriorly. The segment was removed by a posterior approach and then after making the patient supine, the other implants were removed (Fig. 32.18).

Lesson: Such breakage of the wire is observed, even after a fracture has well consolidated and when the wire is less likely to be under load. Hence it is recommended that after union, the implant should be removed in each case, because one cannot predict, which will have a segmental break and migrate to an area, like posterior compartment.

Multiple Undisplaced Fragments

In this case of multiple fractures, the fracture neck and ipsilateral femur was fixed with an AFN and patient was made supine. The patella was fixed with a circlage to assemble all the fragments and a figure of loop added. (In the same sitting a Barton fracture was stabilized and in the next stage the posterior tibial eminence was fixed).

The fracture fragments were not displaced. The circumferential wire held all fragments together and the figure of 8 loop resisted any likelihood of fracture distraction, when the knee was mobilized (Fig. 32.19).

Partial Patellectomy

A patient reported for a problem, unrelated to the knee, along with ache in the knee joint. He has maybe 3- to 4- part fracture of patella few years ago and was treated elsewhere by excision of the distal part of patella. During flexion of the knee beyond 70 deg the edge of the patella, proximal fragment would irritate the joint.

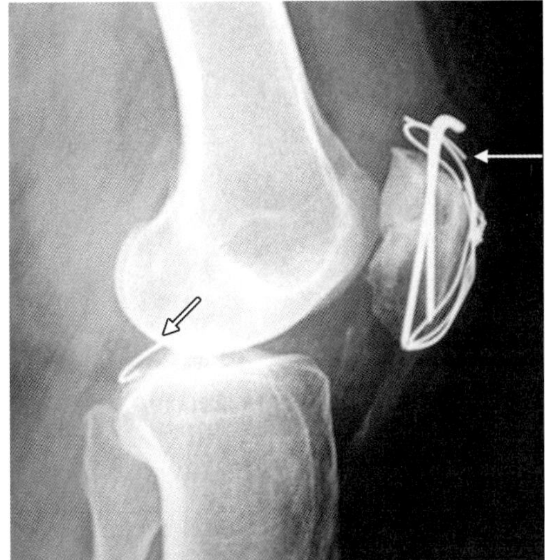

Figure 32.18 Broken and migrated segment of wire

Looking at the earlier radiograph, I feel internal fixation would have been possible with a better outcome. Today, with technical know how and TBW technique, patella preservation is possible and should be attempted (Fig. 32.20).

Avulsion of Ligament Patellae from Tibia

A gentleman past middle age had hemiparesis and sustained a fall. The patella was not fractured and clinically avulsion of ligamentum patellae from the tibia was noted. The reattachment of the tendon was necessary for a good knee function.

A vertical approach was taken and the end of the ligament was sutured to the upper tibia, with help of suture anchors. The extensor expansion needs to be protected from avulsion, till the ligament healed well.

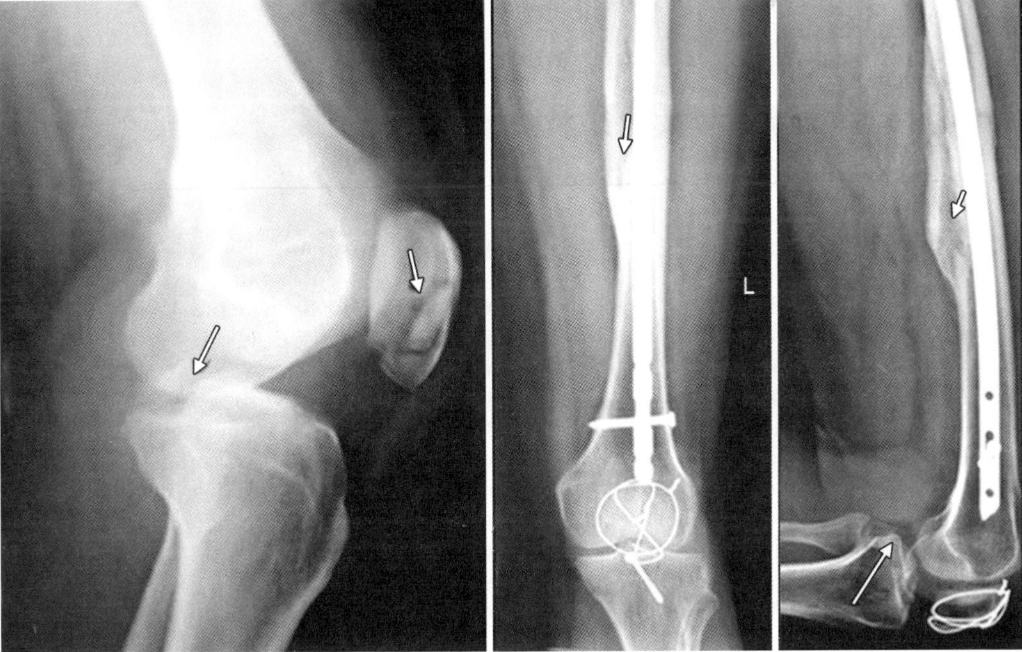

Figure 32.19 Only TBW

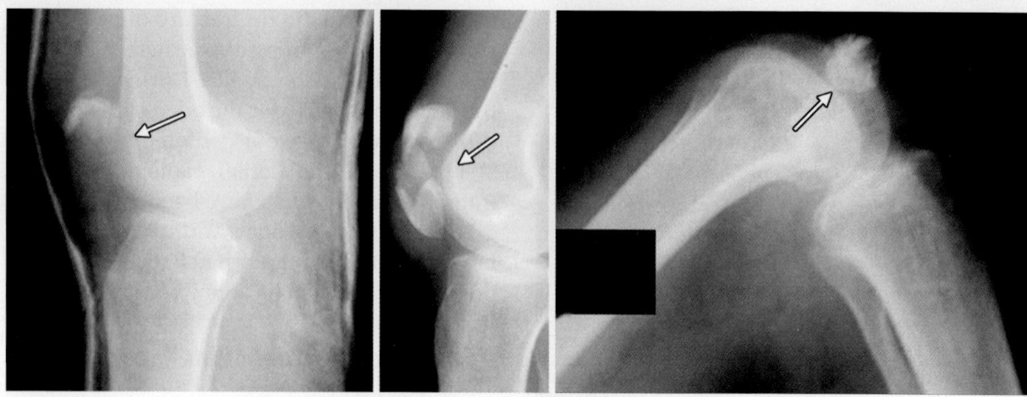

Figure 32.20 Partial patellectomy

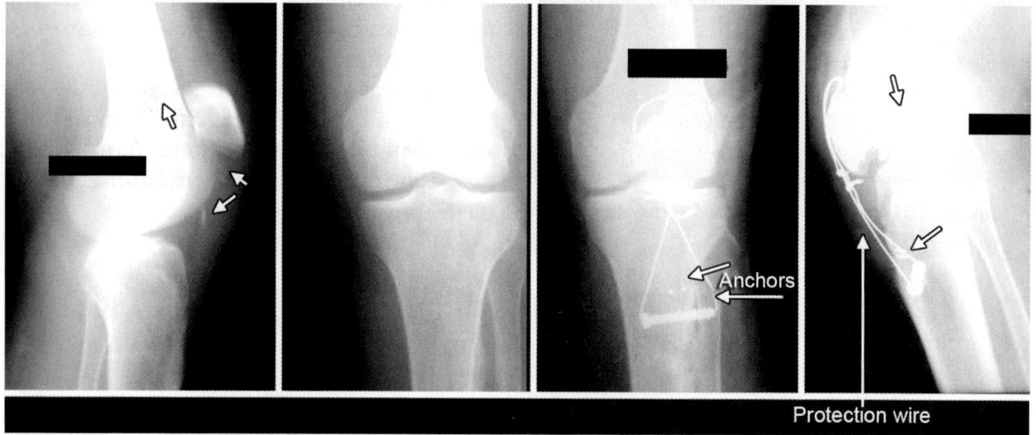

Figure 32.21 Ligament avulsion and protection wire

The protection wire: To take stresses off the suture line, a soft bone wire was passed around the proximal patella and crossed in the middle. If such a wire is passed through a drill hole in the upper tibia, there is a danger of wire cutting out of the bone. Hence a cannulated 6.5 mm screw was drilled at the desired level and the wire was passed through it. The wire was loaded, just necessary, so that the ligament is well-protected and the wire also does not give way. With such an assembly, it is possible to manage the knee with a crepe support only. However, the patient being hemiplegic, did not have good control over the limb and hence a cylinder cast was applied (Fig. 32.21).

Late Infection

In operative management of any bone and joint injury, diabetes is the greatest deterrent to an open surgery. Hence, every care must be taken to exclude this associated condition. If it is a comorbidity, it needs to be taken care of, perhaps more than the injury itself. Prior to surgery, patient needs to be shifted on insulin. During the postoperative phase, one should continue to maintain the insulin, howsoever small may be the dose needed. Often one is advised to stabilize on oral drug only. However, experience tells us that use of parental insulin, in addition to oral anti-diabetic drugs, for a long term, at least a month or so after the surgery would keep the blood sugar well controlled. One may not realize the importance, till one comes across such an unfortunate incidence. Thus, every precaution of highest order must be taken, while operating a patient with diabetes.

A fracture of patella is not a surgical emergency. Hence, the surgery should be carried out, only when the blood sugar is stabilized well.

A Case

This case was managed elsewhere and may be diabetes was not thought of or was uncontrolled. For the vertical fracture, transverse K-wires and a circlage was carried out, indeed very well executed. However, later on patient had persistent pain, especially on weight bearing. Hence the implants were removed. The infection continued, as seen in the X-ray film. As is known, often antibiotics are added in large amount. Still the infection keeps lingering. If the process results in a sound fibrous ankylosis of the knee, the patient is lucky.

At times, the septic arthritis, thus occurred, in an elderly diabetic patient, due to atherosclerosis one faces few technical problems. The atherosclerosis is so extensive, that a pneumatic tourniquet cannot occlude the blood flow and to carry out a knee fusion, without a pneumatic tourniquet, is a difficult task. Due to atherosclerosis, and the infection, the blood oozing is difficult to control.

Even after a successful fusion, the patient, the family, and of course, the treating team are not happy to see a patient with shortening and a stiff knee, which is indeed difficult to live with. This is especially true, while sitting in a public place as in a transport vehicle, auditorium, etc. (Fig. 32.22).

Post-Knee Stiffness Fracture of Patella

Knee stiffness is a difficult condition to live with. Due to reduction or loss of the knee range and quadriceps atrophy, osteoporosis of adjacent area ensues. With a normal supple and mobile knee, as a result of a jerk or a fall, the knee easily bends and often no serious injury occurs. However, in a stiff knee, due to intra-articular adhesions following an intra-articular fracture or extra-articular quadriceps adhesions, following an osteomyelitis of femur, knee cannot bend quickly and forces are dissipated in a bone, leading to a fracture.

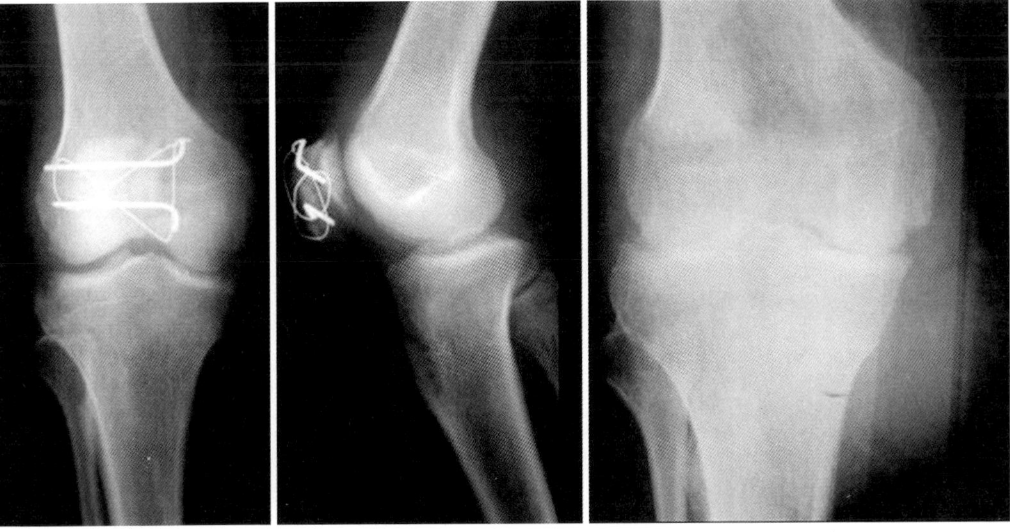

Figure 32.22 Infection

Case 1

Had sustained a Hoffa injury and was managed elsewhere. The knee had limitation of range of motion. After a fall, the patella fractured and she reported to me. It was managed with a TBW and pre-injury range was restored again.

Her misfortune was not yet over. She had later a fracture lower end femur, which was treated with a locking plate. Then she had a fracture of tibial condyle, treated with a buttress plate. I wonder, after union of all the fractures, now if I should recommend her implant removal, to restore the bone elasticity and avoid any further fracture adjacent to the existing plates, which would be a difficult task later on! If she agrees to the procedure of removal of all implants, I wish, she does not get a stress fracture through one of the screw holes, from where a screw was removed.

Case 2

This young lady had a fracture of shaft of femur and ipsilateral acetabulum. Both were operated and unfortunately had infection leading to a stiff hip, with some range of motion and a stiff knee. She reported to me for osteomyelitis of femur, which was appropriately treated. After a nuclear scan examination, a window was made in the bone, over the entire infected area and curettage carried out. The wound was left open with a roller pack and dressings carried out. The wound healed from the depth and had no recurrence for four years.

Later an uncemented THR was done and she enjoyed the hip mobility. However, the knee continued to be stiff, because of the quadriceps adhesions, which are difficult to be overcome. She had a fall, leading to fracture of patella. This was treated with a TBW (Fig. 32.23).

At times, X-ray film of a fracture of patella shows may be 3- or 4-part fracture. However, on exposing the patella, one finds few more fracture lines, not visible in the earlier X-ray films. If the fracture lines are in the coronal plane, then transfixing them is rather difficult and tricky. The antero-posterior thickness of the fragments is often very less, to be able to be pierced by the K-wires. Besides, due to the fracture morphology, adding adequate load by a TBW may disrupt the assembly.

This is an example, where I assembled all the fragments, as much as possible and loaded carefully, to offer good stability. However, the lateral X-ray showed some fracture voids, which, I knew, would require later bone grafting. To carry out it on day 1 would be rather dangerous, because, some grafts may slip in the joint. Hence, postoperative careful mobilization was carried out, with an understanding that at appropriate time a bone grafting would be necessary.

After 5 months, a good range was achieved, with persistent fracture line. Small fragments had well-consolidated, while the major fracture line was seen to be persistent. Cancellous bone grafting was carried out. On exposure, at the

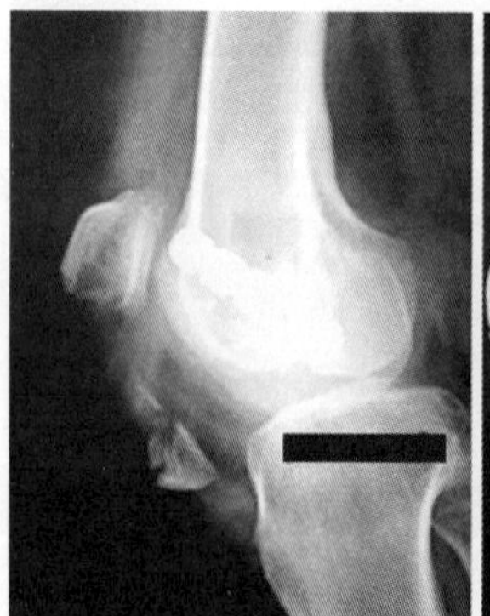
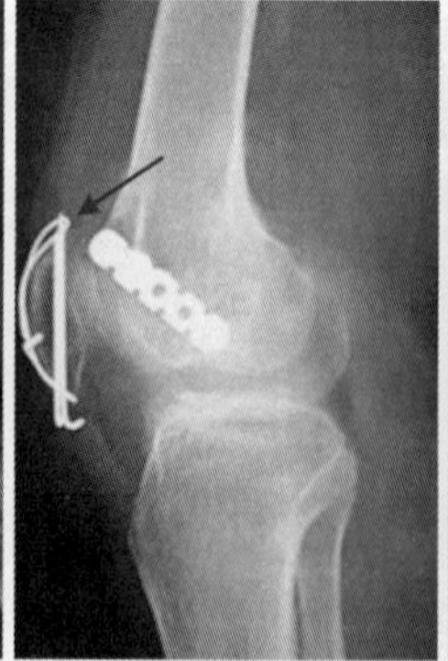
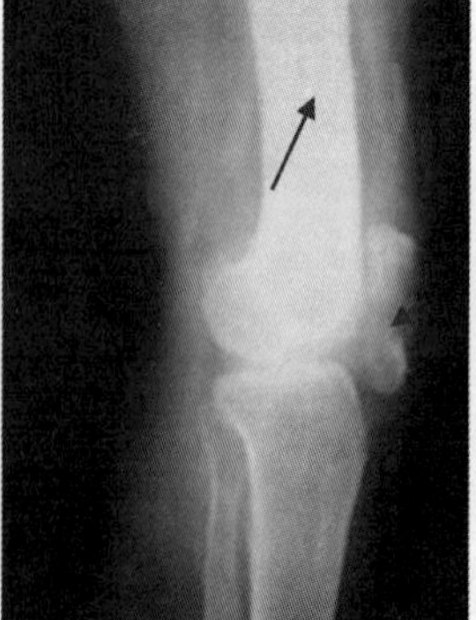
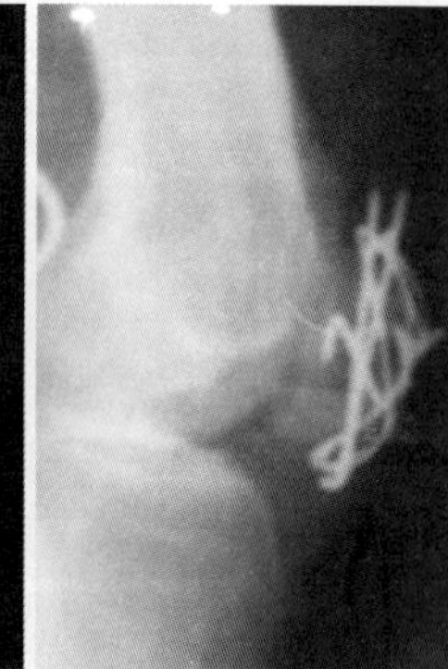

Figure 32.23 Post-stiffness fracture of patella

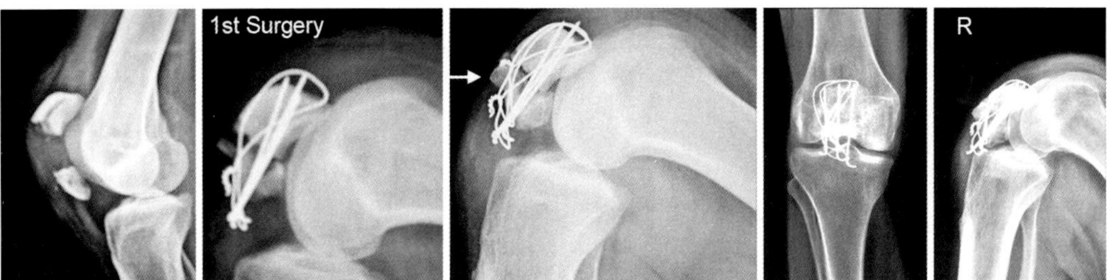

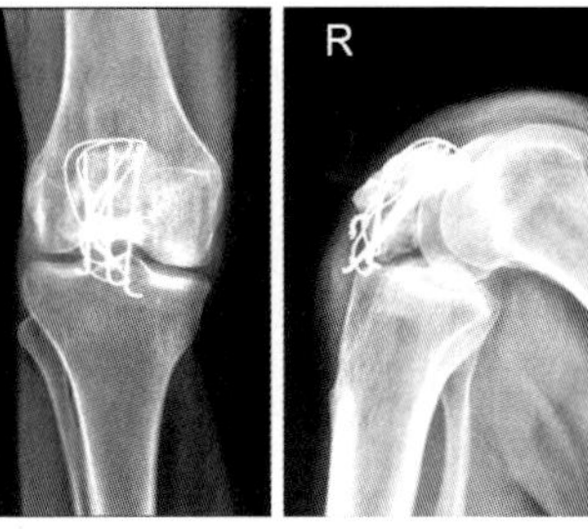

Figure 32.24 Ununited fracture of patella

expected site in the patella, fibro-osseous union was noted. It was gently curetted and cancellous grafts were laid down. At this stage, I expected fatigue of the first tension band, which was kept as such and an additional wire loop was added to it, as a further protection. Mobilization was carried out and at the end of every six months further consolidation was observed. He is advised removal of the implant at appropriate time (Fig. 32.24).

CHAPTER

33

Post-Stiffness Fractures

Case 1: Fracture of Acetabulum and Shaft of Femur

This young lady had fracture of left femur and acetabulum around 1999 and reported to a hospital. She was operated there and both the fractures were fixed: posterior acetabular plate and IM nailing for the femur. Unfortunately had infection at both the sites. The day 1 and postoperative X-ray films and details were not available.

As per the history, the femur IM nail was removed in the year 2000 and the acetabular plate in the year 2001. She had a stiff hip, with a few degree of motion and fibrous ankylosis of the knee.

She had recurrent discharging sinuses on the left thigh and presented for further treatment in 2007. X-ray examination showed cavities in the distal femur. A nuclear scan was done, which confirmed infection in the distal femur.

Left femur 2007: A window was made in the lateral femur cortex and curettage was done. It was washed and a roller pack dressing was done, to permit healing from the depth, to avoid recurrence. Appropriate antibiotics were given. The wound was dressed and it gradually healed from below, without any need of secondary suturing.

She desired to have a mobile hip. An uncemented THR was done and was doing well

Three years later, she slipped and had a fracture of patella on the same side and was treated with a TBW, united well (Figs 33.1A and B).

Case 2

This young lady had an open fracture of lower femur and was managed with an external fixator and then internal fixation. There was some scarring of the skin, with reasonably good function. She slipped and sustained an avulsion fracture of the tibial tuberosity.

The fracture was fixed with a 4 mm shaft screw, through a 1/3 tubular plate, which served as a buttress plate and also resisted the quadriceps forces. Early mobilization could be safely carried out, with return of preinjury function (Fig. 33.2).

Case 3

A young man had a fracture of lower end of femur and was fixed elsewhere. He did not attend for regular follow up, though advised to do so. During rehabilitation, prior to fracture consolidation, he had another injury, causing avulsion fracture of tibial tuberosity.

The fragment was stabilized with a shaft screw with a washer. To protect the screw avulsion, a protection wire was passed above the patella, crossed in the front and then

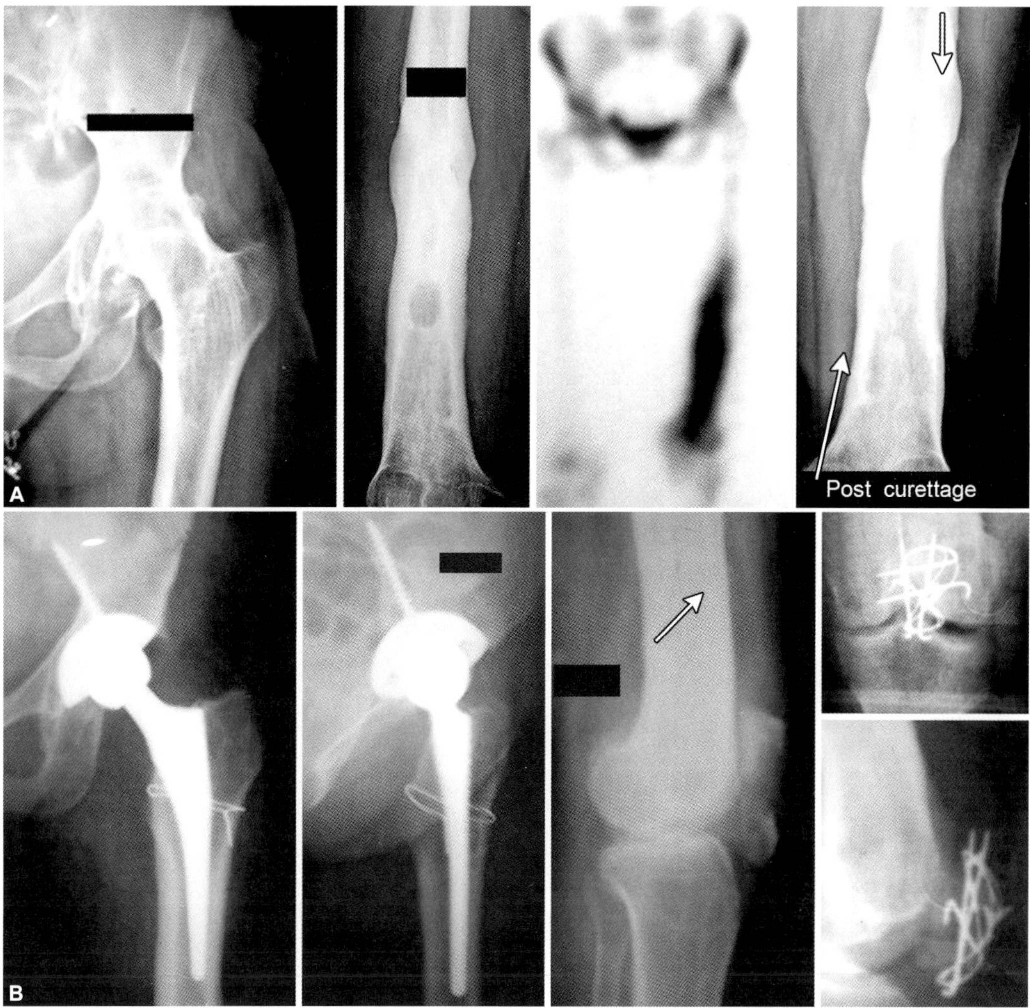

Figures 33.1A and B Post-knee stiffness fracture of patella

threaded through the tibia. To prevent its cutting through the tibia bone, a cannulated 4 mm screw was inserted transversally across the tibia, through which the 1 mm soft wire was passed. Such a protection wire takes all the stress of knee mobilization, while the tuberosity united. The wire is known to break, indicating, it was taking the stress of mobilization, indeed (Fig. 33.3).

Case 4: Post-Knee Fusion SC Fracture of Femur

This gentleman in 20's in 1967 sustained a fracture of a femur in mid/3, fracture of femur condyle and fracture of tibia and fibula. As was the practice then, femur was stabilized with a K-nail and other injuries were treated non-operatively. He was immobilized in a hip

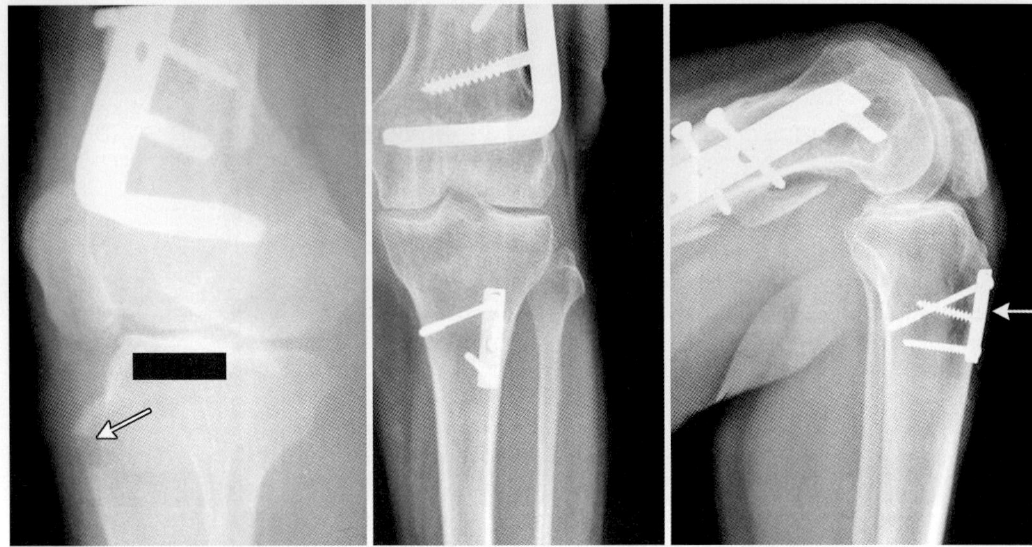

Figure 33.2 Avulsion of tibial tuberosity I

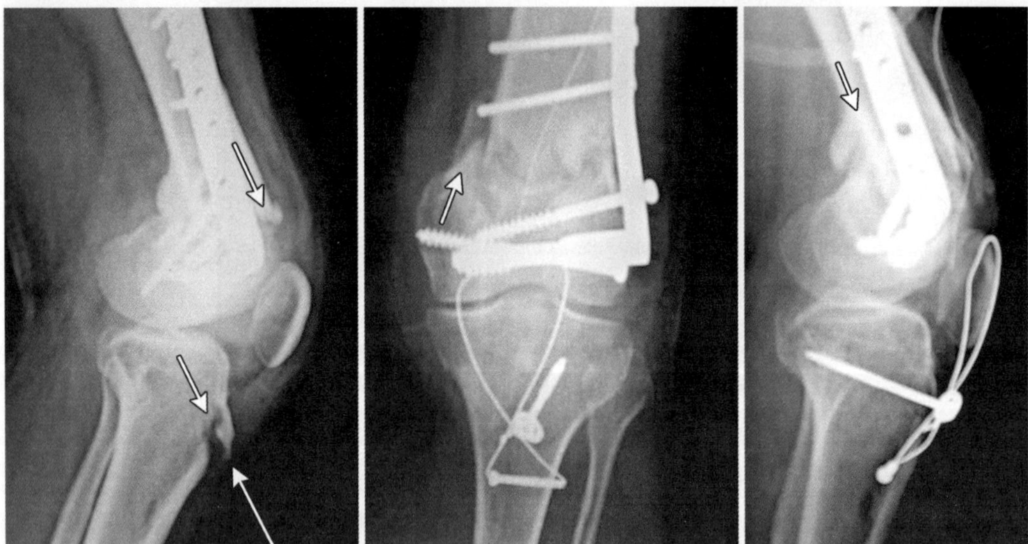

Figure 33.3 Avulsion of tibial tuberosity II

spica and the fractures united with some knee stiffness.

Around 1975, developed fever and local swelling around the knee and subsequently may be infective arthritis. Details are not available. Hence for the painfull knee, a knee arthrodesis was carried out. (This was an accepted and commonly carried out procedure then). With the fused left knee, he had been walking/ climbing hill as well since then. He would get intermittent discharge from the fusion area and a sinogram was done, as seen in a film.

Twenty two years later, around 1997, he had a fall and had an oblique SC fracture of the femur. He was immobilized in a Thomas' splint and then a long leg cast.

The fracture did not unite. There was no local infection then. He was recommended to undergo internal fixation with a long interlocking nail, which was available then, to cross the knee joint. He refused to undergo the procedure, accepted the local status and is using a plastic moulded splint and moves about with a walker/crutches.

Around 2009 he has undergone angioplasty, as per the information received (Fig. 33.4).

Case 5: Multiple Fractures Around the Knee

This lady sustained a Hoffa fracture of femoral condyle. The surgeon did internal fixation, the way it was possible then, and a reconstruction plate was applied. The knee had about 60 to 70 degrees of knee flexion at the end of t reatment.

She had a fall and sustained fracture of patella on the same side. It was fixed with a TBW and she regained the range, as was prior to this injury.

Two years later she had another fall and sustained a supracondylar fracture of femur, which was fixed with a locking plate and recovered, to regain back the range of movement (Fig. 33.5A).

Exercises were carried out to maintain the range and strength in the muscles around. The misfortune continued and another injury, leading to a fracture of tibial condyle. A medial plate was applied and she recovered again (Fig. 33.5B).

Thus she has implants around the knee. The question with us is whether to leave the implants as such or remove them step by step.

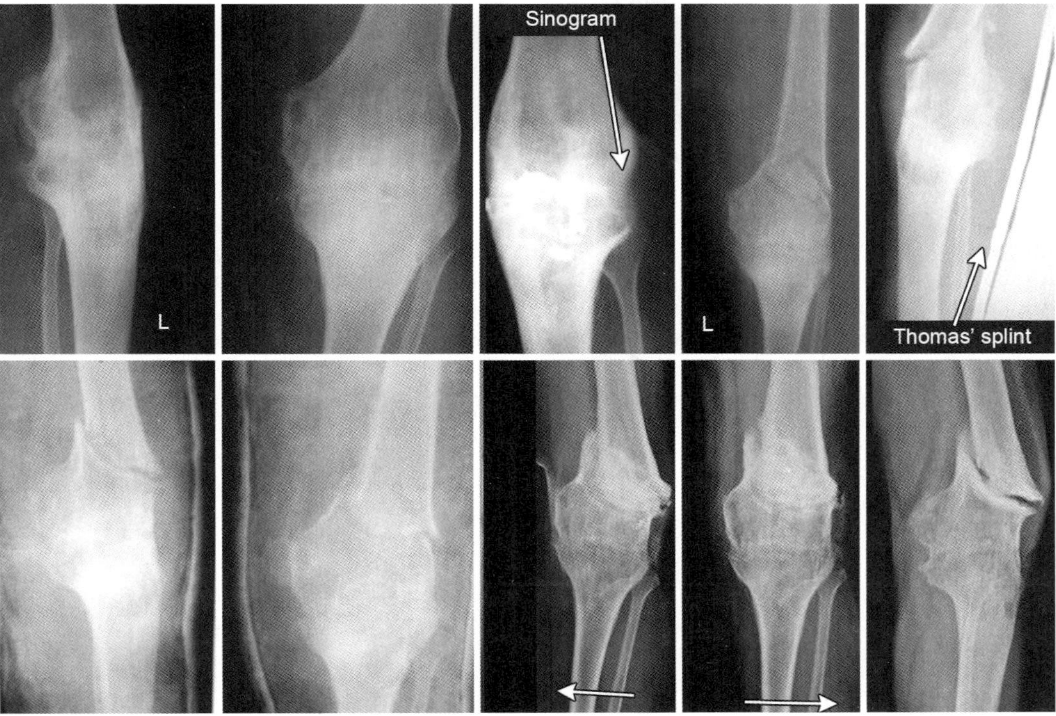

Figure 33.4 Post-knee fusion, fracture of femur

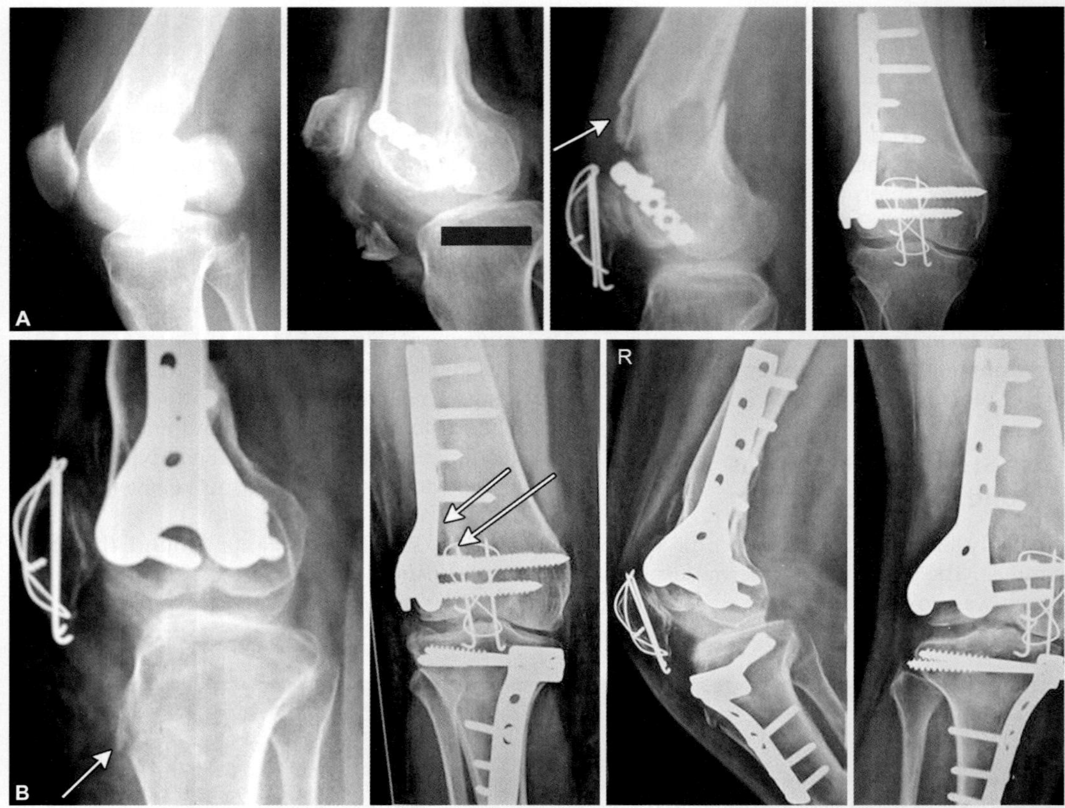

Figures 33.5A and B Multiple fractures around the knee

Message

Any injury around the knee, especially in any part of the femur, needs to be addressed seriously and carried out with precision, to restore good range of motion. Postoperative position of the limb, during soft tissue healing, rehabilitation should be carried out, as a team work, to restore preinjury suppleness of the knee with full range of motion. We should take all the efforts to avoid a situation, as above.

CHAPTER

34

Fracture of Anterior Tibial Eminence

FIXATION WITH A CIRCLAGE WIRE

Case 1

Quite often postoperative pain is severe after this surgery and hence it is preferable to have an epidural catheter in place, to offer postoperative analgesia and help early knee mobilization.

Quadriceps board and tourniquet make the procedure easy.

Incision: Antero-medial from the top of patella, till 4 cm distal to the joint line.

The deep fascia and medial quadriceps expansion is incised. The periosteum is erased from the anteromedial surface of the tibia in the upper end, from where drill holes are to be made.

The Hoffa body fat pad: It is excised, as it comes in the way of vision. The displaced bone fragment of the anterior eminence is located at the distal end of the ACL. Trial reduction with a punch is carried out.

A curved cobbler awl used to pierce the ACL and a 1 mm soft cold drawn wire is threaded through it. In fact, 0.8 mm wire should also do the work as it is more supple and malleable and thus, can be bent and loaded well.

An ACL jig attached and the drill sleeve inserted in its appropriate hole and pressed against the anterior tibia, say, at 5 cm distal to the tibial plateau edge.

The intra-articular tip of the jig is maintained on one side of the avulsed fragment, adjacent to the fracture area. A 2 mm ACL drill wire is inserted through the sleeve. Jig is exchanged with a cobbler awl and one end of the wire pulled down. Similar technique is used on the other side of the displaced eminence. The distance between the holes on the tibial surface should be 10 mm, to have adequate bone in between the two drill holes.

It is also possible to make these two holes by visual judgment, a free hand technique, instead of the ACL jig, using a 3.2 mm drill bit with a drill sleeve.

Prior to pulling down the wire ends, any curves in the bone wire are removed and tensioned manually to prevent any intraosseous bent portion or a loop.

A wire tractor bow is used to gently load the wire and to tie a knot. The load has to be just necessary, unlike that in a fracture of olecranon. This is so, because the anterior eminence bone fragment is thin and small and it has to be just replaced in its crater securely. (Even tensioning the wire ends with two pliers is also adequate). By moving the knee, stability of the fragment is confirmed. Tourniquet is deflated and hemostasis is achieved. On table X-ray is taken, so one can confirm the position of the wire, prior to the wound closure and dressing.

Closure + padded pressure bandage is applied, with knee in 20 deg flexion, so comfortable elevation on a Bohler frame can be given. Pedal pulses are checked.

The limb is elevated on two pillows and later on a Bohler frame. Static quadriceps exercises are begun, which is followed by active knee extension on the Bohler frame. The elevation this way keeps the tissue edema to a minimum, and helps to carryout the quadriceps drill. Since the epidural catheter is in place, CPM machine can be used. This facilitates early restoration of pain-free knee range and prevents knee stiffness as well.

At the end of three days, bedside sitting and active knee extension is encouraged, which is a step forward towards non-weight bearing mobilization. Toe touch weight bearing is permitted at the end of two weeks.

Points to Remember

- Long antero-medial incision
- Excise the Hoffa body
- Thread the wire through the ACL first and then apply the jig to pull down the wire ends (Fig. 34.1A).

Option

Fixation of the fragment by a 4 mm shaft screw is also described. I would prefer the screw direction from backwards to the front. This is so that the screw would be in the same axis as that of the ACL. However, to get this direction of the drill bit and the screw, I find it rather difficult, with a danger of drill bit breakage. The pull out strength of the wire is much more than that of a screw and hence preference for a wire loop (Fig. 34.1B).

Follow Up

- X-ray examination is carried out every month for three months. It is important to prevent any fixed flexion deformity in the knee.
- Active knee exercises need to be monitored, to restore return of full range of motion, which one should achieve by the end of three months.

Future

Having seen breakage of wire loops in fracture patella and in this fracture, I recommend removal of the wire at the end of 4 to 6 months. This needs to be emphasized upon the patient.

FRACTURE OF THE ANTERIOR TIBIAL EMINENCE WITH ASSOCIATED FRACTURE OF TIBIAL CONDYLE

Fracture of the anterior tibial eminence may be associated with fracture of medial or lateral or both condyles. Hence, on clinical examination, one needs to assess, if there is local swelling/ bone tenderness on the condyles. If necessary, an MRI scan is helpful, which may demonstrate a fracture not visible on an X-ray film.

CLINICAL EXAMPLES

Case 2

This lady had sustained a knee injury. X-ray examination revealed a fracture of anterior tibial eminence. However, she had tenderness on the lateral tibial condyle and inability to bear any weight. An MRI was done and confirmed an associated fracture of lateral tibial condyle. During surgery, the eminence was fixed first. This was followed by a screw fixation for the lateral tibial condyle. During making a drill hole, one needs to be careful to plan the direction of the drill and keep the track, different from that of the intraosseous wire, which is inserted first (Fig. 34.2).

Case 3

This patient had a fracture of anterior tibial eminence, fracture of the medial and postero-medial tibial condyle.

He was operated on a quadriceps board. The medial tibial condyle required a medial buttress

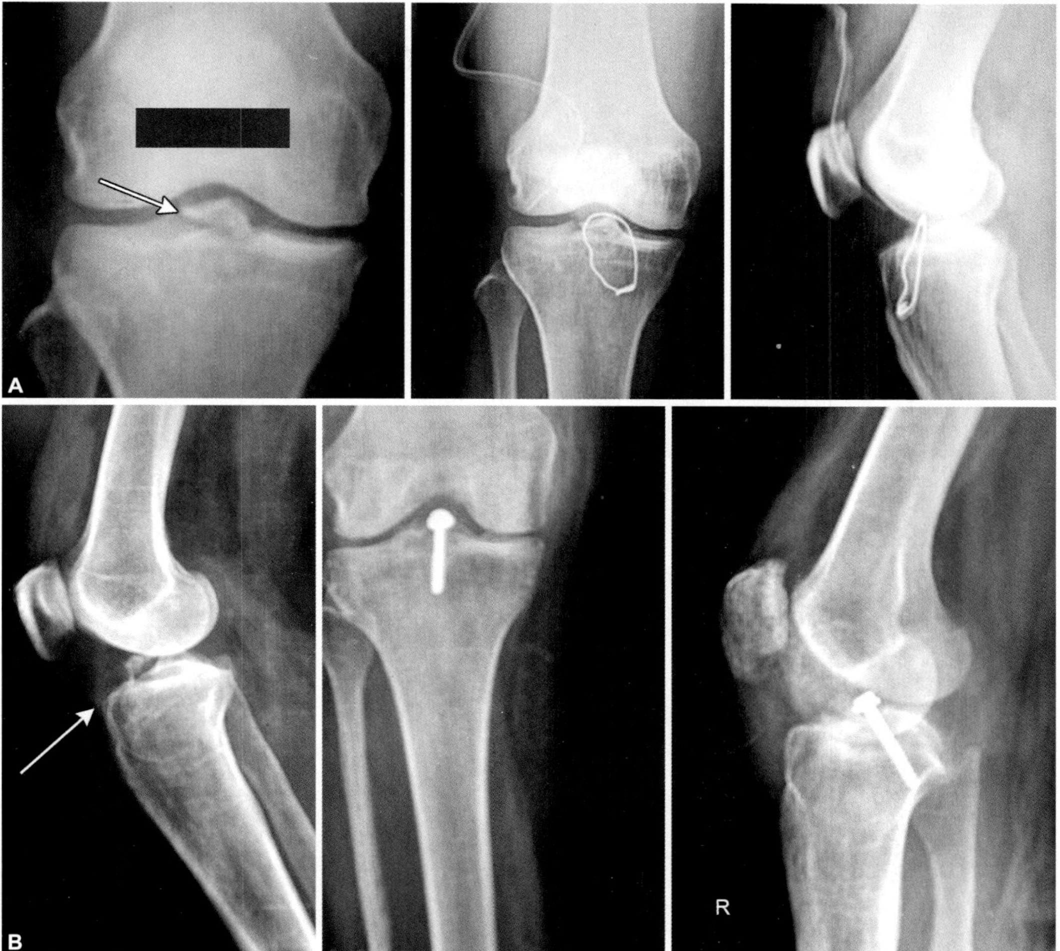

Figures 34.1A and B (A) Anterior eminence fracture; (B) Screw for anterior tibial eminence

plate. Hence, the wire loop was passed from the lateral tibial surface. (The lateral incision being small, blood supply in between skin segments is not a problem).

Then an anteromedial approach was taken. The plateau of medial condyle was reduced and provisional reduction and stabilization of the posteromedial part was done, with a K-wire.

- A 6.5 mm screw was passed from the anterior surface medial to the crest, to fix the posterior condyle.
- From the antero-lateral surface, two drill holes were made and the anterior eminence was fixed, as described above.
- Medially an L plate was fixed to stabilize the medial condyle. The medial to lateral 6.5 mm partially threaded screw was so planned that it would be superior to the AP screw and posterior to the wire loop. Thus the two 6.5 mm screws and the wire loop were in different planes, as seen in the X-ray photo.
- *Postoperative care*: The knee was elevated on a high Bohler frame. Static quadriceps

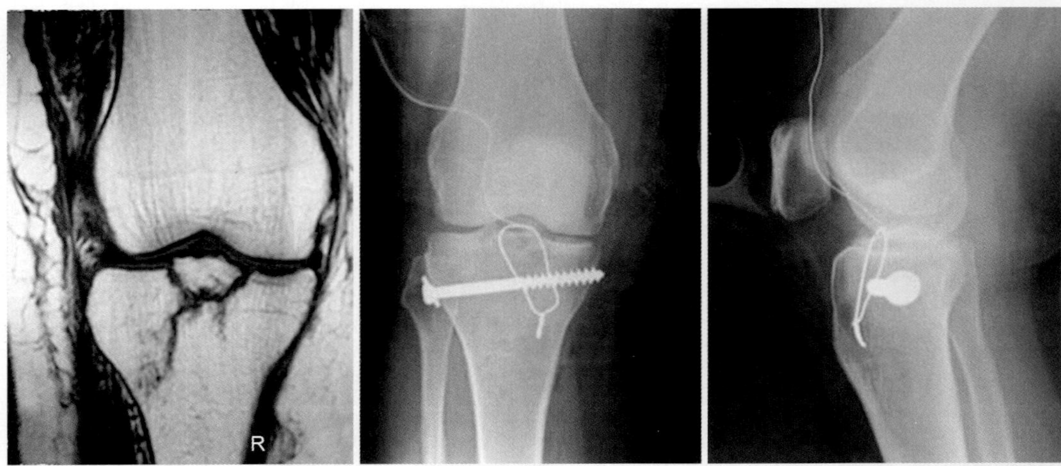

Figure 34.2 Fracture of anterior tibial eminence with a fracture of lateral condyle

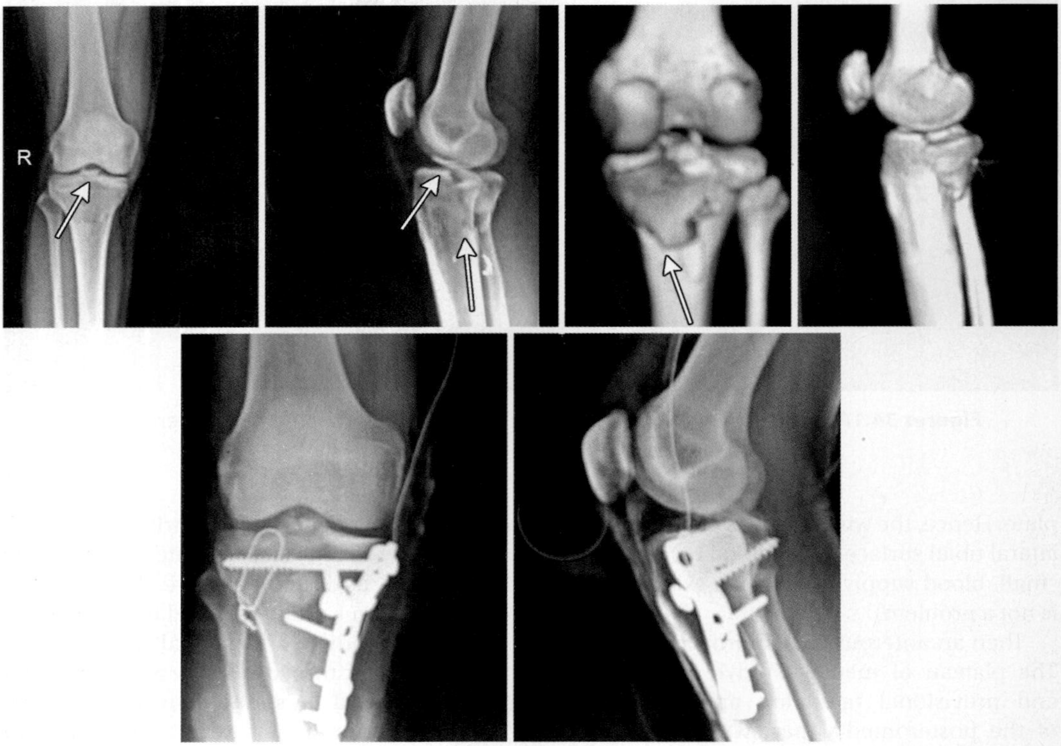

Figure 34.3 Fracture of posterior and medial tibial condyle with fracture of the anterior eminence

exercises and active knee extension was carried out, with a good end result (Fig. 34.3).

Case 4

- The patient had a vertical fracture of *lateral tibial condyle*, with a third fragment and fracture of the anterior tibial eminence. The eminence fracture was stabilized with a wire loop over the medial tibial surface. The bone was locally soft and to prevent wire cut out, the wire ends were threaded through two washers. It is also possible to place a two hole 1/3 tubular plate or a reco plate over

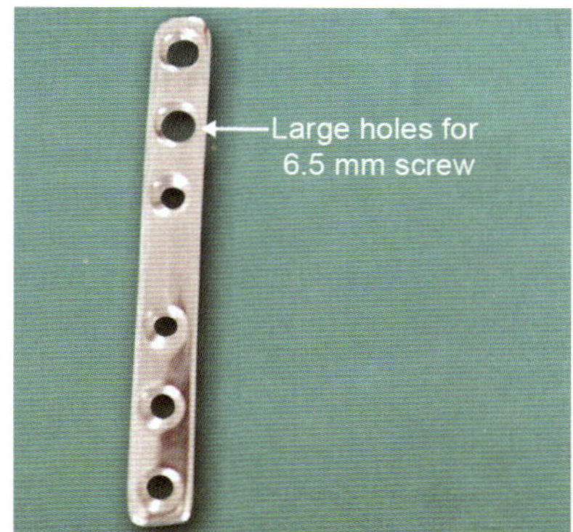

Figure 34.4 Custom-made plate with two large holes for 6.5 mm screws

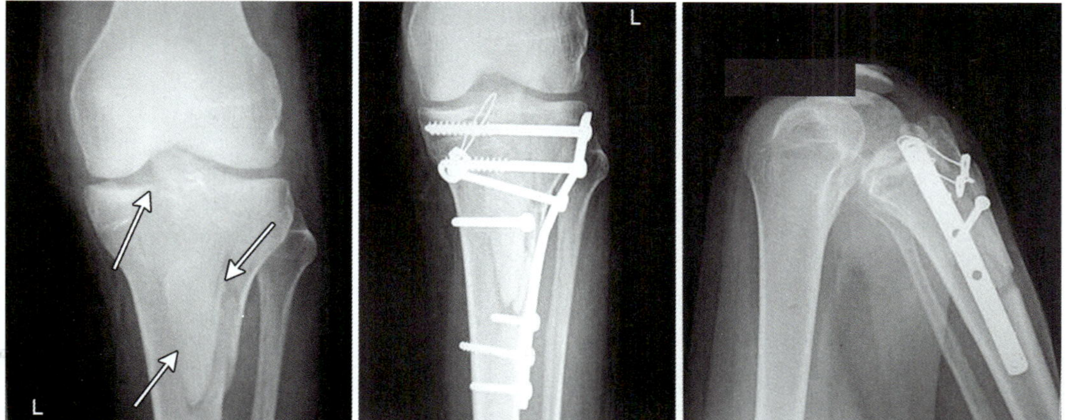

Figure 34.5 Fracture of lateral tibial condyle with tibial eminence

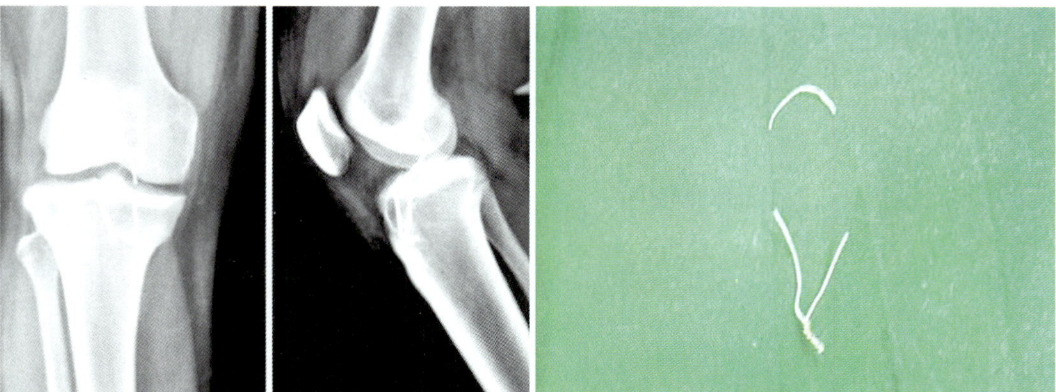

Figure 34.6 A broken wire removal

the two holes, so the wire loop and the knot is over the plate and wire cutting through the bone is avoided.

- Laterally a custom-made 12 mm tibial plate was applied. It was contoured, so that it will fit closely on the lateral tibial surface. The proximal two screw holes in the plate were made adequately large, so, the 6.5 mm screw could be easily passed through them. Use of two 6.5 mm screws at the upper part of the condyle offers more stability (Figs 34.4 and 34.5).

Late Breakage of the Wire Loop

Follow up of every case treated by this method is important. The wire is preferably removed between six and twelve months, from the surgery. This is necessary, as at times, a segment of the wire breaks, separates from the host wire and migrates elsewhere. If it moves away, then to locate it and remove successfully, could be a challenging job (Fig. 34.6).

CHAPTER

35

Fracture of Posterior Tibial Eminence

It is not commonly observed to be associated with fracture of medial and lateral tibial condyle, but seen in conjunction with a fracture of a posterior tibial condyle. In management of multiple fractures, internal fixation of this injury, a prone position is required and hence the timing of surgery has to be appropriately planned.

AN ISOLATED INJURY

The patient may report with a limp, pain and swelling after this injury. The CMO on duty should be aware of such an injury. In an undisplaced fracture, the injury is likely to be missed. If one observes pain during a posterior drawer test and X-ray examination does not clearly indicate the injury, an MRI examination is worthwhile or else the injury may be missed.

Case 1: Undisplaced Fracture of Posterior Tibial Eminence

Treatment in such a case: This middle age lady had a fall from a scooter and could slowly stand and do some weight bearing. X-ray examination raised a suspicion of an undisplaced fracture of posterior tibial eminence and MRI examination confirmed the fracture. The fracture was undisplaced at the end of two days, when she reported for consultation and was already walking about. Hence, the limb was given a padded crepe bandage, a knee brace and was kept off the weight for three weeks. Gradually active mobilization was carried out and toe touch weight bearing permitted. End result—good stability and range of motion (Fig. 35.1).

Late Presentation

This patient reported two weeks after the injury. He was able to walk slowly, without a walking aid and had an abrasion on the patella. Because some weight bearing was possible he reported late.

There was resolving fullness around the knee and posterior drawer test evoked some pain.

X-ray examination showed an undisplaced fracture of the posterior eminence. Since he was able to move about, without any walking aid, a padded crepe was given and was advised to be off the weight for two more weeks. Then gradually partial weight bearing was permitted. Good end result (Fig. 35.2).

In a Case of a Displaced Fracture

Approach and Procedure

One has to get access to the fracture, keeping the neurovascular structures out of harm's way. Hence, it is a good idea to revise the surgical exposure from an appropriate book and pay a visit to the department of anatomy and study

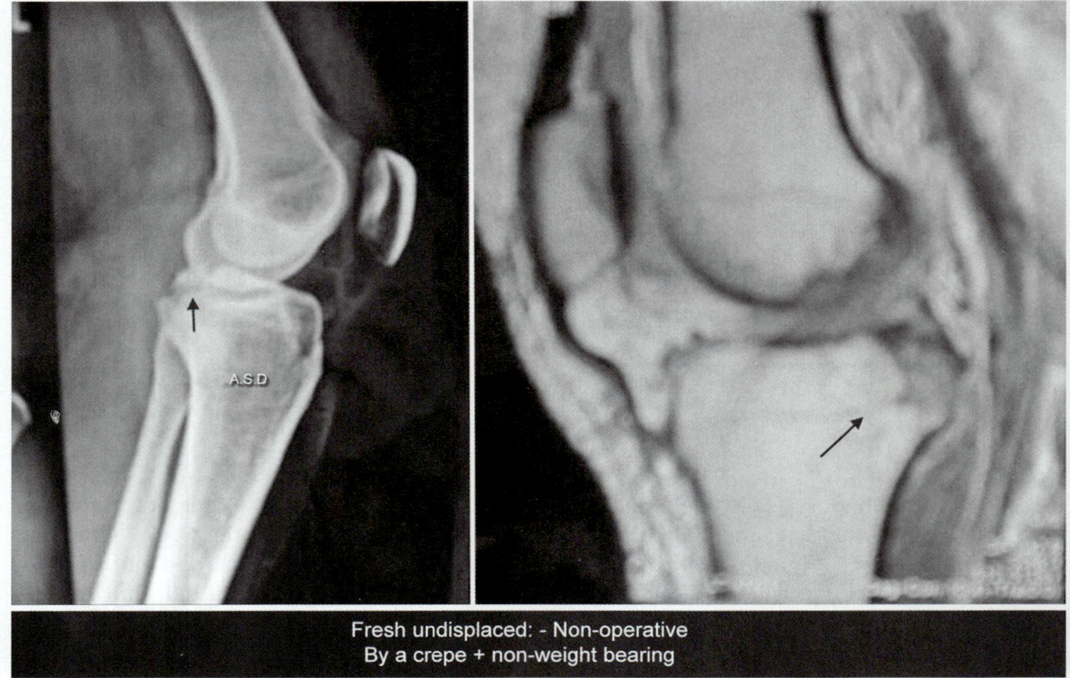

Figure 35.1 Undisplaced fracture of posterior tibial eminence

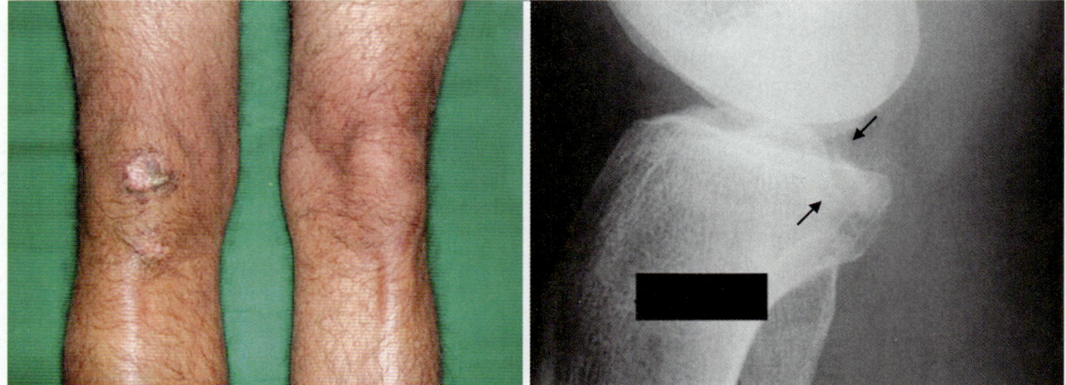

Figure 35.2 Late presentation

the anatomy in a specimen as well. This gives a 3-dimensional idea about various structures and as to how, one can keep the important structures safe.

Patient Position

In a prone position a small pillow is kept under the ankles, which helps to keep the knee flexed to 15 degrees. A pneumatic tourniquet is used and the surgeon stands on the side to be operated.

The posterior transverse crease as is seen during the surgery is 15 mm superior to the anatomical joint line and hence the incision has to be accordingly placed. Locating the posterior cutaneous nerve of the calf and the short saphenous vein helps to proceed further. The standard approach has been a lazy S shape approach, with the superior vertical limb on the medial side. The medial head of the gastrocnemius is erased and moved laterally, which in turn, protects the neurovascular structures. After fixation of the fracture, the medial head of gastrocnemius has to be reattached and the knee needs to be immobilized for three weeks, so the muscle reattachment is strong enough.

(After practising this technique in a few cases, one can expose the area by a different method).

A transverse incision is taken 15 mm inferior to the joint crease and is *extended distally on the medial* side for 10 cm. The skin flaps are raised. The deep fascia is incised close to the midline and the belly of the medial head of the gastrocnemius is well palpated. Incising the deep fascia near the midline offers good access to the medial surface of gastrocnemius and also it can be better retracted laterally. One clears the medial surface of the belly and with knee flexed, can lift it posteriorly. By a careful blunt finger dissection, one can reach the midline area of the popliteal fossa. Presence of fracture hematoma helps to lead to the fracture area. If in doubt, one should not hesitate to deflate the tourniquet, so one can well-palpate the

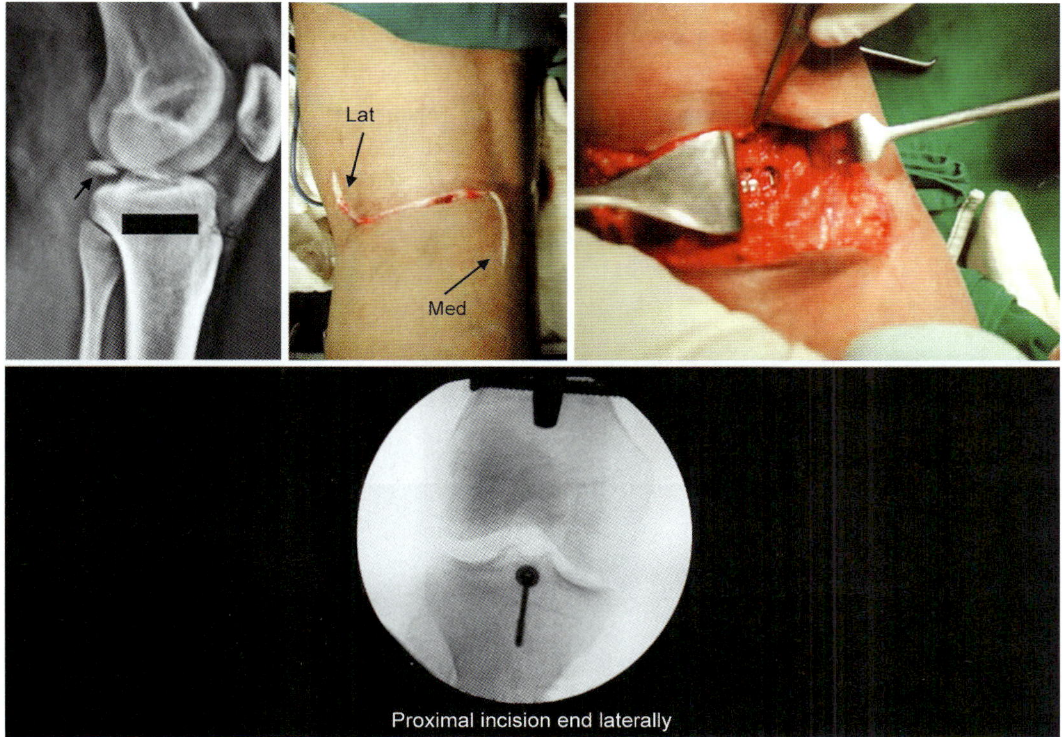

Figure 35.3 Lateral end taken superiorly

popliteal artery. A knife should be sparingly used and a finger and a scissor dissection is a safe method. A medium size Hohmann bone lever inserted on the medial tibial surface helps to keep the soft tissues well medially and use a Langenbeck retractor to keep the medial head towards the midline.

Having thus exposed the fracture fragment, the hematoma in the fracture surface is cleared and the fracture is reduced and kept so with a punch. Using a 2.5 mm drill with a drill sleeve, a track is made in the displaced fragment and for a cm in the parent bone. The drill bit is changed to a 1.8 mm K-wire and further drilling is done with it. Thus the track created in the cancellous bone is adequate enough to accept a 4 mm shaft screw, which has a good purchase in the bone. The K-wire is removed and a (usually a 50 mm) 4 mm shaft (partially threaded) screw with a 7 mm washer is inserted and just tightened, finger tight only. Thus the posterior cruciate ligament is reattached to the shaft of the tibia. The proximal end of tibia has a good strong bone. One may be tempted to drill the anterior cortex of the tibia, to have a good fixation, by passing the tip of the screw, across the anterior tibial cortex. However, one should not attempt to do so. The drill bit tries to enter the hard anterior cortex at an angle and invariably breaks! In fact, because the proximal tibia has strong cancellous bone, a screw inserted for 50 mm has adequate hold (Figs 35.3 and 35.4).

If the fragment is large, it is reduced and kept in place with a punch, and a K-wire is inserted, at a place, where a second screw can be inserted and adequate area is available for one more screw. Adjacent to the K-wire, a 4 mm screw with a washer is passed and the K-wire is later replaced with another screw with a washer. Thus, the large fragment is well-stabilized by two screws (Fig. 35.5).

Multiple Fractures in a Limb

This case had a basilar fracture of neck of femur, an ipsilateral fracture of the shaft femur, with a

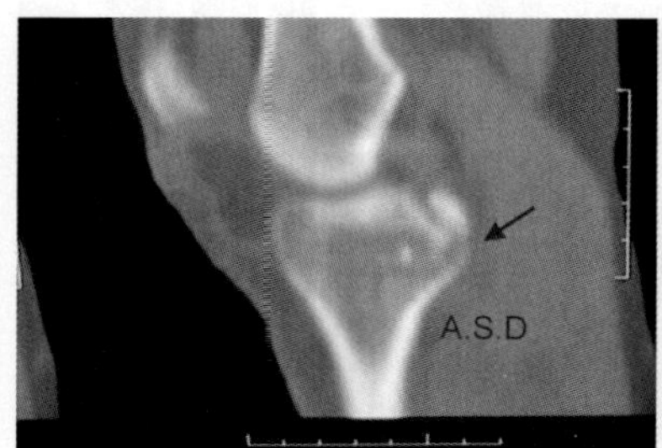

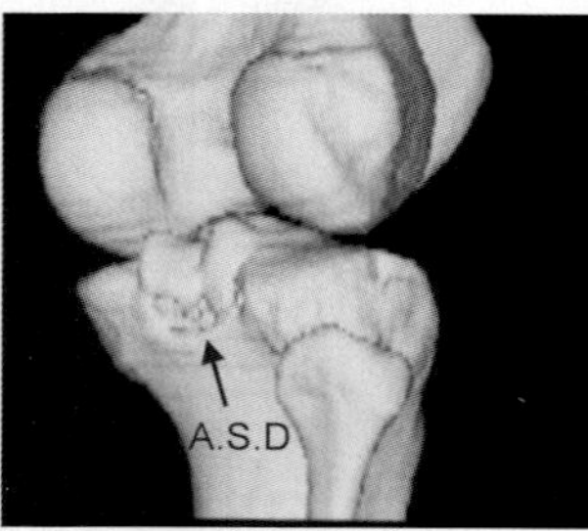

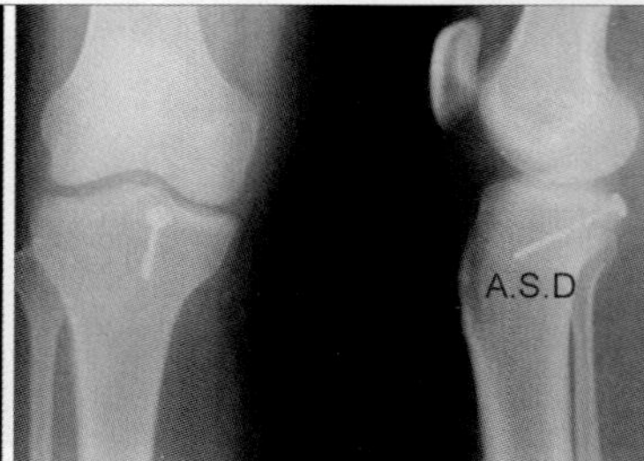

Figure 35.4 1 screw

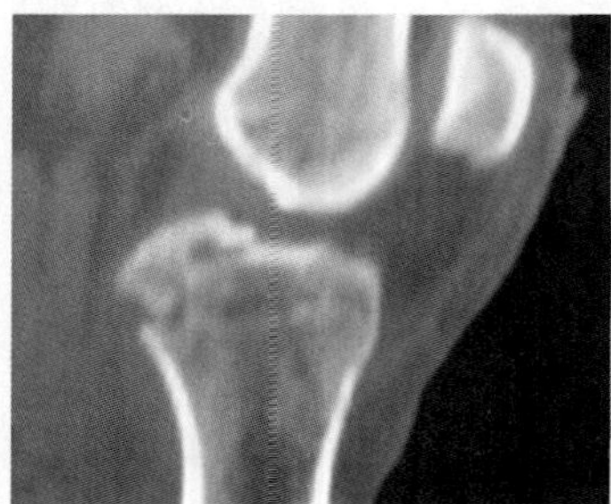
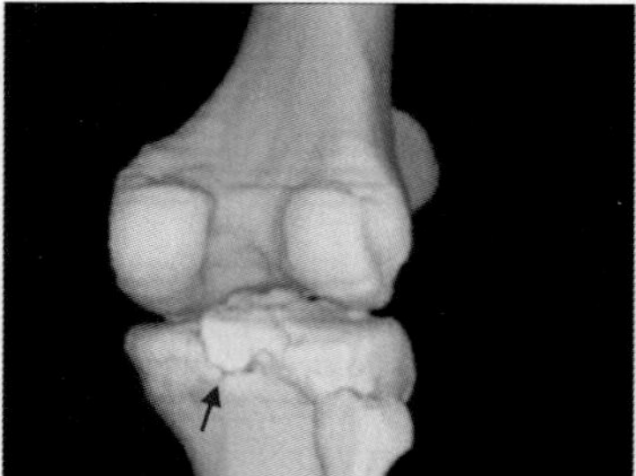
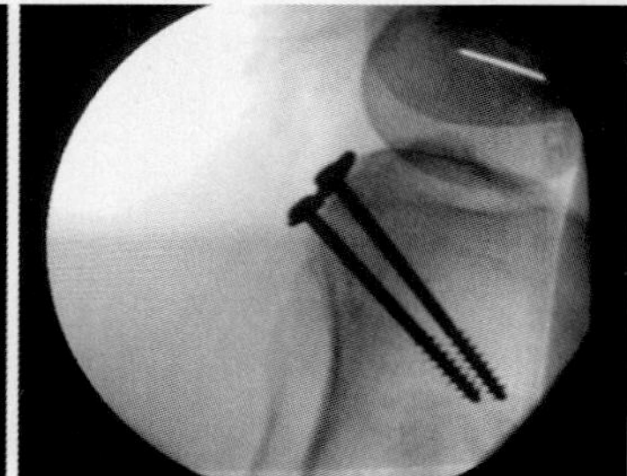

Figure 35.5 2 screws in a large fragment

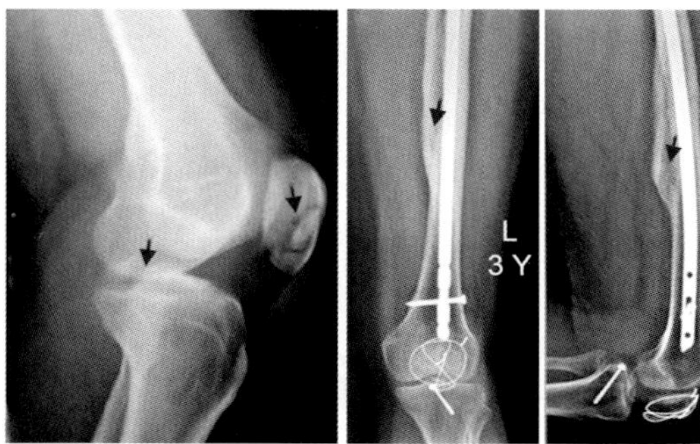

Figure 35.6 Multiple fractures in a limb

3rd fragment, a fracture of patella and fracture of the posterior eminence of the tibia. He also had a Barton fracture of lower end of the radius.

On day 1, an antegrade femoral nail was inserted and patient made supine. The patella was stabilized with a circlage and a figure of 8 loop and the Barton fracture stabilized with a buttress plate. Thus the three fractures were stabilized on day one. After a few days, when he was stable, the posterior tibial eminence was fixed. Good end result with complete restoration of the function (Fig. 35.6).

CHAPTER

36

Fractures of Tibial Condyle

INTRODUCTION TO THE FRACTURE OF TIBIAL CONDYLE

In a crowded city two-wheel vehicles are in large number. The traffic is very dense and often undisciplined. Hence, injuries of tibial condyle are in a large number.

A variety of morphological types are seen. The spectrum is from an undisplaced fracture to a severe fracture dislocation.

I have illustrated examples, which would convey the message and make management easier for the reader.

Fracture of either a medial or a lateral condyle alone, fractures of both the condyles, with or without associated dislocation, make the spectrum very wide and hence the description as per any method of classification difficult. Case illustration should be able to pass the message in a variety of morphological types, in terms of diagnostic problems, first aid and definitive method of management found useful and hence recommended.

It is also observed that, apparently for no fault of the patient, he or she gets an injury and becomes irritable. Often the advice given to the patient is not accepted by him or her, which leads to delayed return of function of the knee and the limb. Hence a good and detailed dialogue with the patient and the members of the family is essential. Often, in addition to a good quality X-ray examination by taking the necessary views, MRI examination is required, to diagnose, if one has a fracture. In a case where the fracture is obvious, the extent of injury, the degree and the type of a depression, is known, only after a CT scan, with a 3D reconstruction. Such a diagnostic procedure helps to plan the treatment and to help to restore an early and close to full return of knee function, considering the initial injury.

In a severely displaced fracture (as in an ankle injury) often emergency closed reduction, padded crepe support and appropriate immobilization in a plaster support or a Thomas' splint or a temporary external fixator is necessary. This relieves the discomfort and prevents likelihood of development of edema and blisters in the area. In case of an internal degloving injury, it is prudent to carry out an emergency closed reduction and wait, till the local skin and soft tissue condition is optimal to carry out a definitive procedure of internal fixation. This is especially true in a patient with diabetes, which needs good pre-operative control of diabetes. In the illustrated case of associated diabetes and vasculopathy, it was necessary to wait for a few days (Fig. 36.1).

If one studies cases, which had wound dehiscence, discharging sinuses in the post-operative period, or infection, often one finds that:

- Adequate first aid like immediate closed reduction, crepe application and plaster

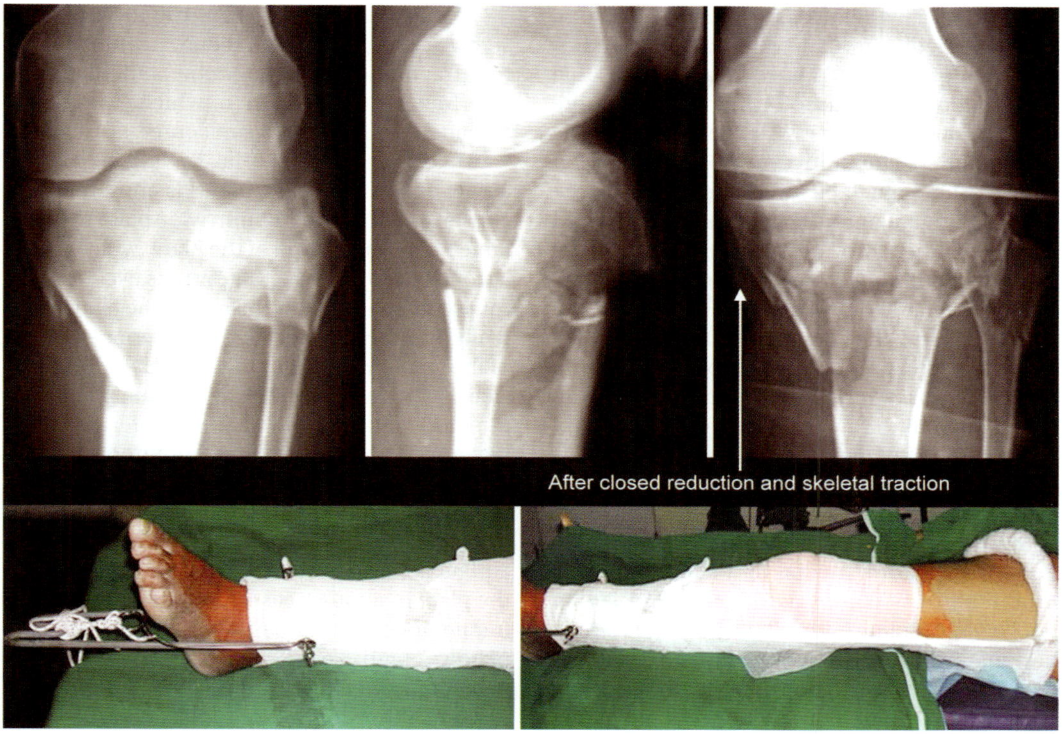

Figure 36.1 Diabetes and fracture of tibial condyle. First aid with Thomas' splint and skeletal traction

immobilization was not done and purposeful delay for surgery was not done, for the soft tissues to recover.

- Definitive internal fixation was carried out, when the limb skin condition was not optimal.

If an immediate closed reduction, application of a pressure support, necessary immobilization was carried out, followed by elevation of the limb for adequate period and then carried out the surgery, the incidence of complication would have been much lower and manageable (Fig. 36.2).

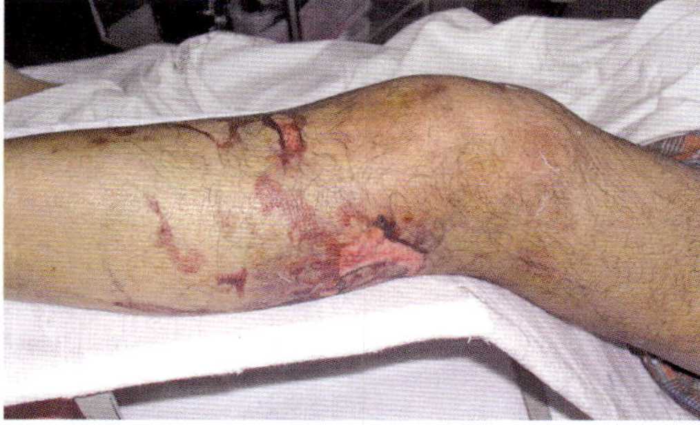

Figure 36.2 Skin injury and edema

FRACTURE MORPHOLOGY AND SITE OF FRACTURE

A fracture just below the condyle, cannot be well-immobilized by external support alone, as with a plaster cast or a Thomas' splint. This is due to various muscle attachments to the bone fragments, which tilt the fragments. Hence, without any consideration of non-operative method, one should proceed with internal fixation (Fig. 36.3A).

Postoperative analgesia is possible with an epidural medication and should be offered. A wide range of Bohler frames should be available for elevation of the limb. A high Bohler frame offers about 60 degrees of knee flexion in the immediate postoperative period. If one can control the pain, active mobilization of the knee is possible at this stage, leading to a good return of knee movements. In cases, where use of a continuous passive motion machine is desirable, it should be used. Training of the ward staff and the therapists goes a long way for a satisfactory outcome. Compared to the hip or ankle, restoration of a good range of motion of the knee, is very necessary in personal and professional life (Fig. 36.3B).

Innovation in Plate Design

For a fracture of a medial or a lateral condyle, L or T buttress plate was designed. Of late, a hockey shape plate and locking plates of various designs are available. For enhancing stability IF. Screw is necessary for the upper part of the condyles. In a L or T shape buttress plate, one has two holes on the transverse limb for 6.5 mm screw. At times, one has to insert the screw at an angle to the plate, to be entirely intra-osseous and be at right angle to the fracture line. This may result in having the screw head slightly more prominent, which is acceptable.

In a locking plate design, the locking head screw being fully threaded, cannot offer interfragmentary compression and necessary interfragmentary stability, which a partially threaded 6.5 mm screw can confer.

In a fracture of medial or lateral condyle alone, one of the above plates is chosen. I have chosen and modified 12 mm wide plate with two large holes on one end of the plate, which would accept 6.5 mm screws. This permits use of two 6.5 mm screws, one below the other. The plate width being less, the required anteroposterior exposure of the condyle on either the medial or the lateral side, is also less. The thickness of the plate is 3.8 mm and enhances the stability conferred by the plate. The plate is not precontoured and one needs to do so on table, as per the morphology. An option would be to contour the plate, prior to sterilization and keep a few plates ready. If a plate is not used in a given case, one can use the plate in another case. Changing the contour frequently, is not to be done, as it reduces the plate strength. Few examples of such plate are illustrated and are self-explanatory.

Here the middle plate is so designed that the two holes on one end would permit easy passage of a 6.5 mm screw. It can also be passed at some angle, as per the direction of the fracture line (Fig. 36.4).

In a fracture of either a medial or a lateral condyle, use of only this plate is adequate.

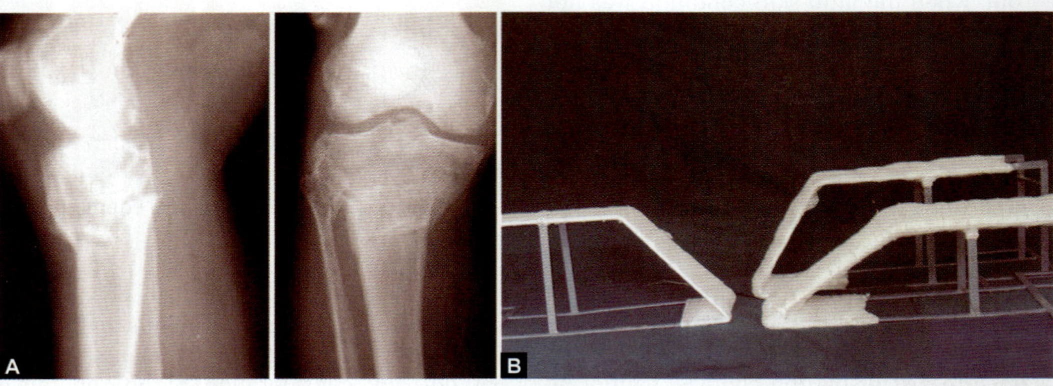

Figures 36.3A and B (A) Must do internal fixation; (B) Bohler frames of various designs

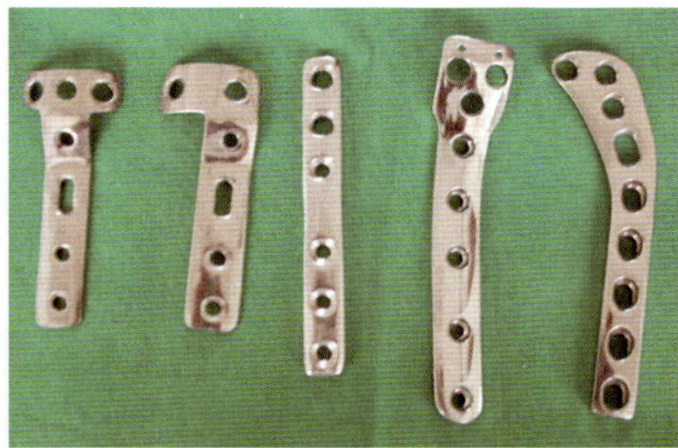

Figure 36.4 Plate design

However, in a bicondylar fracture, where two plates are necessary, this plate applied on the medial condyle, confers adequate stability. The load on the medial column being more, this plate, if used medially, enhances the stability of the construct.

The conventional 'L' shape plate is used for lateral condyle. In small frame Asian persons, the available plate needs excess erasing the soft tissue on the bone rim. Hence a custom-made plate with short transverse limb is useful (Figs 36.5A and B).

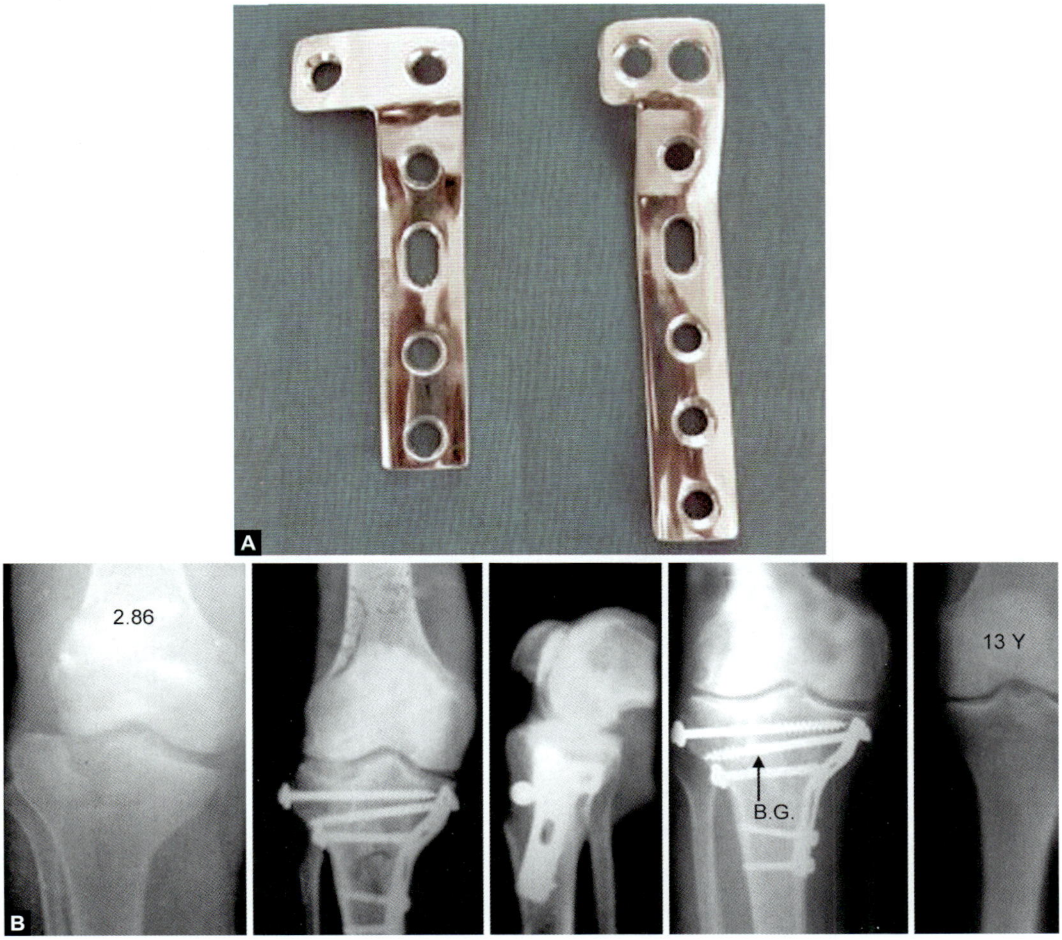

Figures 36.5A and B (A) Plate with a short transverse limb; (B) Early case

THE INCISION FOR A GOOD EXPOSURE

For adequate access to the proximal tibia, a T shape incision was used in early years. However, it had problem of skin edge necrosis and was not extensile (Fig. 36.6).

For an isolated medial or a lateral condyle, a vertical incision on appropriate side is adequate.

For fixation of a bicondylar fracture, where both sides of condyle need to be approached, a generous midline incision is satisfactory. The flaps need to be thick. The closure and wound healing is usually uneventful.

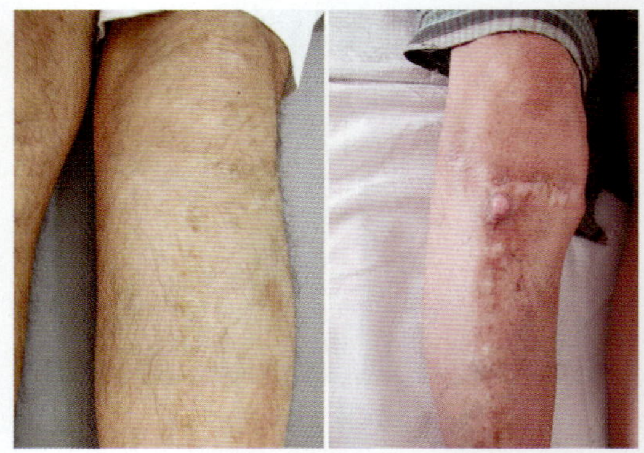

Figure 36.6 T-incision

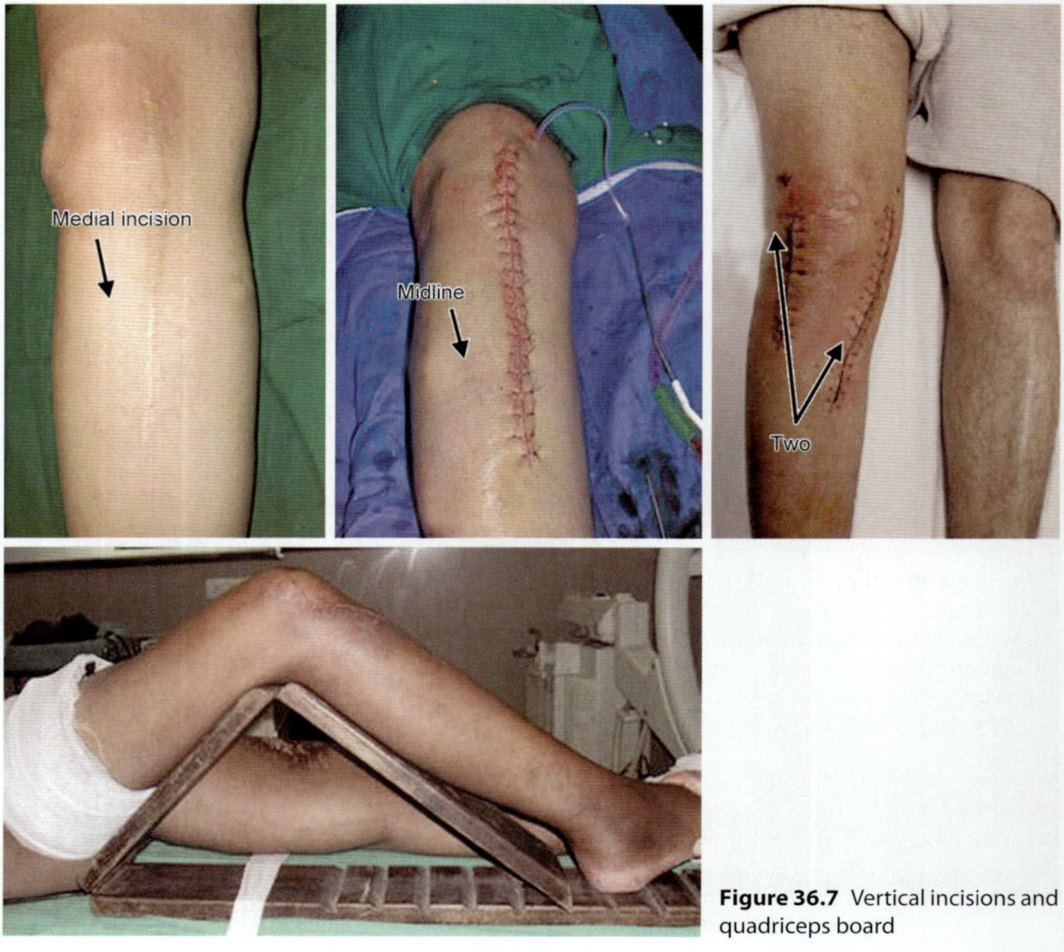

Figure 36.7 Vertical incisions and quadriceps board

In a situation, where one needs to have access to a fracture on either side of the condyle, the distance between the two incisions should be more than 5 cm, so that the blood supply is well-maintained, to the area in between the two incisions.

Use of a quadriceps board offers a comfortable position for the surgeon, so access to either side of the condyle is possible and the knee angle can be adjusted as per the need. Being of wood, use of a 'C' arm is also possible (Fig. 36.7).

Implant Removal

In a young and middle age persons, it is recommended that the plates and wires (for the tibial eminence) be removed, usually 12 to 18 months after fracture consolidation. This:

- Restores the bone elasticity
- Should there be another injury, adjacent to the fracture of condyle, its management is easy
- If the implants are not removed within this period and there is need to remove them at a much later date, the removal of all the implants may not be successful. Late removal of surface implant, leads to more stress shielding and its restoration is rather slow, at that age.
- With advancing edge, restoration of the stress shielding effect takes much more time and may be incomplete. This is especially troublesome, should joint replacement is required at a later age.
- It is observed that the bone wire around the anterior tibial eminence, breaks even after fracture union and the wire pieces may migrate anywhere around the knee. The wire segment may migrate towards the posterior compartment and its retrieval could be a difficult procedure (Figs 36.8 and 36.9).

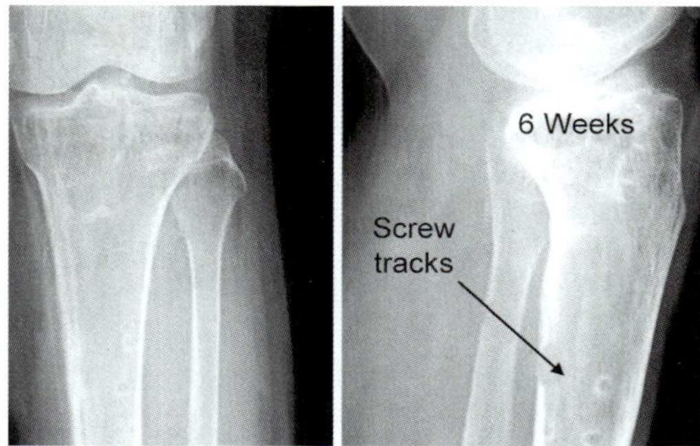

Figure 36.8 After a plate removal

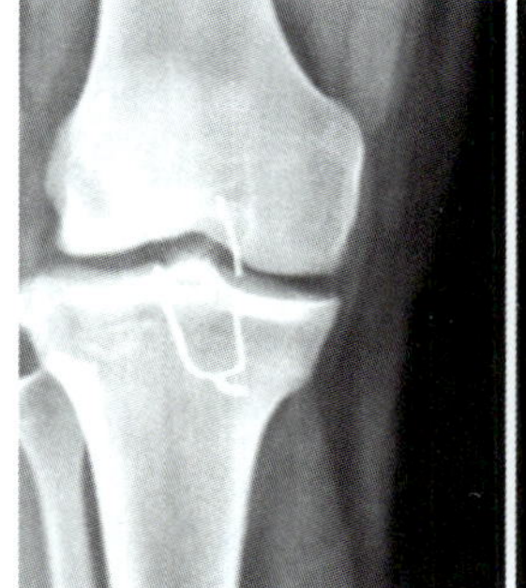

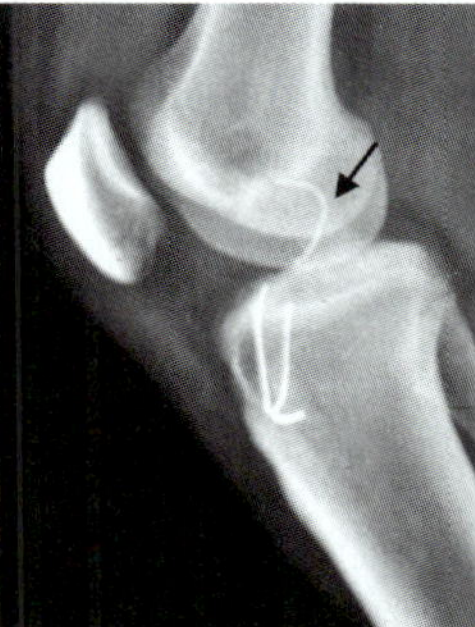

Figure 36.9 Wire migration

FRACTURE OF TIBIAL CONDYLE IN A NEUROPATHIC JOINT

This young man presented with a disorganized left knee joint. He had a fracture of medial tibial condyle and a surgeon had done fixation with cannulated cancellous screws. The fracture failed to unite (Figs 36.10 and 36.11).

Soft Tissue Loss around the Knee

A case with severe injury to the knee with soft tissue loss, needs to be managed carefully. After wound excision and necessary care, minimum internal fixation to align the fragments with complementary external fixation saved the limb. A rotation of a flap, offers a mobile and supple cover for the knee, which does not breakdown, like an adherent scar (Fig. 36.12).

BICONDYLAR FRACTURE OF TIBIA

A bicondylar fracture of the tibia may be associated with subluxation of one condyle.

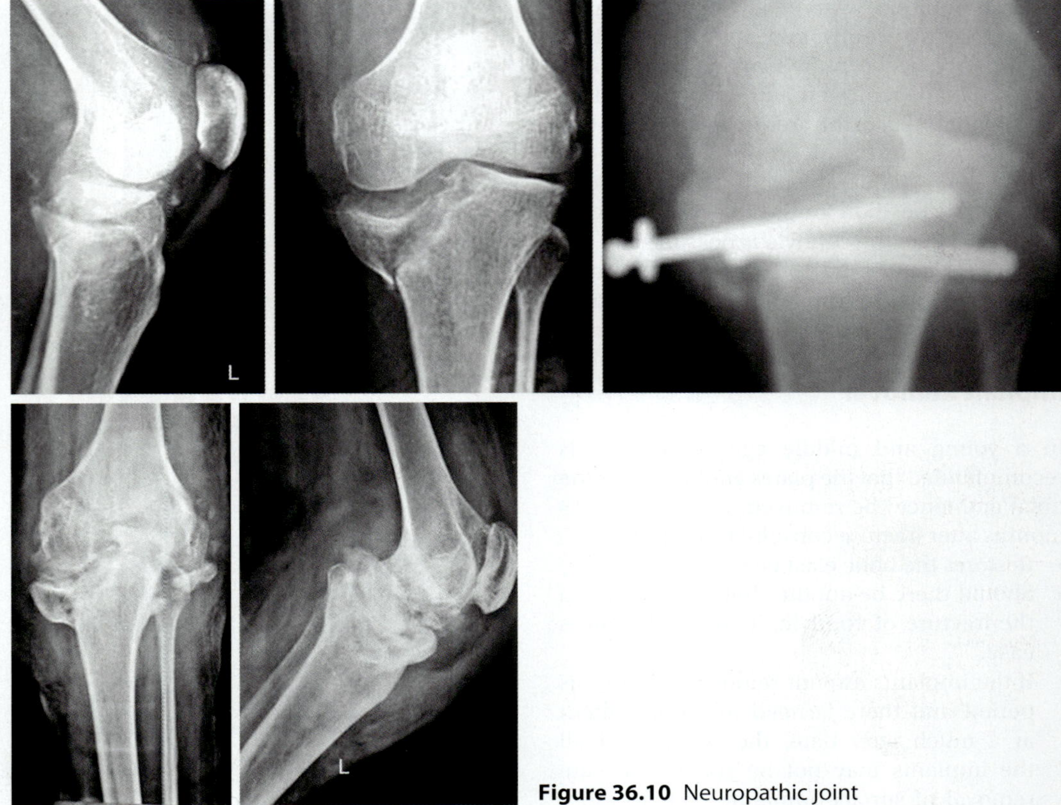

Figure 36.10 Neuropathic joint

This often leads to crushing or extrusion of the eminence area. All such injuries need immediate closed reduction, padded crepe bandage and above knee plaster slab, followed by elevation of the limb. This restores the venous drainage, the cartilage nutrition of the displaced fragments and skin blood supply. If this procedure is not followed, often troublesome local edema and perhaps development of blisters is a common observation.

Being an intra-articular injury in a weight-bearing area, anatomical reduction, a stable fixation and early mobilization help to achieve nearly the preinjury function.

In the last two decades evolution has occurred in the exposure technique and plate design leading to a better outcome.

CASE EXAMPLES

Case 1

Tri-radiate or a star shape approach was recommended in the initial stages 30 years ago. However, at times, difficulty in the wound closure and edge necrosis was seen. In due course of time a midline long vertical approach was found suitable for access to both the condyles, permitted a wide exposure and had very little skin flap problems (Fig. 36.13).

Case 2

In a bicondylar fracture, the medial plate fixation is the most important. A well-contoured medial plate stabilizes the fracture

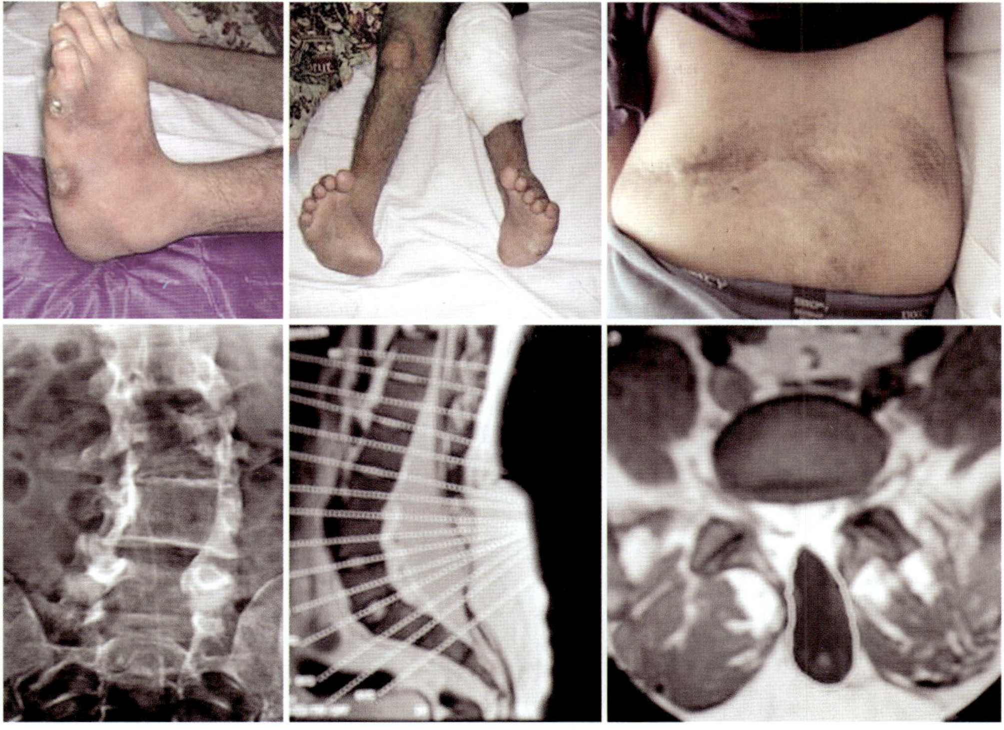

Figure 36.11 Neuropathic joint

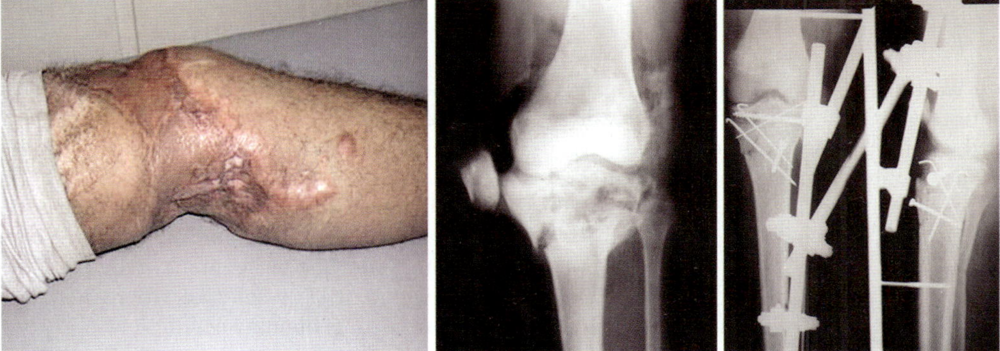

Figure 36.12 Skin loss around the knee

far better and restores a good limb alignment.

The conventional 'L' plate, T buttress plates with different contours have been recommended since early 80's. The transverse limb has two large holes, which accommodate 6.5 mm screws. Still, in some cases, often it needs to be further contoured, so that it fits well on the proximal tibia.

Thirty years ago, when operative method for these injuries was thought of, the L and the T

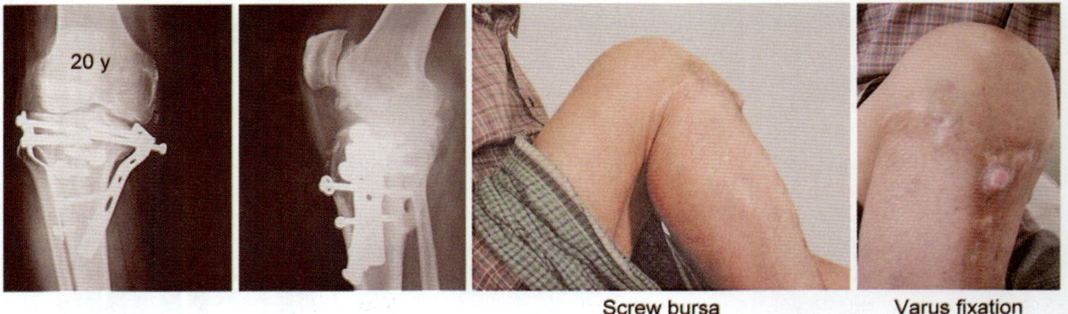

Figure 36.13 Tri-radiate incision (Early days)

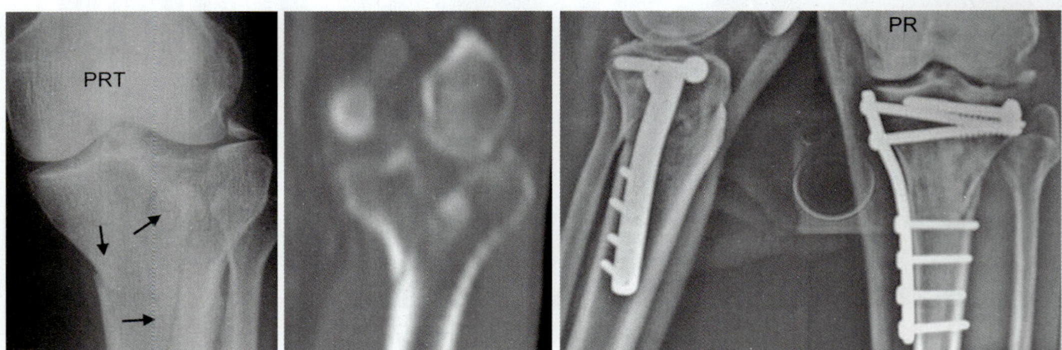

Figure 36.14 Evolution in medial plate fixation

plate were used. Besides, the 'C' arm facility was not available. As the 'C' arm, quadriceps board were available, the speed of surgery, the accuracy of implant placement, etc. remarkably improved (Fig. 36.14).

Case 3

I have used a 12 mm narrow tibia plate (used in the past for shaft of tibia) and found it offers good stability and strength for the fixation. It has only the end hole large enough to accept a 6.5 mm screw. I have made two end holes large to accept such a screw. This permits insertion of 2 × 6.5 mm screws, one below the other. However, both the screws cannot be at the subchondral area, to offer a stability to an elevated depressed and impacted segment. In addition, I have designed different types of plates, in terms of different lengths and different central span distances. It permits its use in various types of fractures.

The advantage of such a plate: Often a screw hole needs to be left void, if it comes over a fracture line. Such a segment of the plate tends to be a potentially weak spot, where mechanical failure of the plate may occur.

In a fracture where medial condyle is displaced and the lateral condyle is nearly in place, one should use the 12 mm plate medially. The 6.5 screws through the plate holes, would adequately stabilize the lateral condyle as well and lateral exposure can be avoided.

In some cases, where there is *a fracture of medial condyle and a depressed fracture near the eminence—*

OPTIONS POSSIBLE

Option A

Elevate the depression in the central area via a window made in the lateral surface, insert bone grafts and apply a medial 3.8 mm straight plate medially. 2 × 6.5 screws inserted through the upper two holes, lag both the condyles. Additional another screw from the lateral condyle towards the medial, below the plateau confers additional stability.

Disadvantage: One needs to expose the lateral surface as well, to make a window, to elevate the depressed fragment.

Option B

Make a window medially only, elevate the depressed segment, add bone grafts and apply a medial plate. This would avoid additional lateral exposure. However, one needs to take the plate little longer, because one may have to leave one or two plate screw holes unused, over the window made to elevate the fragment (Fig. 36.15).

Case 4

Displaced Medial Condyle and Undisplaced Lateral Condyle

A custom-made plate with square head plate permits 3 × 6.5 mm screws in the subchondral area and offers good stability and early mobilization. At the border of the proximal square part, holes are available for insertion of 1.8 mm K-wires, which offer stability for the provisional reduction. Thereafter, the fixation can be rapidly completed (Fig. 36.16).

Case 5

A Split Bicondylar Fracture

The fracture was a split fracture, in both medial and lateral condyles, without any depression. Hence with a midline incision, both the condyles were exposed. The fracture line and the adjacent area were cleared of any interposition and were reduced with a reduction forceps. Medially a 12 mm wide with 3.8 mm thickness plate was applied. Laterally, a 2 mm thick, and

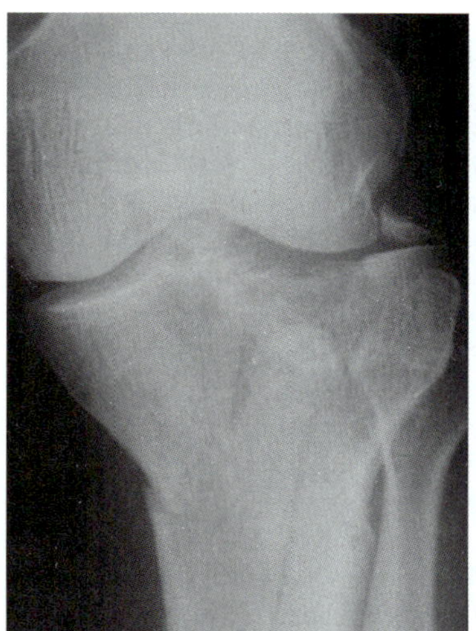

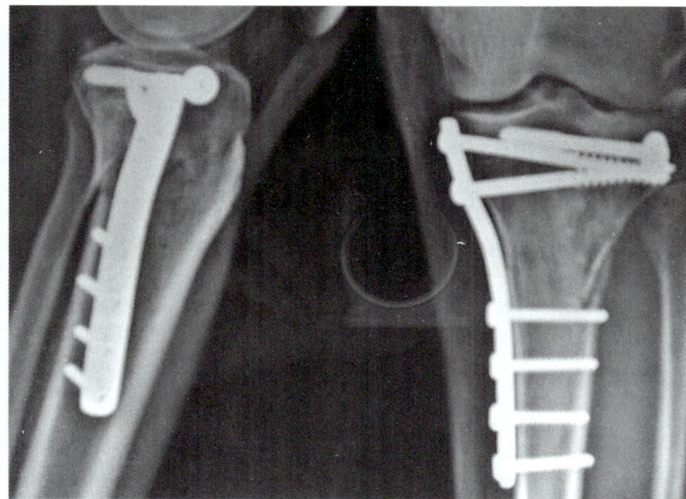

Figure 36.15 Elevation of depression and a medial plate

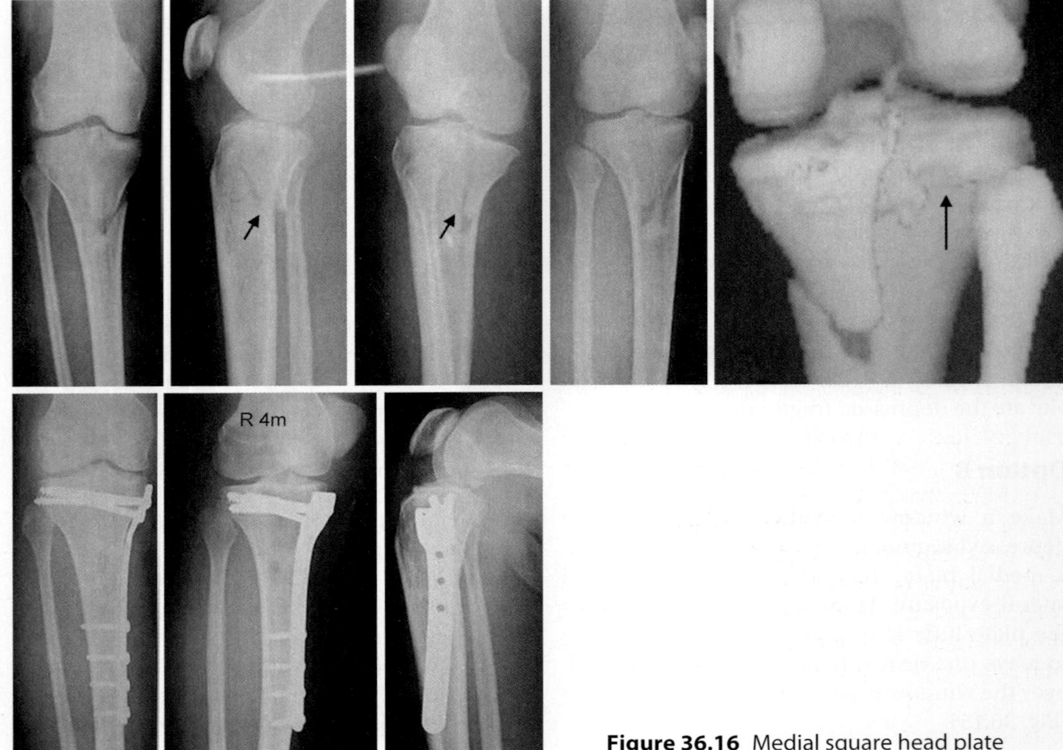

Figure 36.16 Medial square head plate

10 mm wide plate was applied. This plate being thin, can be well contoured.

Medially there is a 3.8 mm plate and hence, in a bicondylar fracture, laterally such a 2 mm plate is adequate.

Steps in Screw Fixation

- The medial plate is more important part of fixation.
- The plate is kept on the medial surface and contouring confirmed.
- A 1.8 mm K-wire is inserted through the upper most hole, as if the final screw is inserted and is confirmed under 'C' arm. Additional K-wire is also passed, through a hole at the edge of the plate.
- The second screw from the distal end is fixed. This screw anchors the plate to the bone.
- The upper most hole K-wire is replaced with a 3.2 mm drill bit, and a drill hole is made. Screw length is taken with a depth gauge and a 6.5 mm screw with 16 mm threads is inserted. As one is completing this screw fixation, one can visualize that the medial and the lateral condyles are well opposed and stable. Thus two screws are holding the reduction and the medial plate.
- At this stage, One can complete the medial plate fixation and then proceed with the lateral plate OR fix the lateral plate with two end screws and then complete the medial plate fixation. I may prefer the second option, because its proximal end hole 6.5 screw will further enhance the stability.
- When such two plates are applied on either side of tibia, the screws—
  - In the distal portion of the plate need to be unicortical. This so, because a long bicortical screw may abut against a screw inserted from the opposite side. The

direction of screws is posteromedial for the lateral plate screws and posterolateral for the medial plate screws and not towards transversely towards each other. Still, preferably the drill hole be made unicortical.

- If a drill bit collides with opposite screw it may break and hence this precaution (Fig. 36.17).

Case 6

Bicondylar Fracture with Depression of Lateral Condyle

Patient had a bicondylar fracture with a central depression in the lateral condyle. The depression was well seen in a CT scan.

A generous long midline approach was taken and thick flaps were raised. Through a window in the antero-lateral surface the depressed fragment was elevated and bone grafts were laid down. Medial and lateral plates were applied and good stability was achieved (Fig. 36.18).

Case 7

This young man had a bicondylar fracture with multiple fragments in the shaft, extending till the lower/3 of the tibia. The lateral condyle had a split fracture and an impacted area with lateral dislocation of the condyle. Immediately after arrival a closed reduction was done and a padded crepe, plaster back slab and elevation was carried out. Calf was tense and was watched for compartment syndrome. We had to wait for six days for the tissue reaction to settle down.

Through a midline approach full thickness flaps were raised, for exposure on either side. The central depression was elevated and grafted. A medial 12 mm plate and few IFS from the lateral side and outside the plate, offered good stability. Continued elevation on a high Bohler frame, helped to keep the reactionary swelling to a minimum. A CPM machine was used for early restoration of motion.

Though the anatomy was well-restored, he continued to have FFD of 15 deg, which settled in due course (Figs 36.19A to C).

Case 8

A Segmental Medial Fracture in a Bicondylar Fracture

On the medial side, there was a segment of bone, which had to be bridged by the medial plate.

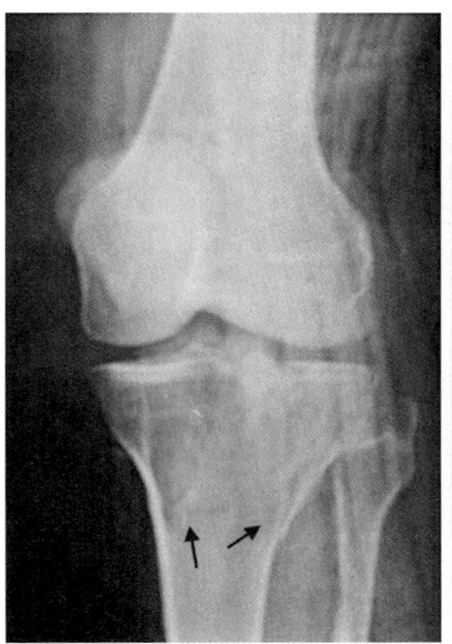

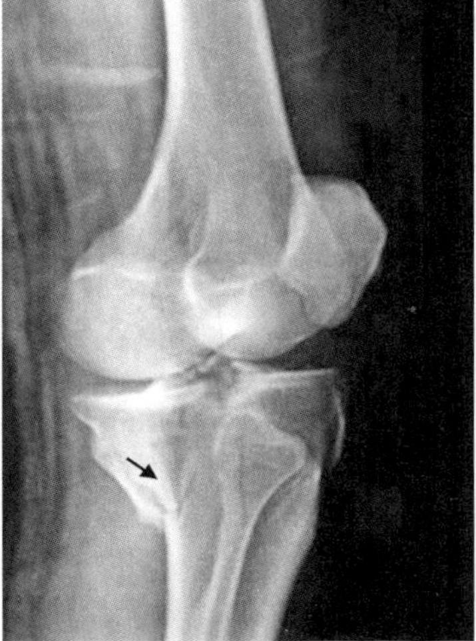

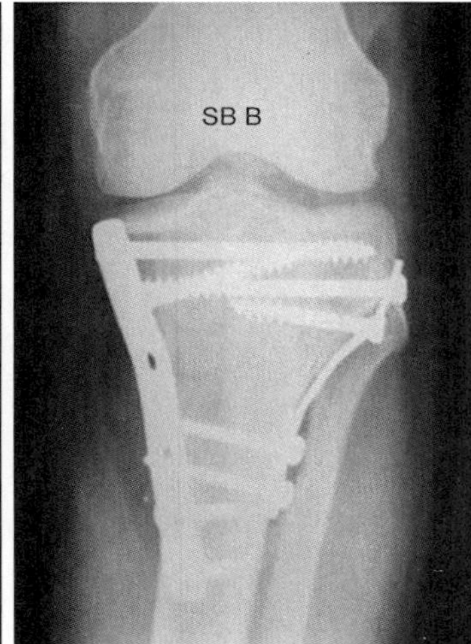

Figure 36.17 Dual plate fixation

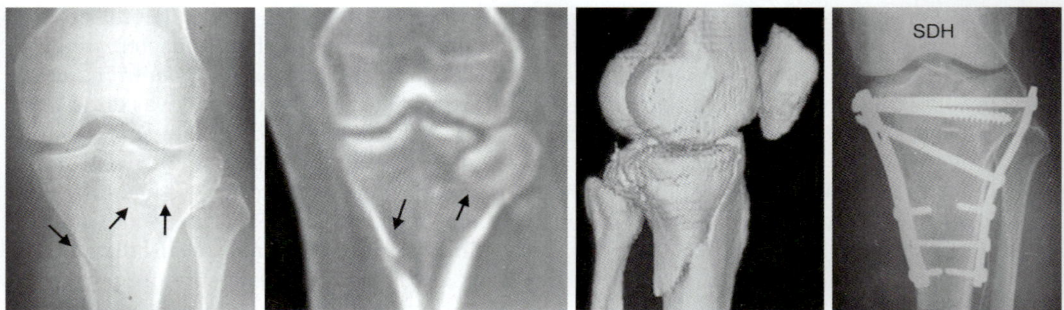

Figure 36.18 Elevation of the depressed segment and medial and lateral plates

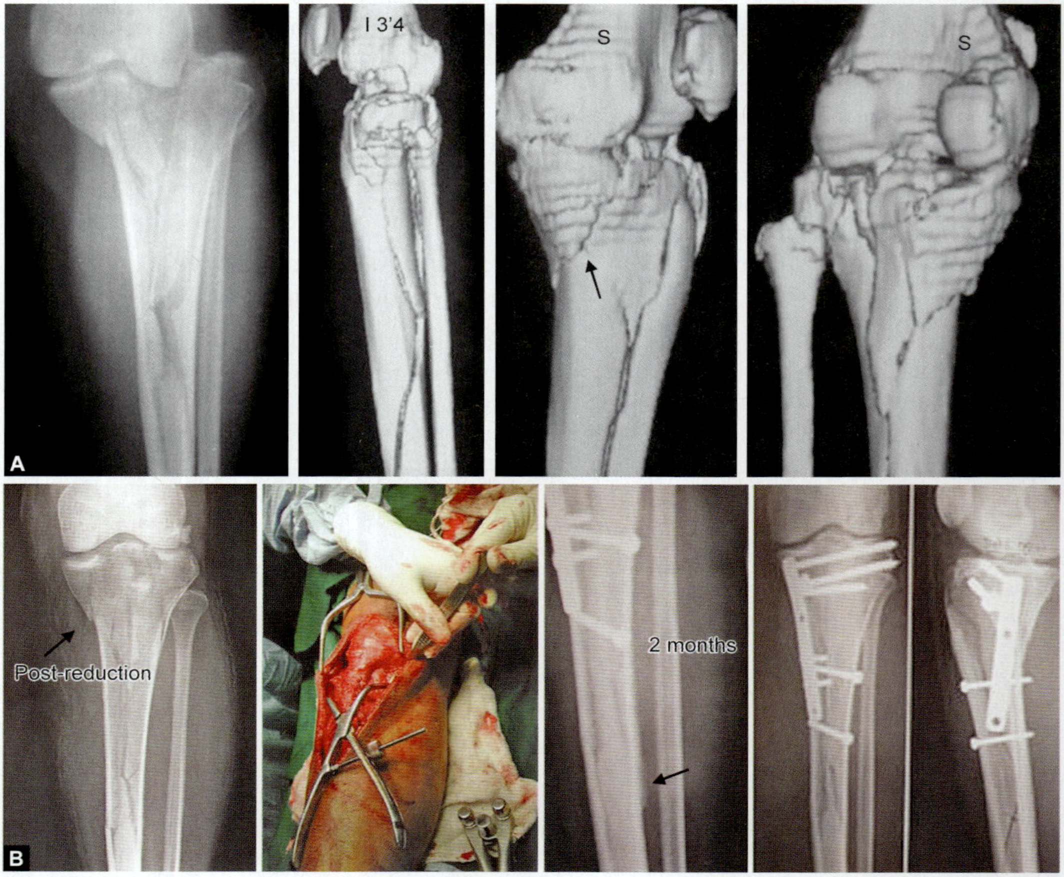

Figures 36.19A and B (A) Bicondylar fracture subluxation, with a long medial fr line; (B) Intra-operative

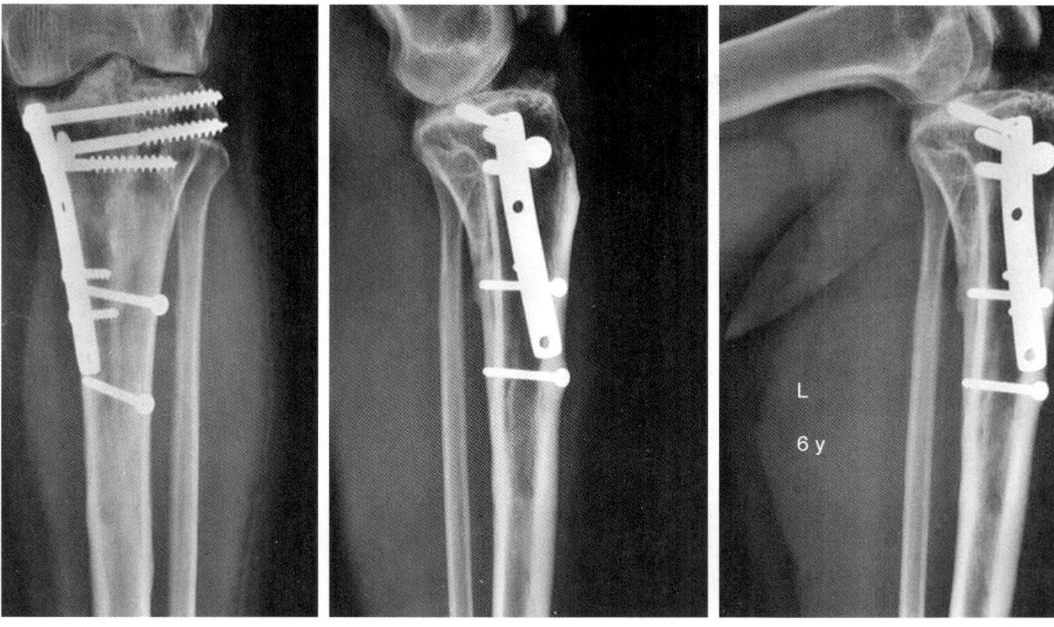

Figure 36.19C 6-year result

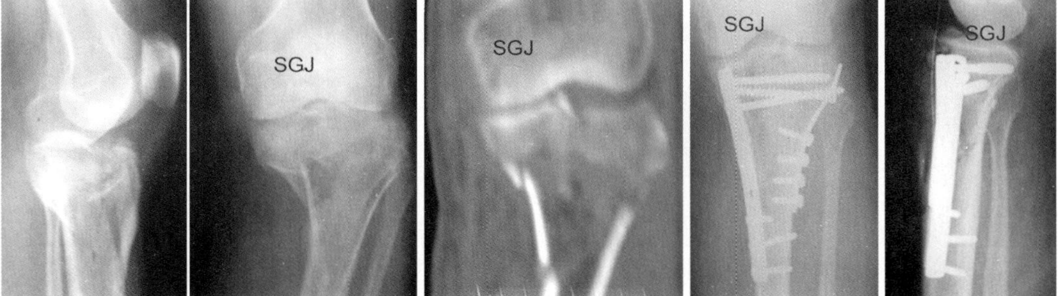

Figure 36.20 Medial and lateral plates

- Elevation of the depressed lateral condyle
- Medial 12 × 3.8 mm plate
- Lateral 10 × 2 mm plate fixation was carried out.

Medial plate had to be long enough, to have three screws beyond the segmental fracture fragment. Since the middle fragment had a good soft tissue attachment and hence blood supply, no screw was inserted in it. The entire proximal tibia consolidated well, with a good outcome (Fig. 36.20).

Case 9

This case of a bicondylar fracture with depression of lateral condyle was managed by elevation of the depression, bone grafting and a lateral plate fixation. Medially a short plate was applied, as the fracture was undisplaced. 'C' arm appearance and X-ray taken on table was satisfactory, with good restoration of the plateau. Postoperative leg elevation and mobilization was carried out, as per the protocol. Clinical follow up showed good range of motion. However, long term X-ray revealed that a part of the lateral condyle showed depression again. Reviewing the lateral X-ray indicated that if the uppermost screws were inserted in divergent mode, they may have supported entire segment of the elevated fragment (Fig. 36.21).

Case 10

Avoid Only a Lateral Plate in Bicondylar Fracture

In a bicondylar fracture, a medial plate is of prime importance. Physiological weight passes more through the medial side and hence a medial buttress plate is mandatory. It supports the medial column well and has major role in preventing a varus deformity. The lateral plate also contributes to the stability, but the load it has to transfer is much less.

In this case only a lateral hockey plate was applied, by a colleague, resulting in a varus deformity. Illustrated cases above have shown that a medial plate alone can stabilize the proximal tibia well. In the given case, In this fracture geometry, both medial and a lateral plate are required. However, even if only a medial plate was applied, it would have maintained the limb alignment and prevented the varus deformity.

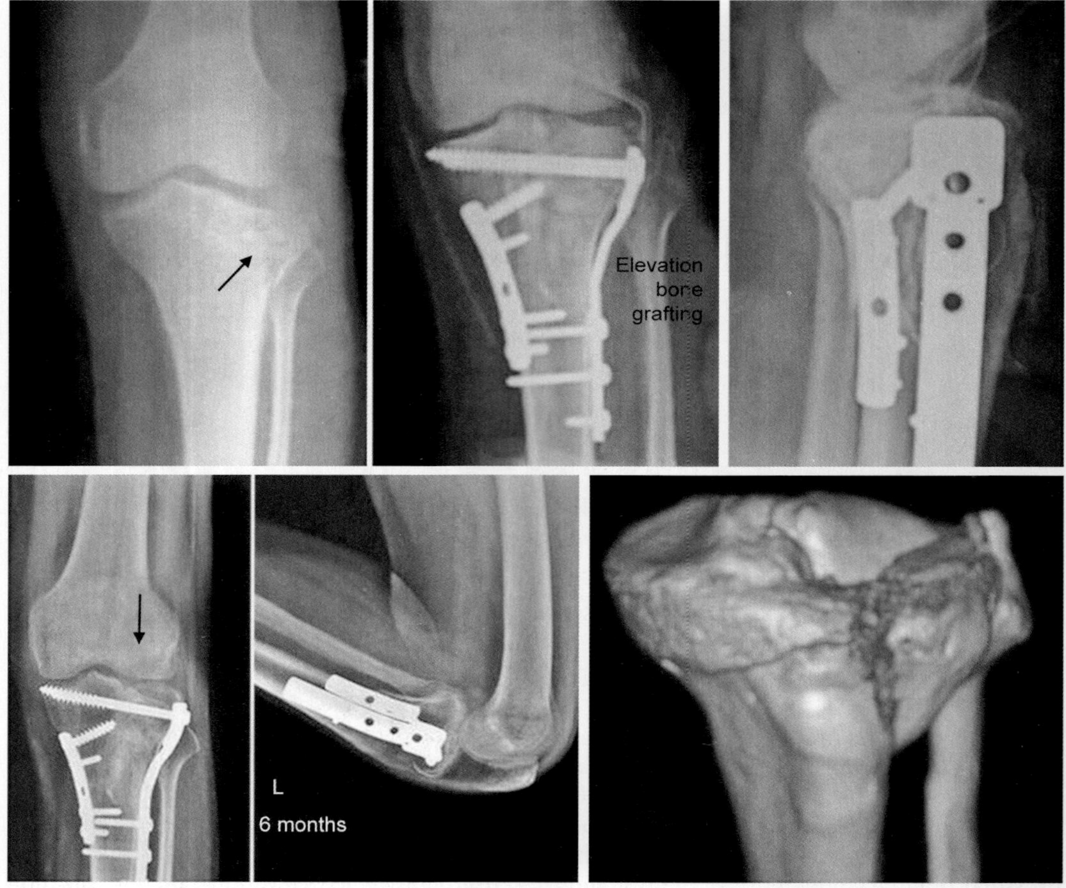

Figure 36.21 Late collapse

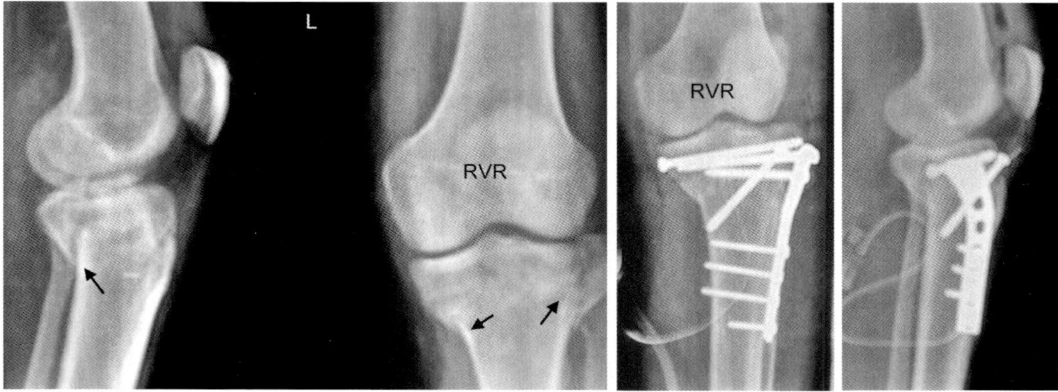

Medial plate less likely to cause varus

Figure 36.22 Lateral plate alone

Time and over again, one comes across such cases, where only a lateral plate is applied, where the medial plate is biomechanically more important (Fig. 36.22).

Case 11

In this case of displaced fracture of lateral condyle, there was an undisplaced fracture on the medial side. The lateral plate offered good stability. To offer stability medially, a tension band wire was applied over two screws with washer and offered a good result. It is important to understand that the tension band wire loop confers stability, only when it is fixed in a figure of eight manner and not as a circlage. Besides, a figure of eight loop forms acute angle around the screw and less likely to slip out. This medial TBW can be practised in an exceptional situation, where the medial column stability is quite good.

In still a rare situation, one should know a possibility that the screws inserted from the lateral side, above and below the medial surface fracture, may be kept 2 to 3 mm long and over the second last threads, the TBW loop can be added and loaded (Fig. 36.23).

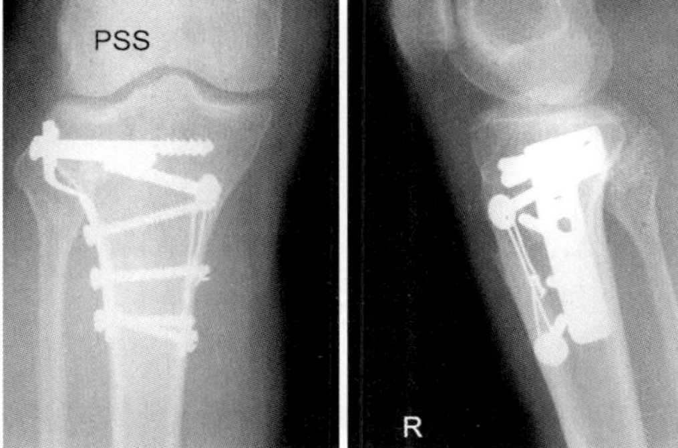

Figure 36.23 Medial surface TBW

Case 12

An elderly lady, with osteoporosis, sustained a fracture of both condyles. A locking plate was planned, to prevent avulsion of the screws and the plate. However, to confer interfragmentary compression, a 6.5 mm screw with partial threads was used. The assembly was neutralized by 3.5 mm LCP system. Good end result (Fig. 36.24).

Case 13

This elderly lady with diabetes had sustained a fracture of neck fibula and a bicondylar fracture. Associated fracture of neck of fibula, adds to the instability. A medial T shape locking plate was applied. This plate has an advantage that, a middle screw is so directed, that it leads to the apex of the lateral condyle and stabilizes it well. Though, the tips of the screws appear to be very close, there is no danger of breakage of the drill bit. This is because the direction of the screws is predetermined and do not cross pathway of adjacent screws, in the same plate (Fig. 36.25).

Case 14

In this young man with a bicondylar fracture, a medial plate with two 6.5 mm screws was applied. A lateral to medial subchondral screw enhanced the stability.

In an attempt to pass, a 3rd screw from the medial side, the drill bit hit one of the screws and gave way. It was made from austenitic steel, we expected that there would not be reaction to it and was left as such (Fig. 36.26).

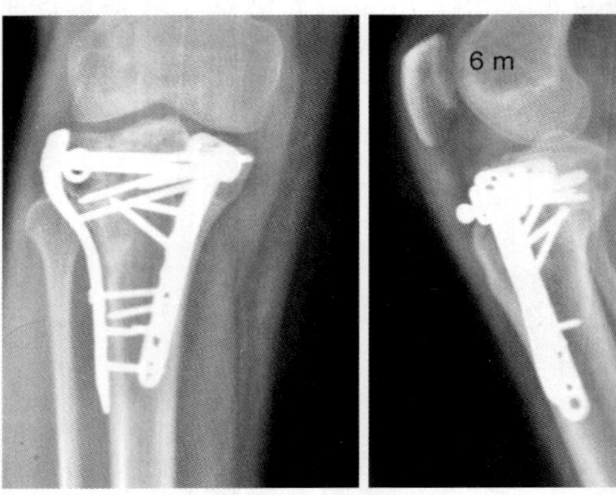

Figure 36.24 Medial and lateral LCP

Case 15

This gentleman over the age of 80 years had sustained a fracture of the proximal tibia and was at home, without any treatment for two months. Due to age and disuse, had local osteoporosis. CT scan defined the injury.

Both medial and the lateral condyles were stabilized with locking plates. Patient had dementia, confusional state and was uncooperative. Hence, a plaster cast immobilization was given. Was followed up well. However, he succumbed to some unrelated illness (Fig. 36.27).

Case 16

This elderly lady presented with some problem unrelated to the earlier knee injury and gave

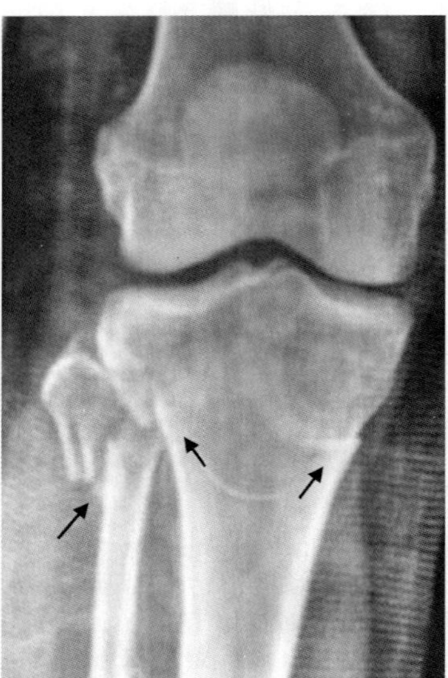

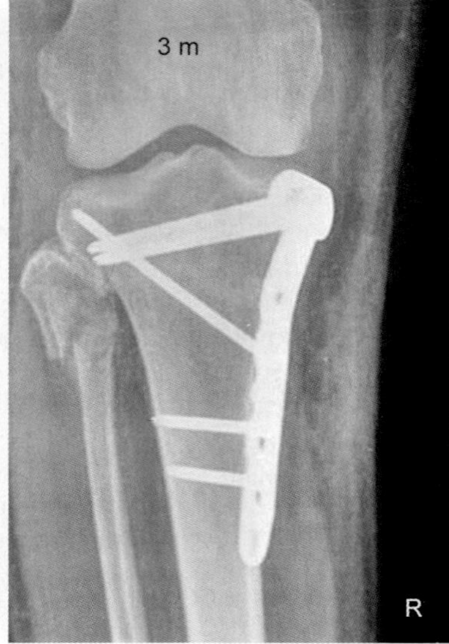

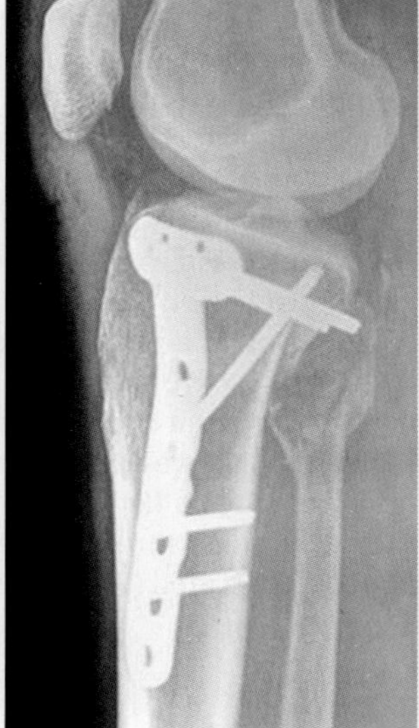

Figure 36.25 Medial locking plate

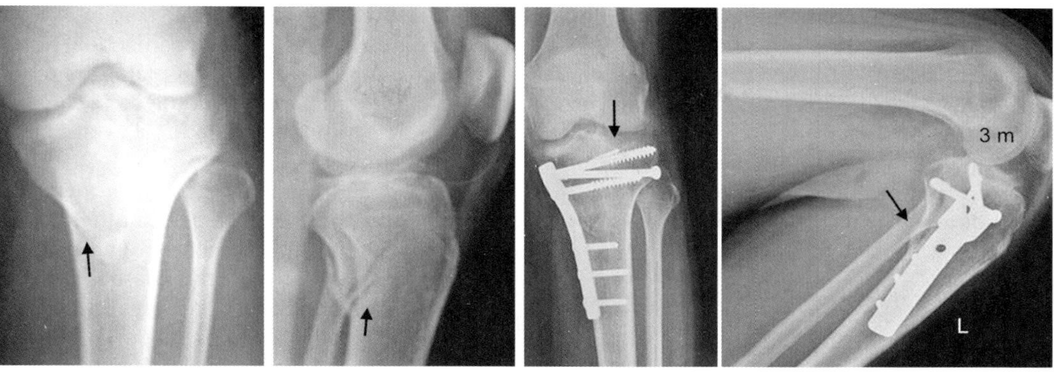

Figure 36.26 Broken drill bit

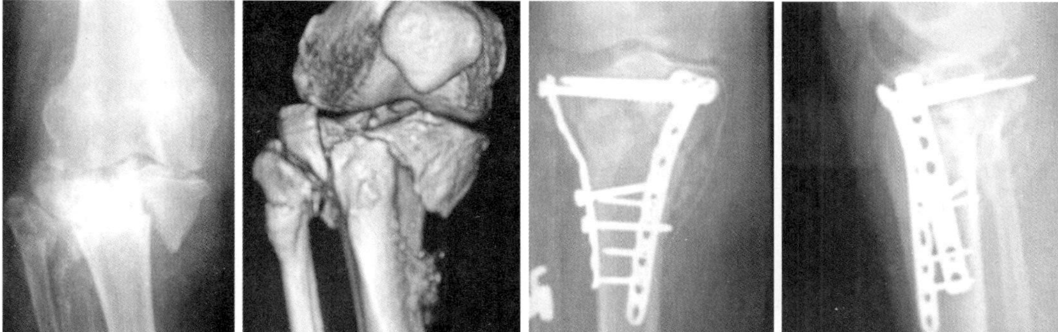

Figure 36.27 Osteoporosis and LCP

history of a knee injury. Having gone in details, I learnt that she had sustained injury to the tibial condyle and was managed elsewhere. The day 1 X-ray film was not available for study. As per information given by her, after the knee injury, she was operated and it resulted in a valgus deformity. May be later developed arthritic changes and the joint was replaced by another surgeon.

One thus learns the importance of restoration of limb alignment, while treating a fracture of proximal tibia (Fig. 36.28).

CHOICE OF A PLATE FOR FRACTURE OF TIBIAL CONDYLE

In the last few years, precontoured locking plates for the proximal tibia are available. The cost may be a constraint, to use it in each case. Besides, it is also important to understand the principles of using a non-locking plate in this site. Once one understands it, then use of a locking plate would be easy.

In internal fixation of a fracture of tibial condyle and nearby area, one needs to have a plate which will accommodate 6.5 mm screw at one end of the plate. 6.5 mm screw has partial threads of 16 and 32 mm length. Being a shaft screw, it exerts interfragmentary compression well.

The conventional T or L shape plate has two such holes on the transverse limb and when 6.5 partially threaded screw is used in IFS mode, a stable fixation is achieved (Fig. 36.29).

In management of a split fracture of a condyle, I have modified a 12 mm narrow straight plate. The plate thickness is 3.8 mm and acts as a good buttress plate, on medial or lateral side.

- Two holes on one end of the plate are made wider, to accept a 6.5 mm screw in each hole.
- Usually after using two holes in the plate, often the fracture line is under the 3rd hole and this hole needs to be kept void. This tends to make the plate strength rather less at this point. (This is especially true in fixation of a diaphyseal fracture, where a hole needs to be kept unused). Hence, plates are made with more span in the middle area. One has to choose a suitable plate for a given type of the fracture (Fig. 36.30).

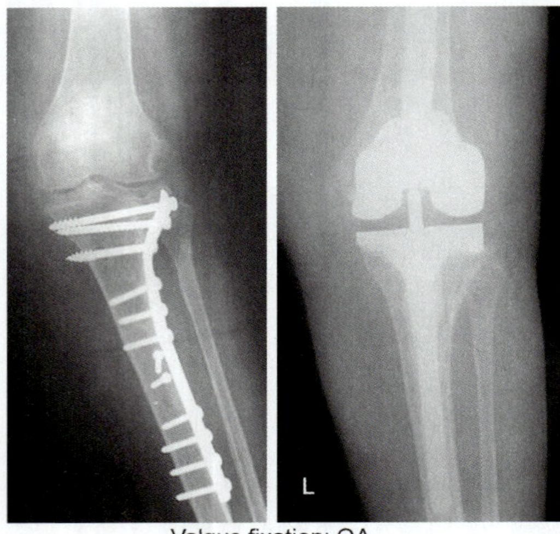

Figure 36.28 Postoperative valgus deformity

Above design permits use of only one screw in the subchondral area. Hence, another design is made, with two holes at the extreme end and one below this. The plate thickness is 3.8 mm (is more thick than the T or L plates). This plate is not side specific and has made possible to have two screws, close to the articular cartilage. It has few holes near the margins, which will accommodate 1.8 mm K-wires, for provisional stability.

It can also be used either on medial or lateral tibial condyle (Fig. 36.31).

Prior to advent of plates and screw design for proximal tibia, as till late 70's, it was advocated to make a window and elevate the depressed segment. The void was filled with bone grafts and the limb immobilized. The depressed segment is thus elevated. However, it was observed, that often late mild recurrence of depression occurred. This late recurrence of the depression, is prevented by a buttress plate fixation. The then newer 6.5 mm screws, besides stabilizing the plate, prevented the late depression of the segment (Fig. 36.32).

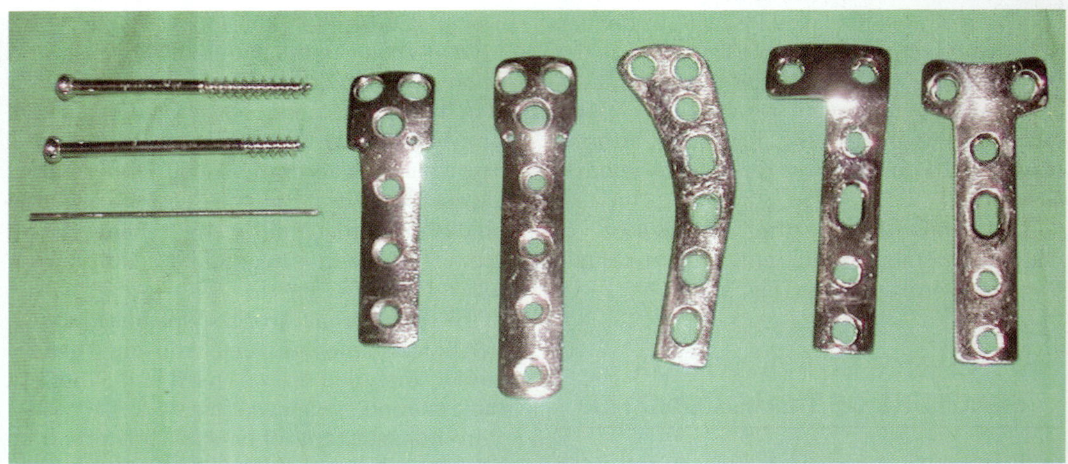

Figure 36.29 Various plates

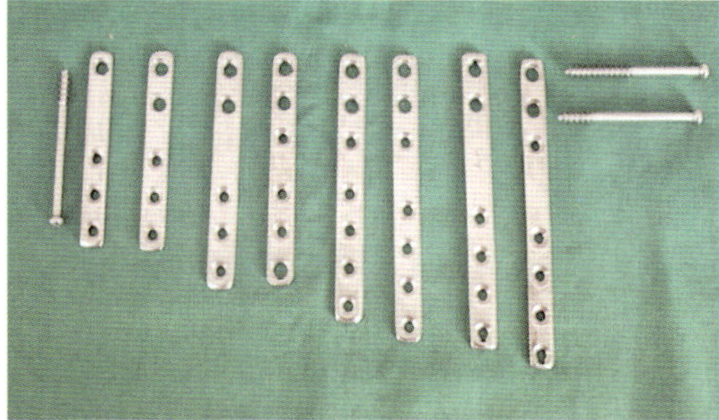

Figure 36.30 Span plates

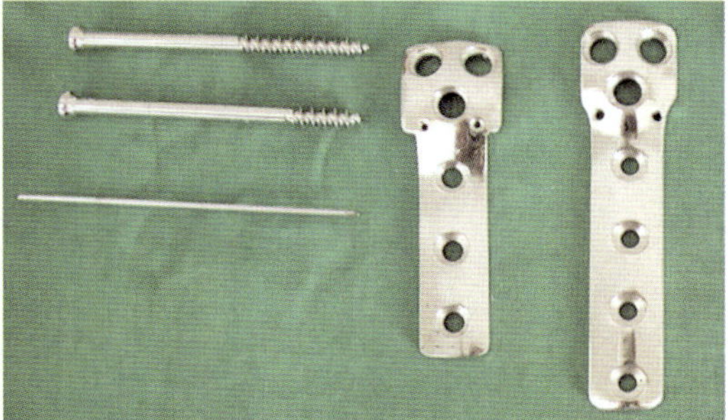

Figure 36.31 Square head plate

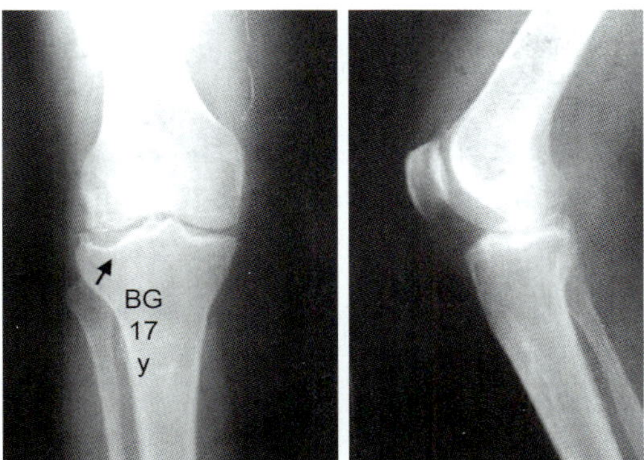

Figure 36.32 Elevation of depression and bone grafts. No plate applied

In a case of split fracture of the lateral condyle, without any depression or impaction of a bone segment, one needs to stabilize it, with interfragmentary compression, to enhance the stability. An L plate can be well used. At times to contour the vertical limb well is often difficult. A 12 mm wide plate, with large two holes on one end, can be safely used. It requires contouring on table. However, with a plate press, a three point plate bender and plate bending irons, it is possible to do so on table. One should do this step by step, increasing the curvature and matching against the bone. One should not over-contour and undo again, as it reduces the metal strength.

TECHNIQUE OF FRACTURE FIXATION

After exposure of the fracture, it is reduced and the reduction is stabilized by temporary fixation with 1.6 mm K-wires.

Three Methods of Temporary Fixation with K-wires

- The wires are so placed, that after they are passed, plate placement is possible and the wires should not come in the way of the drill bit and the screws. The wires are then cut short, to avoid any injury to the operating team.
- Other option is that the wire is drilled ahead, to be taken out from the opposite side, till it is flush with the bone, on the side from which they were inserted. The portion which has come on the other side of the condyle, is cut short, to avoid injury to the assistant's hand. This technique permits temporary stabilization of the fracture and a plate can be applied over the bone surface. The K-wire can be retrieved from the opposite side.
- The chosen plate is placed over the condyle and is held with a self-centering forceps. The small holes near the edges on the plate are used for insertion of K-wires, for provisional stability. The direction of these small holes is such that the screws can be safely inserted, without abutting against the K-wires, already in place.

The alignment of the plate to the proximal tibia is confirmed in both the views. First, a 4.5 mm screw in the middle area is passed, so the plate is well-opposed to the bone. After this screw, the important screw is inserted through the uppermost hole of the plate. Prior to directing the drill bit through a drill sleeve, the point at which the K-wire tip has come out from the opposite side and its relation with tibial plateau is studied and then the direction of drill sleeve decided. This method should be able to place the uppermost 6.5 mm screw, 5 mm below the tibial plateau. Then alternate upper and lower screws are passed. In a fracture of only the lateral condyle, one can use a 6.5 mm screw with 32 mm threads, so that it has a good purchase in the medial condyle (Fig. 36.33).

A patient had an *old injury to the posterior tibial eminence* and was asymptomatic. If it a fresh injury, the patient is turned prone and the eminence fixed with a 4 mm shaft screw (Fig. 36.34).

Split Fracture of Lateral Condyle

In a case of depressed fracture of lateral tibial condyle the void to be filled, depends upon the degree of depression and the void occurring during the elevation. My preference is for

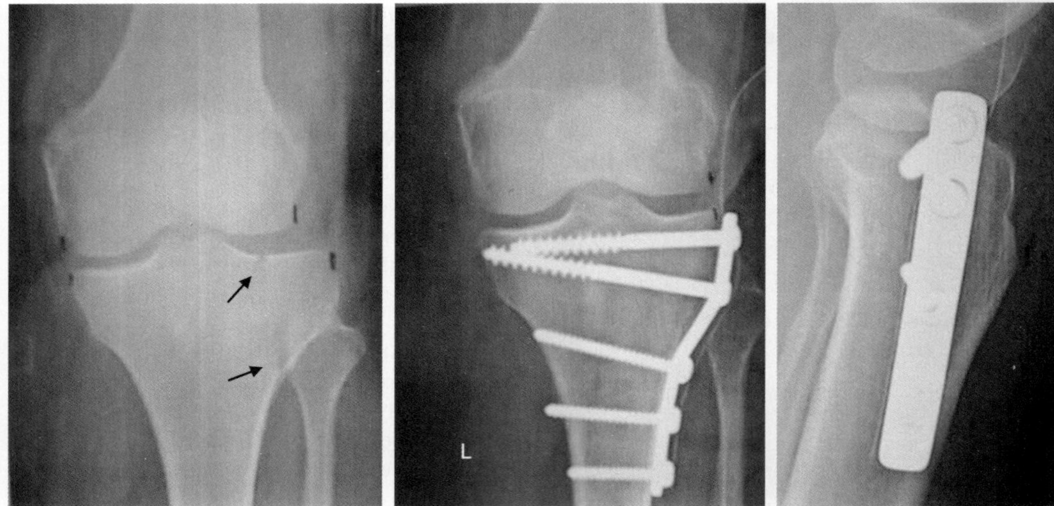

Figure 36.33 A split fracture fixed with a 12 mm plate

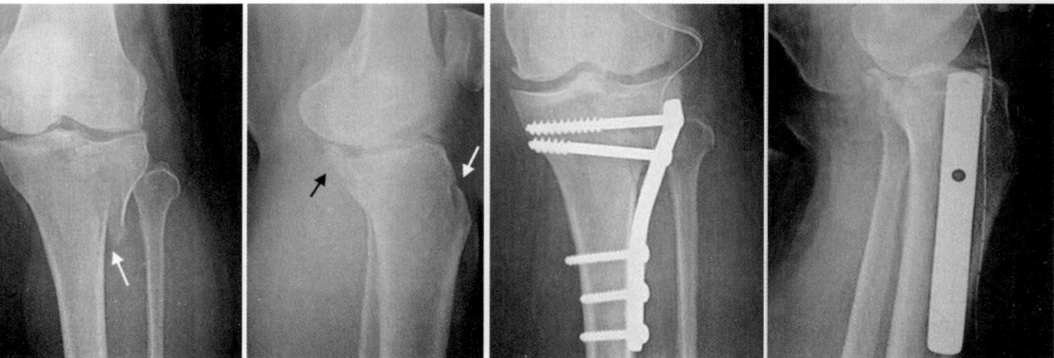

Figure 36.34 Old injury to the posterior tibial eminence, with fresh split fracture of lateral condyle

autologous iliac bone grafts, as they consolidate rapidly. However, in exceptional situation, one may use chemical bone substitute, as seen in the case. It being more dense, stands out more in the X-ray film (Fig. 36.35).

In bicondylar fracture with depression in a condyle, elevation of the depressed segment, bone grafting and stabilization is a standard method. In the available plates, there are two holes at the upper end of the plate, which accommodate 6.5 mm screws. The screws are passed, at right angle to the plate. It is possible to pass a screw at some angle, directed either anteriorly or posteriorly. Care needs to be taken, so it does not penetrate the posterior limit of the bone and injure posterior structures.

As per the area of depression, whether it is anterior or posterior part of the condyle, one should direct the screw. This will support the bone grafts and the depressed segment and prevent late collapse. In most of the cases of depression/impaction of the lateral condyle, one sees two plateau surfaces in preoperative AP views. The one which is not depressed, usually remains as such. The one which was elevated is rather a floating and mobile one and may get depressed in the postoperative period. May be prior to getting re-displaced, some cartilage growth may have occurred, which may be preventing a step offset. Since, one part of the lateral condyle continues to be at anatomical level, weight bearing through it continues and valgus deformity and related sequel are less (Figs 36.36 and 36.37).

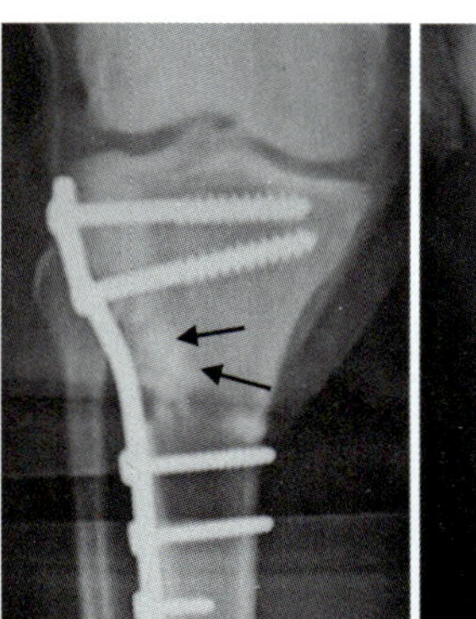

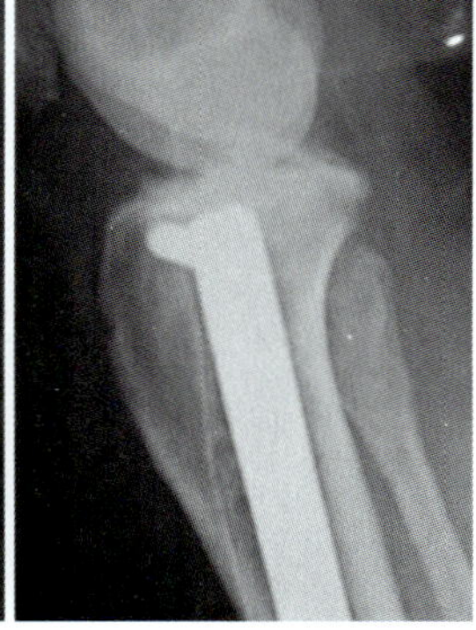

Figure 36.35 Synthetic bone substitute

Multiple screws are inserted through the uppermost edge of a precontoured locking plate. The locking screws may not confer interfragmentary compression. However, since they are placed at the subchondral level, they prevent collapse of an elevated segment (Fig. 36.38).

A fracture with more than four parts, in proximal tibia, involving the joint, is an unstable injury and needs a stable fixation. This is important, to prevent slow union and implant failure. In the given case, the neck of fibula is also fractured, adding to the instability.

Medially a curved (hockey shape) plate and laterally a straight 12 mm plates were applied. It is observed, that unless accurate reduction is obtained, when a curved plate is used, often anterior angulation is observed in the postoperative X-ray. Hence, every care needs to be taken to prevent this. It is possible to achieve this by extending the limb over the quadriceps board and confirming by a 'C' arm image.

HOW CAN ONE ACHIEVE THIS?

First two 6.5 mm screws are inserted medially through the curved plate in the uppermost holes. Then the leg is extended to maintain the reduction of the fracture and confirm in both the AP and the lateral view, that the alignment is well restored. Then two screws are inserted in the distal fragment. This would make the fracture stable. Then, on the lateral condyle, a straight plate is applied, with one screw on either side of the fracture. Now, if the posterior cortices are well aligned, it indicates good reduction (Fig. 36.39).

DIAGNOSIS AND MISSED FRACTURE OF TIBIAL CONDYLE

In a junctional fracture (fracture in metaphyseal area) often the fracture is an impacted fracture and quite often the patient is able to take a few steps with support. When the patient reports early, knee hemarthrosis may not be fully formed. Clinically, it is necessary to detect a

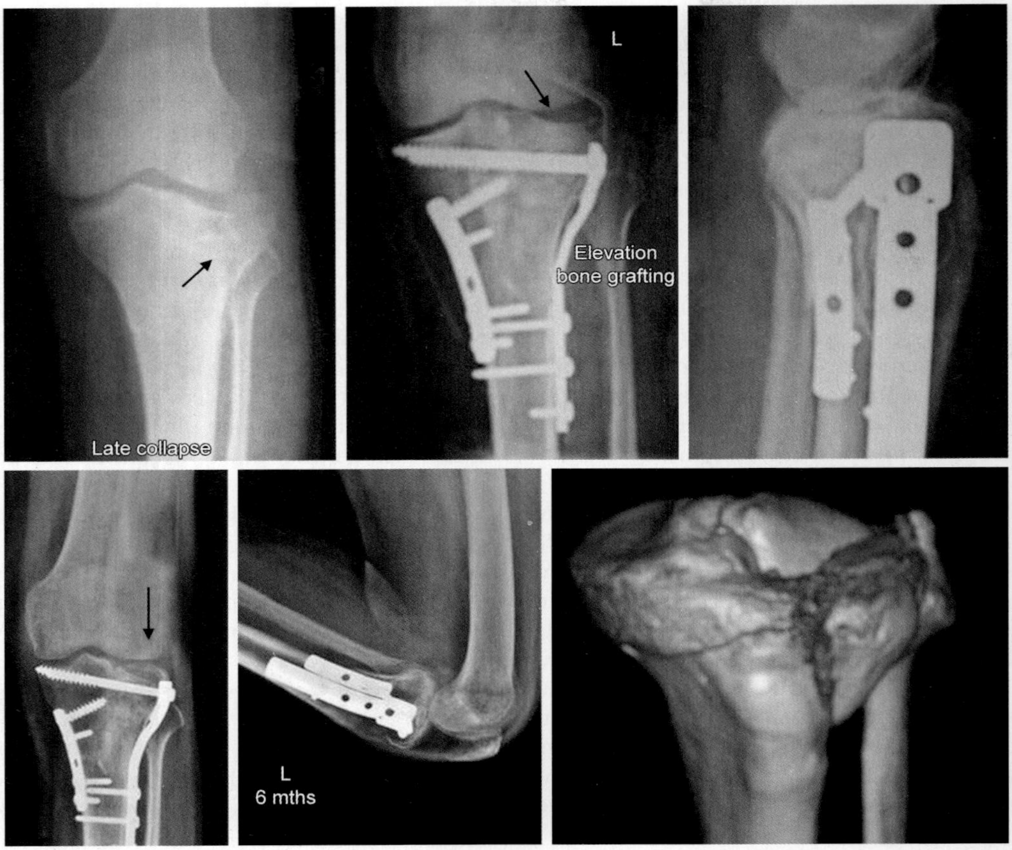

Figure 36.36 Partial recurrent depression

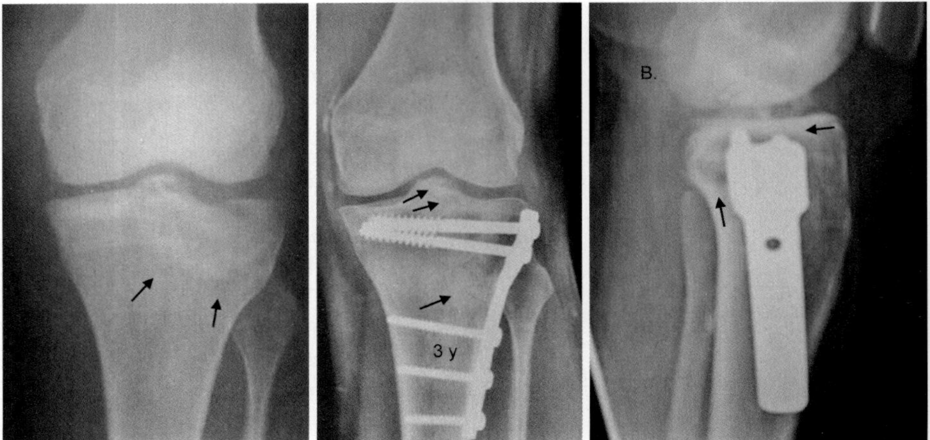

Figure 36.37 No late collapse

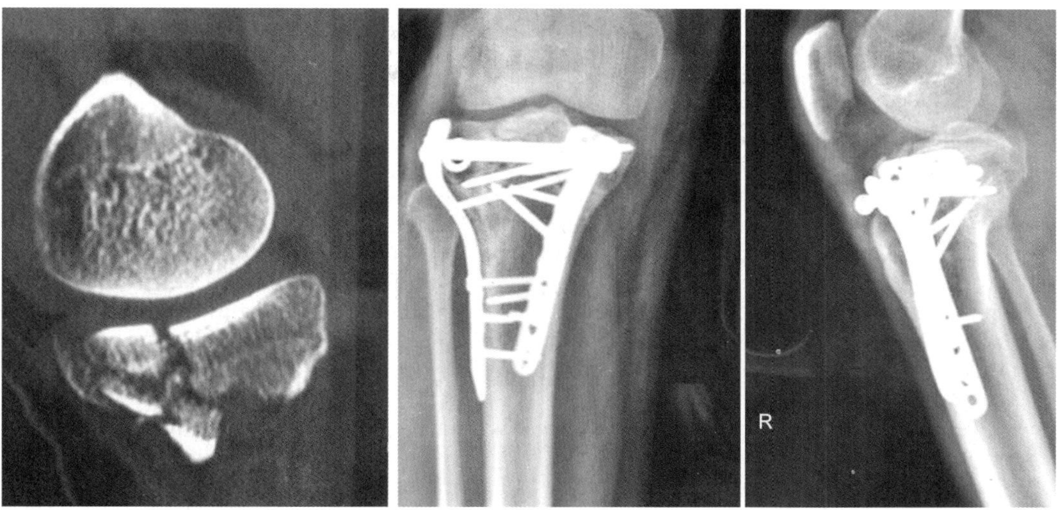

Figure 36.38 Raft screws in locking plate

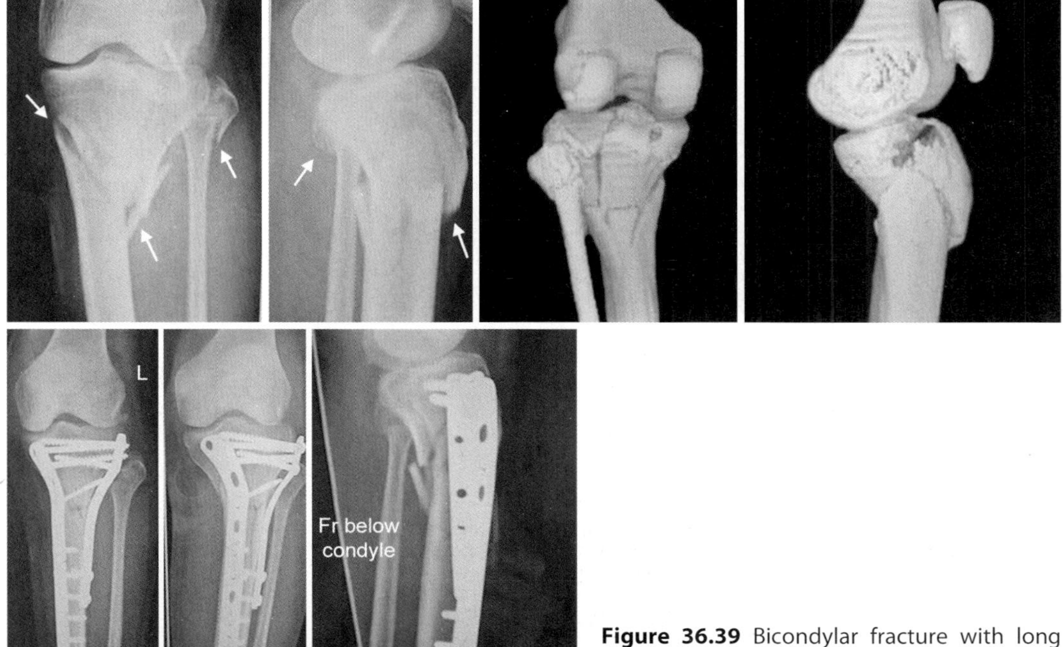

Figure 36.39 Bicondylar fracture with long beaks

bony tenderness, as an aid to clinical diagnosis. An X-ray examination may not very clearly and convincingly indicate presence of a fracture.

In such a depressed fracture of *lateral* condyle of tibia, the patient may be able to take a few steps, when reports to the clinic. (More weight passes through the medial condyle and in a fracture of the *medial* tibial condyle, taking even a few steps is usually not possible. Thus, a fracture of the lateral tibial condyle is more often diagnosed late or is likely to be missed, than a fracture of the medial condyle).

If the clinician and the radiologist are not watchful and unaware of such an injury, the diagnosis is likely to be missed. The usual observation in such an X-ray:

- Slight depression of the lateral tibial condyle
- Disturbed trabecular pattern in lateral condyle (Figs 36.40 and 36.41A).

At times, the patient may present after few days, even after X-ray examination done elsewhere and the fracture may be missed. Local bruise around the knee is a good indicator of a bone injury. If a crepe bandage is applied, prior to coming to you, the bruise is seen beyond the crepe bandage (Fig. 36.41B).

TREATMENT

Non-operative treatment by a plaster cast immobilization is usually accepted by the patient. An above knee plaster cast for four weeks from the injury is adequate. It is necessary to confirm that the patient does not bear weight on the cast, and use of a walker or a pair of crutches is being done. I have seen some clinicians using a knee brace, instead of the cast. I feel, a cast offers undisturbed immobilization and offers strict and rigid rest to the part, which is very necessary. At the end of this period, the cast is bivalved, clinical and X-ray examination is done. The knee is usually pain free.

Now, if the fracture alignment is well-maintained, then:

A crepe support is given to the knee. It is a good idea to reapply the posterior part of the bivalved cast, over the crepe support.

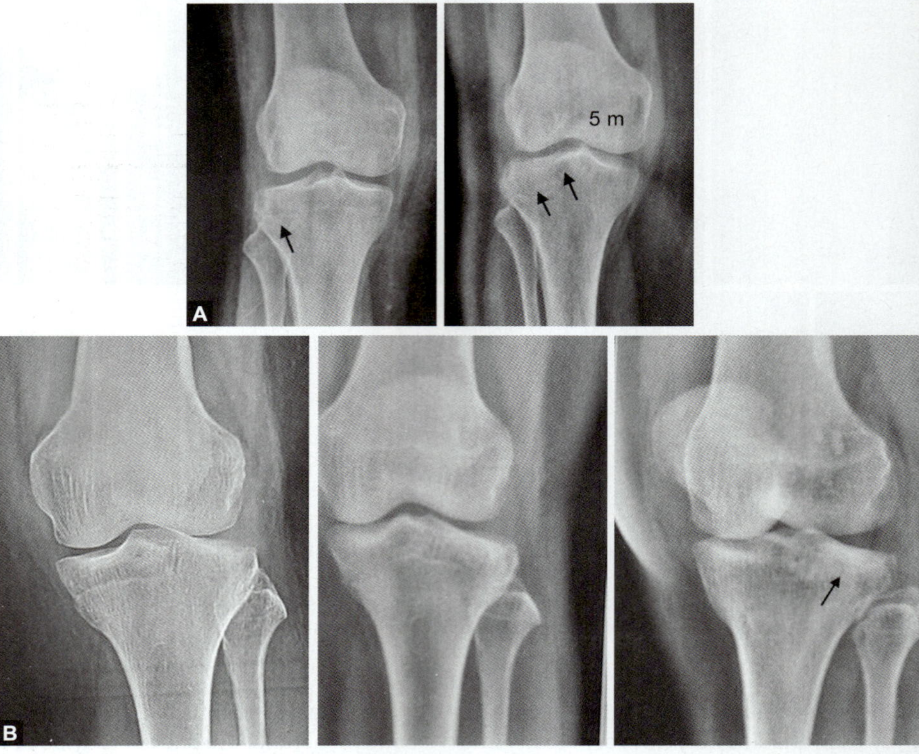

Figures 36.40A and B Plain X-ray diagnosis

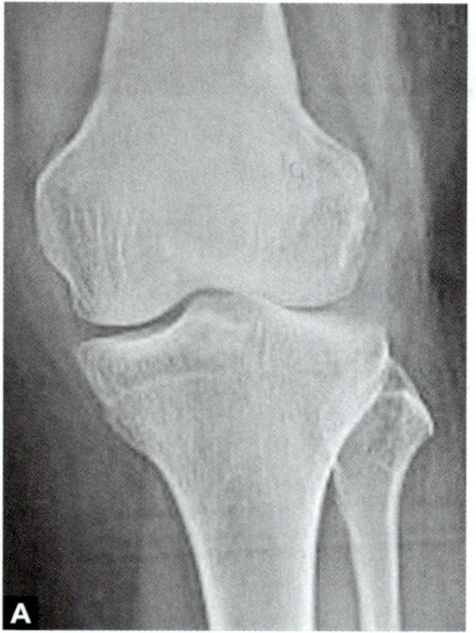
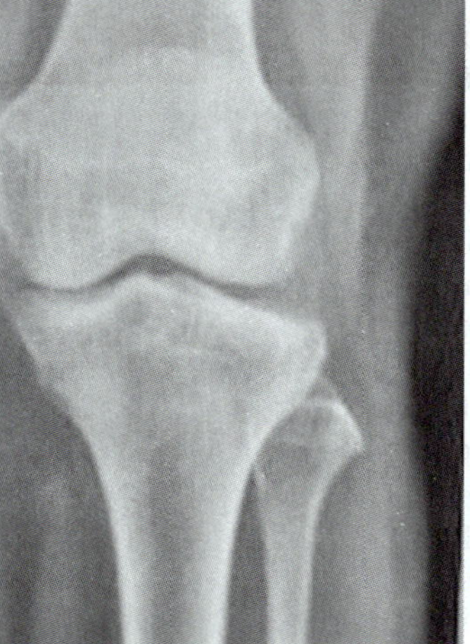
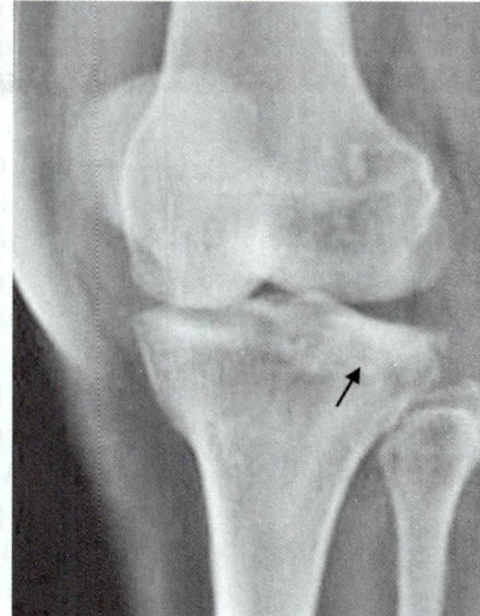
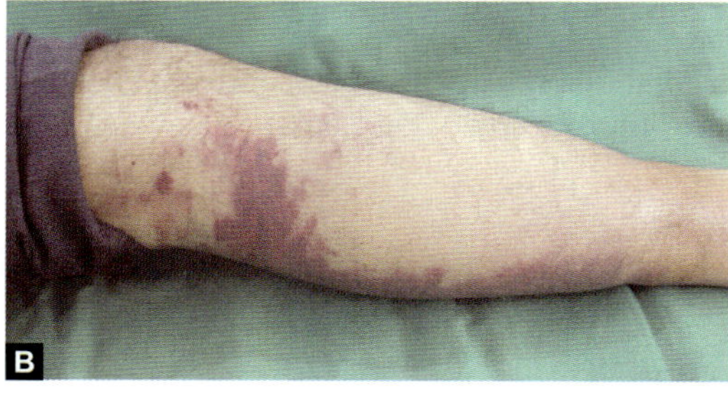

Figures 36.41A and B (A) Oblique view diagnosis; (B) Bruise

Especially, if a synthetic material is used for the cast, the posterior part is adequately strong enough to offer support. This back support does not permit accidental flexion of the knee and the pain which may arise.

Everyday, the back slab and the crepe bandage are removed for bath and the knee is actively mobilized. The crepe and the back slab are reapplied. After a week, partial weight bearing is permitted with the back slab on. Gradually the back slab is discarded and progressive more weight bearing is permitted. Within further two to three weeks, the patient regains good range of motion and is able to bear the weight on the injured limb. If after bivalving the long leg cast, one observes that the back slab portion is weak, one may use a knee immobilizer for support.

At times, the family physician or a casualty officer takes an X-ray of the knee. An undisplaced contusion crack fracture is missed and a crepe is applied and the patient sent home. At the end of, say, two weeks, he is unable to put any weight on the leg and develops *a fixed flexion deformity* and hence reports to the orthopedic surgeon. One should advise both internal and external oblique views of the knee. If one suspects a depressed segment, a CT scan is necessary to ascertain the degree of depression of the fragment.

Often only an undisplaced fracture of the lateral tibial condyle is observed. One needs to offer an indoor care and a traction is applied. Usually in a few days, the muscle spasm is overcome and good range is restored. One may advise a push knee splint, to prevent recurrence of the FFD. If the spasm is more, one should consider a cast immobilization for appropriate duration, and then mobilize the knee. During this period and later on, quadriceps exercises need to be advised and supervised, as it is a key to return of a good function.

CONTUSION FRACTURE OF LATERAL TIBIAL CONDYLE

This lady in 50s had a fall from a scooter pillion and could climb a stair with support. Clinically and radiologically, an undisplaced fracture of the lateral tibial condyle was noted. However, for documentation and patient satisfaction (to accept the treatment offered), MRI scan was done. It confirmed the stellate fracture appearance in the lateral tibial condyle. An above knee cast was applied for four weeks and nonweight bearing mobilization was carried out. Static knee exercises helped to maintain a good muscle tone and prevent intra-articular adhesion formation. Good outcome was noted.

Option of fracture fixation in situ could be considered, so early knee mobilization is possible and inconvenience of the cast is avoided (Fig. 36.42).

FRACTURE OF LATERAL TIBIAL CONDYLE IN THE ELDERLY

This retired lady, medical practitioner, had sustained a mild to moderate depressed fracture of the lateral tibial condyle on the right side and type A fracture of the lateral malleolus on the left side. The knee had changes of osteoarthrosis. Having had injuries on both the legs, she was offered elevation of the depressed segment of the lateral tibial condyle with internal fixation and a cast immobilization for the ankle on the opposite side. She chose to have non-operative treatment for both the fractures. She accepted above knee cast for the right knee and a below knee cast on the other side, in spite of the inconvenience and likelihood of bed sores, etc. Fortunately, she had no complications and had a good union and function of both the knee and the opposite ankle (Fig. 36.43).

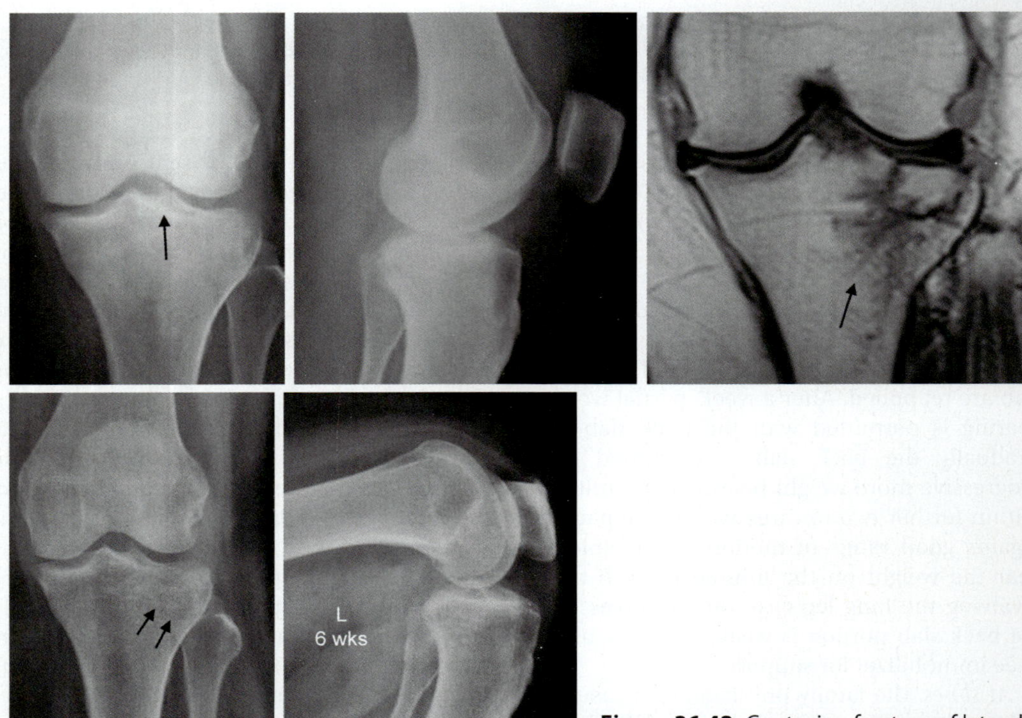

Figure 36.42 Contusion fracture of lateral condyle

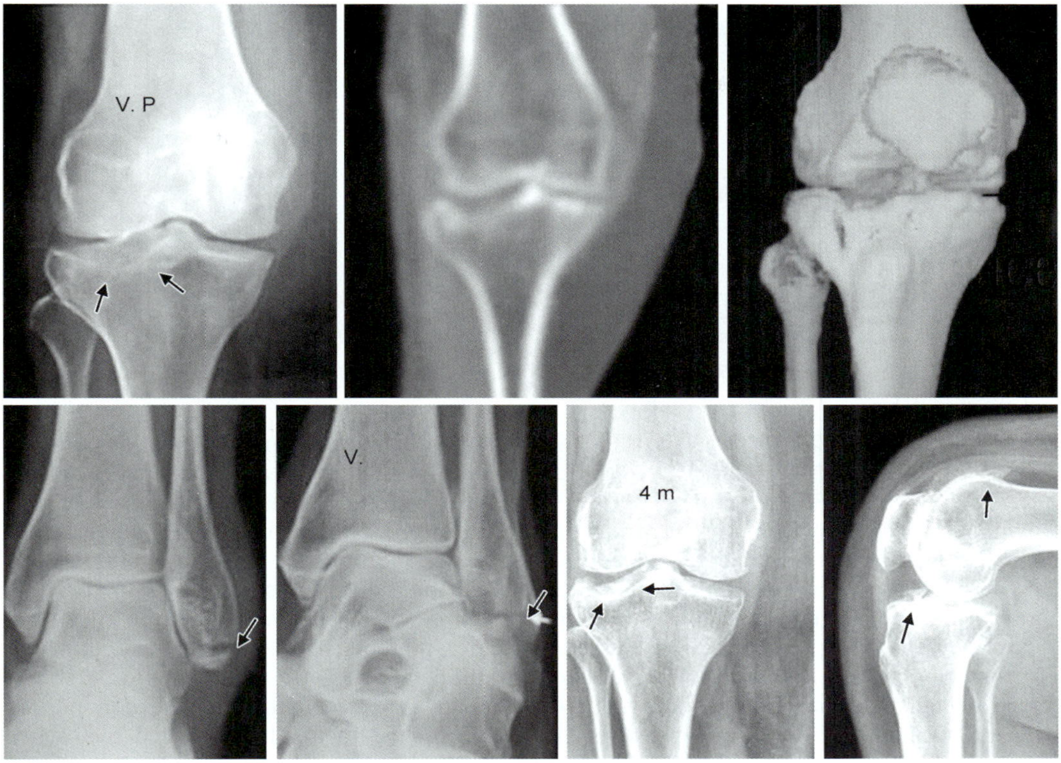

Figure 36.43 Opted non-operative method

WIDENING OF THE LATERAL TIBIAL CONDYLE

This patient had a fracture of the lateral tibial condyle with some widening of the lateral plateau. Intercondylar screw and a buttress plate would have been a good method to treat. This would have restored the width of the tibial condyle. However, she chose a non-operative method (Fig. 36.44).

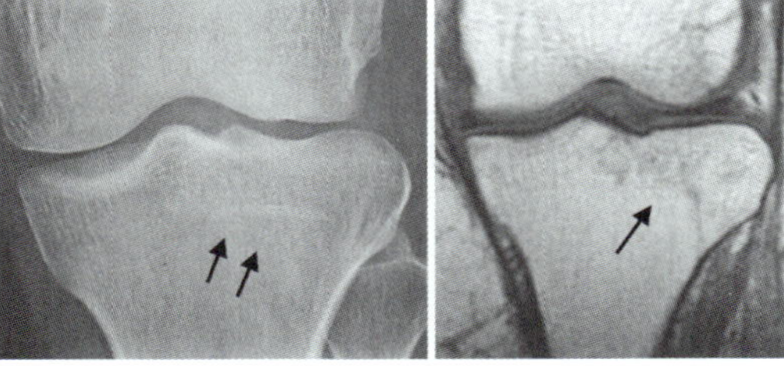

Figure 36.44 Widening of the lateral tibial condyle

FRACTURE OF ANTERIOR TIBIAL EMINENCE AND UNDISPLACED FRACTURE OF LATERAL CONDYLE

This lady had a fall from a scooter and inability to walk about. An X-ray examination was done in a nearby hospital and presented to us for a definitive treatment. The fracture of the eminence was clear, while that of the lateral condyle was uncertain. MRI confirmed both the fractures. The eminence was fixed with a wire loop and the lateral condyle was fixed with a screw and a washer. Good stability was achieved and early mobilization was carried out. Good outcome (Fig. 36.45).

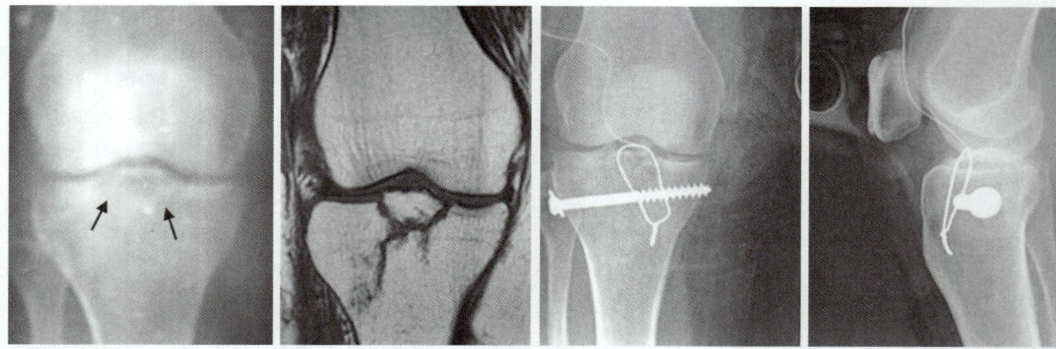

Figure 36.45 Fracture of anterior eminence and lateral condyle

INCORRECT HISTORY AND FASCIOTOMY

A young man came with a history of having jumped from four-feet height a day before and pain and swelling in the left shin and the knee. X-ray revealed a split fracture of the lateral condyle. The swelling and tense calf was out of proportion to the duration and nature of injury of a fall and not a run over injury. There were no vehicle tyre marks or abrasions as well. Doppler study indicated absence of blood flow beyond the popliteal bifurcation. Hence a fasciotomy was done on either side, opening all the compartments. The medial incision showed dark muscle mass, which was excised. Since the bone was exposed, the lateral condyle and the 3rd fragments were stabilized and wound left open. Later split thickness skin grafting was done. The limb survived. Later on the patient came with the story that the injury was a few days old and he had been to a bone setter, who manipulated the knee ten times and gave a vigorous massage and then he had reported to us (Fig. 36.46)!

FRACTURE OF LATERAL TIBIAL CONDYLE

In tibial condyle, more body weight passes through the medial condyle. Hence, in injury to the medial condyle, weight bearing is painful and difficult. The patient reports to the clinician soon and hence an early diagnosis is done. As against this, in an injury to the lateral condyle, with a contusion crack fracture, with very mild depression or displacement, the patient is able to move about with some limp or support of a stick. The injury is so subtle, that a plain X-ray taken on day 1, may not reveal the injury and there is possibility of diagnosing it as a contusion of the knee. It is only when, due to persistent inability to bear weight, that MRI examination is done and the fracture is recognized. In absence of MRI facility, in addition to a good quality AP and a lateral view, two oblique views may be able to detect this injury (Fig. 36.47).

A SPLIT FRACTURE OF LATERAL CONDYLE WITH MINIMUM DISPLACEMENT

A split fracture of lateral tibial condyle with minimum displacement needs internal fixation for a stable fixation and early mobilization of the knee. A well-contoured 12 mm tibial plate with large end holes offers a good stability. Early mobilization and full return of function is possible (Fig. 36.48).

CASE EXAMPLES

A Mild Depressed Fracture Requiring Elevation

A fracture with mild depression, confirmed by a CT scan required elevation of the depressed

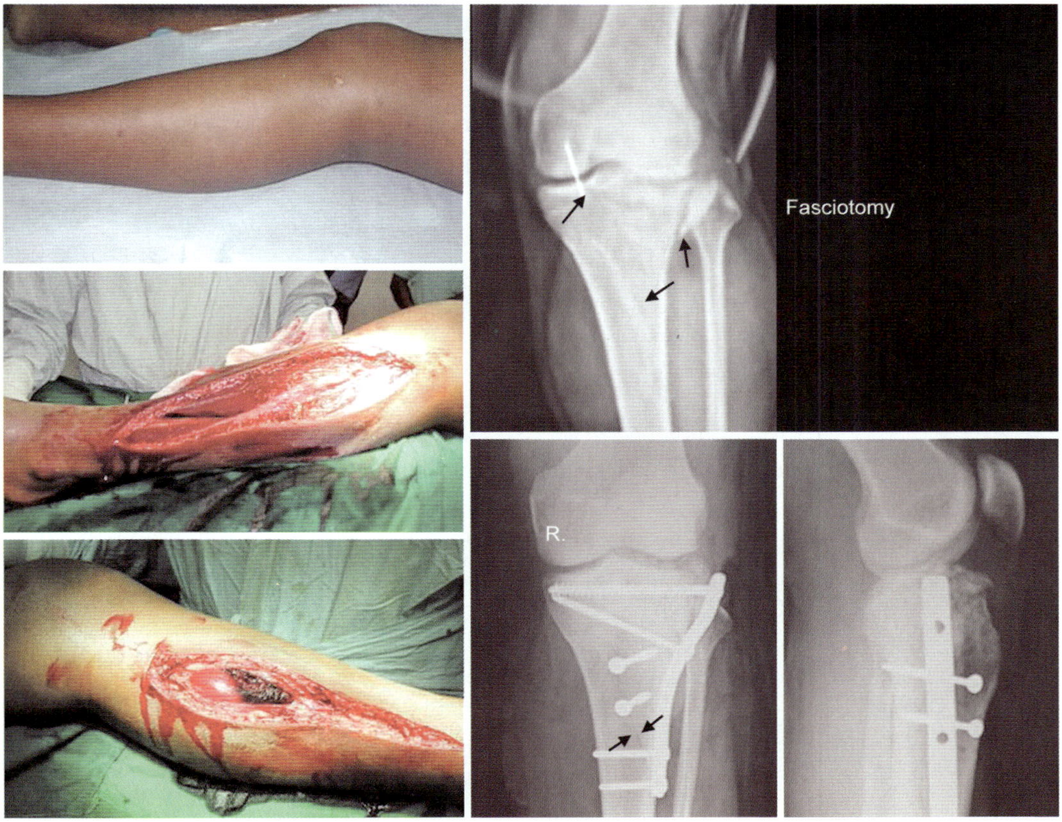

Figure 36.46 Fasciotomy

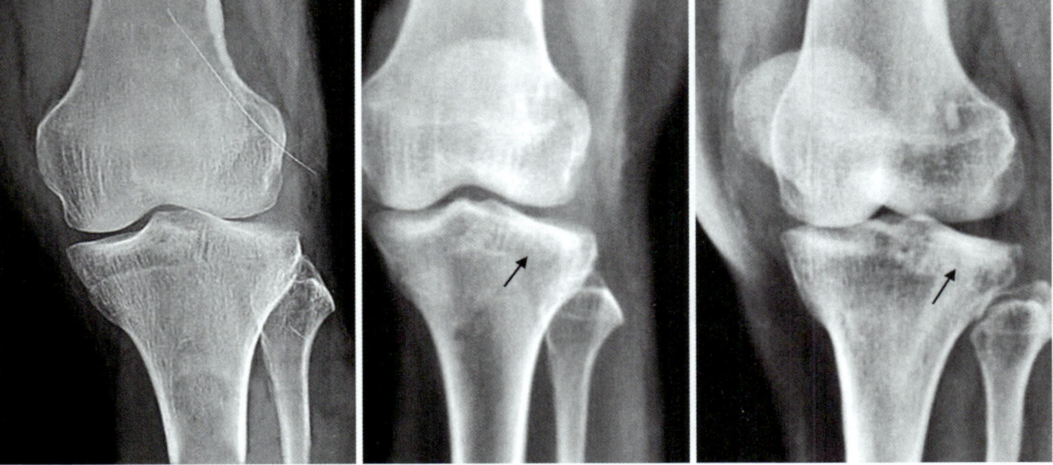

Figure 36.47 Oblique view detects a depressed fracture

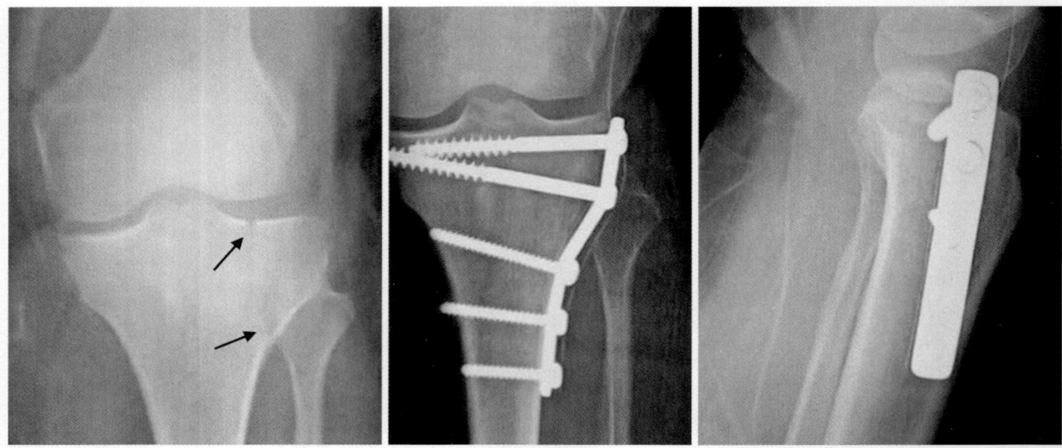

Figure 36.48 A split fracture with minimum displacement

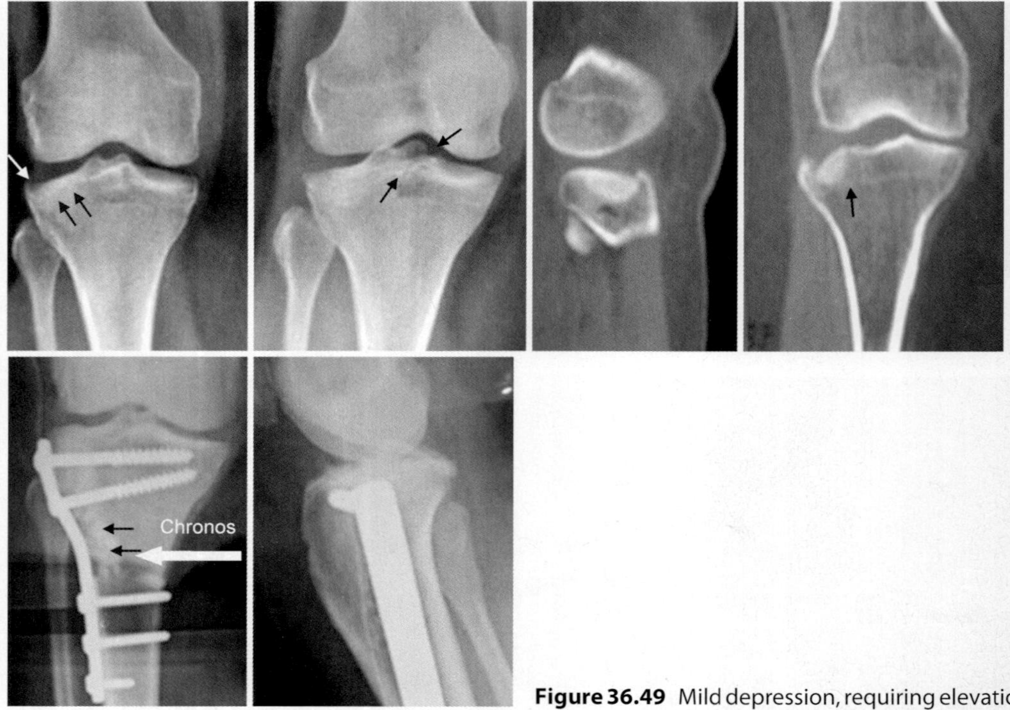

Figure 36.49 Mild depression, requiring elevation

segment. The elevation was carried out through a window in the lateral cortex. The void was filled with a synthetic bone substitute and was stabilized with a lateral 12 mm custom-made plate. Good union and return of range of motion was achieved. However, I would always prefer to use an autologous iliac graft, to build the defect, because the consolidation and remodeling is more sound. Besides, one can clearly observe the trabeculi crossing the injured area, when autologous bone grafts are used. With synthetic bone substitutes, the X-ray appearance cannot indicate for sure, if the fracture has consolidated well (Fig. 36.49).

A Moderate Depression

A moderate degree of depression is elevated through a window made in the lateral surface of the tibia. One needs to make a window and have an access through an uninjured area till the depressed segment. The bone void occurring during the procedure is rather more and hence, it is packed with corticocancellous iliac grafts. The elevation is carried out by a punch under 'C' arm control and the void is filled with grafts. The grafts are gently tapped with a punch upwards and additional grafts are laid down and so on. These steps are carried out alternately, till the void is well filled. This reconstructed condyle is stabilized with a lateral plate. The upper most screws through the buttress plate, help to support the elevated segment. Knee elevation on a high Bohler frame and active mobilization is carried out (Fig. 36.50).

A Severe Depression: Technique of Elevation

In a case where a large segment is depressed in the proximal tibia, it is seen in a plain X-ray film. A CT scan helps to identify the degree of depression, direction of the tilt and the exact place of the depression. It may appear logical to make a window on the medial side of the shaft and elevate the fragment, so that the articular surface is exactly elevated to be at the same level as of the medial condyle. This requires a more generous incision, elevation of a thick flap, etc. It is possible to elevate it through an oblong window on the lateral surface of the tibia only.

Through this window, the depressed and impacted segment is first made loose from the adjacent bone and then gently tapped upwards. Care needs to be exercised to tap alternately the

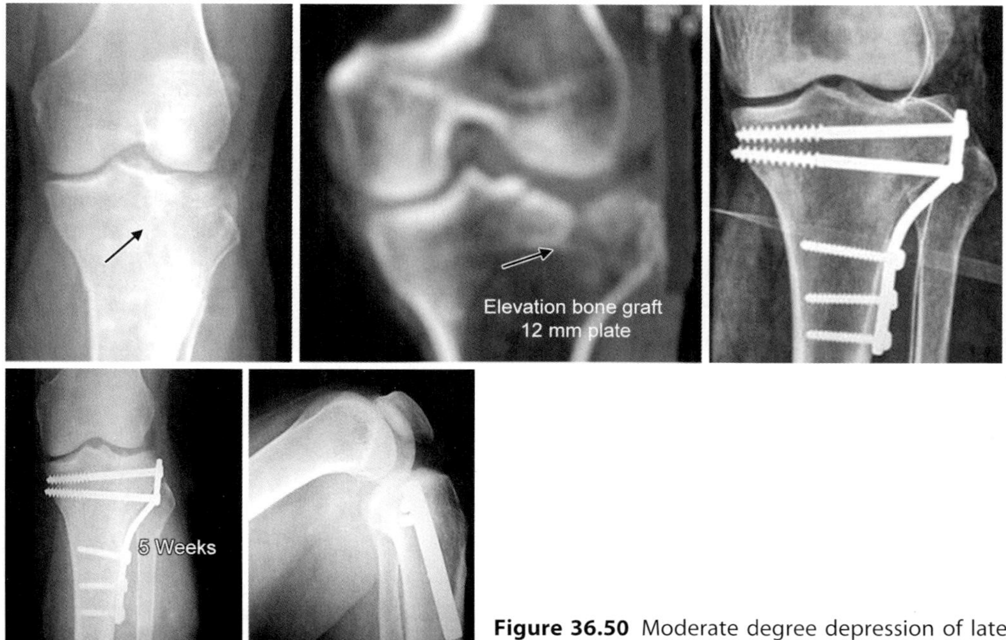

Figure 36.50 Moderate degree depression of lateral condyle

medial and lateral edges of the segment. One should be careful, not to rupture the articular surface and keep the articular surface intact. It is important to maintain some hinge attachment to the depressed fragment, to keep its blood supply intact. Besides, the elevation needs to be just adequate and accidentally, if it is elevated too much, may lie free in the joint. Under correction is better than this complication. One should confirm the elevation in both AP and lateral views. The void is first filled with cancellous bone, which is gently tapped upwards. While this is tapped upwards, one notices elevation of the articular surface well. With advent of 'C' arm, arthrotomy is not required to confirm degree of elevation of the articular surface. Below this cancellous layer, cortical vertical strips are laid in, which would confer additional support like a prop, to the elevated fragment. Finally the cortical window flap is replaced and the lateral condyle is stabilized with a lateral plate (Figs 36.51 and 36.52).

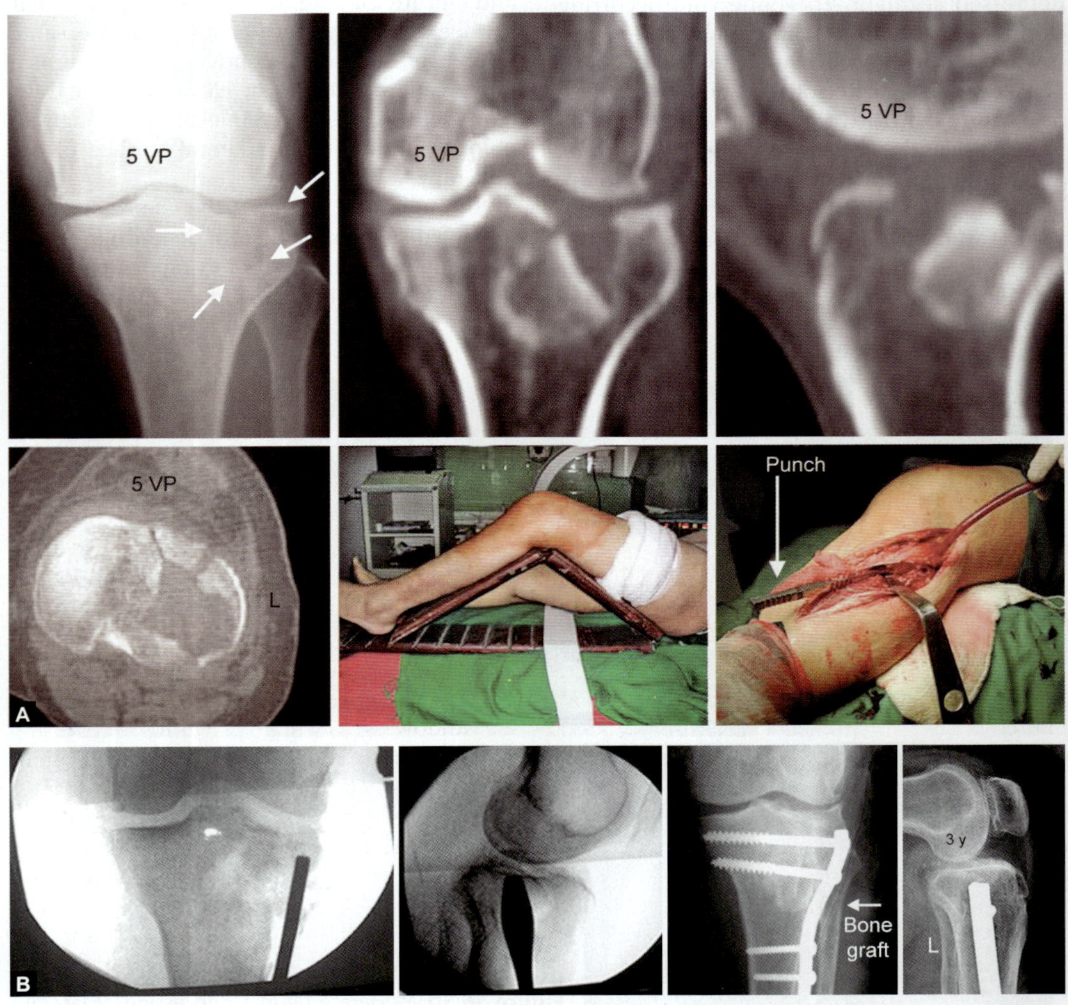

Figures 36.51A and B Lateral condyle elevation technique

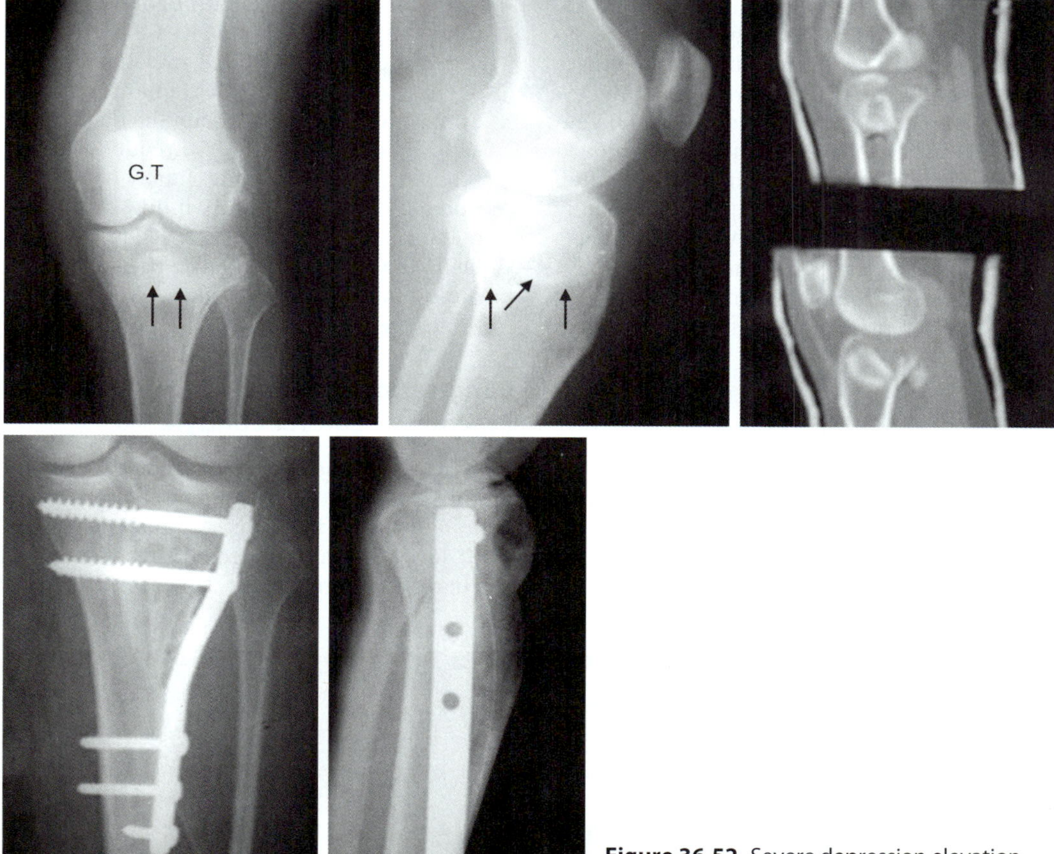

Figure 36.52 Severe depression elevation

LATERAL CONDYLE ELEVATION FROM MEDIAL SIDE

The leg to be operated is placed on a quadriceps board and in addition to the knee, ipsilateral iliac crest is also draped. Prior to the application of an adhesive transparent sheet on iliac crest, saline adrenaline infiltration is done and then the adhesive sheet is applied. By the time, one exposes the crest, its effect is observed.

In a depressed fracture of lateral condyle, at times, the depressed fragment is so displaced that, elevation through a window from the lateral side may not be successful, to bring it back to the anatomical position. Approach from the *medial surface,* assures good repositioning of the depressed segment and restoration of the articular surface. However, it requires additional exposure of the medial tibial surface. One has to draw a line from the depressed fragment, obliquely, medially, where the window is to be made. A window of 10 mm × 20 mm is marked and drill holes are made along it and with 5 mm thin osteotome, the window is completed. The window hood is elevated and kept aside, to be replaced back, at the end of the procedure. Under 'C' arm control, with a punch of appropriate size, the depressed segment is gently tapped and elevated. One needs to tap on either ends of the fragment, to elevate it *en masse.* A lateral view is also seen under 'C' arm, to confirm that the segment to be elevated is exactly above the punch. Having done so, bone grafts are taken from the iliac crest. To act as a strut, few oblong bone blocks are specially taken with this purpose in mind. Few cancellous pieces are first inserted in the void and with the help of the punch, they are moved to the subchondral area. Second layer is then added and pressed upwards (may be gently tapped and not hammered). As the cavity gets filled, finally the strut grafts are kept in place. The window lid removed earlier, is replaced again. Now the plate on the lateral surface is to be fixed.

Steps: Vide Figures 36.53 and 36.54 for the Steps

- Contour the plate well, to adapt to the lateral surface.
- Provisional fixation with K-wires through the upper two holes of the plate.
- A 4.5 mm screw is fixed through the 3rd hole from the top, which achieves a good plate to bone contact. Then 6.5 mm screws with 32 mm threads are inserted through the uppermost plate holes. Then the distal most screw and finally, the full threaded 6.5 mm screw is inserted. Having, finally confirmed under 'C' arm the medial window lid piece is laid back.
- Deflating tourniquet and closure of both the donor and the recipient sites, over drains is done (Figs 36.53 and 36.54).

Long-term Outcome of a Depressed Fracture of Lateral Condyle

Thus if a depressed fracture of lateral condyle of tibia is elevated and adequate bone grafting is done, usually, the joint continues to have a good function and chances of post-traumatic osteoarthritis are less. However, besides

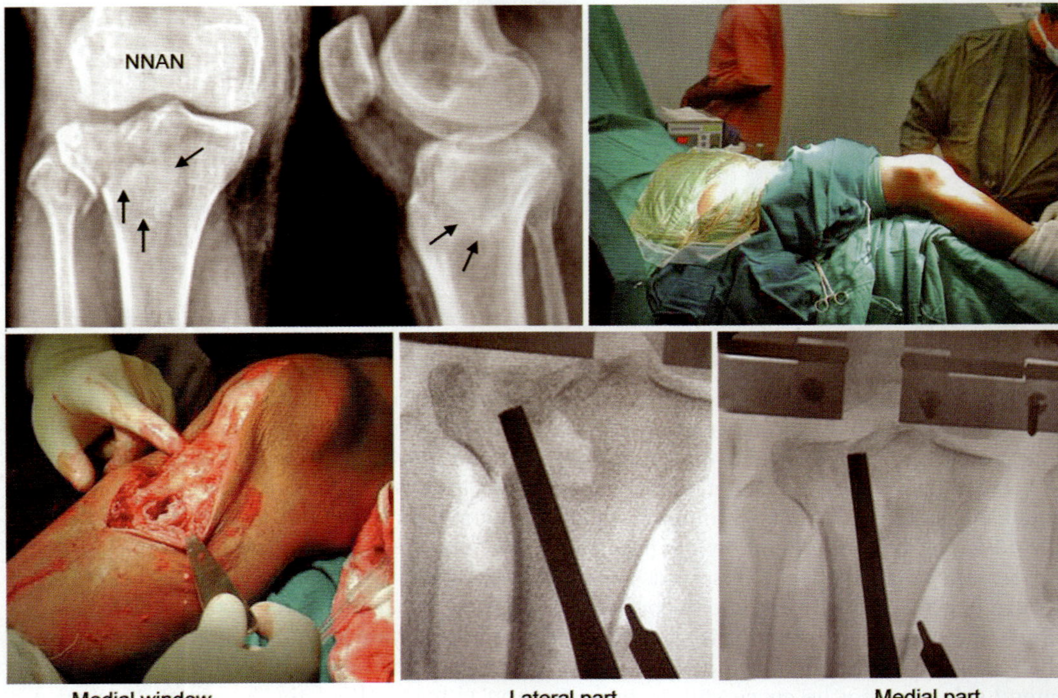

Figure 36.53 Elevation of lateral condyle from medial surface

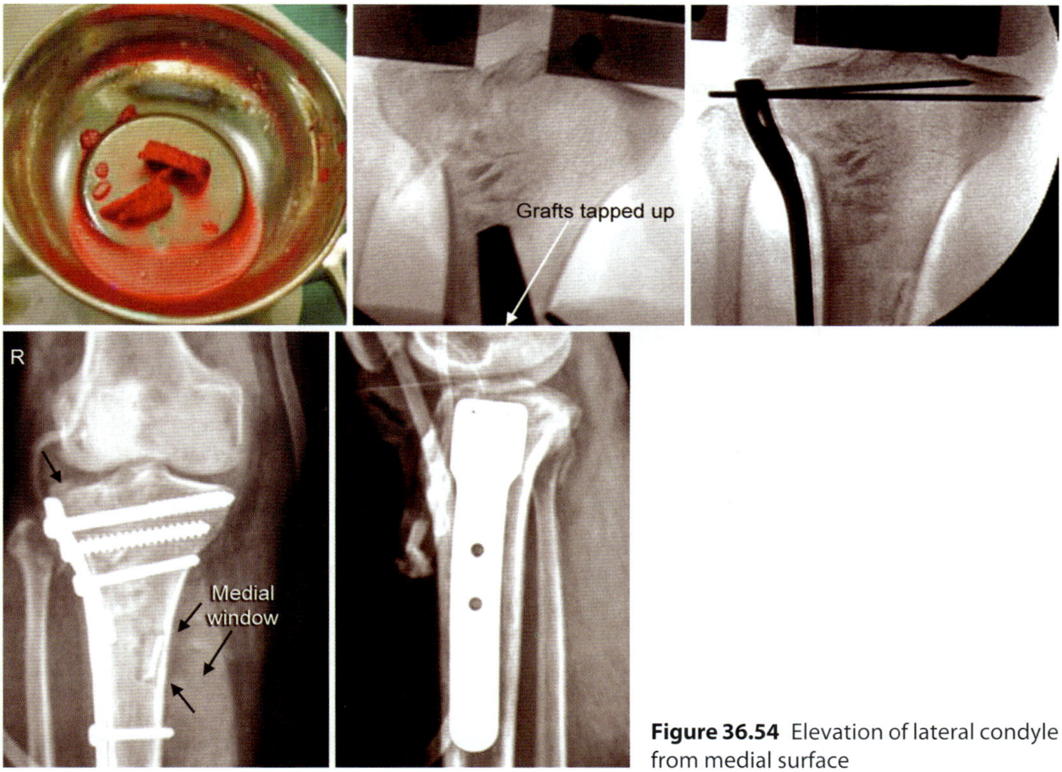

Figure 36.54 Elevation of lateral condyle from medial surface

restoration of the joint surface, the severity of injury to the articular cartilage at the time of initial injury plays an important role (Fig. 36.55).

If a depression is left as such, by the surgeon or if a patient did not accept the advice of surgical elevation of the depression, then chances of developing late osteoarthritis are high (Fig. 36.56).

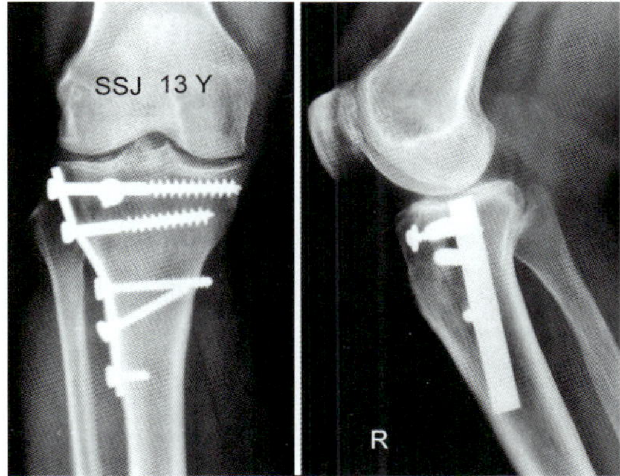

Figure 36.55 13 year's follow up of a case

Fracture of Lateral Tibial Condyle with Fracture of Anterior Tibial Eminence

In a case with a severe injury to the knee, in addition to a condylar fracture, associated injury to the anterior tibial eminence is also observed. Both the injuries can be managed in one stage.

In this case, there were few fragments on the antero-lateral side of the tibial condyle, along with a fracture of the anterior eminence:

Exposure

- For the wire loop, a short medial incision is required, keeping a distance of 5 to

6 cm between the two incisions, so the vascularity of the intervening skin area is well maintained.

- The antero-lateral approach on the proximal tibia helps to approach the lateral tibial condyle.

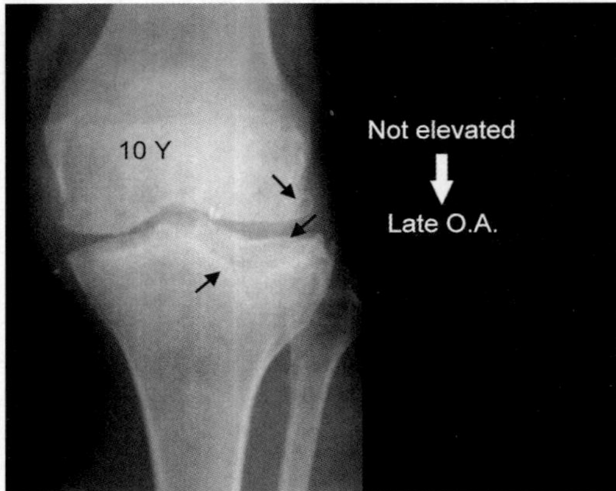

Figure 36.56 Late osteoarthritis in untreated case

The plate and interfragmentary screw fixation has to be done from the lateral side. The eminence is to be fixed with a wire loop. In such a situation, the *eminence has to be fixed first*, by a technique described in other chapter. It is safe to drill two holes for the wire loop and bring down the wire ends from *the medial tibial surface, as a first step*.

This is important, because after fixation of the plate of the lateral surface, there are screws present in the proximal condyle. With their presence, to drill the holes to pass a wire is difficult, with a danger of drill breakage. However, when the wire is drawn first from the medial surface, the wire usually does not interfere with the drill bit or the screws, which would be inserted later on.

On the medial surface, the distance between the two holes was less and hence, to prevent wire cutting through the bone cortex, two large washers were threaded over the wire. The wire was loaded gently with a tractor bow and a knot was tied. With the presence of the wire in the

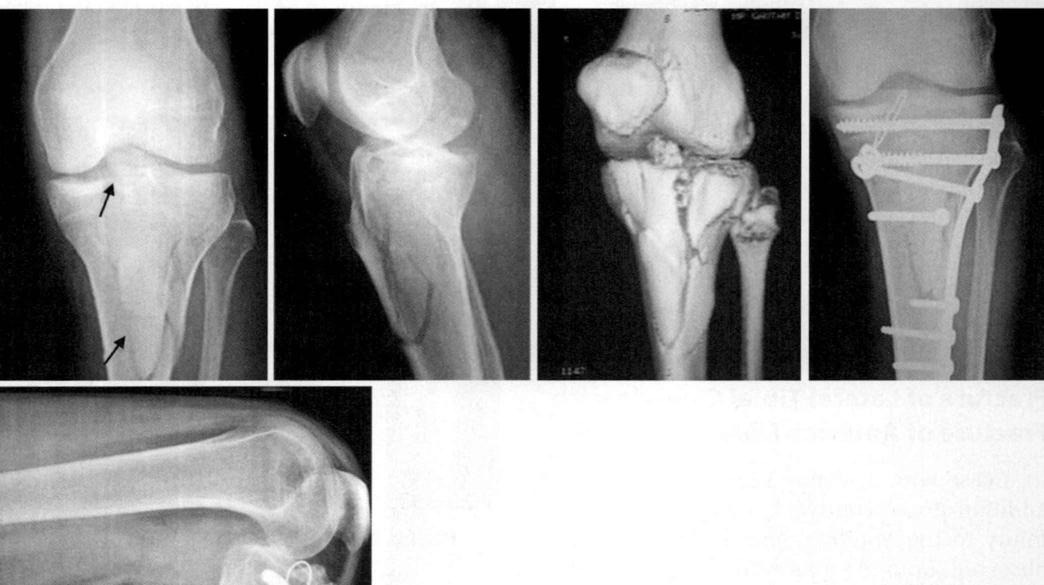
Figure 36.57 Fr of lateral condyle with fracture of anterior tibial eminence

anterior part of the condyle, it is possible to make drill holes for the screws from the lateral side for the necessary screws. One can slightly change the drill hole direction, keeping away from the wire. The wire strands are in the anterior segment of the proximal tibia. Hence the proximal 6.5 mm screws are directed slightly posteriorly. The X-ray photo is self-explanatory, as to how the stabilization was achieved (Figs 36.57 and 36.58).

IMPLANT REMOVAL

In young patients in their 20s and 30s, the fracture consolidates in a year or so. Once the full range of the knee motion is restored, it is preferable to remove the implants. This is especially true regarding the wire loop, as documented cases are presented, which have shown wire breakage and migration of that wire segment.

What Happens if a Plate Continues to be on a Bone?

- Bone overgrowth on the plate
- Stress shielding of cortex under the plate
- Reduced bone elasticity under the plate and differential elasticity under the plate and adjacent to it, which may lead to a likely fracture.
- More the delay in plate removal, more the stress shielding and delayed recovery from it. Besides there are more chances of mechanical problems in plate removal.
- Any subsequent bone injury, next to the plate, makes management of that injury more difficult, than a case, where the plate was timely removed (Fig. 36.59).

LEARNING FROM CASES

Knowledge and experience is gained by observing and studying various cases and as to how they were treated.

Reading Gives Knowledge, while Practical Training and Observation Gives Experience

Keeping the eyes open and mind alert, one can learn from many things in clinical practice.

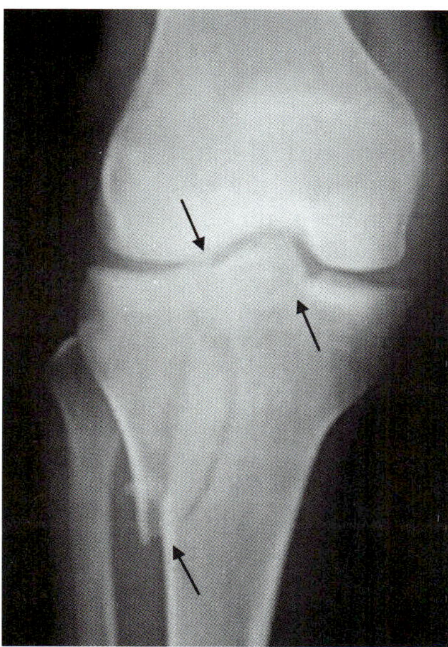

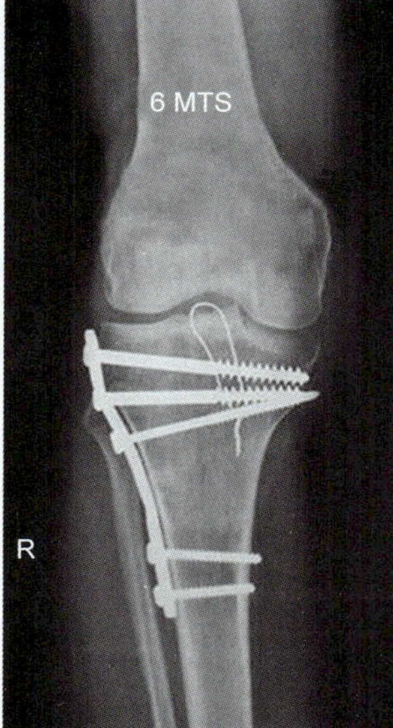

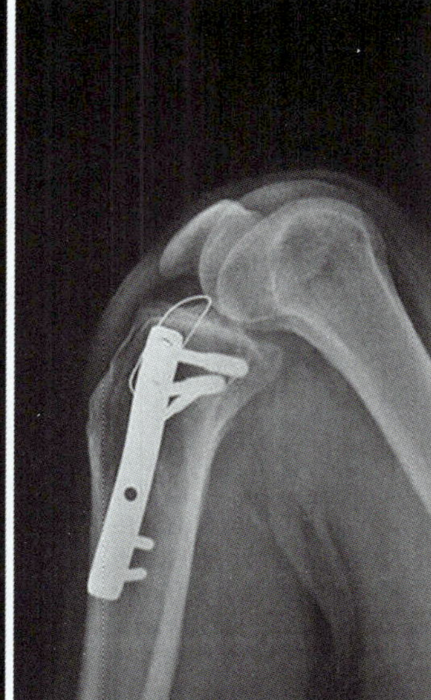

Figure 36.58 Fr of lateral condyle with fracture of anterior tibial eminence

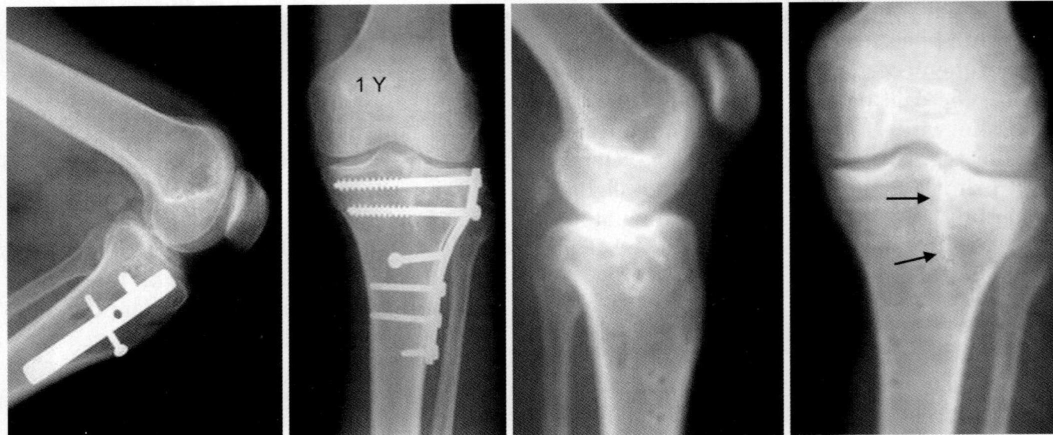

Figure 36.59 Plate removed from lateral condyle

Experience is remembering one's (and other's) failure. It is still prudent to learn from all the cases one comes across in a clinical practice, may be managed by our colleagues as well. When a case comes to a clinician for a second opinion for a given illness or for some other illness/problem, and if one goes through the history and radiographs brought by the patient for unrelated problem, one can see them and still learn a lot.

In this chapter, one would be able to study many cases managed elsewhere. When they come to another clinician, he should give a thought to few things:

1. What may have been the situation then?
2. What is done and if I was in charge, what would I have done?
3. If in the given case, if the result is less than satisfactory, considering all aspects of the case, why this happened?
4. What can I do now? By offering a secondary procedure, will the result improve reasonably?
5. What message do I get from this case?

Thinking this way would add to one's knowledge and planning capacity, which I think is important. I have observed, that time and again:

- In a bicondylar fracture of the tibia, only a lateral plate is applied.
- In a fracture of medial condyle, with dislocation of lateral condyle, again, a lateral plate is applied, where medial buttress plate is mandatory.
- Often internal fixation is done, by percutaneous screw fixation, without a buttress plate application.
- Elevation of the depressed segment and bone grafting is not carried out—may be the depression was not detected. Even if it is detected, its importance was not realized.

I have given my comments on each case, which one should carefully study, think and manage a similar case in the future.

After going through the cases, one would realize, what not to do is perhaps more important than what to do! If one learns from all the cases presented, one should be able to manage next case that one comes across, logically and more efficiently.

Case 1

Thirty years ago, for the proximal tibial fractures, the specific implants and exposure was advocated. In the initial case the importance of alignment was not understood and had residual varus. The triradiate or a T shape incision too had some problems. With learning and experience, we realized the importance of postoperative limb positioning and elevation, which improved the end result (Fig. 36.60A).

Prior to advent of the specific plates for proximal tibia, usually the non-operative method was used. The proximal tibia has muscle attachments, such that, mere cast/Thomas' splint immobilization cannot control it fully. Besides, being a juxta-articular injury, joint stiffness is a common occurrence, which is very annoying for the patient. Hence internal fixation, is a preferred method of treatment (Fig. 36.60B).

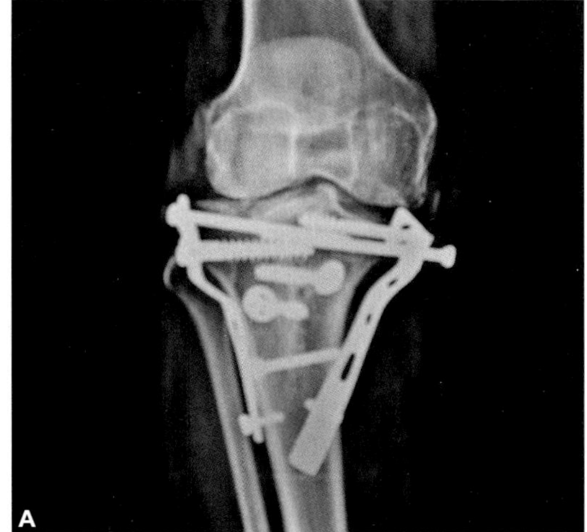

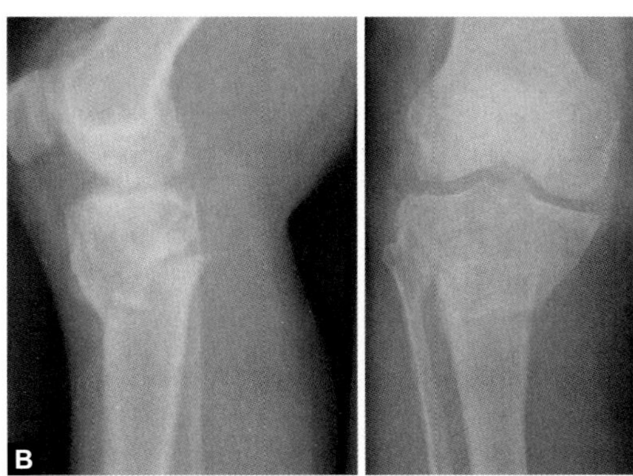

Figures 36.60A and B (A) Evolution. The first case done 27 years ago! Must do internal fixation; (B) Must do internal fixation

Case 2

The arrival X-ray showed a fracture of the lateral condyle with local depression on the analogue film. Perhaps a lateral view was not taken or may be of a poor quality. Lateral to medial percutaneous screw fixation and a cast immobilization was carried out. In fact, the injury was:

- Bicondylar fracture with a depressed fracture in the lateral condyle.
- The neck of fibula was uninjured, contributing to the stability, if correct procedure was carried out.

The fracture fixation was inadequate and as expected, resulted in varus deformity with persistent depressed segment in the lateral condyle. Should one desire to correct it now, with osteotomy, correction of the varus is possible. The depressed segment in the lateral condyle would have well united (being an impacted fragment!) After a few weeks, accurate elevation of that segment and restoration of the tibial plateau would not be possible.

Message

- The day 1 X-ray quality needs to be good for decision making.
- Whether CT scan facility is available or otherwise, internal and external oblique views should be taken, which would help to define the fracture morphology and should be a standard protocol (Fig. 36.61).

Case 3

Depressed Fracture of Medial Tibial Condyle

In this case of a depressed fracture of medial condyle, a percutaneous screw was inserted from the lateral condyle and a cast immobilization was carried out. As expected, resulted in a varus deformity.

Message

A fracture of the medial condyle needs a medial buttress plate fixation and a mere percutaneous screw fixation is inadequate (Fig. 36.62).

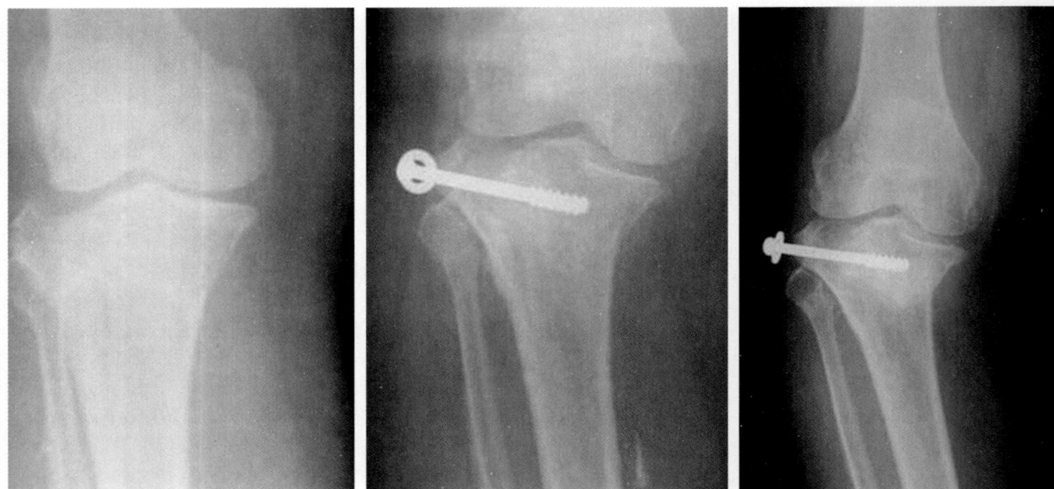

Figure 36.61 Only percutaneous screw and a cast lead to varus. Lateral condyle depression not elevated

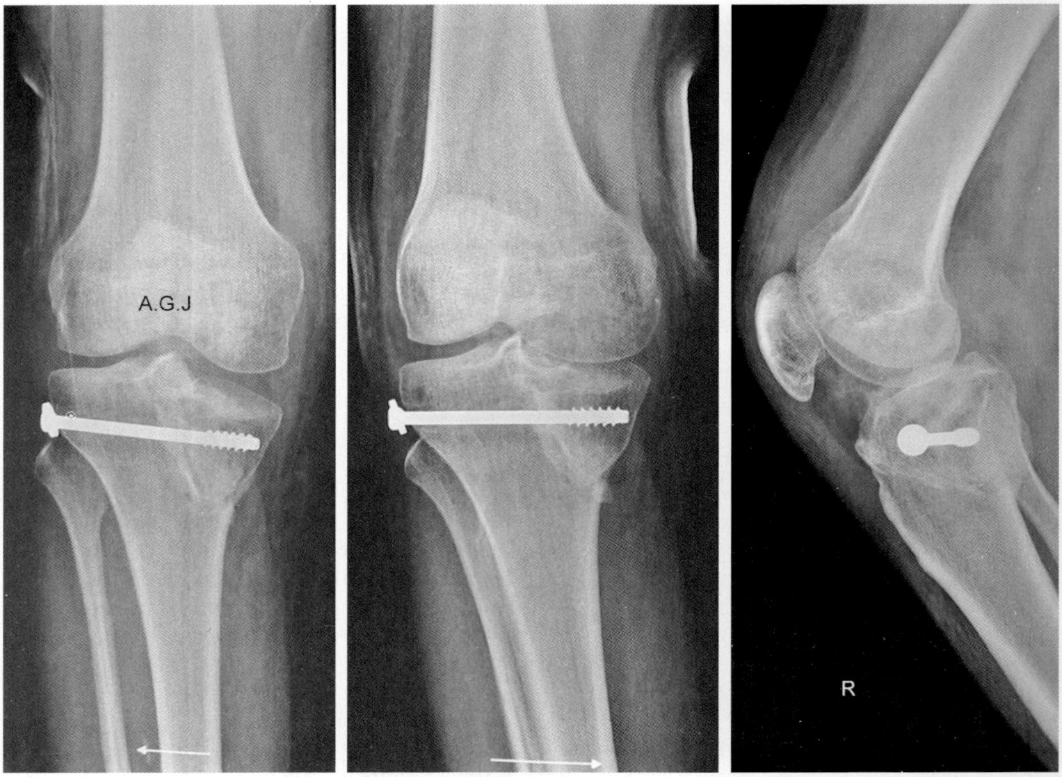

Figure 36.62 Lateral to medial screw inadequate

Case 4

Only Interfragmentary Screws

This case had intercondylar fracture with fracture of both condyles. Percutaneous cannulated screws were inserted form both medial and lateral side and immobilized in a long leg cast. Thus the intercondylar fracture was well-reduced and stabilized. However, the subcondylar fracture was not stabilized and hence late varus occurred.

The patient presented soon after cast removal, before, the fracture consolidated. Medial buttress plate was applied and alignment restored well (Fig. 36.63).

Case 5

A bicondylar fracture with fracture of proximal fibula needs absolute stability in the fracture fixation. In this case, with minimum displacement of the fragments, without any depressed fragment, fixation with a *medial* 12 mm buttress plate would have conferred a good stability. Even today, with availability of precontoured locking plates, mechanically, a medial plate is far superior in terms of stability it offers (Fig. 36.64).

Case 6

Bicondylar Fracture: No Elevation and Only a Lateral Plate

This case had a bicondylar fracture with depressed segment in the lateral condyle. It appears, only lateral plate application was done without elevation of the depressed segment. The end result was as expected—late varus.

The next surgeon revised the fixation by removing the lateral plate and applying a medial

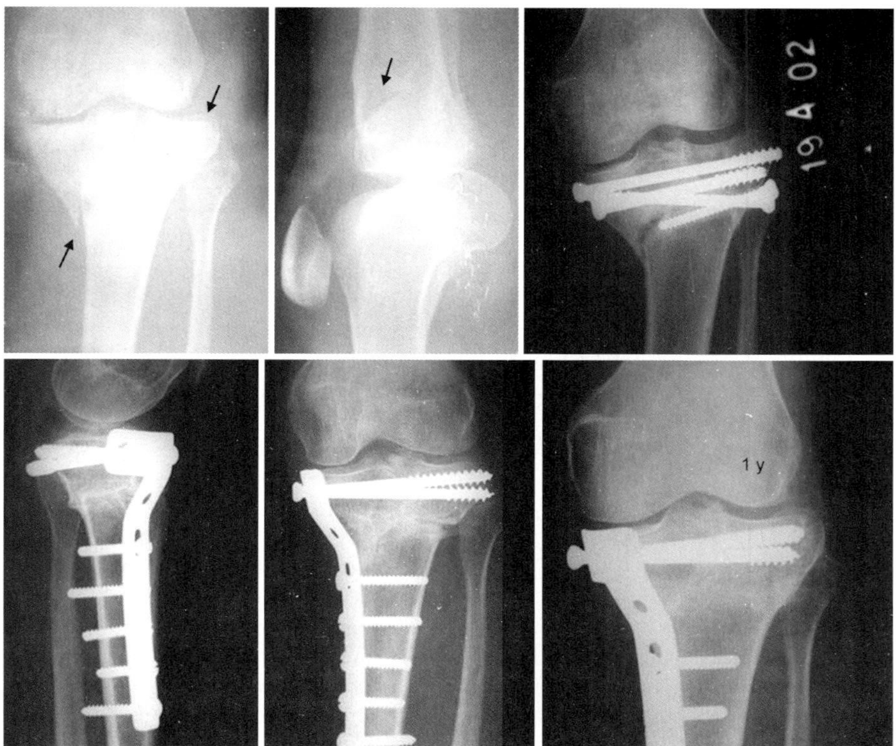

Figure 36.63 Medial buttress plate a must!

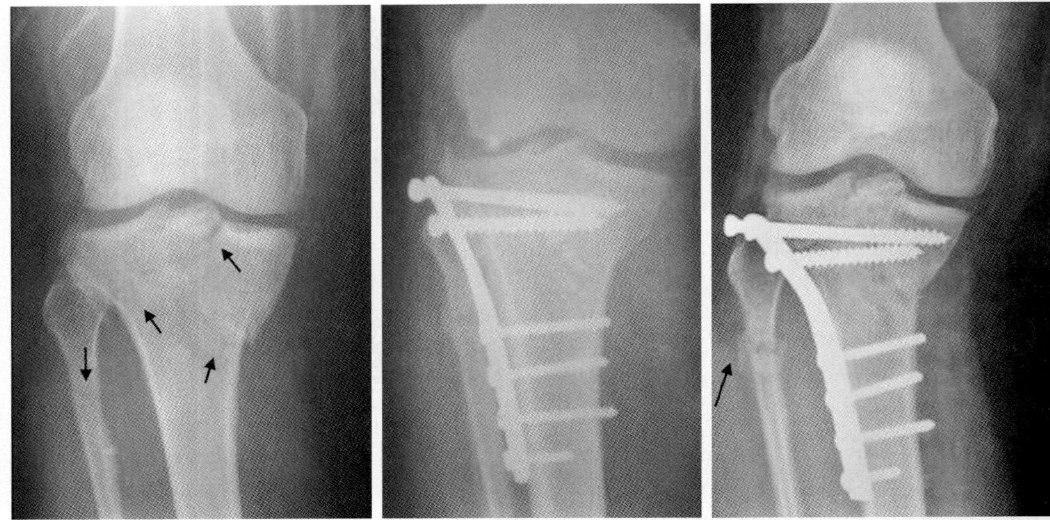

Figure 36.64 Plate be on medial surface in a bicondylar fracture

plate. As is known, the depressed fragment unites rapidly in situ and then its elevation is very difficult. Fortunately, due to intercondylar IF fixation, the lateral condyle could be brought under the lateral femoral condyle and weight bearing on the lateral compartment was possible. The alignment was well restored and patient had a reasonably good outcome. One cannot exclude possibility of late osteoarthrosis (Fig. 36.65).

Message

In such an injury, a midline incision with elevation of lateral depressed segment, bone grafting and stabilization with both a medial and a lateral plate is necessary (Fig. 36.65).

Case 7

A Fracture Dislocation of Lateral Condyle with Split Depression

In this case of fracture dislocation of the lateral condyle with depression in the intercondylar area, the limb was left as such, without immediate closed reduction, crepe application and plaster immobilization. Only a knee brace was applied and was operated after three days. One can well imagine, amount of local knee swelling and tissue edema, that must have occurred and the situation on table. As seen on the X-ray, the staples are seen on two surgical incisions, indicating possibly an MIPO technique was used in fracture fixation. Only a lateral plate was applied.

What would I have considered in this severe injury?

1. Immediate closed reduction: The displaced lateral tibial condyle should be brought well below the lateral femoral condyle. Application of a padded crepe support and immobilization with an above knee posterior POP slab.
2. Elevation of the depressed segment near the intercondylar area and bone grafting to fill the void is necessary.
3. Application of both medial and a lateral plate or at least a medial plate was indicated. This is especially needed when there is associated fracture of the proximal fibula, which requires more stable fixation.

In such a situation, a long generous incision with thick skin flaps is needed. I would have preferred a medial 12 mm wide plate × 3.8 mm thickness. This would have offered a good

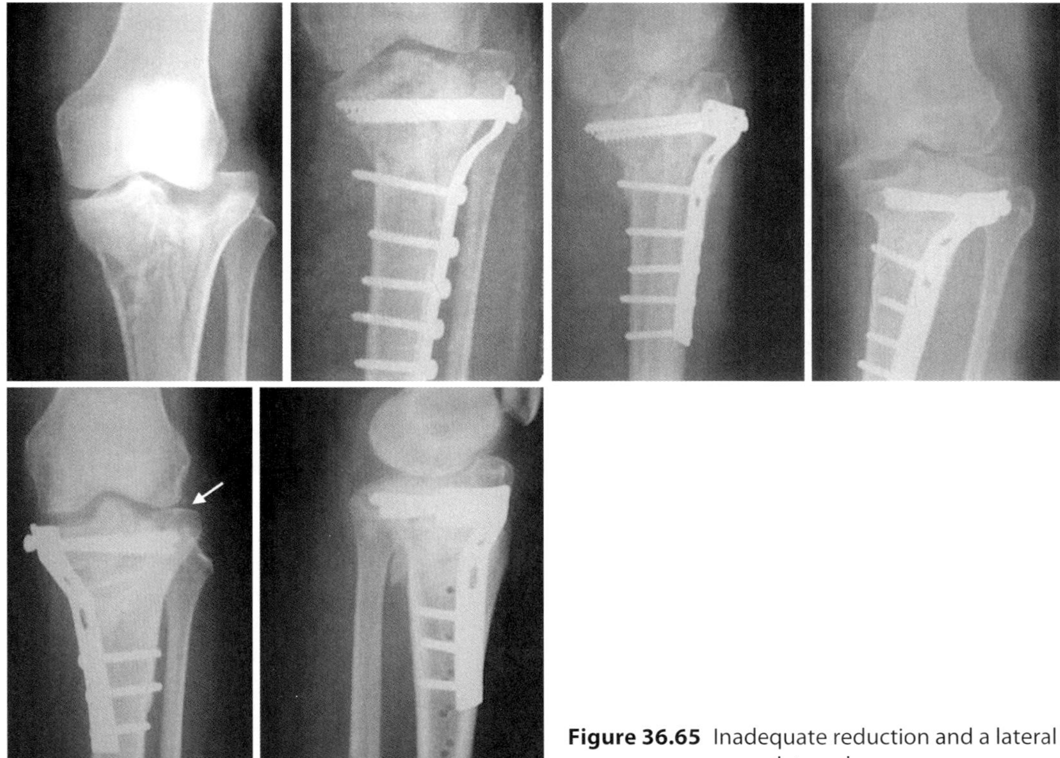

Figure 36.65 Inadequate reduction and a lateral plate only

stable fixation. Elevation on a high Bohler frame, with hip and knee flexed to at least 60 to 70 deg, would have helped to keep the tissue edema to a minimum and to regain good knee range of motion. In a long-term follow up, when reported for a II opinion, there was persistent FFD in the knee with restricted knee flexion and some varus deformity in the knee (Fig. 36.66).

Case 8

In this case of intercondylar fracture of tibial condyle, a lateral plate was applied elsewhere. At the end of three months, the fracture line continued to be seen in both the views. The plate was a curved hockey plate, applied laterally. If one would have left it as such, the mechanical failure of the plate was expected. Hence, it was revised by a medial approach. The lateral plate was continued as such. The fibrosis at the fracture area removed, edges freshened and cancellous grafts were added. Medially a 12 mm plate was applied for additional stability. The fracture united in due course.

Message

- A fracture with this morphology essentially needs a medial plate.
- Whenever, there is local bone crushing and bone defect, primary grafting is helpful.
- An additional lateral complementary plate adds to further stability. This plate is also designed, which is 10 mm wide and 2 mm thick, especially for such a situation.
- If such a correct procedure is thought of, planned and executed on day 1, the result is satisfactory and in an expected duration. Besides, a secondary procedure is also saved. In proximal tibia, subcutaneous

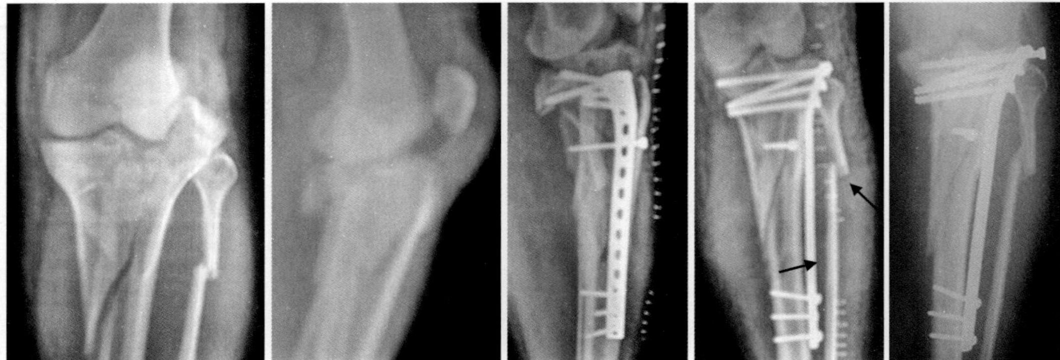

Figure 36.66 Fracture dislocation of lateral condyle with a split depression

tissue is sparse and any revision procedure, requiring raising flaps, is fraught with danger of skin flap necrosis (Figs 36.67A and B).

Case 9

A fracture of both condyles and associated fracture of proximal fibula, needs a special mention. An intact fibula offers a complementary support to the proximal tibia. If it is fractured, then the tibia stabilization needs to be more precise and stable.

The example shows a plate applied laterally, leading to a varus deformity. Even if the plate was a locking plate, there would have severe stress on the upper screw heads and perhaps mechanical failure. Application of a lateral plate is a disregard to biomechanics. (A medial plate offers more stability and resists the deforming forces better) (Fig. 36.68).

Case 10

In a fracture just below the condyles, associated with a fracture of fibula at the same level, it needs to be carefully stabilized. The muscle forces are more and hence stabilization has to be carefully planned. In such a case a lateral plate was applied, with more number of screws with a long plate segment distal to the fracture area, which is not so effective to stabilize the fragment. Later a stress view indicated abnormal mobility at the fracture area. May be the plate was fixed by an MIPO technique.

Message

In such a fracture morphology, the plate proximal end should have been at the subchondral level, so that adequate number of screws are above the fracture line. In IFS in appropriate plane would enhance the stability. A better option would be:

- A midline incision, with thick skin flaps
- Few intramedullary cancellous grafts
- A well-contoured *medial and a lateral plate*. If one prefers only one plate, it should be on *medial* side. The upper most screws should be in subchondral level of the condyle, for a good hold, with fully threaded 6.5 mm screws. IFS fixation enhances the stability.
- Fibula is left as such (Fig. 36.69).

Case 11

In a depressed fracture of either a medial or a lateral condyle, often exact elevation is achieved under a 'C' arm control. The depressed segment may have two fragments. I elevated the fractures well and stabilized with medial and lateral plates, with good intra-operative appearance on the film. To support the elevated fragments, screws are required to be in correct planes. In this case, X-ray taken after a few weeks shows depressed fragment, which could be anterior or a posterior fragment. As seen, the lateral femoral condyle is opposite a part of the lateral condyle, and is transferring the weight.

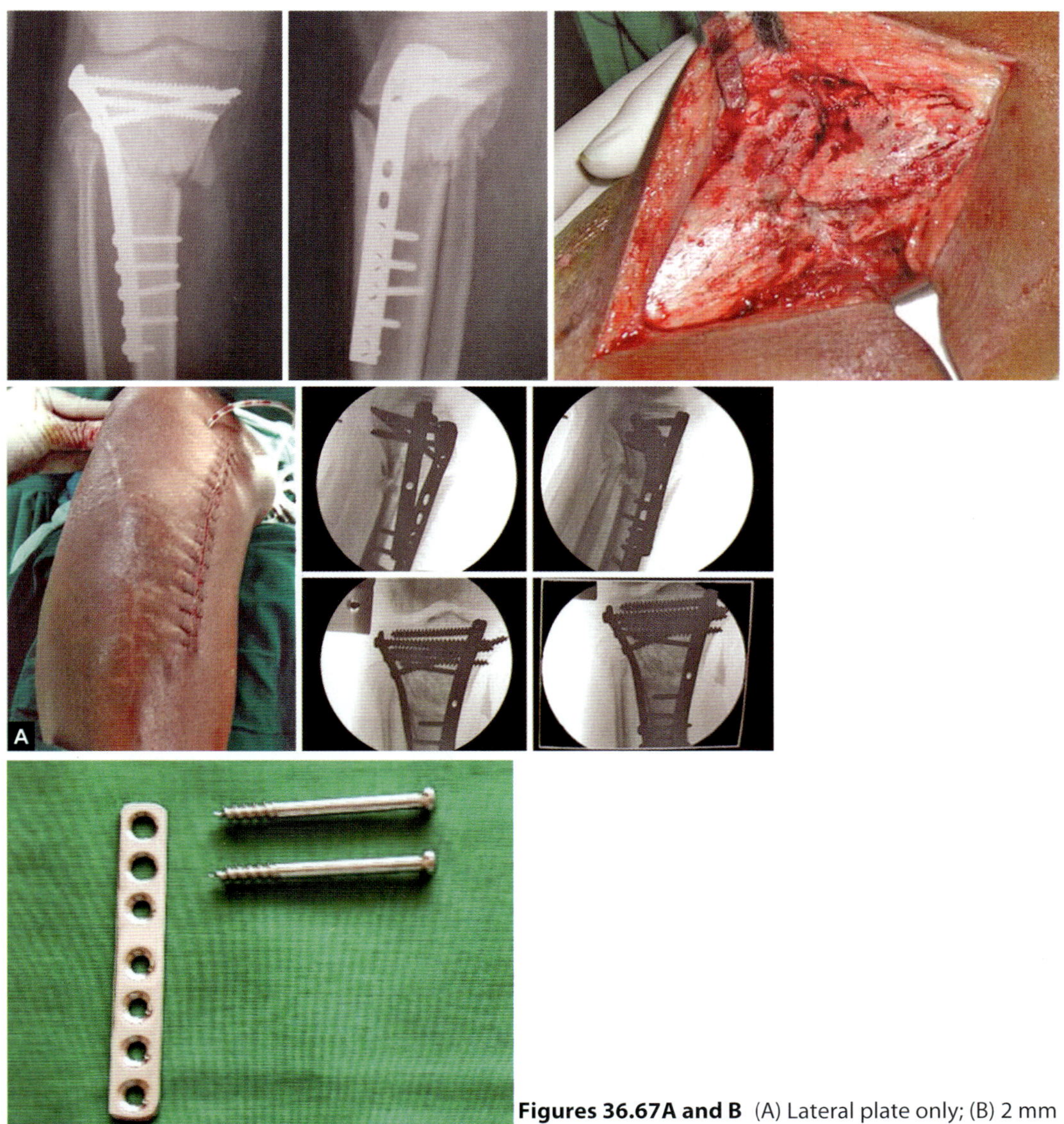

Figures 36.67A and B (A) Lateral plate only; (B) 2 mm thick plate for lateral surface

Message

The two upper screws should be in different planes, angulated about 30 degrees at least, with respect to each other. This would support the elevated fragments well and prevent late inferior migration as well. Raft screws of a locking plate do this (Fig. 36.70).

Case 12

In a bicondylar fracture of tibia, with minimum displacement or after a good reduction in a displaced fracture, stabilization must be done by only a suitable plate. The screws required should be 6.5 mm screws in the uppermost zone and should pass through the upper most

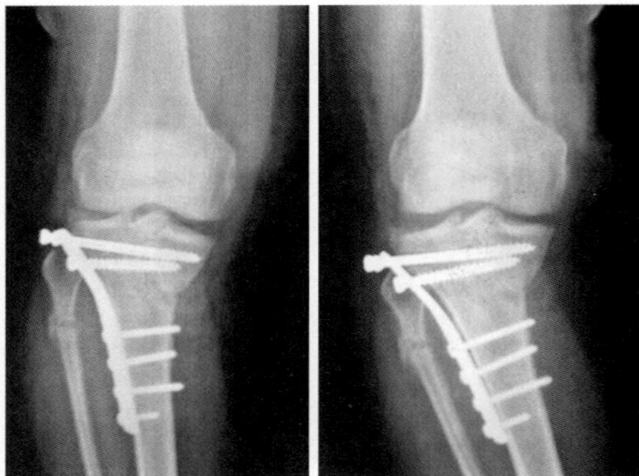

Figure 36.68 A lateral plate leads to a varus

hole of the plate to make a stable construct. Use of a malleolar screw be in exceptional situation and only as a complementary to other standard implants. The buttress plate needs to be of correct physical properties. Needless to predict, that the fixation would fail (Fig. 36.71).

Case 13

In this case of a bicondylar fracture, perhaps the fracture morphology was not understood well. Even if a CT scan facility was not available, study by internal and external oblique views would have defined the morphology and then the treatment planned.

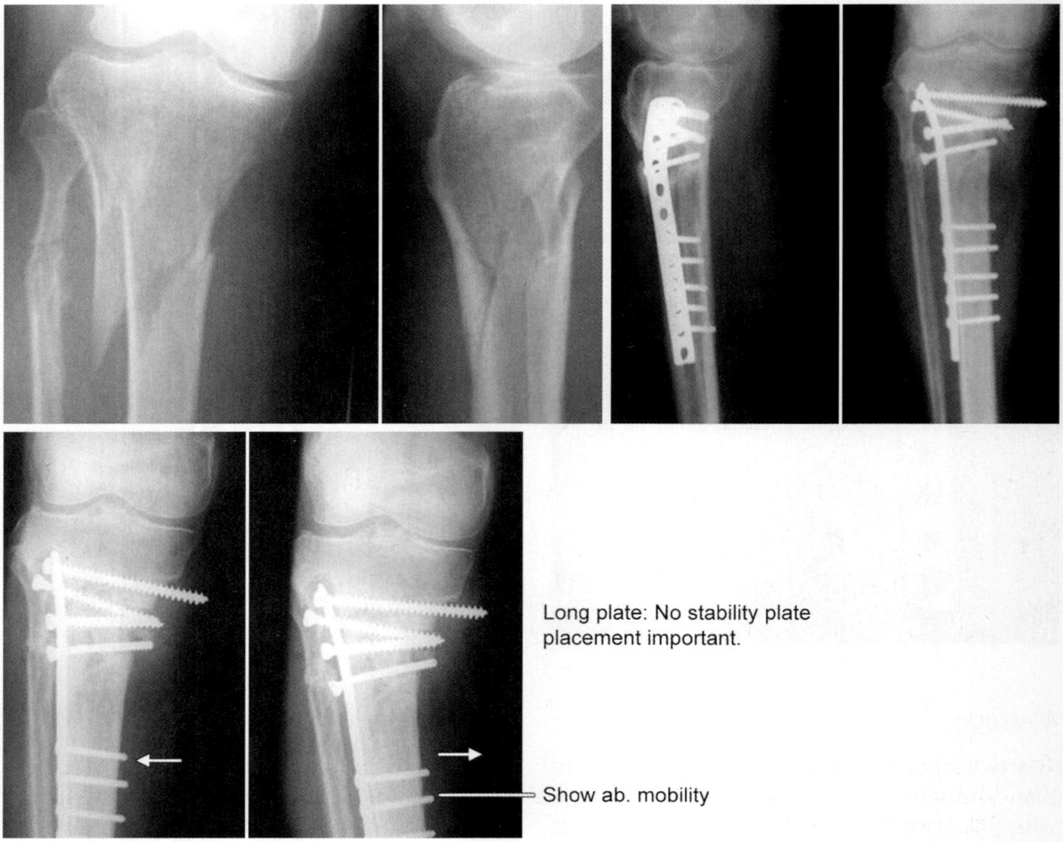

Long plate: No stability plate placement important.

Show ab. mobility

Figure 36.69 Stress views

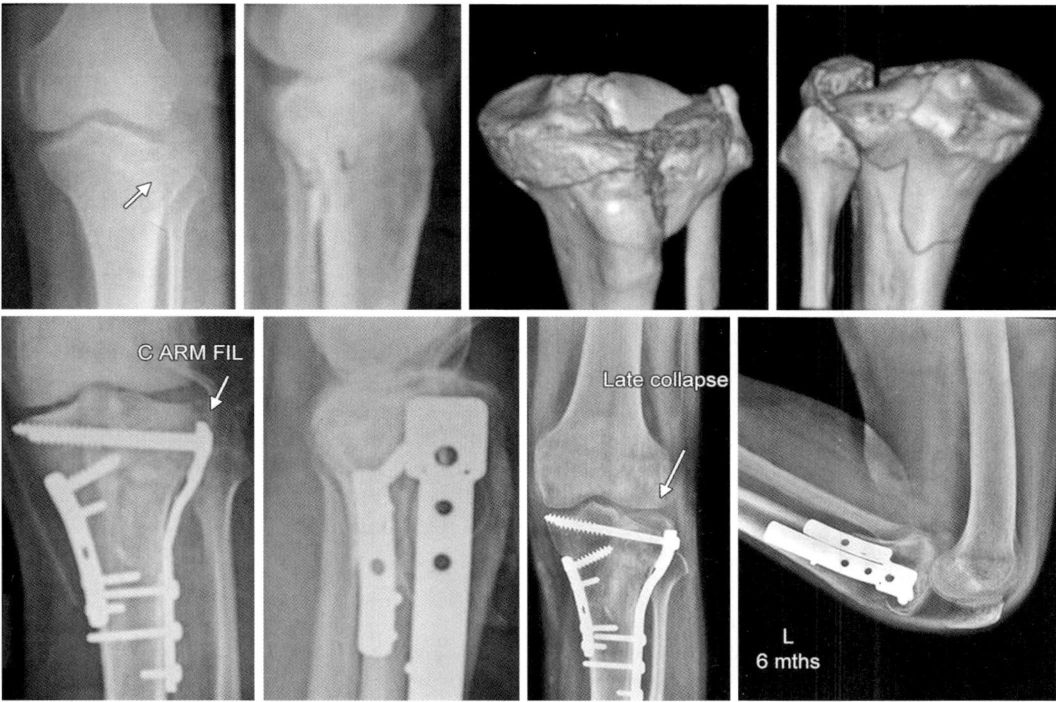

Figure 36.70 Late collapase

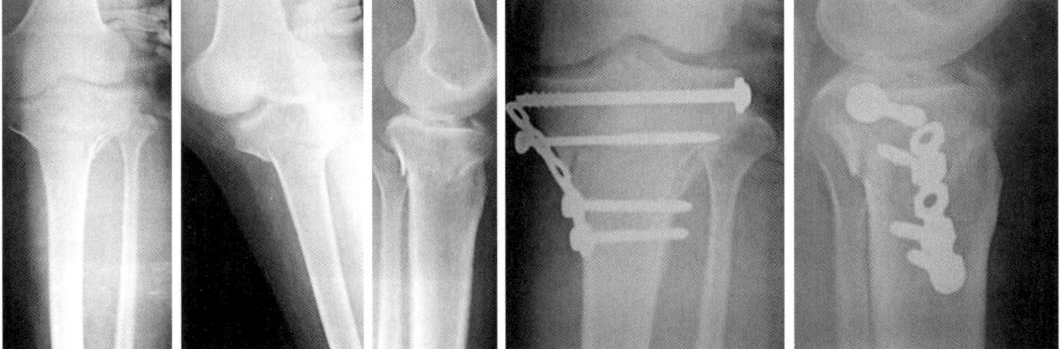

Figure 36.71 Poor choice of implants

How this could have been managed: In absence of a CT facility:

Under anesthesia, with traction reduce the fracture and examine under a 'C' arm and take AP and lateral films. Study the morphology. If possible, the proximally migrated lateral condyle fragment can be kneaded to bring down.

If the posteromedial fragment is quite wide, first one operates in a prone position and with an inverted L approach, reduce and fix the posterior fragment with a buttress plate. Which plate?

- A 1/3 tubular plate. The proximal two holes should be modified, to accept 6.5 mm screws. Now new design of locking plate for this area is available.
- A T long buttress plate used for distal radius can be used, with 4 mm shaft screws in the subchondral area, with 4 mm cancellous screws distally. Deflate the tourniquet and the wound is closed.

Patient is turned to a supine position and with a lateral approach, the displaced lateral fragment is reduced and stabilized.

Such fracture tends to become sticky quite fast and hence an early surgery is preferred (Fig. 36.72).

Message

Looking at the common fracture pattern in the above cases, one observes that:

- The medial condyle usually stays in place and the lateral condyle gets dislocated laterally.
- There is local comminution in the intercondylar area, which may need to be built up with bone grafting. The IFS put across the upper part of the condyle, should be just finger tight, to avoid condylar stenosis developing.

It is necessary to apply *a medial plate* for stability.

MEDIAL TIBIAL CONDYLE FRACTURE

In the knee, more weight passes on the medial side and hence, the medial cortex of the condyle is more thick. In this chapter, isolated fractures of the medial condyle alone or associated with its dislocation or of the lateral tibial condyle are presented.

In a case with associated subluxation/ dislocation of the joint, primary closed reduction, knee aspiration and padded crepe application is absolutely necessary. For pain relief and reduction of the edema, plaster support and elevation is mandatory. One should wait for three to six days for the tissue reaction to reduce, so the skin flap problem is kept to a minimum.

Case 1

Here is a fracture of medial tibial condyle, with some medial displacement. The fracture was reduced, by giving a valgus stress on the limb. Provisional stability was achieved by a K-wire, such that it was anterior to the proposed place of the plate. A five-hole custom-made 12 mm wide narrow straight plate was contoured to the bone and fixed. Good stability was achieved.

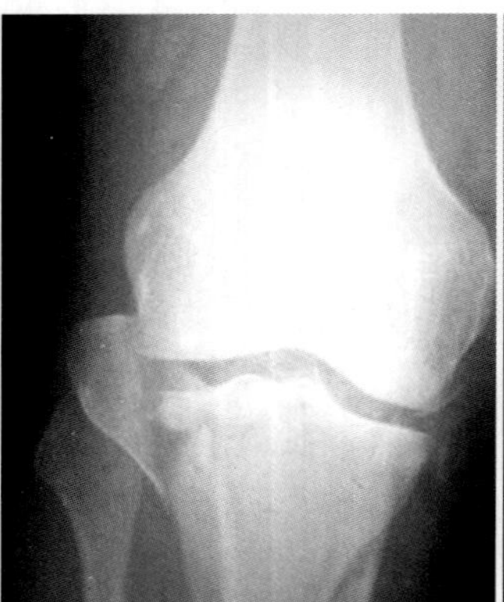

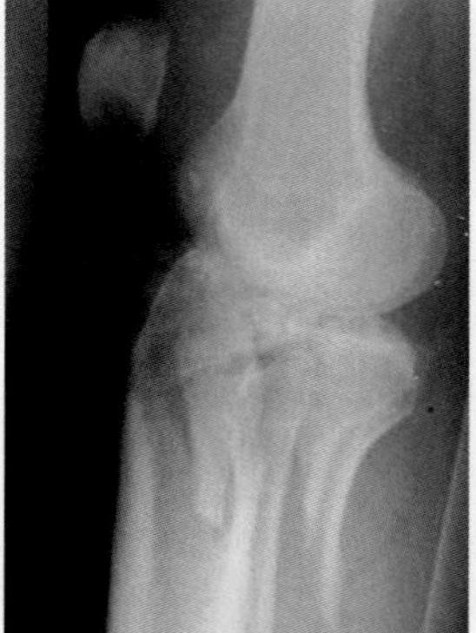

Not realised that medial condyle had a posterior component also.

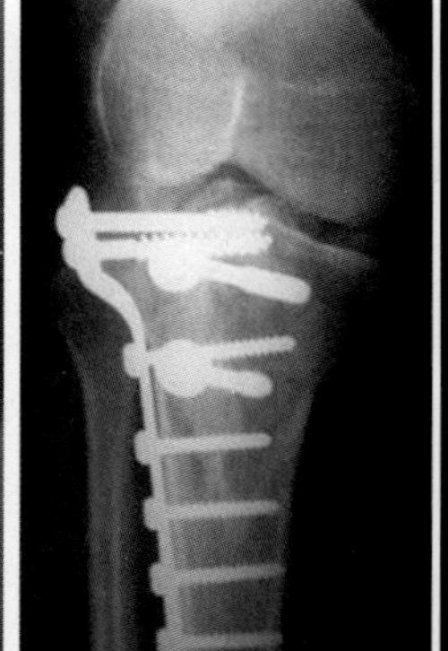

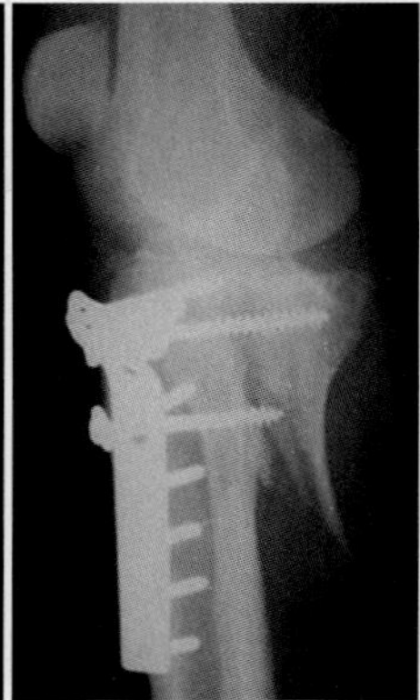

A postero-medial plate was of more importance

Figure 36.72 Bicondylar displaced fragments

Postoperative Position

Till the effect of spinal anesthesia is over, elevation on two to three soft pillows and then on a high Bohler frame is carried out. (In the immediate postoperative period, while the effect of spinal/epidural anesthesia is still present, the leg rolls out laterally. At this stage, if the leg is placed on a Bohler metal frame, as it rolls laterally, the common peroneal nerve is compressed against the metal bar and foot drop is the result). Static quadriceps exercises and active assisted mobilization of the knee was carried out: Good outcome (Fig. 36.73).

Case 2

- A split depression fracture near the tibial eminence
- Lateral subluxation of the lateral condyle.

The medial condyle fracture line extended quite lower down. The tibial eminence area was slightly depressed. Incision was taken, slightly medial to the crest and thick skin flaps were raised. The fracture morphology was studied. The fracture was purposefully opened and with a narrow punch, the eminence area was pushed upwards, to bring it in line with the tibial plateau. The fracture was reduced and the lateral tibial condyle was brought below the lateral femoral condyle. A 12 mm special plate was gently contoured and placed on the anteromedial surface. A provisional fixation was achieved by a K-wire, passed through the second hole from the top. A 4.5 mm screw was passed in the distal fragment, so the plate would be well opposed. A 6.5 mm partially threaded screw was passed through the top hole and finger tightened. This is important, to prevent stenosis of the tibial plateau surface. (The split fracture has a local comminution and applying excess torque to the IFS, often leads to plateau stenosis, as seen in AP view).

The lateral view showed that the fracture line was oblique and hence a malleolar screw was inserted from the anterolateral surface of the tibia. This screw was passed through the same incision, by elevating the skin flap, slightly laterally. If the necessary point of entry required for the malleolar screw comes to lie more laterally, excess retraction of the flap is avoided. Instead of this excess retraction, another short incision is taken 20 mm lateral to the first incision, so the blood supply to the intervening skin area is well preserved. After making a drill hole, one should slightly countersink the drill hole area or one may use a large 13 mm washer, as per the bone surface geometry. A 2 mm K-wire is passed through the drill hole, to remember the direction and is replaced by a malleolar screw. (A malleolar screw can be inserted without tapping. If a 4.5 mm screw is to be used, gliding and threaded hole technique needs to be followed).

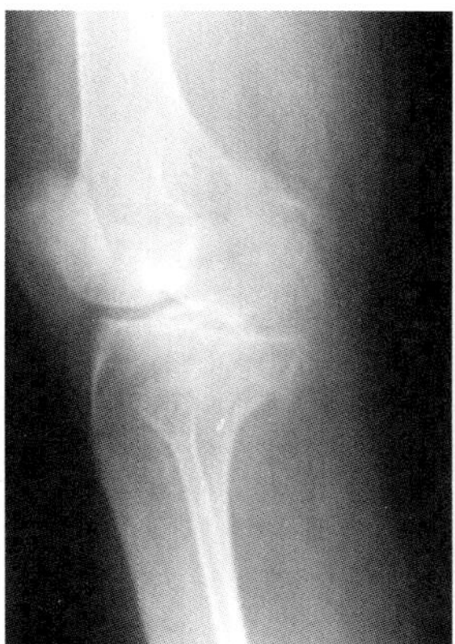

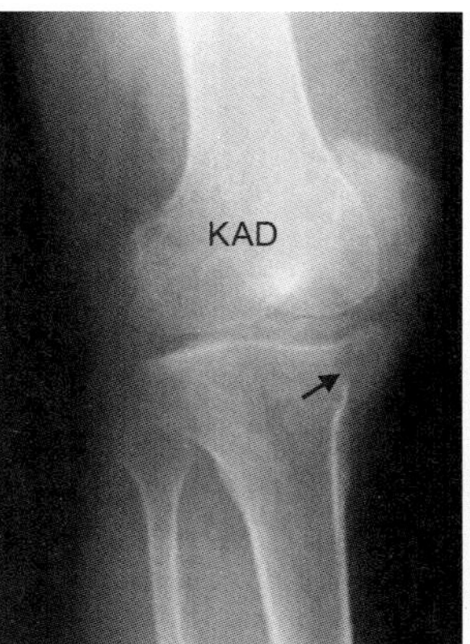

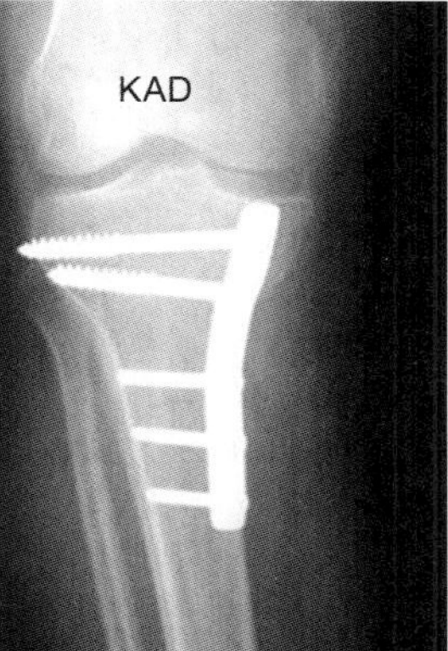

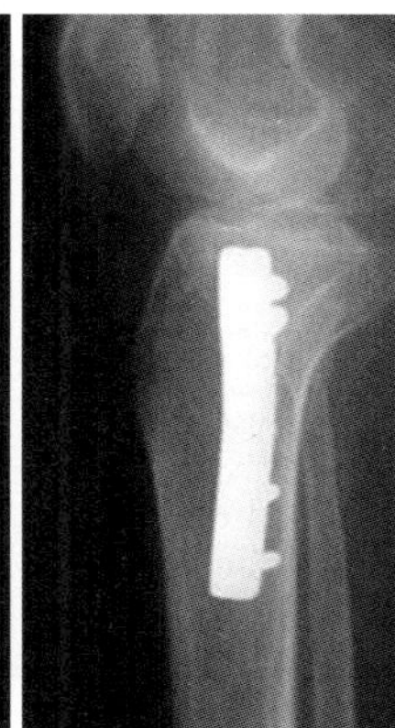

Figure 36.73 Medial condyle plate

The position of the implants was checked under 'C' arm and the fixation was completed by passing a 6.5 mm screw in the second hole from the top and the lower 4.5 mm screws. The fixation was stable. Wash: Release of the tourniquet, closure on a drain was done. The medial buttress plate holds both the condyles well and acts as a buttress also (Fig. 36.74).

Case 3

The lady had a fracture of the medial tibial condyle with few undisplaced fragments. This area has local bone fragments and would not hold any screw. Hence a plate was used, which had a span of 40 mm in the central area. The fracture had anterior angulation, with a small cortical fragment, angulated in the posterior cortex. On reduction of the fracture by traction on a quadriceps board, the alignment was restored and the posterior fragment fell in place.

In a standard 12 mm wide straight plate the distance between the two central holes is 26 mm. If such a plate was used, then at least two holes lying over the fracture lines of comminution, would have to be left unused. It is observed that, a mechanical failure of a plate occurs over a fracture site through the plate hole.

As seen in the X-ray photo, such a span plate was used. However, still one hole was left unused, as it was over a fracture line (Fig. 36.75A and B).

Case 4

Comminuted Fracture of Medial Tibial Condyle with Lateral Dislocation

This middle age gentleman had a severe injury to the knee joint, with a tense knee. The medial tibial condyle was comminuted, with lateral dislocation of the knee: Soon after arrival, the knee was reduced and a padded crepe bandage applied. The limb was immobilized in a Thomas' splint. The splint was elevated and static quadriceps exercises were encouraged. The adhesive skin traction and the Thomas' splint maintained the reduction well. Thomas' splint permits X-ray examination in all the angles. As seen in the X-ray photograph, *in the pre CT scan era*, one could have a 3-dimensional view with the four views through the splint and can have a good preoperative planning, prior to the surgery.

The fragment was quite large and hence in addition to the custom-made plate a 1/3 tubular plate was used, to confer more stability to the assembly (Fig. 36.76).

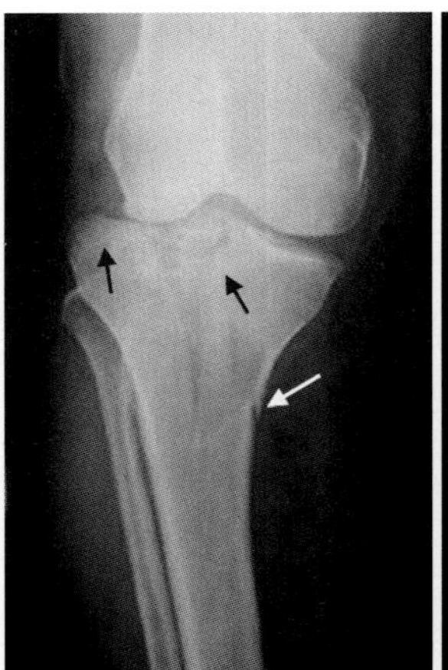

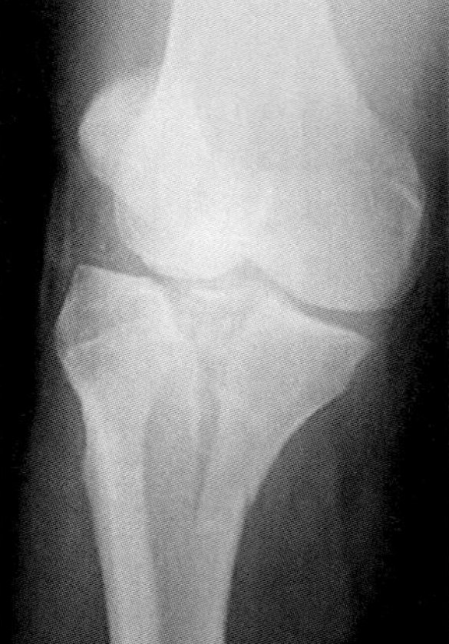

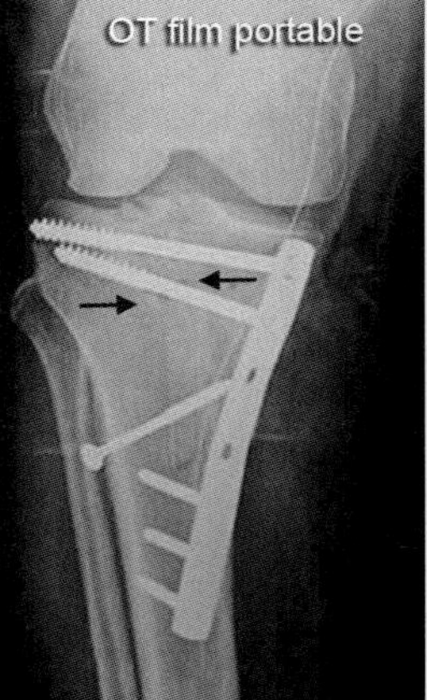

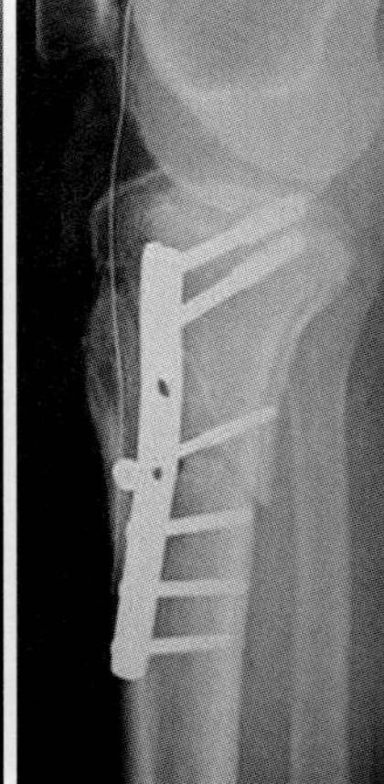

Medial custom plate for 2: 6.5 screws use of a malleolar screw as IFS

Figure 36.74 Medial condyle plate

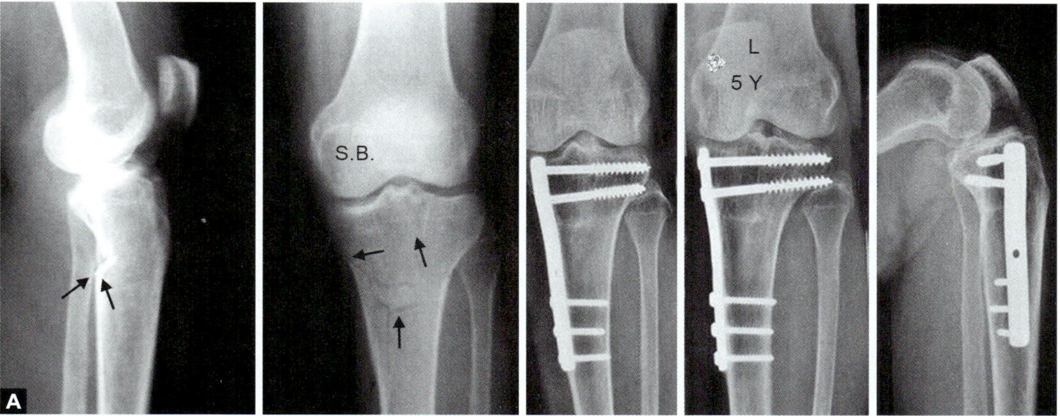

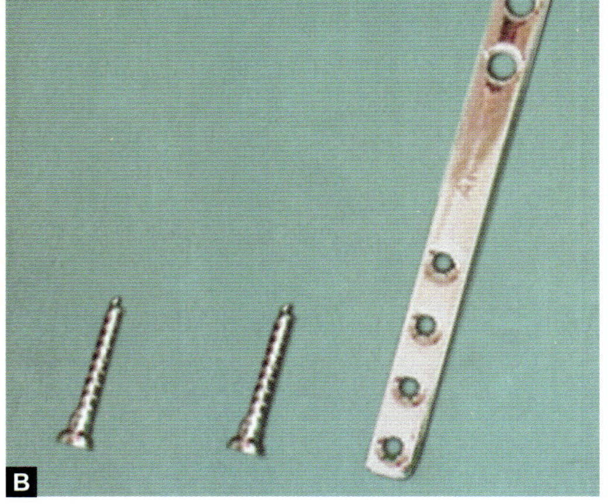

Figures 36.75A and B (A) Medial condyle span plate: Span plate; (B) Span plate

Case 5

This middle aged gentleman had a two wheeler accident and sustained a segmental fracture of medial tibial condyle and lateral dislocation of the lateral tibial condyle. Local pain and swelling was quite severe. Soon after arrival, the fracture dislocation was reduced under anesthesia. A padded crepe bandage and plaster immobilization was carried out. It took about six days for the tissue reaction to settle down, which is the usual period taken.

It is extremely important to educate both the patient and the team to observe patience during this period. The skin nourishment is restored, tissue edema reduces, the surgical procedure is less stressful and smooth and recovery uneventful.

Surgery with the knee on a quadriceps board and manual traction to the ankle, makes the fragments fall in place. A 12 mm tibial plate with proximal large holes was used.

The proximal condyle fragments were stabilized with 6.5 mm screws. The middle segment had fracture lines under the screw holes of the plate and hence the screw holes were left as such. Distal most 3 holes of the plate were occupied by 4.5 mm screws. Post-

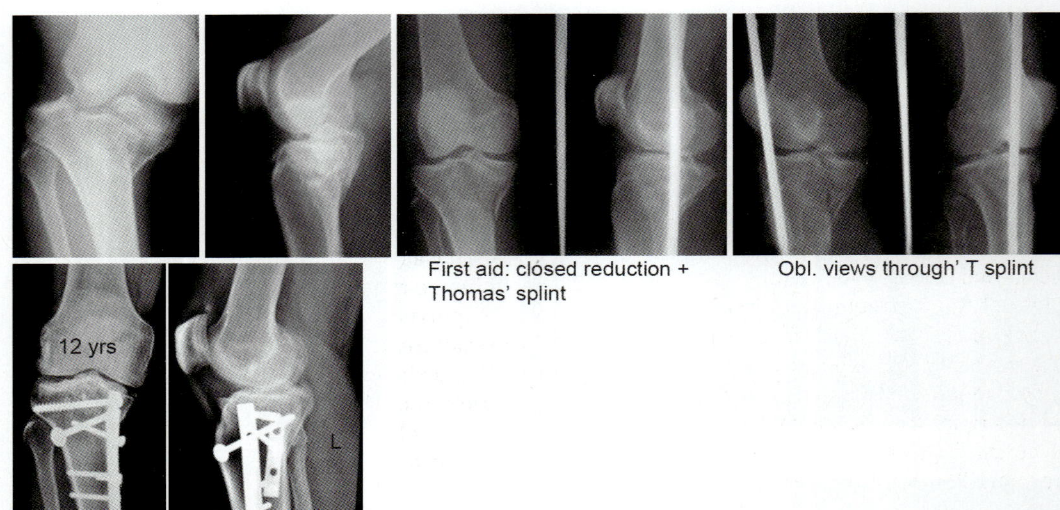

Figure 36.76 Fracture dislocation and Thomas' splint

Figure 36.77 Medial condyle fracture dislocation and a long plate

operative recovery was satisfactory and non-weight bearing ambulation was carried out for 2 months. During this period, active mobilization and muscle strengthening was carried out. Good end result (Fig. 36.77).

Case 6

This patient had a fracture of medial condyle. The medial condyle was small in term of vertical height of the fragment. Required stabilization. Since the height of the fragment was small, only one screw could be accommodated in that plane. Hence a T buttress plate was chosen. It has two holes on the horizontal limb and both the screws were passed. The fixation conferred good stability with a good end result (Fig. 36.78).

Case 7

This tall, obese, elderly person had a severe knee injury.

- Fracture of the medial condyle
- Dislocation of the lateral condyle
- Fracture of the anterior tibial eminence.

There was local bone crushing in the central area. The eminence area was elevated and bone grafting was done. It was fixed with a wire loop. On the medial condyle, two plates, one 12 mm and other 1/3 tubular plate as a complementary fixation was applied. There was collateral laxity and hence required cast immobilization. Later on supervised mobilization was carried out. The fracture united and the knee was stable.

The flexion achieved was till 90 deg only and he preferred to walk with a stick for the last 18 years. No changes of osteoarthritis yet, which was likely to occur (Fig. 36.79).

Case 8

A young man had a fracture of medial tibial condyle and a small fragment adjacent to it. A custom-made 12 mm plate with large holes at

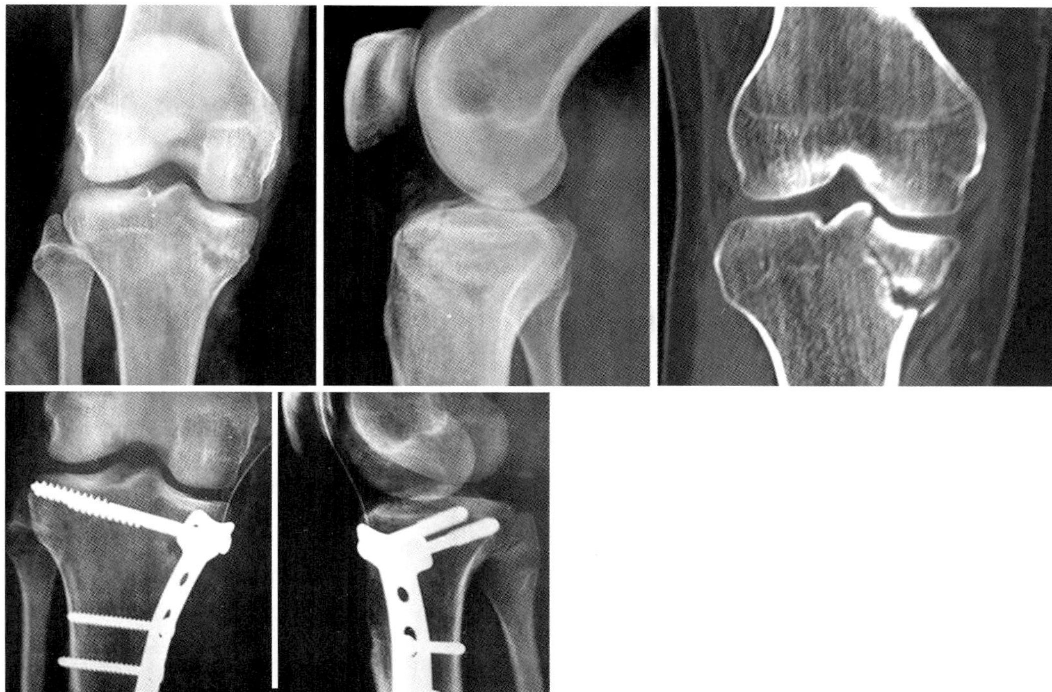

Figure 36.78 Medial condyle small fragment

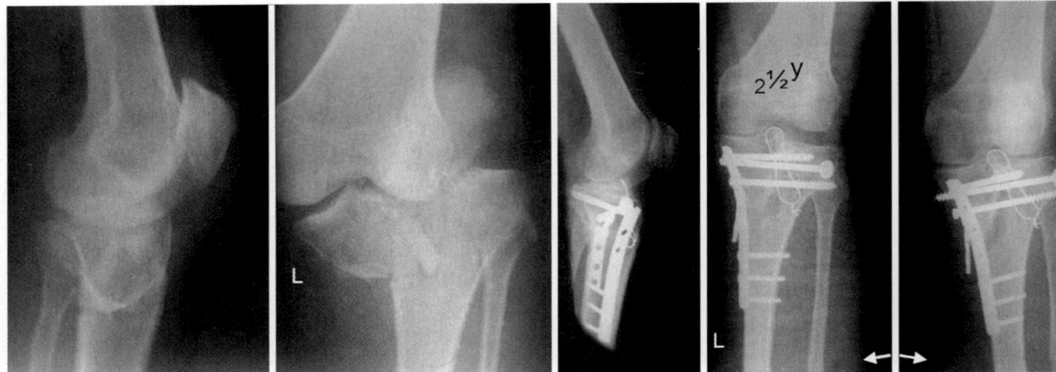

Figure 36.79 Fracture medial condyle and lateral dislocation

one end was used. Adjacent fragment was fixed with a 1/3 tubular plate. Good postoperative outcome.

After a few months local inflammation and a sinus developed, indicating a late infection. As expected, would respond to antibiotics for a short while and would recur again. The fracture had consolidated well, with good range of motion. The implants were, therefore, removed and the screw tracks were well curetted. The wound healed well and good knee function continued (Fig. 36.80).

NONUNION IN FRACTURE OF TIBIAL CONDYLE

Case 1

In this fracture a long plate is seen to be applied laterally. Fracture continues to be ununited.

Observations

- Plate should have been applied medially.
- The screws are away from the fracture line: less stability.

How was managed?

- Removal of the lateral plate and application of a medial plate
- Though the plate was short, mechanically was a stable construct, because screws are close to the fracture line, resulting in union (Fig. 36.81).

Case 2

In a similar fracture morphology, a lateral plate was seen.

Observations

- The plate should have been placed much higher, so the 6.5 mm screws would have a good fixation in the subchondral area.
- The screws are too close to the fracture line, may be through the fracture as well. Result: united fracture.
- Stress views confirm abnormal mobility at the fracture area.

Solution

Revise and apply a medial plate, may be with bone grafting.

Message

- In such a fracture morphology, a medial plate offers more stability.
- The screw placement, should be close to the fracture, but not through it.
- IFS with intraosseous bone grafts would assure fracture union (Fig. 36.82).

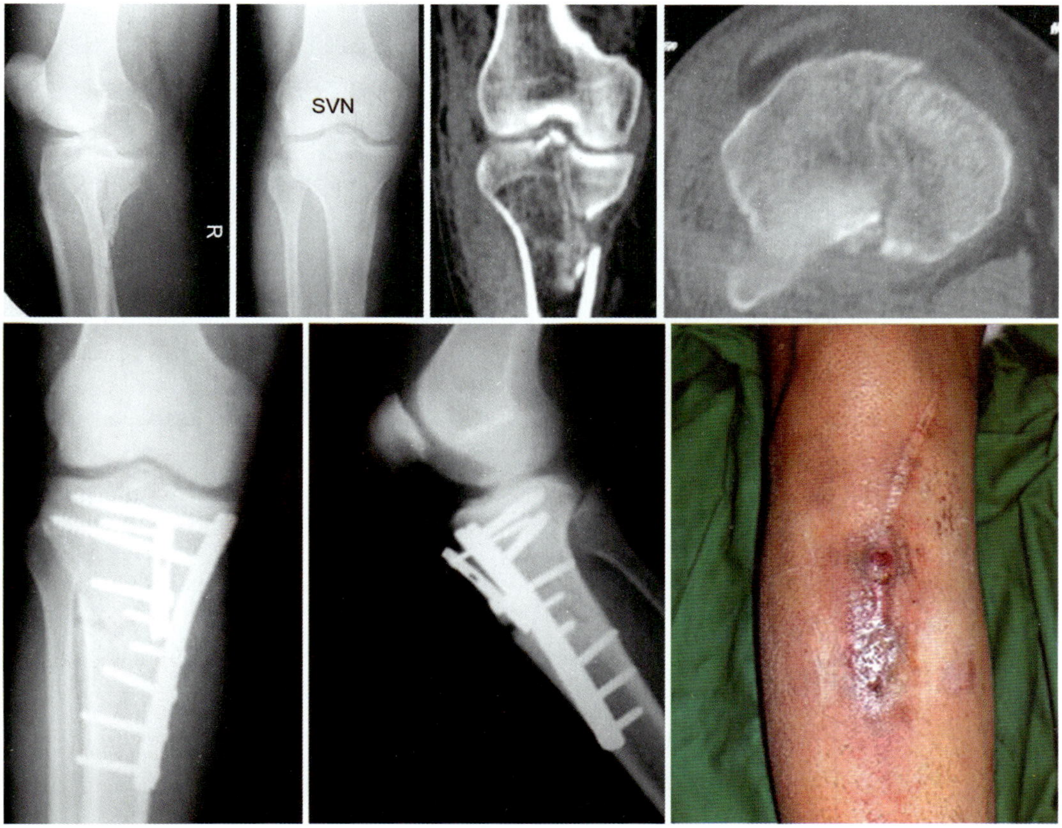

Figure 36.80 Medial condyle and late infection

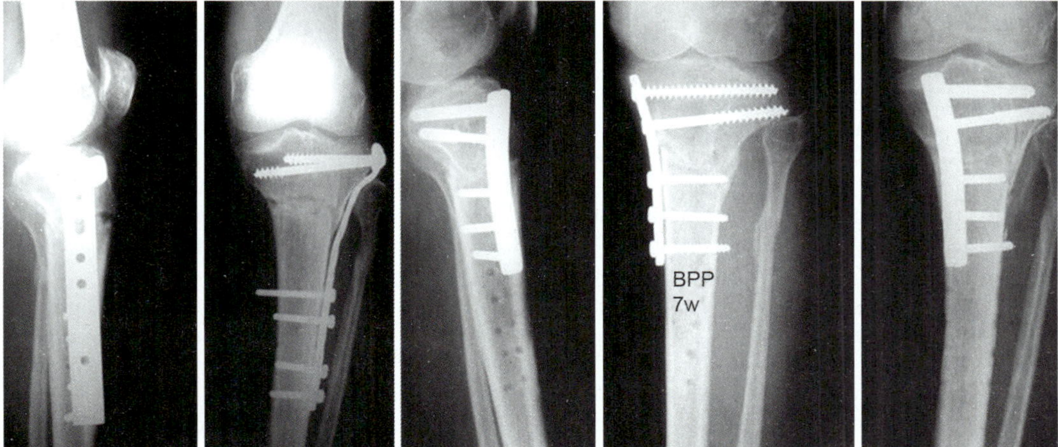

Figure 36.81 Medial plate is stable

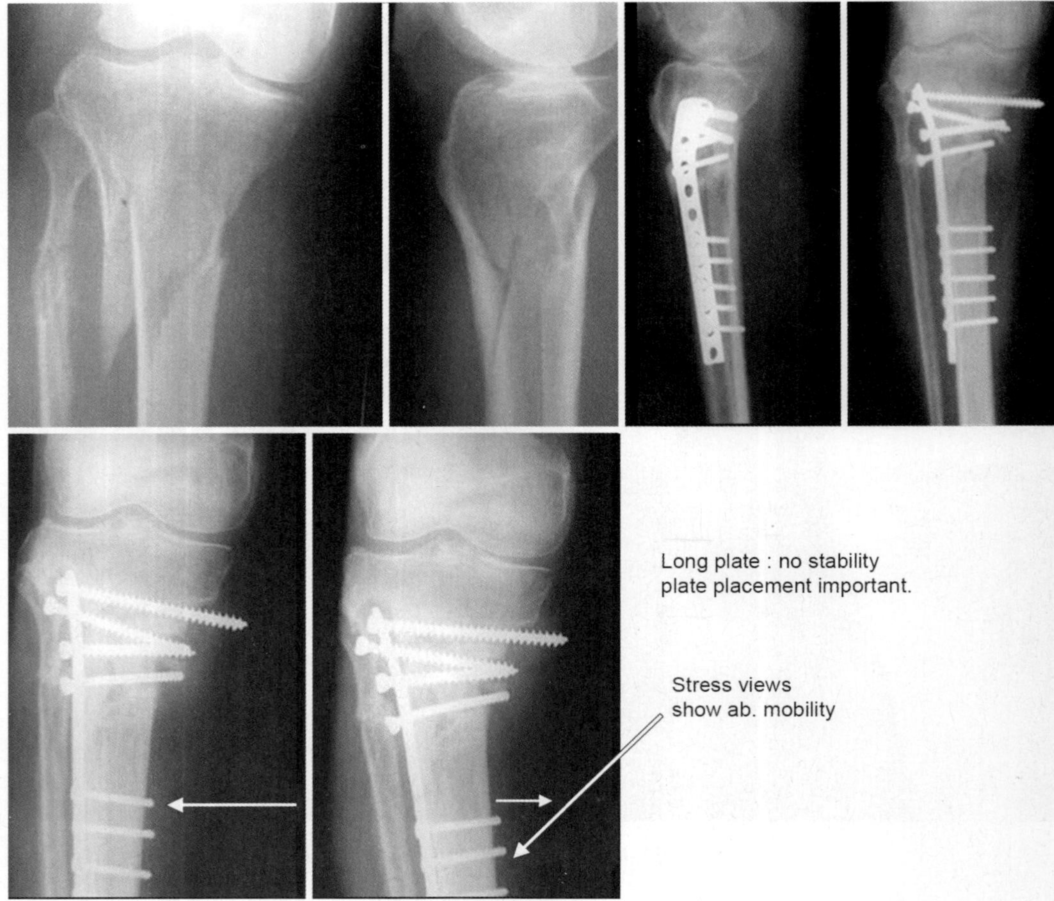

Figure 36.82 Stress views in nonunion

POST-STIFFNESS FRACTURE OF TIBIAL CONDYLE

Stiffness of a knee joint, after a disease or injury, is a very unfortunate situation. It is very inconvenient in activities of daily living. More than this, it tends to make the person susceptible for another injury.

This lady had a possibly a Hoffa fracture in the knee joint. It was managed by a colleague, by a reco. plate application as seen in the photograph. As per the history, neither postoperative 90–90 elevation of the knee nor a CPM was advocated. This resulted in restriction of motion of the knee.

She had a fall and since the knee could not bend, to absorb the forces, the patella gave way. At this time, I was involved for further treatment. A tension band fixation was done and patella united.

A few years later, with another episode, sustained a supracondylar fracture of the femur on the same side and a locking plate was applied, leading to union.

Later, again had an unfortunate injury, leading to a fracture of tibial condyle. This was stabilized, with a medial T plate and the fracture united. Following the last three injuries and surgeries, the knee was elevated to at least 60–60 deg, to maintain the pre-injury range of motion. Fortunately, we could maintain the knee range of motion, to what was prior to the fracture of patella (Figs 36.83 and 36.84).

Message

It is thus important to strive to achieve a full range of knee motion, after any injury near the knee joint.

My dilemma is whether to let the implants be as they are or should they be sequentially removed, to avoid any subsequent injury, adjacent to the implants. We all should realize, what she has gone through, due to the knee stiffness.

POSTERO-MEDIAL AND POSTERO-LATERAL CONDYLE FRACTURE OF TIBIAL PLATEAU

There is a rise in injuries associated with two wheel vehicles. The morphology of fractures of tibial condyle is naturally varied. One comes

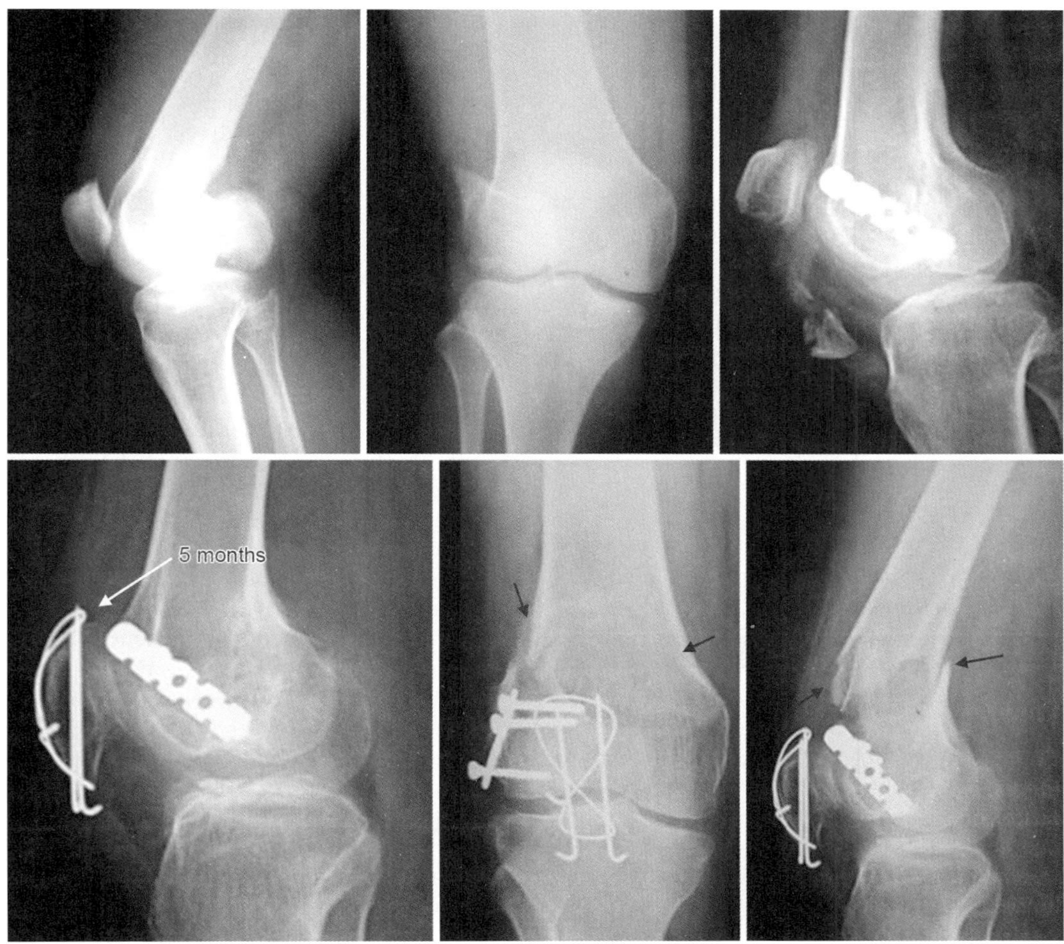

Figure 36.83 Post-stiffness fracture i

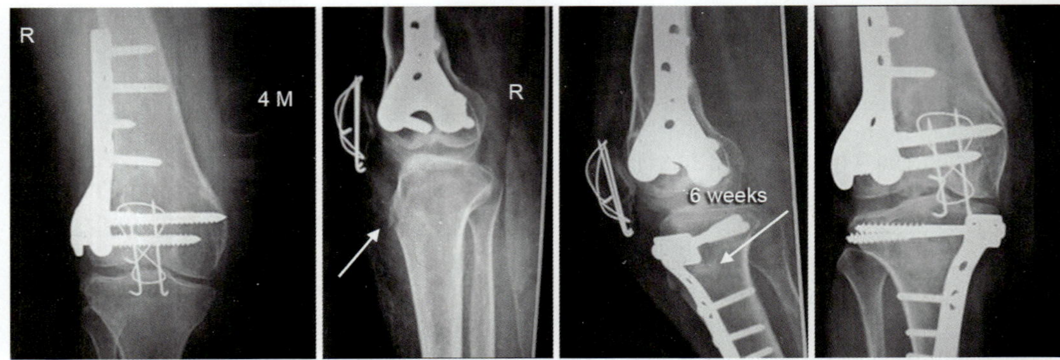

Figure 36.84 Part-stiffness fracture ii

across fracture of medial condyle, which has more component of posterior rather than a medial condyle. Similarly, fracture of posterior of the plateau is also seen more often, than two decades ago. Availability of CT scan helps us to define an injury better.

Fractures of posterior tibial eminence and its fixation is commonly done, than few years ago. Thus, one becomes more conversant with the posterior surgical approach.

A decade ago, for a fracture of medial tibial condyle, with more of posterior component, one would apply a medial plate and an antero-posterior screw, for further stability. In most of the cases, this leads to a good stable fixation, early mobilization and a good functional outcome.

With experience, a direct approach to the posterior fragment is carried out. This approach helps reduction under vision and fixation with a buttress plate.

CLINICAL EXAMPLES

Case 1

This middle age person sustained a fracture of medial tibial condyle, with a long beak on the posterior area. The medial condyle was reduced and held with a pointed reduction forceps and checked under 'C' arm. It was stabilized by a T buttress plate, placed, slightly posteriorly on the medial surface. Then, anterior to the plate, an antero-posterior screw was passed, to enhance the stability. One has to be extremely careful in making this AP drill hole, as neurovascular structures are in the posterior area (Fig. 36.85).

Case 2

This young man had a fracture of medial tibial condyle as in the earlier case. With a medial approach, the fracture was well-reduced and held with a reduction forceps. A medial plate was applied. While the reduction forceps was in place, a 6.5 mm screw with 16 mm threads was passed from anterolateral area, towards, posteromedial part of the condyle. Having had three screws in place, I tried to insert one more screw. As happens in the presence of screws, the drill bit hit a screw present in the condyle and gave way. Being made of austenitic steel, it was left as such and did not cause any reaction. The fracture united well (Fig. 36.86).

After three years, the plate and the screw were removed. A wide track was made along the direction of the bit, but was unsuccessful in removing it. Was left as such. May be use of a crocodile forceps or the like instruments, may have been successful in retrieving the bit (Fig. 36.87).

Case 3

This young lady sustained a fracture of the posterior part of the tibial plateau. She was treated elsewhere. A transverse incision was taken and as seen in the X-ray picture, six

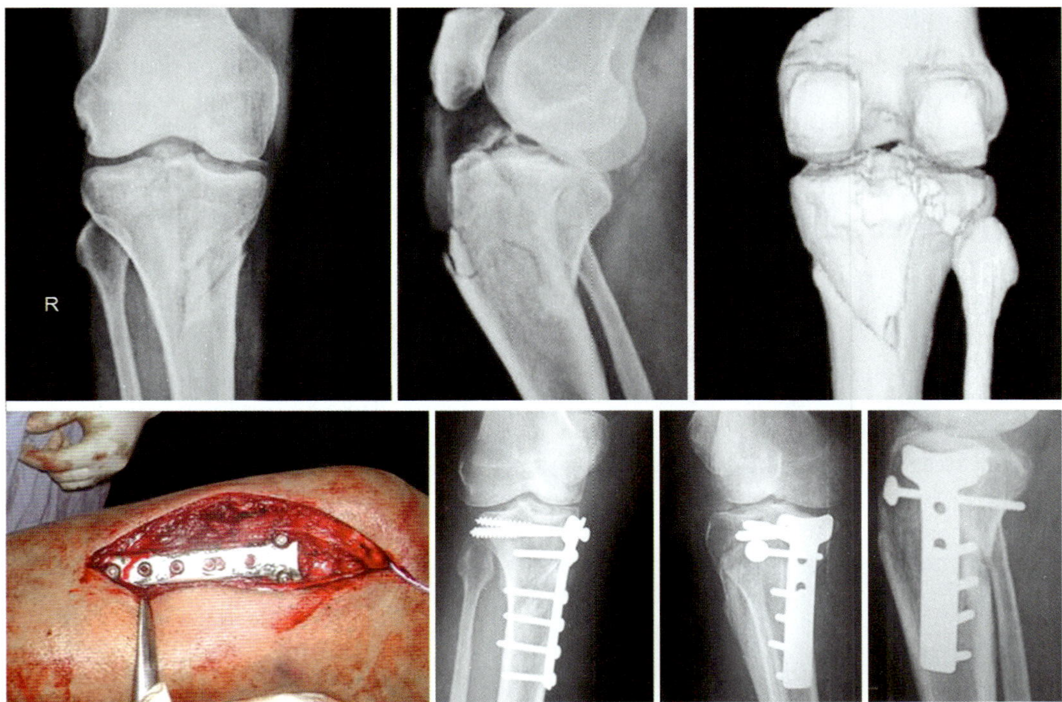

Figure 36.85 Medial plate and AP screw

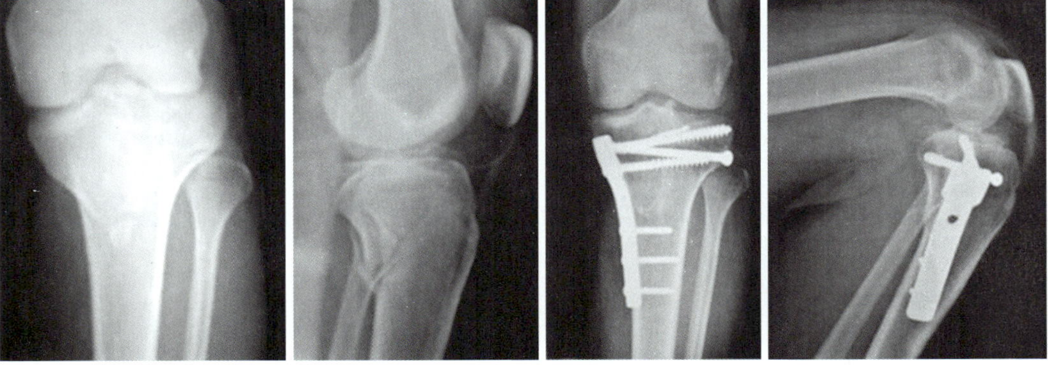

Figure 36.86 Medial plate and broken bit

cannulated cancellous screws were inserted and a long leg cast was given.

As one is taking a posterior approach, I would have preferred to take a lazy S incision, with distal limb on the medial side. It is possible to retract the neurovascular structures, laterally. Having done so, my preference would have been to apply a buttress plate. The plate and the IFS together offer a good stable fixation and one can dispense with plaster immobilization.

Which Plate?

A T buttress plate, used in distal radius, would need use of 3.5 and 4 mm screws. While, if a T buttress plate of tibia is used, a 4.5 mm system needs to be used (Fig. 36.88).

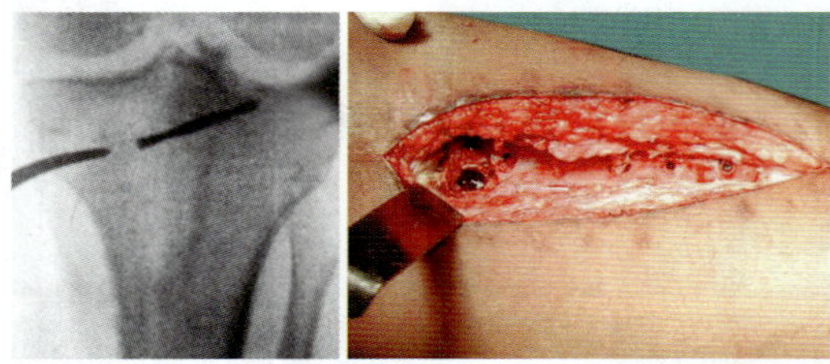

Figure 36.87 Removal of the plate and a track for the bit

Case 4

This lady had a fracture of the medial condyle. The fracture line was above downwards and anterior to posterior side. Looking at the lateral view X-ray film, it is clear that a posterior buttress plate is logical. This was carried out and a T buttress plate was applied.

Tips in Posterior Approach

It is necessary to study the anatomy of this area again, looking at diagrams in the exposure technique and atlas of anatomy. A visit to anatomy hall to see a specimen, is the time well invested.

- Prior to prone position, due care of patient's eyes needs to be taken, especially for a

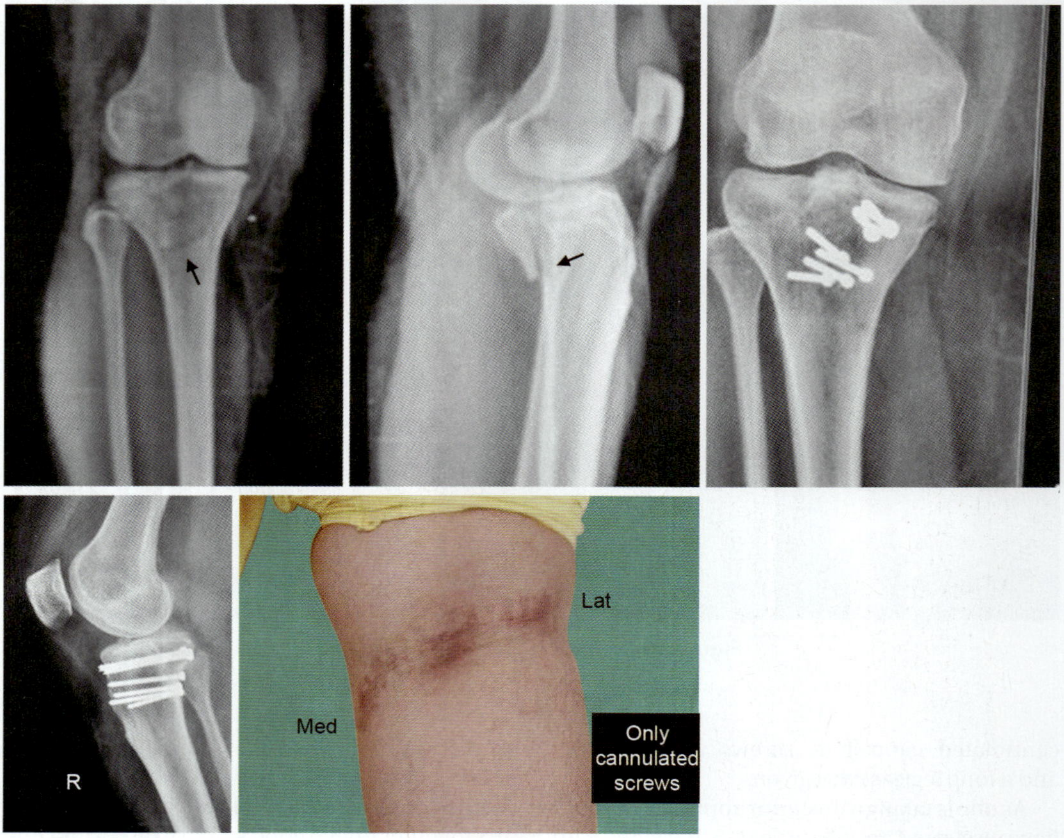

Figure 36.88 Connulated concellous screws only

procedure under GA. A tourniquet is applied on the thigh, with the air tube so placed, that it will not kink in prone position.

- Two long bolsters are placed vertically under the torso, with comfortable space for chest movements. Adequate padding is kept under the ASIS for protection.
- A draped pillow is kept under the ankle, to keep the knee slightly flexed.
- Check that a good AP and Lateral 'C' arm image is possible.
- The conventional and a modified approach is described in fixation of the posterior eminence of tibia. In the transverse limb of the incision, one comes across the short saphenous vein and long cutaneous nerve of calf. A thick flap is raised, just superficial to the deep fascia.

Having exposed the posterior fragment, it is reduced and assistant holds it with a punch. Provisional fixation is done with a 1.8 mm K-wire, at such a place, so that it does not come in the way of the plate placement.

The posterior border of the plateau is seen covered with the capsule. A T shape proximal tibia buttress plate is placed over the fragment and may need some contouring. The upper most edge of the plate is so placed, that the proximal most screw will remain entirely intra-osseous and not penetrate the joint cartilage. It is necessary to understand the direction, which a screw would take, when passed through the uppermost hole in a T buttress plate, when placed on the posterior upper end of tibia.

A K-wire is inserted through the distal most hole, of the plate, to keep the plate stable. A 4.5 mm screw is inserted through the oval hole and not fully tightened. The placement is again checked under 'C' arm and the possible direction of the uppermost screw is remembered. A 6.5 mm screw with 32 mm threads is passed through the uppermost hole in the plate and the progress is checked under 'C' arm. The oval hole screw is tightened and the rest screws are inserted. Finally the fixation is checked under 'C' arm, tourniquet deflated and closure over a drain carried out. Prior to the closure, it is safe to palpate the pulsation in the wound (Figs 36.89 and 36.90).

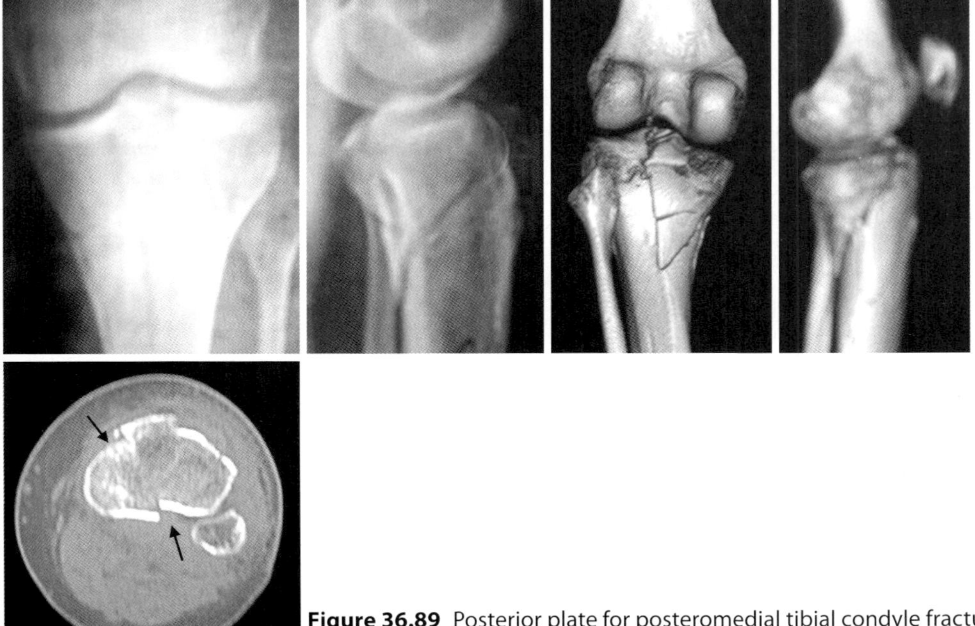

Figure 36.89 Posterior plate for posteromedial tibial condyle fracture i

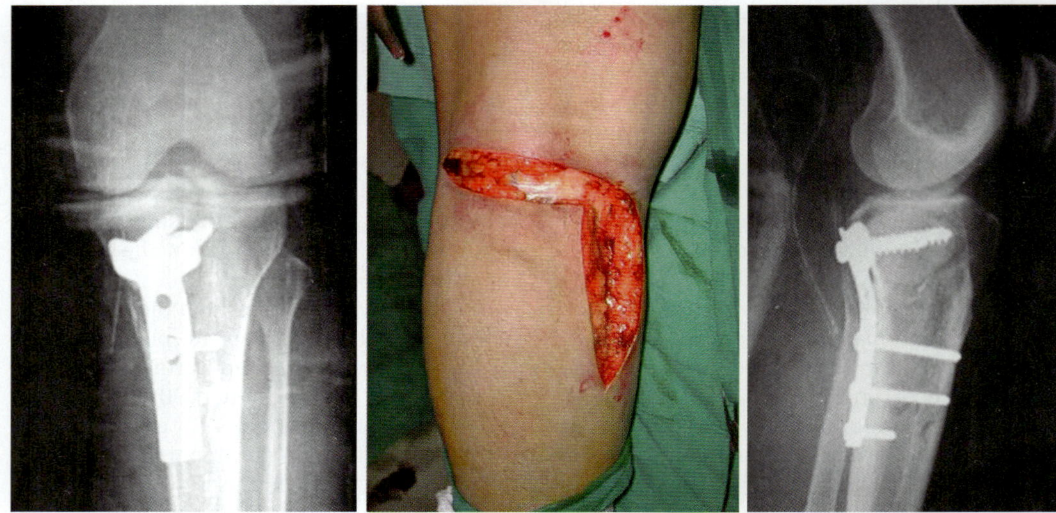

Figure 36.90 Posterior plate for postero-medial tibial condyle-fracture ii

Case 5

This girl had a fracture of posterior part of the medial condyle, with posterior tibial eminence. A CT scan with 3D reconstruction showed few small fragments at the posterior eminence area.

Exposure

A posterior exposure was taken, with the vertical limb medially. The medial head of gastrocnemius was identified, and the deep fascia incised vertically. The medial head was freed from deeper structures with blunt finger dissection and with the knee slightly flexed could be moved laterally. One can reach the midline area safely, as the neurovascular structures are taken laterally.

The posterior fragment and the posterior eminence were stabilized with K-wires.

The eminence was fixed with a 4 mm shaft (partially threaded) screw, with a washer. The following method is useful:

The trick: A drill hole is made with a 2.5 drill bit, through the posterior eminence, till it enters the host tibia. It is changed to a 1.8 mm K-wire and further drilled. This creates a track for the screw to be passed. The K-wire is removed and a 1.2 mm K-wire is inserted, till it goes easily. A hemostat is attached to it, where it emerges from the bone and the wire is removed. The length of screw is thus determined. Thus in the proximal tibial cancellous area, there is a track of 1.8 mm and now when the screw is advanced, it gets a good purchase. The proximal tibia structure being cancellous, the shaft screw can advance well and have a better hold than when the entire drill hole would have been made with a 2.5 mm bit.

The large fragment was fixed with a T plate, which is used for proximal tibia, medially.

Postoperative Care

Postoperative elevation on a Bohler frame was carried out as usual and static quadriceps exercises started at the earliest. Active knee mobilization and non-weight ambulation was done at appropriate time. Weight bearing needs to be withheld for at least 8 weeks, since the fracture was in weight bearing area.

It is observed, that if a plaster immobilization is carried out, even for three weeks, later on, to regain the flexion is rather difficult, so much that, one may need manipulation under anesthesia (Figs 36.91 and 36.92).

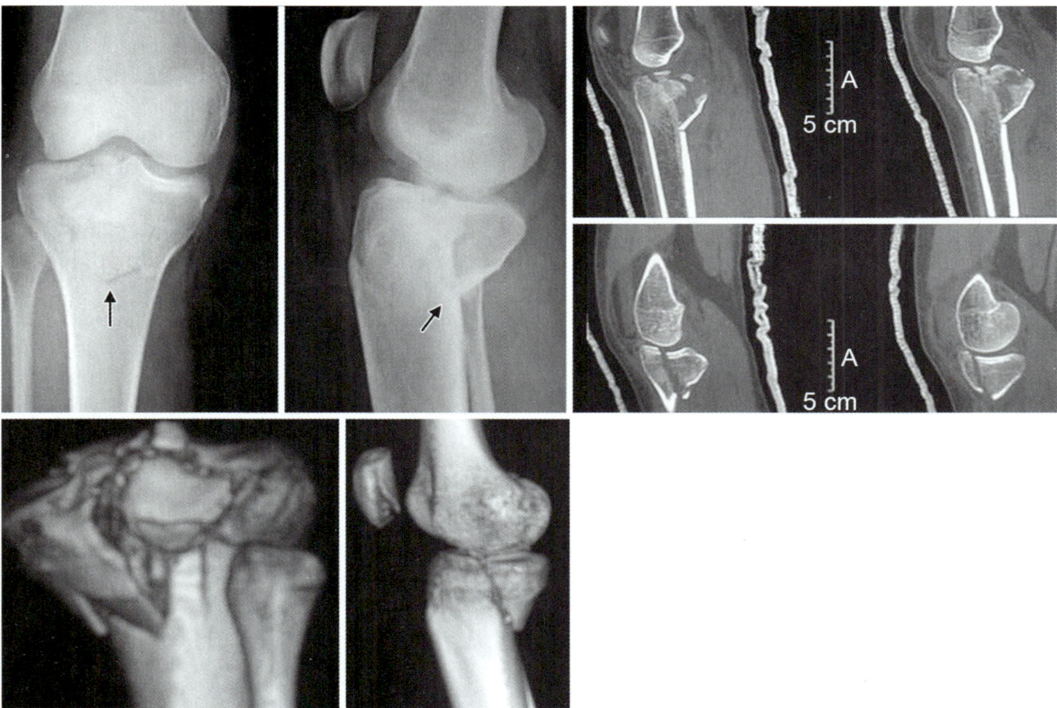

Figure 36.91 Posterior tibial condyle and posterior eminence fractures

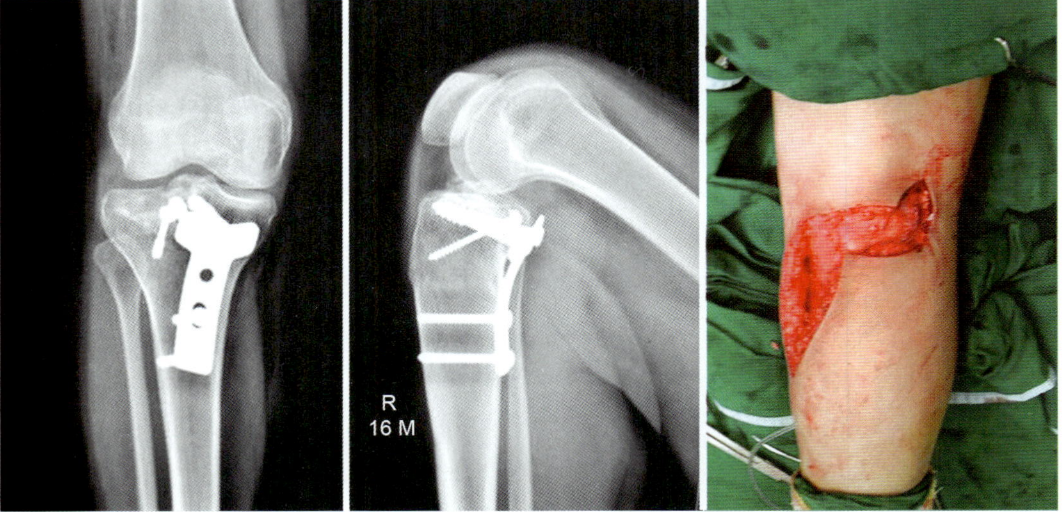

Figure 36.92 Posterior tibial condyle and posterior eminence fractures

Case 6

This person in late 30s sustained an RTA with injury to the right proximal tibia. Both the medial and lateral tibial condyles were fractured. The fracture lines extended more posteriorly and inferiorly, especially on the medial side. CT scan confirmed this and made the fracture morphology clear.

Planning

- The posteromedial fragment required stabilization, using a locking plate, especially designed for this area.
- The lateral condyle had less of posterior component and hence, a laterally fixed 12 mm custom-made plate would be adequate.

Steps Done

First he was made prone and the posteromedial fragment was fixed with a locking plate. The incision was a lazy S with medial limb inferiorly.

He was then made supine and a quadriceps board was used. With an anterolateral exposure, the lateral condyle was fixed with a 12 mm wide custom-made plate. The proximal two large

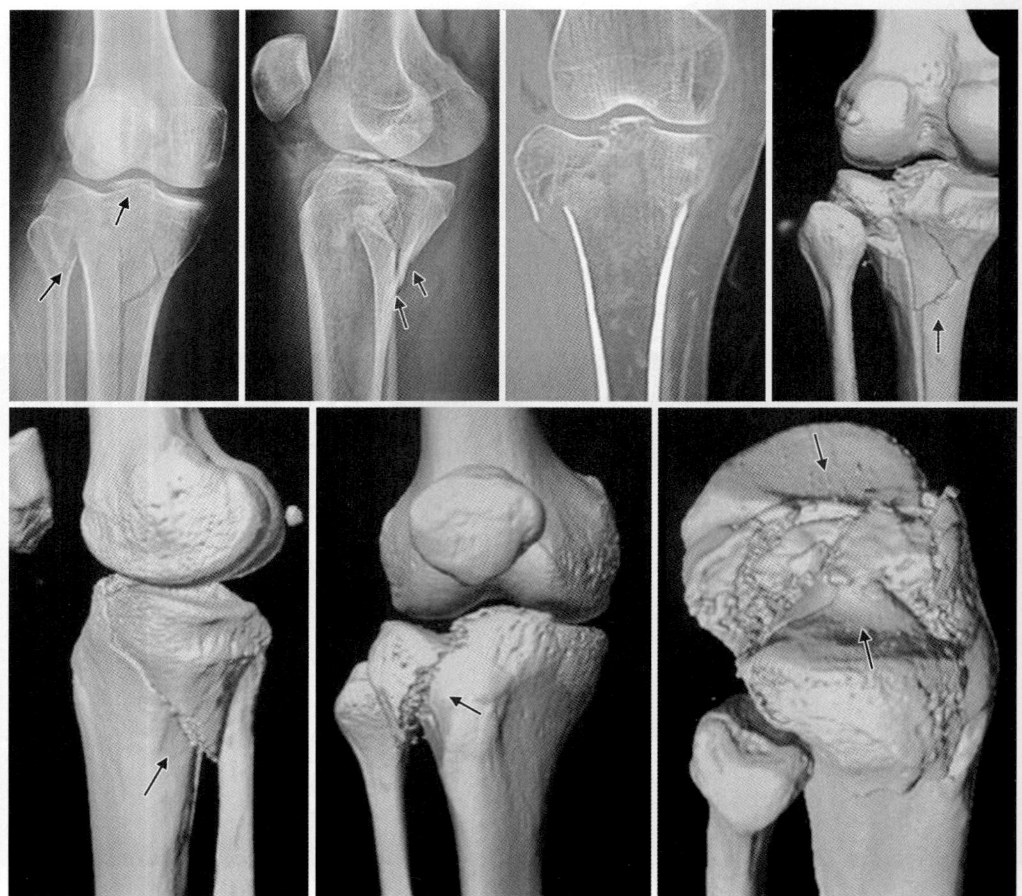

Figure 36.93 Posterior condyle

holes were used to pass 6.5 mm 32 mm threads screw. The drill bit negotiated, so that it did not strike the locking screws. The distal most screw was bicortical, while, the middle ones were unicortical, as the locking screws were located at the same level.

Release of tourniquet, drains and a padded crepe completed the procedure. The day 1 plaster slab was continued for two days. Then the removal of drains and elevation on a high Bohler frame was done. Postoperative recovery has been uneventful and has regained flexion till the 90 deg. and is improving further (Figs 36.93 and 36.94).

Case 7

This elderly lady had sustained injury to the right knee having had fractures of posterior and lateral part of tibial condyle and head of fibula. On arrival, a padded crepe and elevation was carried out. A CT with 3D reconstruction defined the fracture well.

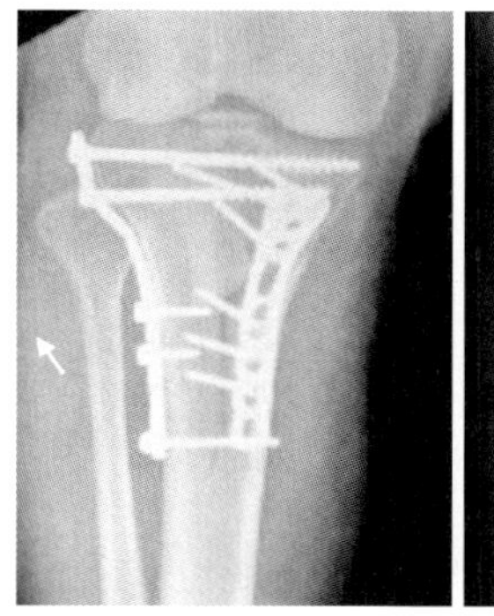
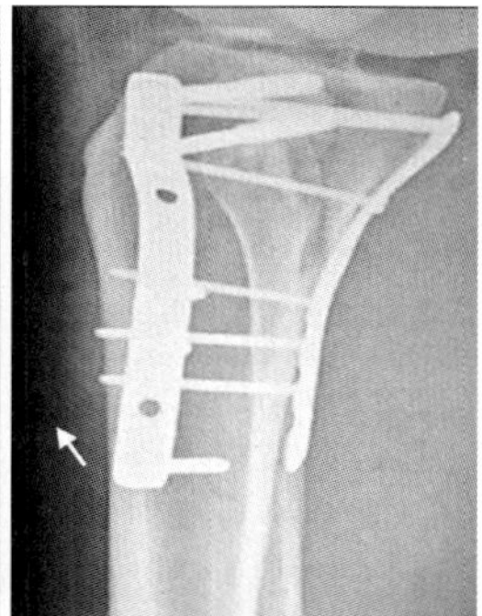

Figure 36.94 Posterior candyle

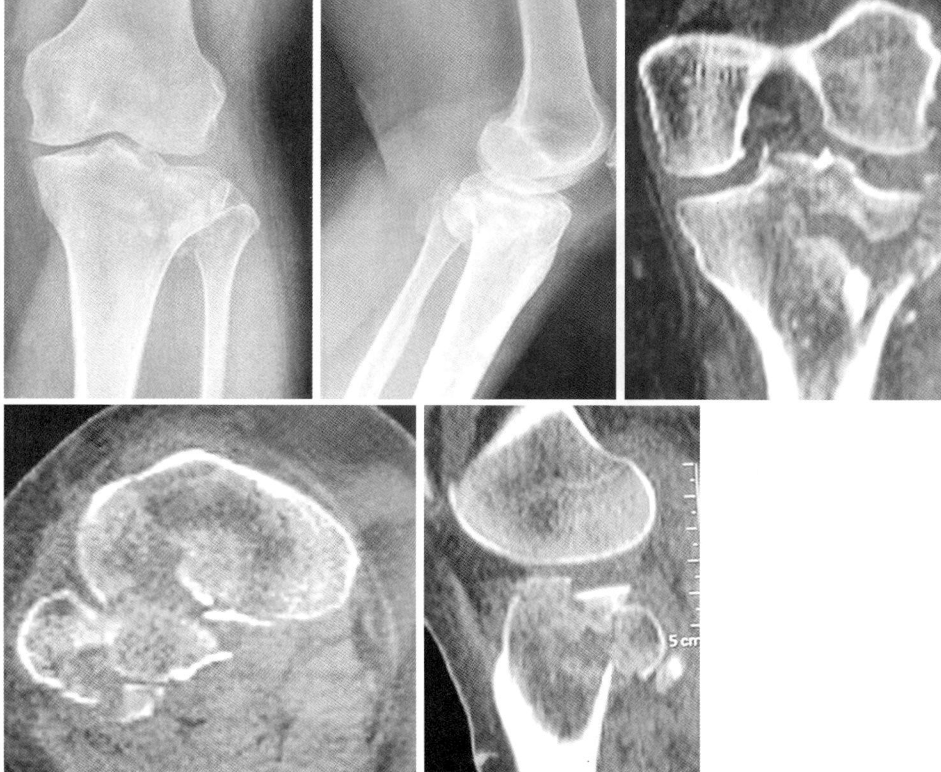

Figure 36.95 Post-lat condyle

Described Positions and the Techniques

- Both prone and a lateral positions are described.
- Approach has been posterolateral, exposing the common peroneal nerve and retracting it well.

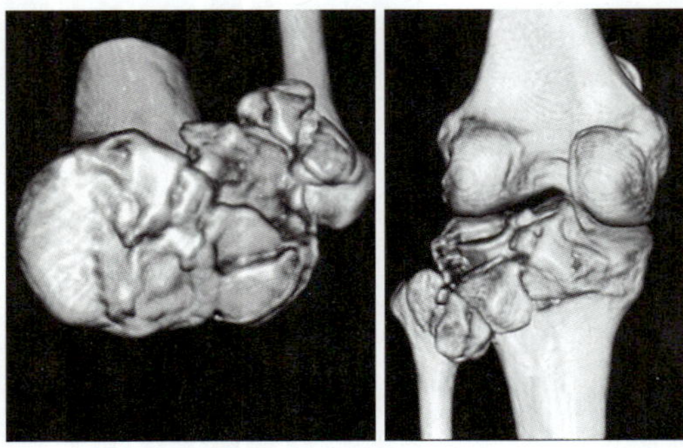

Figure 36.96 Post-lat condyle

- Osteotomy of the head of fibula taking the insertion of lateral collateral ligament is said to offer more exposure.

In the given case, the lateral condyle had a fracture and had widened as well. There was a central depression, such that, it required elevation from the lateral side and a lateral plate. Hence a lateral position was preferred, so that, one can have access to the posterior part as well as the lateral part through the same approach and in the same position.

The incision was slightly posterior to the lateral surface of the fibula. The common peroneal nerve was palpated and accordingly exposed. The fascia over it was incised in the same line and the nerve was tagged with an umbilical tape. It was slightly taken forwards and one could have access, along the posterior surface of the fibula, to the posterolateral part of the tibia. The muscles over the postero-lateral part of the condyle were erased and with

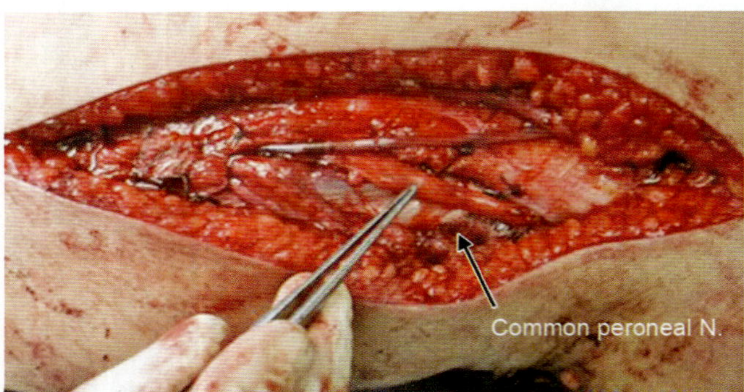

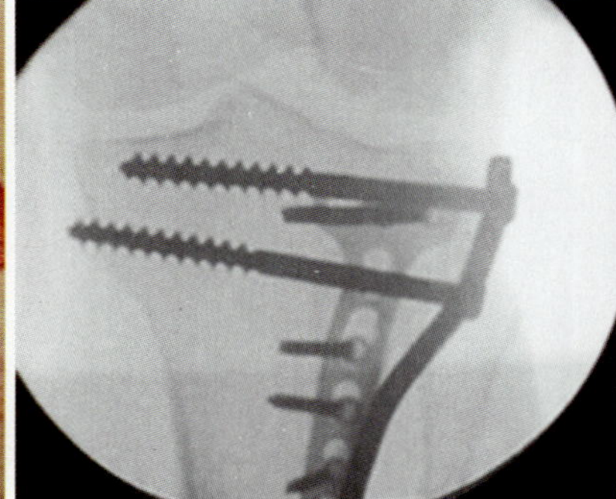

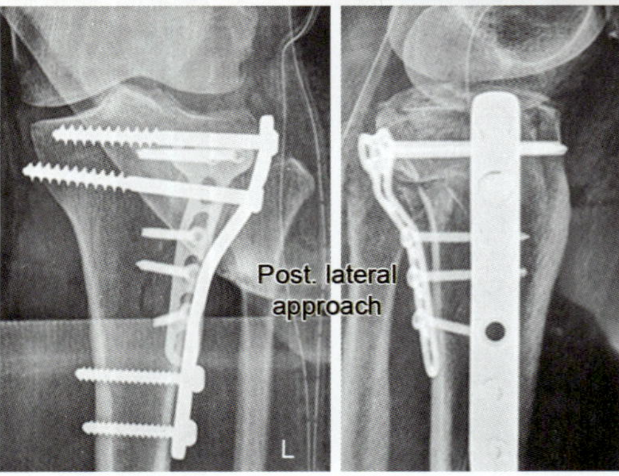

Figure 36.97 Post-lat condyle

the knee flexed, could get access to the superior part of the condyle. The fracture hematoma leads one to the fracture area. The lateral belly of the gastrocnemius was elevated and one can have access to the fracture area.

The fragments were fixed provisionally with K-wires and were stabilized with a distal radius locking T plate. It had to be slightly contoured.

Then the lateral surface of the tibia required to be exposed. The anterior skin flap was erased and the tibialis anterior was erased from the lateral surface of the tibia. Then making a window in the lateral surface, elevation of the depression, laying in left iliac grafts was done. A 12 mm custom made tibial plate was contoured for the lateral condyle and the fragment was fixed. Release of tourniquet, drains and closure was done. In the anterolateral exposure in the second part, the deep fascia over peroneus longus is incised. This fascia cannot be well opposed (as can be done after a closed wedge HTO). This was loosely opposed and left as such, to avoid any danger of possible compartment syndrome, after such an exposure.

Postoperative pain relief was good, due to the continued epidural catheter and she could start active knee range of motion exercises. There was slight weakness on dorsiflexion of great toe and recovered in due course of time (Figs 36.95 to 36.97).

CHAPTER

37

Fractures of Tibial Shaft

After a fall, a child may sustain a fracture of the lower/3 of the tibia. Usually, it is an undisplaced spiral fracture. Refusal to touch the foot to the ground and inability to bear weight on the affected leg is the hallmark of such an injury. X-ray confirms such an injury and an above knee cast for a few weeks settles the problem. This injury, like a pulled elbow, needs more discussion with the parents and the grandparents, who are quite anxious and concerned and naturally so. After three to four weeks, as the fracture starts uniting, the child himself starts to bear weight on the cast. At this stage, an X-ray through the cast is taken and if the alignment is satisfactory, which is almost always, a watchful neglect should be done. This weight bearing in the cast on his own helps to consolidate the fracture and makes it pain free.

Occasionally, the child is very anxious and the pain is so much, that immobilization in a cast (without manipulation,) is difficult. This procedure of application of a cast only, may need anesthesia and is justified (Fig. 37.1).

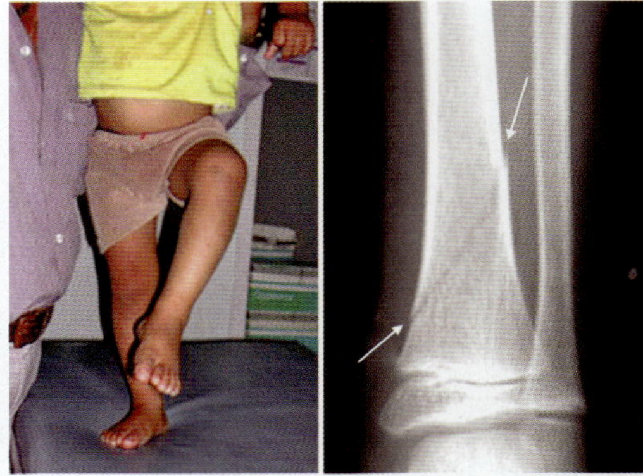

Figure 37.1 Typical presentation of fracture of lower end tibia in a child

A greenstick fracture in the upper end of a tibia, needs special attention to assess and plan the treatment. Clinical assessment of the deformity is equally important. The fracture is in a coronal plane and the angulation does not remodel itself, with time because, it is not in the plane of motion. Being a greenstick fracture, it tends to unite rapidly and hence early closed reduction under anesthesia is necessary. This child had sustained such an injury and was treated with a cast immobilization, without manipulation (Fig. 37.2).

In a transverse fracture in mid/3 tibia, the fibula sustains a greenstick fracture and needs to be reduced under anesthesia to align the tibia correctly (Fig. 37.3).

A short oblique fracture in lower/4 of tibia, may have a medial 3rd fragment. The fibula has a greenstick fracture and needs to be reduced well. Gradual and progressive three-point manipulation is done to reduce the fracture of fibula. Once, the fibula deformity is corrected,

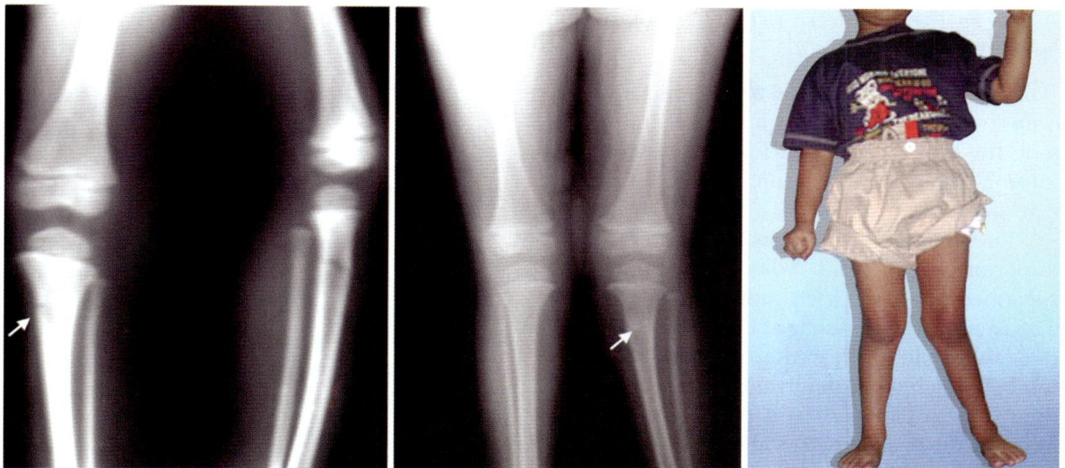

Figure 37.2 Correct the valgus deformity in upper end tibia

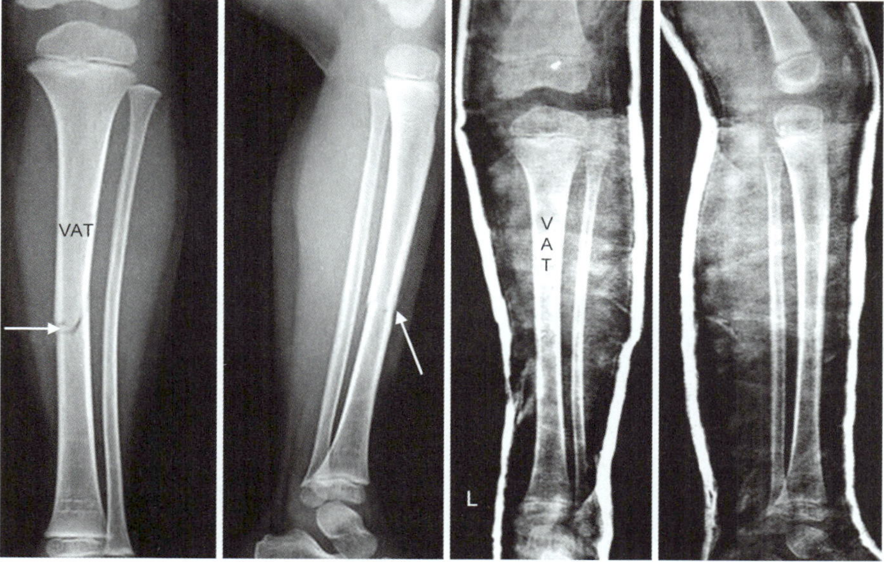

Figure 37.3 Greenstick fracture of fibula

the tibia is aligned well. A closed reduction is thus successful and the length of the limb is usually well maintained.

While the limb is immobilized, the second assistant holds the thigh in internal rotation and the surgeon, sitting on a stool, maintains 10 degree of physiological external torsion. He then hands over the foot to the first assistant and himself proceeds to apply a padded plaster cast. This first assistant has to keep the foot and ankle in neutral position, maintain the slight external rotation and at the same time, with three-point fixation, maintain the varus of the leg. When one takes specific efforts to hold the leg in varus, the leg within the cast stays in neutral position. The surgeon, thus, has to supervise the job every person is doing and apply the plaster as well.

Warning: If above method is not followed and only one person, sitting on a stool holds the foot, the foot and hence the distal fragment is internally rotated, while the thigh rolls out in external rotation.

The maintenance of varus is especially important in a child, where the fibula has sustained a greenstick fracture and tends to offer a resistance to its reduction (Figs 37.4 and 37.5).

A long oblique fracture of tibia alone, the intact fibula may be deterrent to achieve a good opposition of the fracture ends. The overlap may lead to a shortening of 8 to 18 mm or so in a child age 7 to 12 years. Being in the second growth spurt, usually the growth takes care of the limb length discrepancy. However, if in doubt, an open reduction and internal fixation with a small fragment instrumentation and use of a 1/3 tubular plate and a plaster slab immobilization, followed by a cast may be considered. Once the fracture consolidated, it is necessary to remove the implant in the next vacation or else bone growth over the plate makes the procedure difficult (Fig. 37.6).

A girl age about 12-year-old, close to puberty, sustained a long oblique fracture in the lower/3 tibia. The tibial epiphyses were open then. She was treated non-operatively. The closed reduction was done. However, being a long oblique fracture, overlap occurred. The fracture united, with shortening of about 20 mm. While a closed reduction and cast immobilization is carried out, one cannot compare the leg length with the other leg. It was thought, that she may have further two years of growth and the discrepancy would at least partially correct. However, it did not correct and she has to use a raised foot ware, which is not so convenient, indeed.

What could have been done? The X-ray at the end of a two to three weeks showed more overlap in the fragments. Even at this stage of fracture healing, may be an external fixator, with some distraction or an open reduction and internal fixation with a plate may have reduced the shortening.

Lesson: In a case nearing puberty, though the physes are still open, one should strive to achieve reduction by surgery, to restore the leg length. My preference in a case at this age,

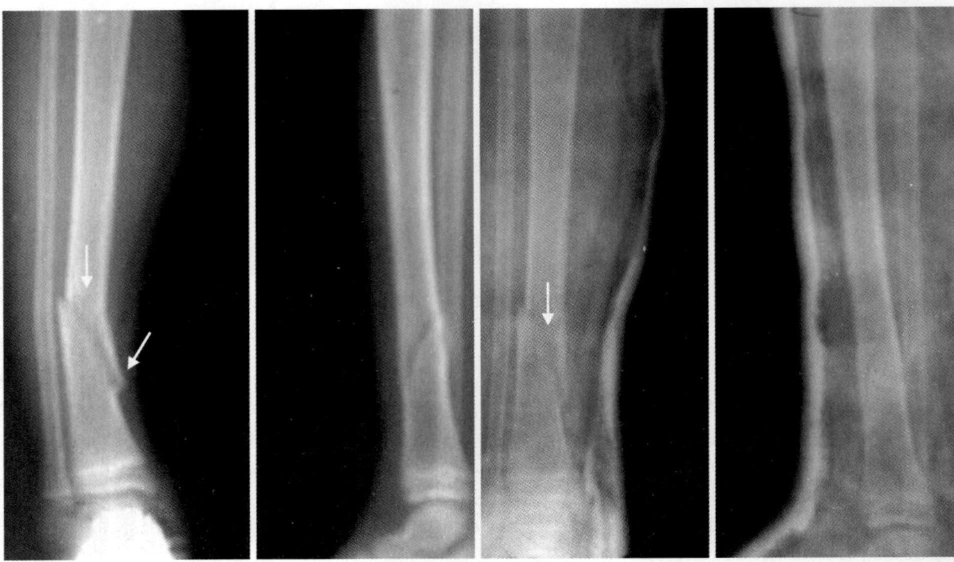

Figure 37.4 Short oblique fracture of tibia lower end

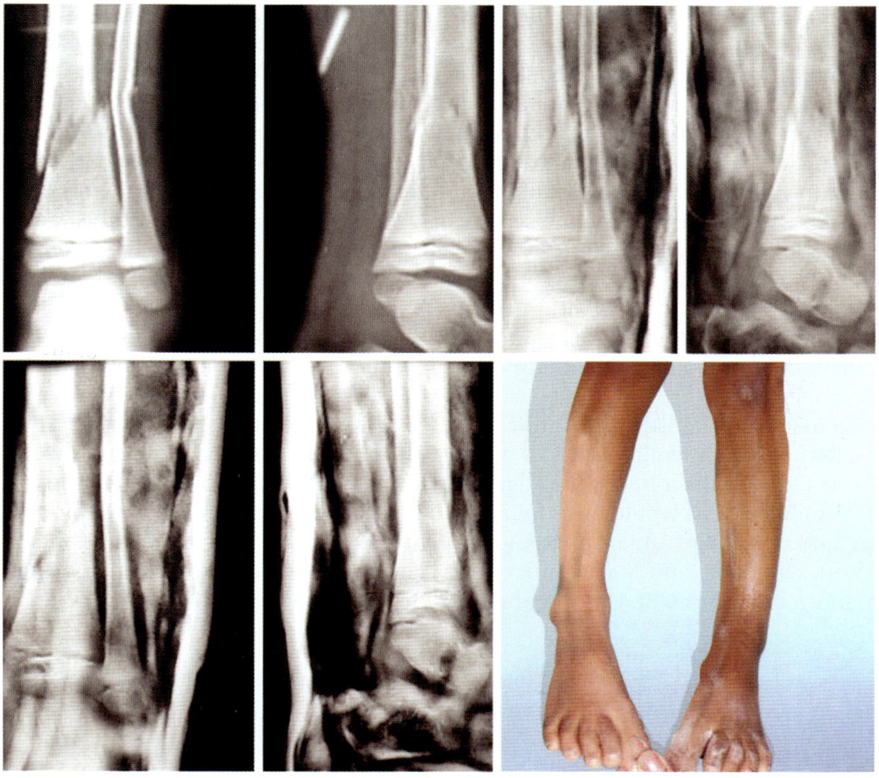

Figure 37.5 Oblique fracture: Restore alignment

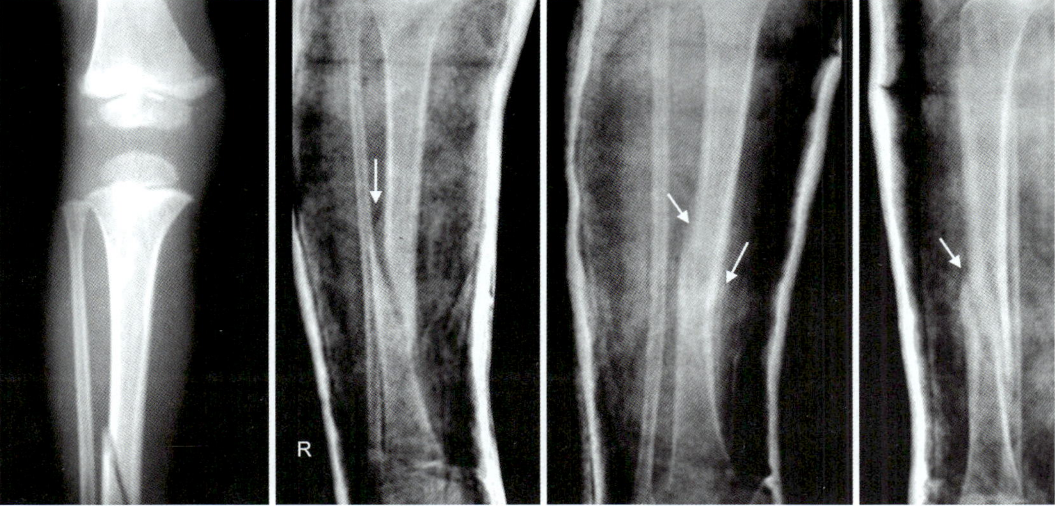

Figure 37.6 Oblique fracture: achieve valgus position

would be to carry out an open reduction. The apices of the fracture ends need to be broken by at least 5 mm on each side or else, reduction is not achieved. This has been aptly emphasized by our teachers. At this age, the patient well tolerates a long leg cast and hence, rather than using a 12 mm plate, I would prefer to use a 1/3 tubular plate with an IFS as a bone suture. This would be followed by a plaster cast, as if the fracture is treated non-operatively. The purpose of the plate is to prevent fracture ends overlapping, rather than achieving a stable fixation and to manage without any cast immobilization.

Someone may also choose an IFS crew and a tubular external fixator, which is also a good option. If one chooses this option, the steps in which this should be done would be as follows:

- Reduce and align the tibia—proximal to distal end clinically and pass transverse Steinmann pins, may be of 4 mm diameter near the ends of the bone, some distance away from the epiphyses. Pass 3.5 mm Schanz's pins on the antero-medial tibial surfaces, above and below the fracture area. Keep 11 mm tubes of appropriate lengths with adjustable clamps mounted, ready.
- Then expose the fracture and carry out IFS fixation. Then add the tubes and prestress the pins and complete the fixation.
- If one does IFS first and then insert the Steinmann and Schanz pins, the stresses of drilling and insertion of the pins would unnecessarily put stress on the IFS which may become loose.

Thus one may carry out an IFS or a 1/3 tubular plate fixation and neutralize with either an external fixator or a cast. If one has used an external fixator, at the end of say four weeks, the fixator should be removed and a long leg cast applied for further union and consolidation of the fracture (Fig. 37.7).

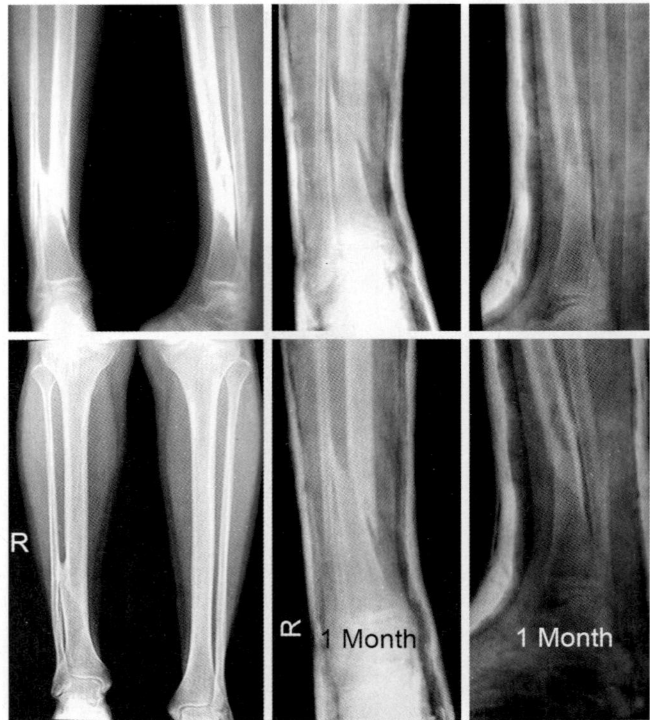

Figure 37.7 20 mm shortening by a non-operative method

Some children are accident prone in some part of their life. This young girl had a fracture of lower tibia, every successive years on three occasions (Fig. 37.8A).

NON-OPERATIVE METHOD

Closed method of management of a fracture is a time honored method. It is both an art and science. However, in the past twenty years or so, with advent of internal fixation, this method is not practised. If unfortunately, the operative method fails to reduce a fracture and stabilizes well, the outcome is less satisfactory and further treatment demanding. In fact the repeat surgery, the cost, duration of absence from work, stay in hospital, the cosmetic appearance , delay in weight bearing is far more than the nonoperative method. In fact a book on operative method of fracture management does mention that the method of treatment of an isolated fracture of humerus and tibia, is non-operative, unless there is some specific indication, to carry out internal fixation. This is conveniently forgotten. In fact, today, if one takes a data from a surgeon in practice, very few surgeons would have cases treated non-operatively. As a matter of fact, having talked to them, I observed, they have not been exposed to this method of fracture management. After going through the cases shown, it is up to them, whether to manage a few cases non-operatively, what was called a conservative method in yester years. I feel, at least in a teaching institute, selected cases should be managed by a non-operative method, to perpetuate the art and to train the students.

Few Tips in Non-operative Method of Management of Fracture of Tibia by a Plaster Cast

Since, the non-operative method is not commonly practised, necessary steps are mentioned here, which the reader may find useful: Besides the adults, it will be of use in children, who are often treated non-operatively.

- Soon after arrival, an X-ray examination is done from the knee to the calcaneus. If the fracture displacement is minimum, as in a spiral or a 3-part fracture in lower/3 of tibia, application of a plaster cast by using this method would help:
  - If the pain is tolerable, it is preferable to apply the cast without anesthesia. The patient being conscious, the muscle tone maintains the fracture alignment. When

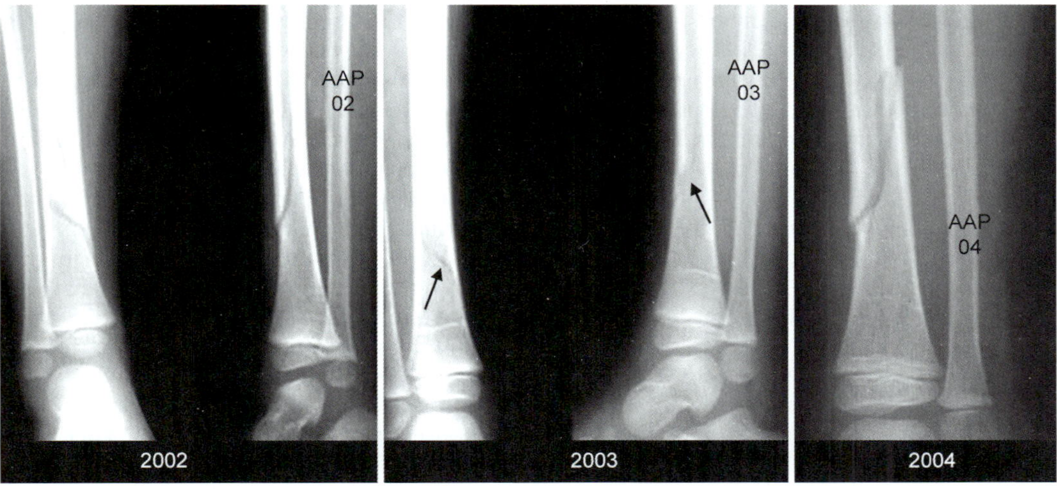

Figure 37.8A Accident prone child

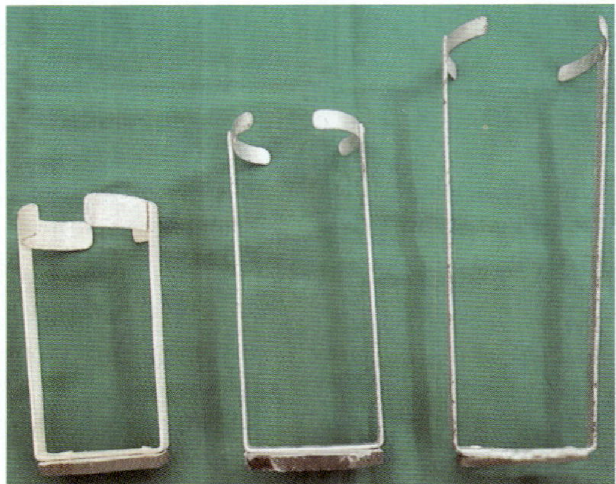

Figure 37.8B Weight-bearing caliper

anesthetized, the muscle tone and spasm is no more and the bone fragments are free to move about and to keep them aligned is rather a difficult job.

- The patient is administered parenteral analgesic and explained as to what co-operation one needs from him. The clothes covering the leg are removed. The patient is brought at the edge of the table. The surgeon must have a operation theatre or a plaster outfit on, which may get soiled with the plaster material. He has to sit on a low stool and gently put a hand behind the fracture area and with the other hand, hold the middle three toes. The patient is asked to relax and gradually bend the knee, so the knee is at 30 deg. of flexion or so. Let the leg hang comfortably. The gravity helps to reduce the fracture and aligns it well. Some muscle spasm, due to pain, help to keep the bone ends aligned.
- A second assistant puts his pronated hand below the mid thigh and the fingers rest on the edge of the table. This helps to internally rotate the thigh. At this point, the surgeon maintains the foot (and hence the distal fragment) in 15 deg. external rotation. This aligns the tibia well. The shin is gently palpated to know the side to side alignment. If the thigh and hence the proximal fragment is not purposefully internally rotated, it falls in external rotation and the foot being held in neutral position, the end result is an internal rotation deformity. If the fracture of both tibia and fibula is at the mid and lower/3 junction, one should study the tibio-fibular interosseous space and the thickness of fracture cortices. If the space above and below is the same and the thickness of bone ends is the same, the rotational alignment is correct. It is possible to study this in a 'C' arm image.
- One hand of the surgeon should support the fracture site and gently tend to give an anterior angulation to the fracture. The other hand supports the foot and keeps in neutral position, with respect to planter and dorsiflexion. Gentle varus alignment of the limb is maintained. If these steps are not followed, almost always, the limb goes in recurvatum, valgus and an internal rotation deformity.
- Today, since a 'C' arm is available, one may confirm the fracture position by rotating the X-ray tube.
- On the day 1, a stockinet is not used, as the limb is expected to swell. I prefer to use cotton rolls made from a large roll, rather than a readymade available compressed rolls. The former offers more cushioning and accommodate the edema better than the precompressed rolls. More padding is needed on the malleoli and the heel, to add to comfort and prevent pressure sores. It is preferable to have little more padding, than a need to bivalve the cast because of a burning pain on the heel. A bivalved cast is less fitting, than a padded and contoured cast.
- A trained assistant applies few rolls over the below knee portion, while the surgeon changes the hands, as the roll has to go a round the limb. This cast is permitted to set and is moulded at this time. Thereafter, a thin anterior and a thick above knee posterior slab are added. A check image is taken through the cast. Having confirmed the position, the above knee portion, keeping the knee at 15 degree flexion is completed. The patella and the second web be in a line. The cotton

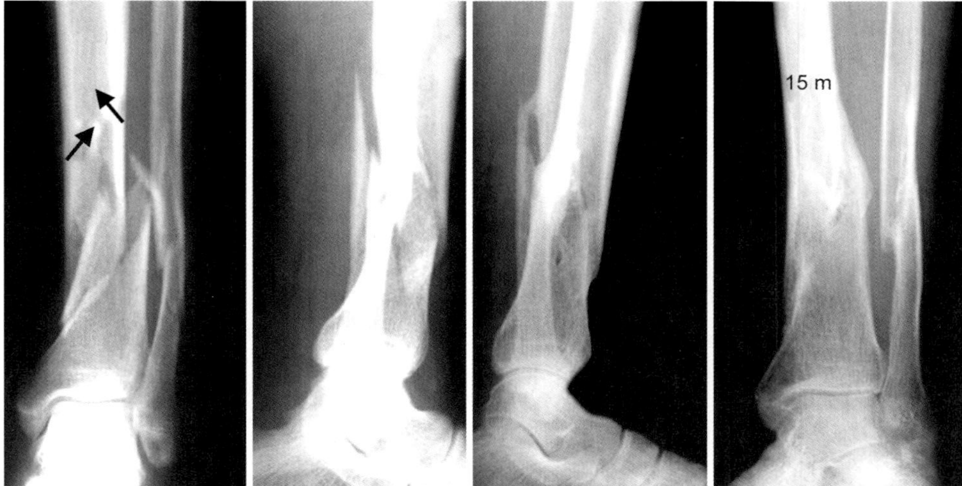

Figure 37.9 Non-operative method in spiral fracture of tibia in lower/3 area

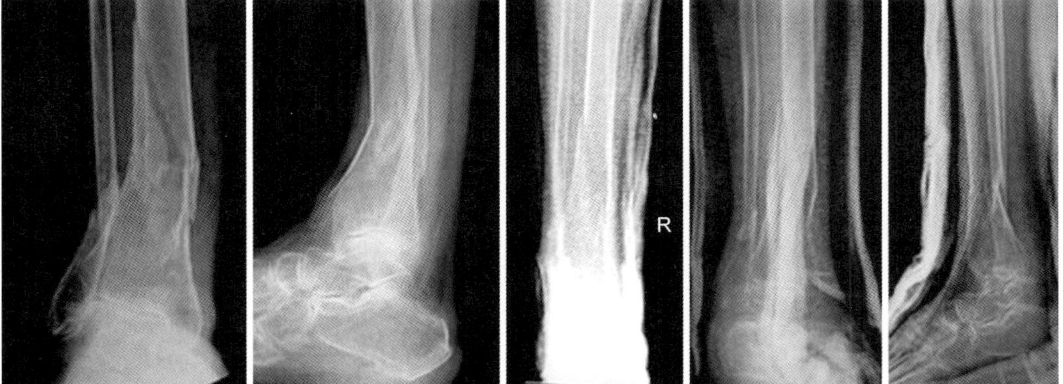

Figure 37.10 Non-operative method in spiral fracture of tibia in lower/3 area

padding in the mid thigh should be rather less, for better fitting. Till this stage of plaster application, my preference is to use a plaster of Paris material. Once an above knee cast is completed and the position of the fragments is acceptable, one may add a synthetic roll for further strength.

- If the fracture is a transverse or a short oblique, with displacement, then under anesthesia, it needs to be reduced and telescopic stability assessed. The cast is completed. If the limb edema is too much, one may achieve the same result by using a posterior and an anterior slab, which are kept in place by a wet roller bandage roll. A wet roller bandage keeps the cast strength good and becomes homegeneous with the plaster of Paris material.
- Elevation on a Bohler frame keeps the patient comfortable and reduces the edema and hence the pain. Further management is as usual.
- When and whether to change a plaster cast? A weekly X-ray examination is carried out, to

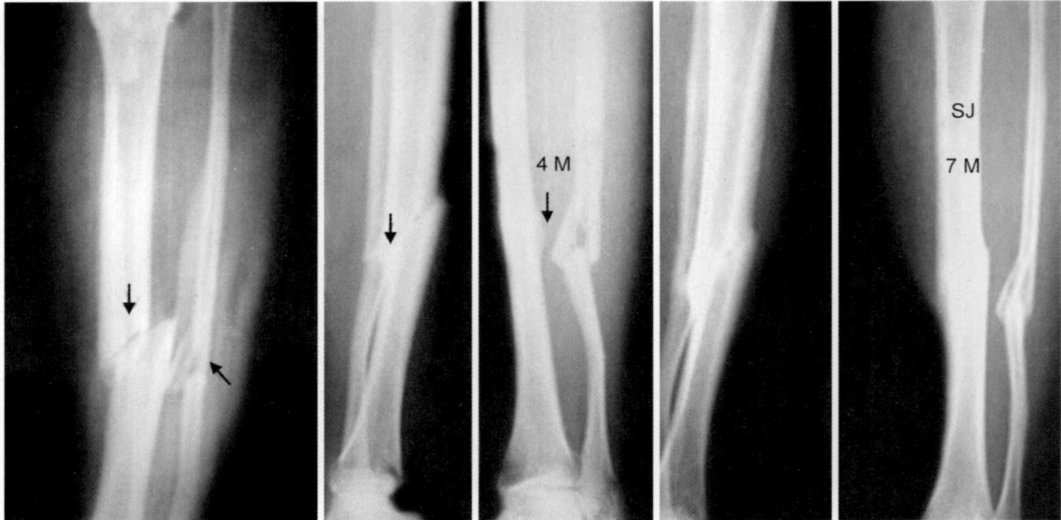

Figure 37.11 Non-operative method in spiral fracture of tibia in lower/3 area

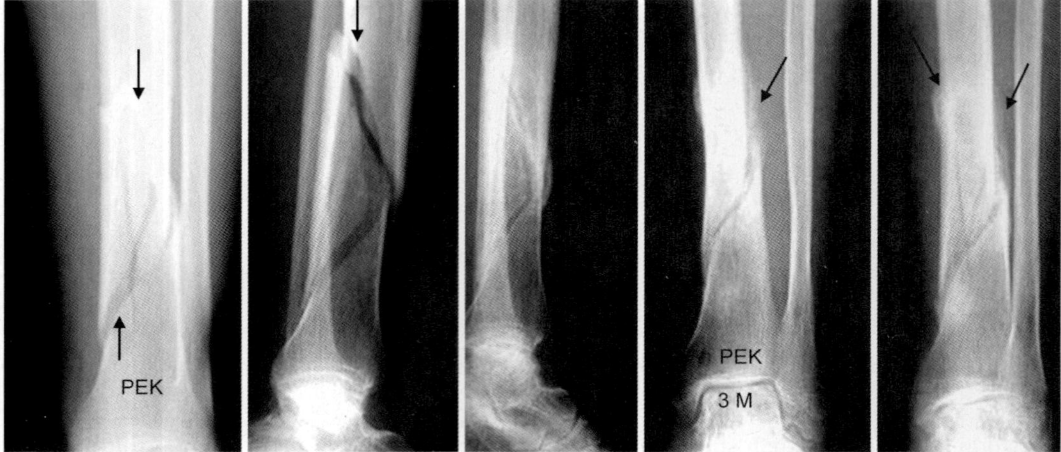

Figure 37.12 Non-operative method in spiral fracture of tibia in lower/3 area

confirm that the position is maintained well. As the edema reduces, the cast fitting may need to be changed. If the fracture position is maintained well, the same cast may be continued for at least four weeks. Due to a soft callus formation, the pain reduces. At this stage, during a change of plaster the fracture is less likely to get displaced. Now, the cast may be applied over a stockinet and compressed cotton roll, for better fitting.

- During the change of cast, degree of clinical union is noted and recorded, so one can estimate further duration of immobilization in the cast. At the end of eight weeks from injury, X-ray examination would show some callus appearance. Prior to availability of the

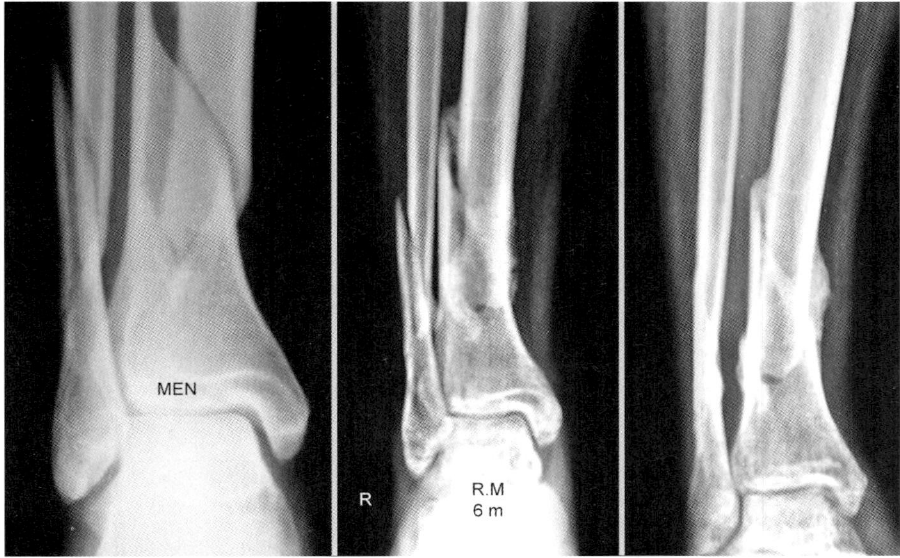

Figure 37.13 Non-operative method in spiral fracture of tibia in lower/3 area

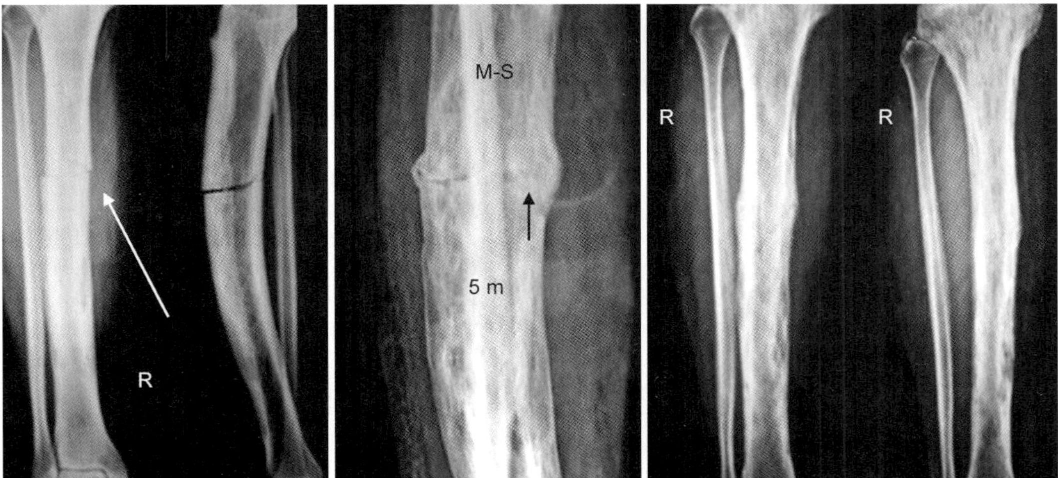

Figure 37.14 Non-operative method in spiral fracture of tibia in lower/3 area

synthetic material is/was a practice to change the cast, with less flexion at the knee. Since the fracture has become sticky and X-ray shows some callus appearance, the above knee cast is applied in one stage. At the end of 80% application of a cast, a metal walking caliper was added. The proximal transverse strap of the caliper should be either below or much above the fracture area. If it is at the fracture site, the weight bearing force is detrimental to fracture consolidation. Few plaster layers are added where one expects the transverse strap and only after this area has hardened well, the caliper is added. If

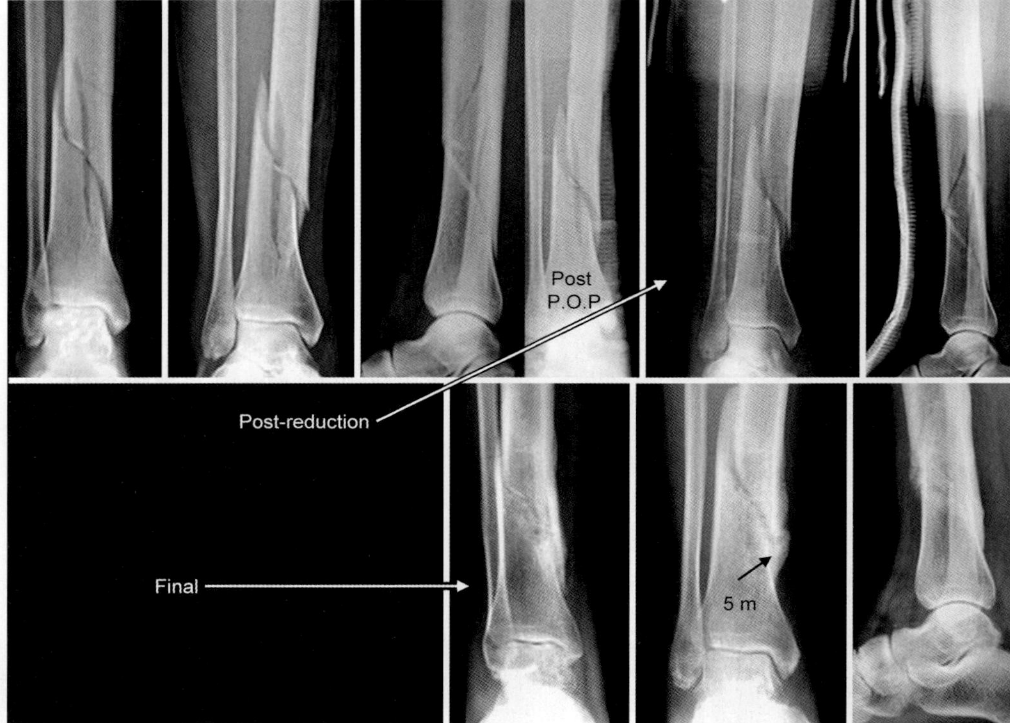

Figure 37.15 Non-operative method in spiral fracture of tibia in lower/3 area

the caliper is added, while the cast is soft, it is known to bite in the skin and cause sore and wound in the skin (Fig. 37.8B).

- Today, with availability of synthetic material, which is quite strong, though brittle, there is no need of a caliper. Use of a cast overshoe keeps the cast clean and prevents chipping under the sole. When callus bridge across the fracture is adequate, progressive walking on the cast must be practised. This helps fracture consolidation and restores the weight bearing reflexes. Having walked with nearly full weight bearing, the cast is removed, clinical assessment and X-ray examination is done.
- Having had the cast on for 10 to 12 weeks, it is necessary to add padded crepe support and elevate the leg for a few days. If this is not followed, ankle and leg edema appears, which is difficult to get rid off.

Examples illustrated below aptly indicate that a spiral fracture in lower/3 tibia, may have a fracture of fibula at the same level or much higher or not at all.

- *A spiral fracture is a stable one,* while an oblique one is not so, and usually needs internal fixation. If an internal fixation is to be carried out by a plate, it is preferable to have an open surgery, with primary bone grafting. Plating by a MIPO technique has its own limitations, described elsewhere.
- All the cases of spiral fracture treated by a non-operative method united in due course. They did not require a secondary procedure of internal fixation and/or bone grafting.
- Anesthesia was required in few cases only. Problem of wound dehiscence, infection, skin cover, removal of implant, etc. were naturally absent. In this anatomical area, the skin cover is important. Once the skin problem begins, then even secondary bone grafting is difficult and one has to take to

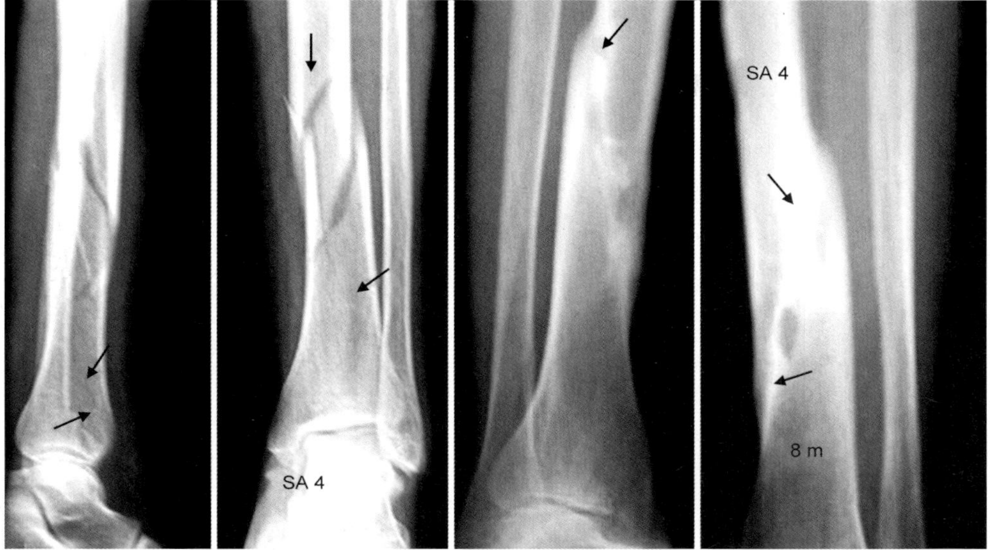

Figure 37.16 Non-operative method in spiral fracture of tibia in lower/3 area

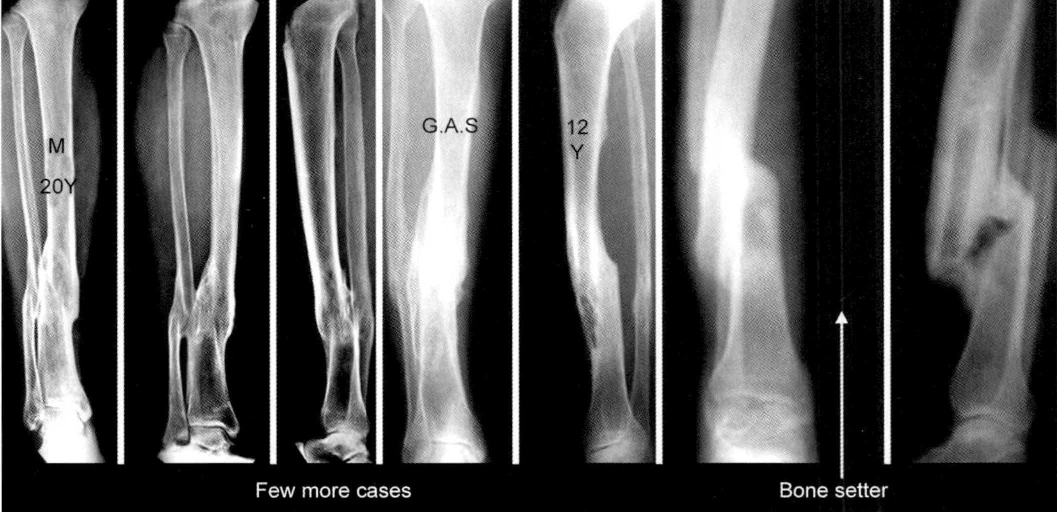

Figure 37.17 Non-operative method in spiral fracture of tibia in lower/3 area

a ring fixator, etc. (Still the fracture may remain ununited, as depicted elsewhere).

- A drawback of a closed method is that, there is some translation or angulation of the fragments. The medullary cavity of both fragments may not be in one line. Hence, later if he has another injury, use of an IM nail may be difficult.

Few Clinical Examples

Figures 37.9 to 37.17: Non-operative methods in spiral fracture of tibia in lower/3 area.

CHAPTER

38

External Fixator

The modern external fixator was invented about 30 years ago. The fixator with threaded bars or the tubes, fixator with clamps and discs have their own advantages. Currently with a better understanding of internal fixation, availability of early medical and surgical care after an accident, has changed the type of treatment offered to a patient with an open fracture and soft tissue injury. Besides its use in open fracture, it has a place in procedures such as osteotomy and arthrodesis. Today, its use is more in open fractures, where primary internal fixation is not advisable, due to contamination, the fracture geometry, segmental bone loss and extensive loss of soft tissue cover at the time of arrival.

If the soft tissue damage, especially due to crushing and associated comminution of bone fragments, the chance of infection is high. This is especially if a primary internal fixation is done. Often there exists internal degloving injury, which should be kept at the back of mind.

REVIEW OF THE PRINCIPLES AND TECHNIQUE OF APPLICATION OF EXTERNAL FIXATION

An external fixation does not offer absolute stability necessary for primary bone union and is too rigid to offer physiological stimulus for a bone union by callus formation. Hence, if it is continued to be used as a definitive mode of fracture management, the bone heals very slowly or may not unite. Hence, when adequate soft tissue cover is achieved, a secondary procedure of bone grafting or change to an internal fixation is necessary to offer a good union in an expected duration. Therefore, when external fixation is carried out on day 1, the place of Schanz pin insertion is so planned, that Schanz pins are inserted rather away from the fracture site, so that a secondary internal fixation can be carried out at appropriate time. When, a secondary procedure of internal fixation is planned, one should allow an interval of three weeks between removal of the fixator and carrying out an internal fixation. This permits soft tissue healing of the pin tracks.

An exception would be an oblique fracture, where an interfragmentary screw is inserted on day 1 and it is neutralized by external fixation, so a primary union could be expected.

In an infected nounion of a long bone fracture, one may need to do excision of the dead fragments, which may lead to a gap nonunion. In such a situation, one needs to apply a stable frame, with triangularization to offer absolute stability. Once the local infection is cleared, one can consider addition of cancellous grafts for union.

If the trauma surgeon requires help of a surgeon, who does reconstruction of soft tissues, then it is necessary to involve him on the day 1, when the external fixator is applied. This colleague can guide, as to which is a better site for insertion of a Steinmann or a Schanz pin. This planning is of immense help to carry out secondary procedure like split thickness skin grafting or a flap rotation, etc. This can be done at a later date, with a minimum of temporary removal of the assembly tubes, to gain access to the wound.

Thus application of an external fixator helps to:

- Ease the wound care and dressing
- Assists in limb elevation, to keep the reactionary edema to a minimum
- Helps to mobilize the adjacent joints
- Offers stability to the limb, even in presence of local bone loss and defect
- Permits insertion of bone grafts, keeping the external stability
- Allows a possibility of changing the method of management to that of an internal fixation, subsequently.

THE COMPONENTS OF ASSEMBLY

The Tubes

The tubes are available in 10 and 11 mm diameter. One should have a policy to have either a 10 or a 11 mm system. This is important, so the tubes and clamps match each other. My preference is to an 11 mm diameter system. This offers optimal strength and rigidity required in all the limb segments, viz. the femur, the tibia and the humerus. It is observed that a tube has a light weight and more rigid than a threaded bar, which was used earlier. A tube permits ease of clamp sliding over it. It also permits addition of an open clamp, should it be needed during or after a procedure, without a need to remove the tube from a pin, to which it is fixed.

The Clamps

The commonly used clamp is called an adjustable clamp, though some call it a universal clamp. The clamp should be naturally be matching the 11 mm tube. Early design had an option to have a clamp useful for either a 4.5 mm or a 3.5 mm pin. If this matching was not done, then the pin clamp composite was not stable. Today with engineering help, there is a possibility to use a pin of either diameter in the same clamp. The new design of the plate component of the clamp, has made this possible, which is of a great help to reduce the inventory. The central threaded bolt of a clamp, should accept an 11 mm nut. This permits to have only an 11 mm combination spanner (open spanner on one end and a ring spanner on the other end). Besides a socket wrench for an 11 mm nut is necessary and very useful for ease and the speed to the surgery. This remarkably reduces the operative time and increases the comfort and efficiency (Figs 38.1 to 38.3).

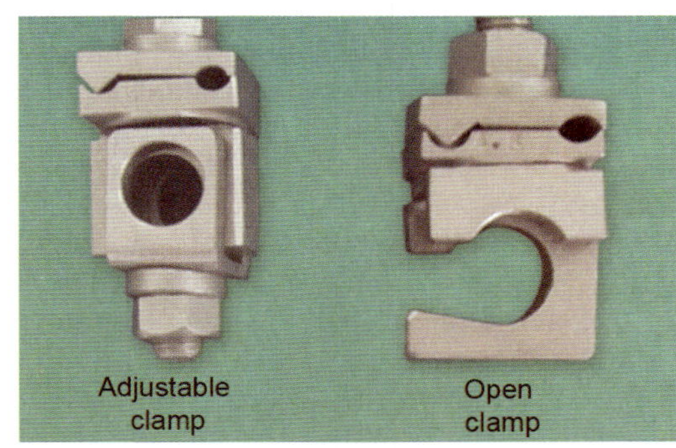

Figure 38.1 Clamps

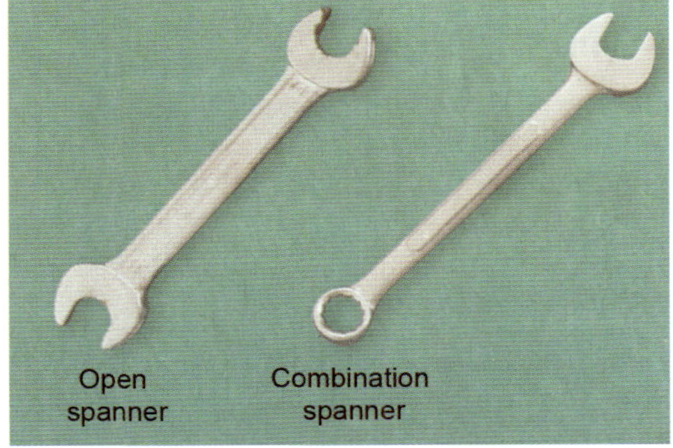

Figure 38.2 Spanners

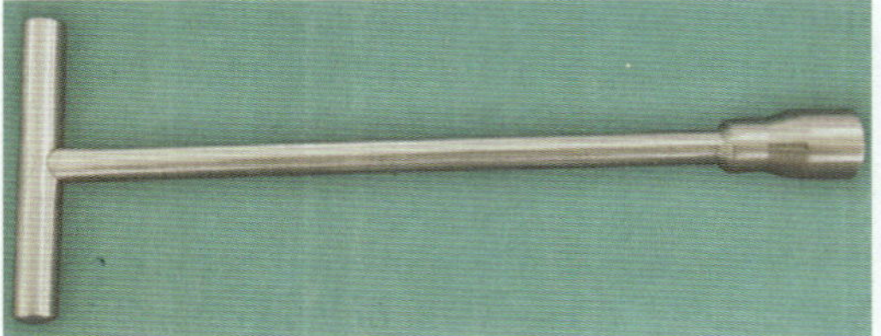

Figure 38.3 Socket wrench

Steinmann Pins

In external fixation of a tibia, with local bone loss or a segmental fracture, I prefer to have a 4.5 mm Steinmann pin inserted mediolaterally at the upper and lower ends of tibia. In addition to these, I prefer on either end, a second pin towards the midportion of tibia, making two pins on either end. These additional second pin, near the 4.5 mm Steinmann pin, be of 4 mm diameter. This is especially necessary for a person with small skeleton. Today, both the 4.5 mm and 4 mm drill bits are available, which makes insertion of these two different diameter pins easy. I prefer to make a drill hole by a 4.5 and 4 mm drill bits respectively and then pass the corresponding Steinmann in the hole, with a T handle. The pin passes easily. Since the drill hole and the pin diameter is the same, there is no possibility of bone splintering. This is especially true in a cortical bone area, adjacent to the metaphysis. While the tubes are attached and the pins are prestressed, they remain stable and do not slide on either side, in the bone.

Schanz Pin (Screw)

They are available in various length, as per the soft tissue mass on the bone. I prefer a 4.5 mm diameter pin, with 18 mm threads (short threaded).

Technique of Insertion

A triple trocar is a useful tool. The commonly available triple trocar has the following components:

- Outer sleeve has an inner diameter of 5 mm

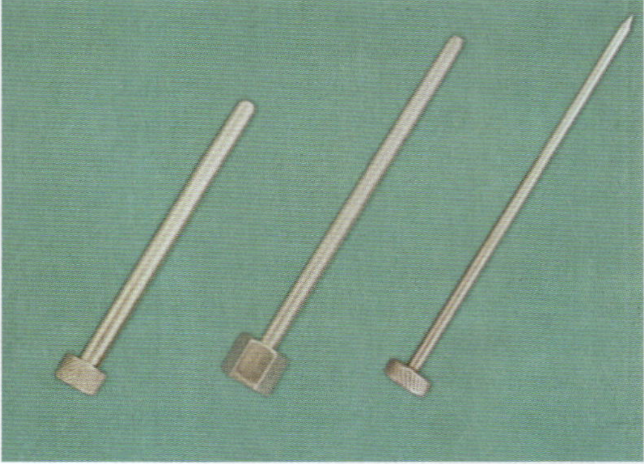

Figure 38.4 Triple trocar

- The insert sleeve goes easily in the outer sleeve and has an inner diameter of 3.5 mm and hence accepts a 3.5 mm drill bit.
- A central trocar, which passes through the insert sleeve (Fig. 38.4).

A triple trocar with this specification is made for use of a 5 mm Schanz pin. I prefer a 4.5 mm pin, because of following reasons:

- The corresponding 4.5 mm drill bit is available everywhere.
- The strength offered by a 4.5 mm pin is useful in all the three segments, viz. the humerus, the femur and the tibia.
- The near cortex is occupied by the broad 4.5 mm portion of the pin and offers good resistance to the bending forces. It is also observed, that such pin does not break, because a 4.5 mm segment of the pin has adequate strength to resist the bending forces. If one uses a long threaded pin, both the cortices are held only by the threaded part of the pin and the pins are observed to break through the threaded portion, making its removal painstaking. (One should strive to remove it, because should any intramedullary device is required to be inserted at a later date, it would be difficult).

In spite of the fact that, an external fixator is not recommended as a definitive method of treatment in a fracture pattern, which can be adequately treated by other method of internal fixation, some surgeons prefer external fixator as a method of choice. In such a method,

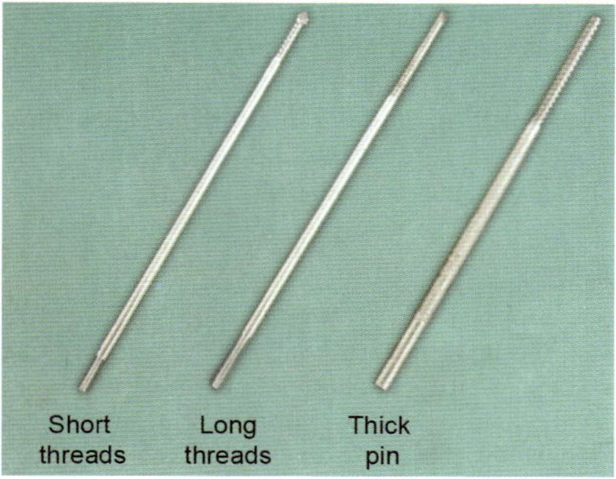

Figure 38.5 Pin types

the pins used are of more diameter, may be 6 mm diameter or so. The entire assembly becomes quite strong, so much that that with a uniplaner, unilateral patient is able to put some weight before the fracture unites. However, the fracture unites very slowly (Fig. 38.6).

- The triple trocar assembly is placed over the desired place and is gently tapped on the bone. The trocar makes a mark on the bone. Then with a 3.2 mm bit a drill hole is made through both the cortices.
- This bit and the inner sleeve are removed from the outer sleeve and the bit is changed to a 4.5 mm bit. Now, only the outer cortex is drilled with 4.5 mm bit through the outer sleeve.

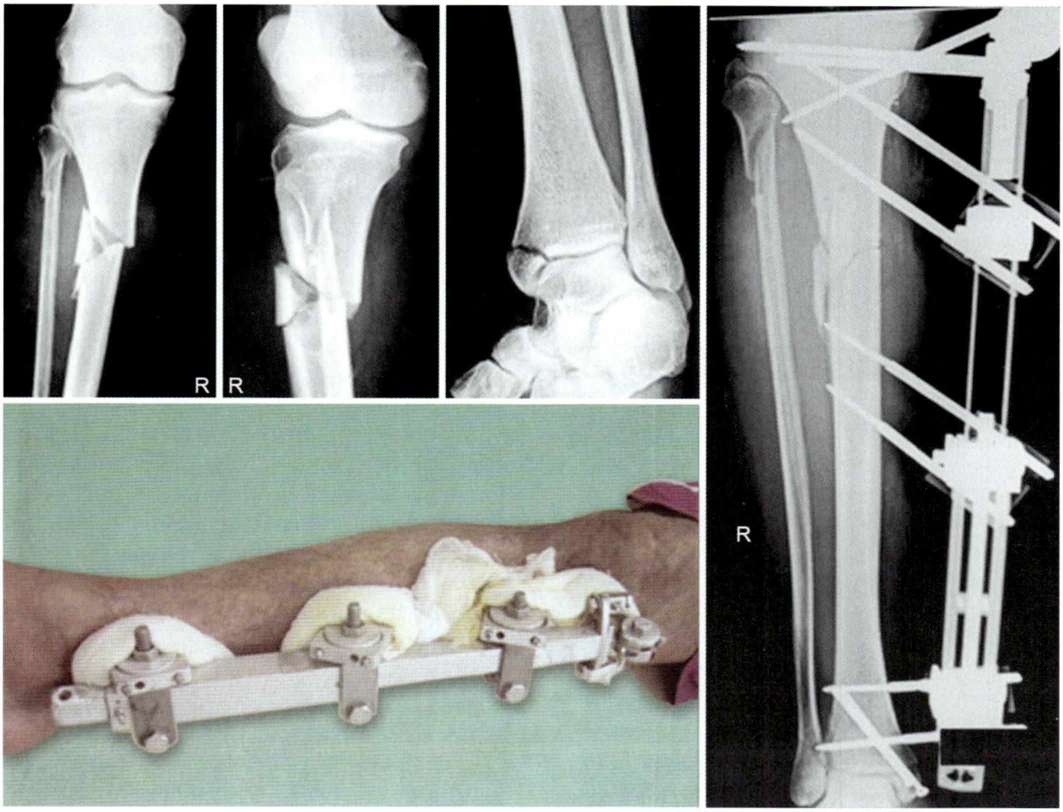

Figure 38.6 External fixator as a definitive method

(Alternatively, first, one can make the 4.5 mm hole in the outer cortex and then after using an insert sleeve from the basic set, make a 3.2 mm hole in the far cortex). It is up to the surgeon, with what technique he is comfortable. A Schanz pin depth gauge is inserted through the outer sleeve and the length of the Schanz pin required is noted. This much length + 2 mm of the pin is kept outside the T handle (Fig. 38.7).

The outer sleeve is kept against the bone and a 2 mm K-wire is inserted in the holes, to know the direction. It is removed and then through outer sleeve, a 4.5 mm Schanz pin is inserted in the bone. Now, as the threads engage the far cortex, one gets a feel and resistance. The pin is advanced, till the T handle touches the outer sleeve. Thus, one can do this procedure without the use of a 'C' arm. However, since, it is available, one can take a view in it. The outer sleeve is removed. The pin is slightly angulated to confirm that it has pierced the far cortex. If so, the pin is quite stable and does not tilt, when angulated. The shaft of the Schanz pin thus fits well in the near hole and is stable, when prestressed. Thus, a short threaded Schanz pin offers a good anchorage in the bone.

UNIPLANER, UNILATERAL FIXATOR

In the early days, this configuration was commonly done. In an open and stable fracture in mid/3 of tibia, all the four Schanz pins were inserted from the antero-medial surface of the tibia. The surface being a flat one, insertion is easy. Besides, if the pin tip penetrates little more, it is in the soft tissues on the lateral side of the tibia and is acceptable.

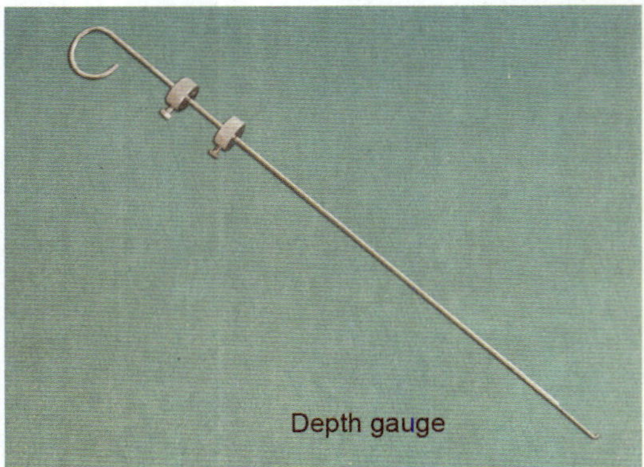

Figure 38.7 Depth gauge for a Schanz pin

Steps

- First the uppermost Schanz pin is inserted.
- The fracture is aligned and the lowermost pin inserted above the plafond, keeping it parallel to the first one.
- An 11 mm tube with four clamps is attached to the two pins. In fact, it is necessary to attach two tubes, one above the other, in a mirror image fashion. The length of the tubes be such that both the ends of the tube are at least 3 cm beyond the end pins. This segment of the tube is used for attachment of a tube to tube clamp, required for dynamization of the fracture. (This is also called a universal clamp by some).
- The 3rd pin is planned to be inserted 5 cm below the first one. A triple trocar is attached to the second clamp from above and is kept in the same plane as the first pin. The third pin is inserted through the triple trocar.
- Then the 4th clamp, above the lowermost clamp is utilized to insert the 4th pin, as per the 3rd pin.
- Attaching the pins with only one tube does not confer good stability. Hence a second tube is attached on the first pin only at the beginning and then carry out fixation of rest of the pins. This is relatively an easy method. The clamps of this second tube are fixed in mirror image, so the tubes are on either side of the bar.

A better technique: After the two pins are inserted, then both the tubes are attached at this time only and the 3rd and the 4th pins are inserted through two clamps, placed, one above the other.

Another method: Pin aligner device: A possibility: Imagine, the device has only four sleeves. (Six sleeves are needed for the femur).

- The first pin is inserted at the upper most end of the tibia.
- The upper most sleeve of the aligner device is threaded over the first pin and is aligned over the tibia at desirable level from the bone and the screw on the first sleeve is tightened.
- A triple trocar is inserted through the fourth sleeve and the screw is hand tightened to maintain the level of the aligner from the tibia. Through it the lower most pin is inserted. The second and the third pins are similarly inserted. The aligner sleeve screws are loosened and the aligner is removed.

It is preferable to practice this on a bone model as a training, so it adds to ease, in real life situation. In the real life situation, the fracture fragments are mobile and one needs help of an assistant to stabilize the distal fragment, well aligned (Fig. 38.8).

PRESTRESSING AND FINAL FIXATION

In a stable transverse fracture, prestressing is done across the fracture. (In a comminuted fracture or in a fracture with bone defect, two pins in a fragment are prestressed against each other).

The assistants are trained in the mechanics. The surgeon should maintain the reduction, The nuts of each two clamps over the 1st and the 4th pins are kept slightly loose, just short of tight and the pins are prestressed across the fracture. The total four nuts on the two pins are tightened. While doing so, the distance between the two tubes should be about 2 cm, so that, as the pins tilt, the clamps do not brush against each other. The reduction is studied under 'C' arm image.

Then the 2nd and the 3rd pins are prestressed against each other. The extra lengths of the Schanz pins are cut off with a heavy duty cutter and protection tubes are attached to the cut ends, to avoid injury to the team and to the other limb, during recovery and follow up.

The incision at each pin insertion is closed, without tension. The pin sites are dressed with tulle gras, antiseptic cream, etc. After 3 to 4 days, these sites may be left open and the discharge is wiped away, as needed.

Option: All the pins are placed *in the sagital plane*. The first pin is inserted through the tibial tuberosity and the fourth one above the plafond. This exposure is as in distal locking in AP direction. The tendon of tibialis anterior crosses at this area and hence, it is safe to make a formal incision and keep it out of harm's way. If the 4th pin insertion is done percutaneously, the tendon is likely to get impaled. The 2nd and the 3rd pins are inserted in the middle area.

Dynamization of the Unilateral Assembly

Mechanically it is possible to dynamize the unilateral fixator with two tubes, one above the other and is useful in a transverse fracture with good bone to bone contact.

The prerequisites:

- The fracture be transverse and well opposed
- Relatively painless fracture union
- May have some appearance of callus around.

At this stage, if controlled weight bearing is permitted, the union advances well in further expected duration (Fig. 38.9).

The Principles and Technique

- On the upper ends of both the tubes, the tube to tube clamp of type ii shown above, is added.

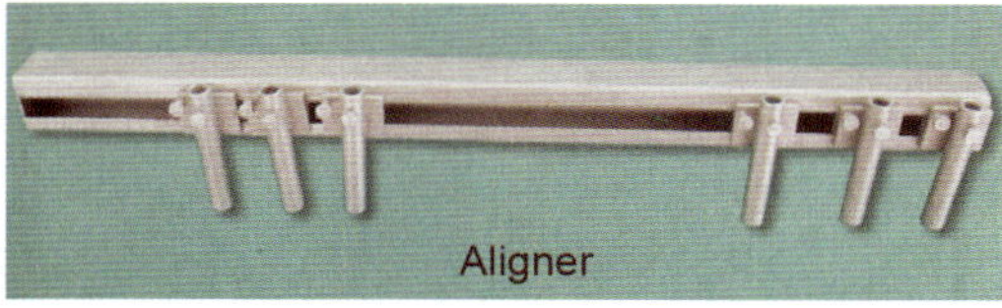

Figure 38.8 Pin aligner device

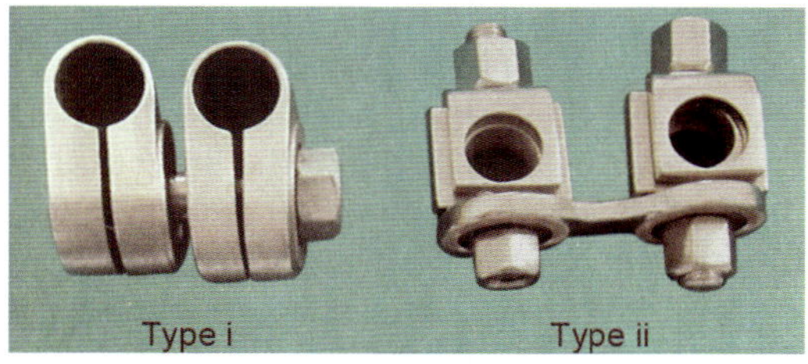

Figure 38.9 Tube-to tube clamp

- The two adjustable clamps on the superficial tube, at the proximal end, and the two clamps on the deeper tube at the distal end, are made loose by loosening the nuts on each clamp, which grip the tube. This reduces their hold on the tubes. Hence, the clamps are able to slide over the tubes and achieve fracture cooption.
- *Nuts in the tube to tube clamps:* On the superficial tube, the proximal clamps are made loose.

When one studies the geometry and mechanics of the assembly, one will notice that, both the fracture fragments are able to come across each other to some extent, when partial weight bearing is started. The presence of the tube to tube clamp helps to prevent twisting of the tubes, during dynamization.

Uniplanar/bilateral frame: I prefer a 4.5 mm diameter Steinmann pin of 9" length. In case of an obese person, a longer pin is necessary. This diameter is suitable for both proximal and distal end of the tibia. A 4.5 mm drill bit is commonly available. Prior to drilling, a Steinmann pin mounted on a T handle is kept ready. The bone should be drilled with a 4.5 mm drill (and a drill sleeve) and then the Steinmann pin mounted on a T handle can be passed with rotary motion. After making the drill hole, a 2 mm K-wire is inserted in the hole by the assistant, to visually know the direction of the drill hole track, while the surgeon picks up the Steinmann pin mounted in a T handle. The K-wire is removed and the Steinmann pin is passed through the drill hole by a rotary motion of an arc of approximately 40 deg. Two 11 mm tubes of adequate lengths are taken and four adjustable clamps are mounted on them, the end ones are finger tightened, while the middle ones are left mobile. The fracture is reduced and kept so. It is necessary to have a correct rotational alignment, while the surgeon inserts the second Steinmann pin in the lower end of the tibia, by the above method. At this stage, if the fracture is an oblique one and one desires to insert an IFS across it, it is done so. When the fracture is well-opposed and IFS is inserted, usually the rotational alignment is achieved.

One the tube is attached to both the upper and the lower Steinmann pins, on either side of the limb, the clamp nuts are finger tightened, keeping the tubes as close to the skin as possible, with necessary distance for dressing. The pins are prestressed across the fracture area. Additional Steinmann pins are inserted adjacent to the previous ones, at a distance of 5 cm or so, towards the fracture site as follows: The adjustable clamp is placed at this level and a triple trocar is held in its jaw, so that the pin would be parallel to the previous one. Both the cortices are drilled with 4.5 mm drill bit and a 4.5 mm Steinmann pin is passed. The procedure is repeated at the lower end of the tibia. The adjustable clamps are fixed over the pin ends, on either end of a Steinmann pin. Both the pins are prestressed across the fracture and fixation completed. (It is desirable that, the assembly is triangularized: vide infra).

Pin loosening is a common phenomenon. A pin which is not prestressed, tends to be loose and local discharge and infection is likely. Straight pins are under no load and cause bone resorption. Hence *prestressing* them is necessary.

In a fracture with good contact opposition, the prestressing is done across the fracture, while in presence of bone loss at the fracture site, the prestressing is done in the bone fragment only (intrafragmentary prestressing)

Such an assembly, using two Steinmann pins on either side, may not resist torsional stresses. Hence, lateral end of the 1st pin and the medial end of the 4th pin can be linked with cross tubes, using twin clamps. (This method leads to not so stable a triangularization) (Fig. 38.10).

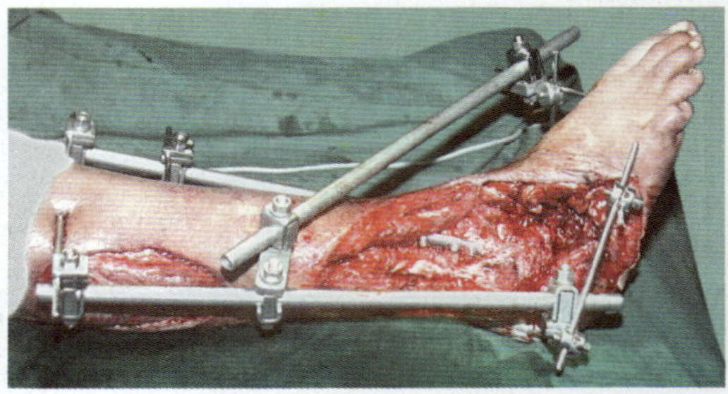

Figure 38.10 Triangularization: less stable

TRIANGULARIZATION

Steps

- One mediolateral Steinmann pin on either end of tibia, with a tube medially and laterally (in coronal plane).
- One Schanz pin proximally on the anteromedial surface.
- Second Schanz pin on the distal fragment on the anterolateral surface. This surface, being more rounded, the pin may have to be passed in AP direction.
- These two Schanz pins are attached to a tube and prestressed across the fracture.
- Open clamps are added on all the three tubes, one each on the medial and lateral tubes and two on the third tube. The third tube is liked to both the tubes, with a connecting bar (which is a Steinmann pin).

This completes the triangularization and adds to the stability in all the planes, immensely (Figs 38.11 and 38.12).

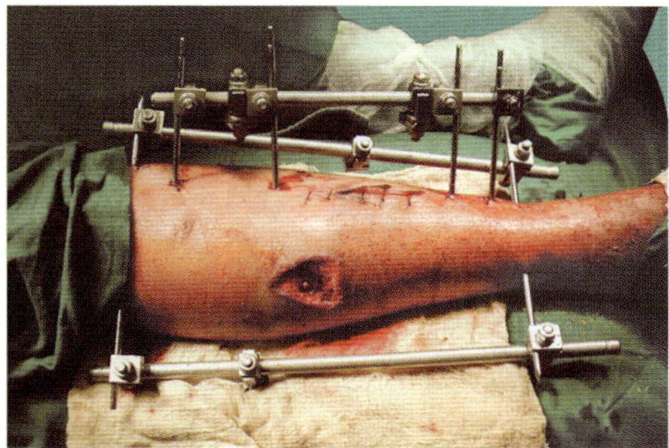

Figure 38.11 Triangularized: connecting bars removed

Application of Principle of Prestressing in a Skeletal Traction

In an upper tibial skeletal traction, in a young person, with good bone density, a single Steinmann pin is adequate. It continues to be well-fitting for a few weeks. A pin is known to loosen, if:

- The bone is osteoporotic, as in elderly person
- The swivel of the stirrup is not freely rotating and hence, with the movement of the knee, the Steinmann pin rotates within the bone
- The pin is inserted in a bone, without prior appropriate drilling, some fragmentation of the adjacent bone occurs, in cortico-cancellous junctional area. If the pin is passed without predrilling in metaphyseal area, being cancellous bone, the bone is compressed around the pin and the fitting continues to be good.

Therefore, in elderly persons or in an osteoporotic bone, it is necessary to pass two pins. They are attached to a Charnley clamp and prestressed by compressing against each other. The appearance of a parabola is seen and the assembly continues to be stable for few weeks and the pins do not loosen (Fig. 38.13).

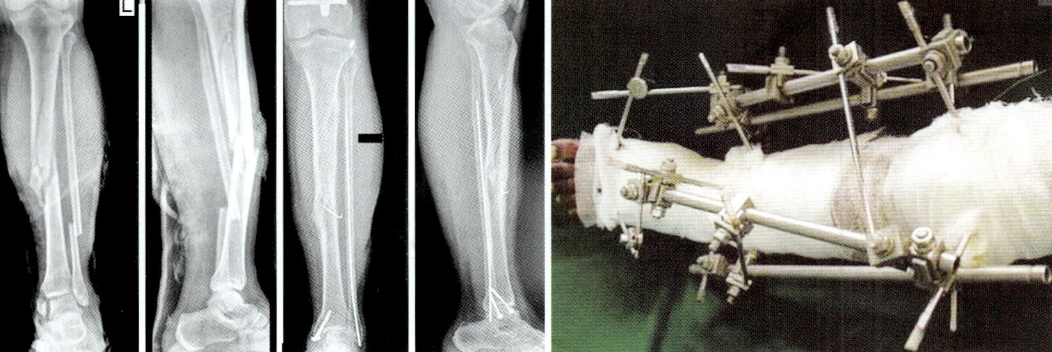

Figure 38.12 Triangularized: segmental fracture

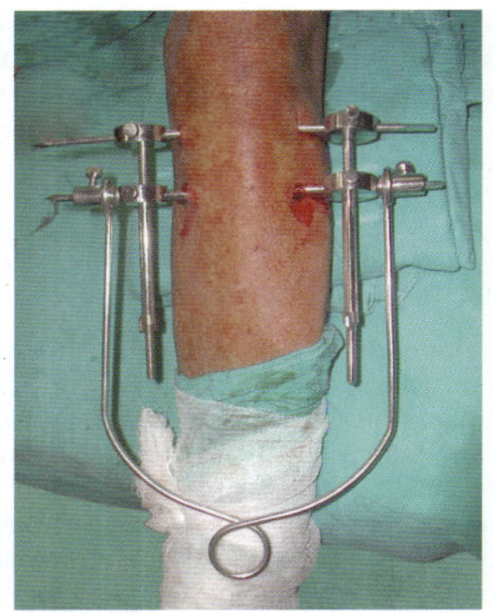

Figure 38.13 Twin pins traction technique

CASE EXAMPLES: USE OF AN EXTERNAL FIXATOR

Case 1

This young adult had a bike accident and sustained open 3-part fracture of tibia and fibula. In the town of injury, wound cleaning and suturing was done and was referred to a larger town for further management. The limb dressing was opened and revealed a primarily sutured wound with abrasions and blood clots dried on the skin.

On examination under anesthesia, the fracture was found to be unstable and hence local plate application to keep contact opposition, was necessary. This was done and the wound was kept open and after a few days, loose opposition was done. An above knee POP

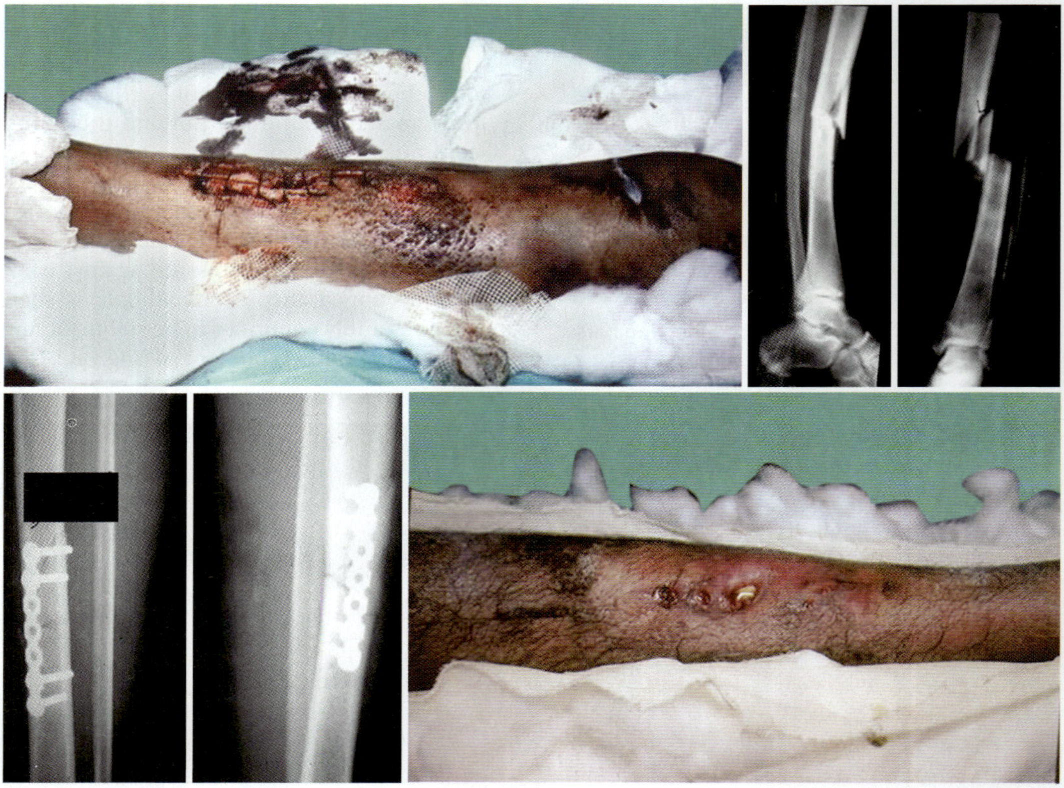

Figure 38.14 External fixator

slab was applied and window dressing was carried out (Fig. 38.14).

At the end of about two months, the wound did not heal. The plate made its appearance through the wound and there was no indication of union on X-ray film. During this period, fibrosis had occurred around the bone ends and the plate could be removed. Hence, the plate was removed. There was no evidence of local sequestrum formation. To offer good stability, a tubular external fixator was applied at the same time. In due course, the discharge reduced and infection cleared out.

After a month, a bone fragment was seen to be appearing in the wound. It was a sequestrum and confirmed in X-ray film. It was removed (Fig. 38.15).

Two months later, there was no local infection, but the wound required reconstruction to have a soft tissue cover the area. Hence, a colleague plastic surgeon, raised a flap and rotated it. The local condition was healthy without any indication of infection. At the same time, *bone grafting* was done. The external fixator was stable and continued. In due course of time, the flap was taken up well and gave a good wound cover (Fig. 38.16).

Two months later, the fixator was made loose and the fracture was noted to be uniting well. Hence, the fixator was removed and an above knee cast was applied. No weight bearing was permitted still (Fig. 38.17).

Gradually weight bearing was permitted on the limb and the fracture consolidated. Still, at

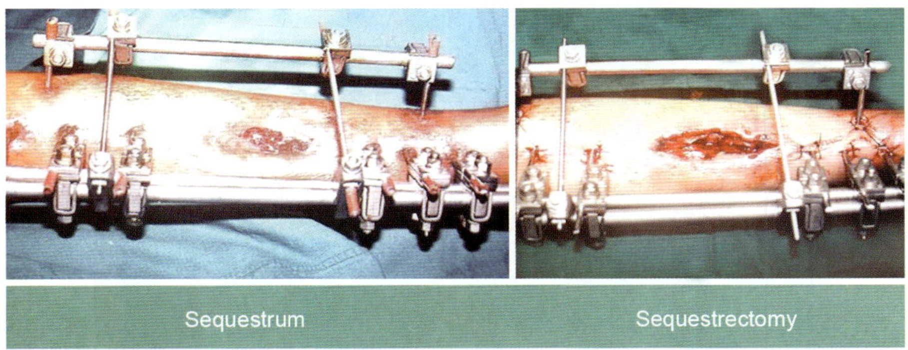

Figure 38.15 External fixator sequestrum

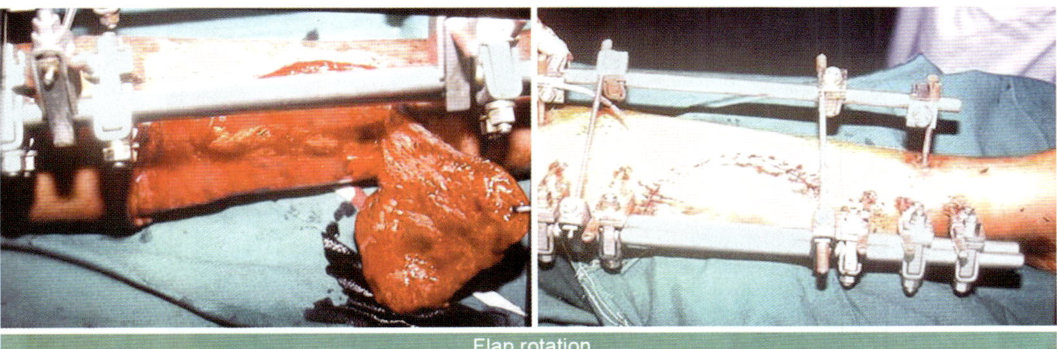

Figure 38.16 External fixator flap

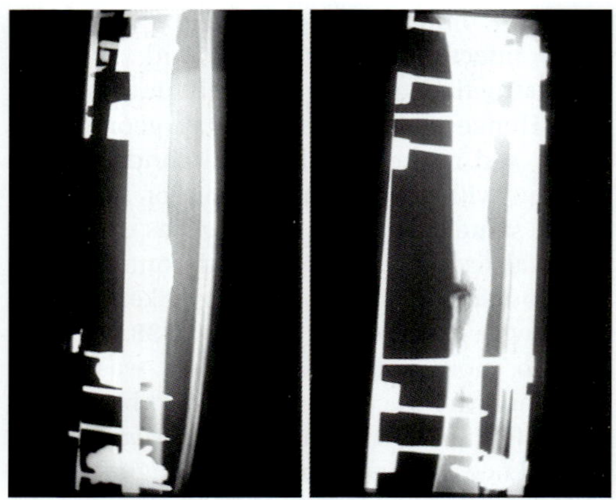

Figure 38.17 External fixator fracture uniting

times, he would get some discharge through the wound and discharge small flake of bone.

Case 2

The patient had an open fracture in the mid/3 tibia and fibula, with some skin loss. On arrival, wound excision, thorough lavage, etc. was done. Fracture ends were stabilized with a plate and a complementary fixator was applied anteriorly with two tubes. The wound was loosely opposed and there was no infection.

To offer a skin cover, colleague plastic surgeon carried out a local flap rotation.

The rotation flap united well, so also the fracture. As is known, once, a fracture is well

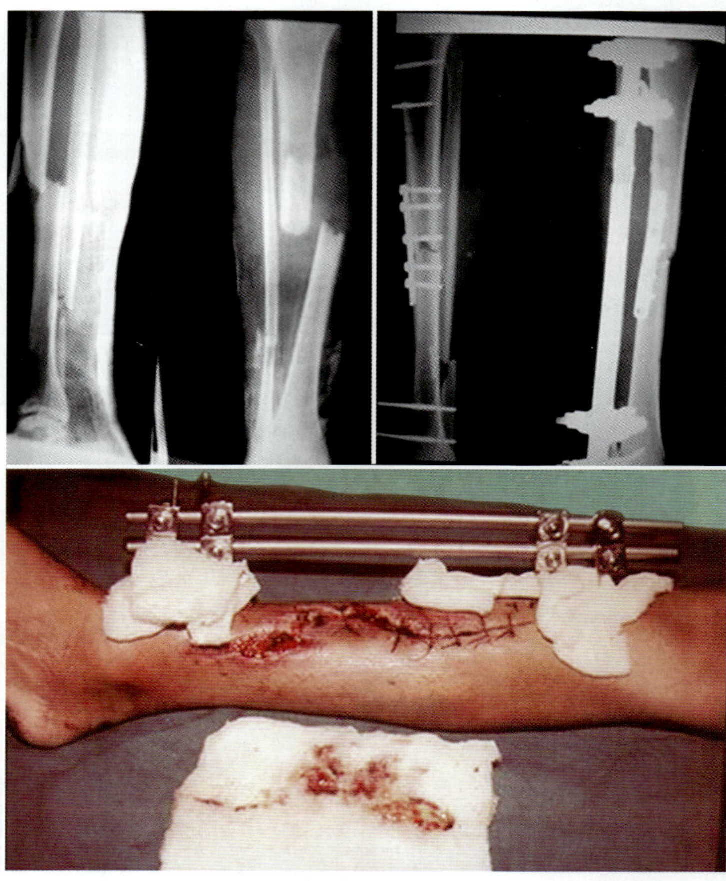

Figure 38.18 Plate with a fixator

covered, the tissue perfusion improves and the fracture unites in an expected duration. The fracture was uniting, well and hence, the fixator was removed. A posterior long slab was applied and after 10 days, when the tracks were dry, a final weight bearing cast, with a caliper on was applied. (This was prior to the availability of synthetic cast material and hence a walking caliper was used. The clamp needs to be extended above the fracture area, so the weight bearing occurs from an area above the fracture. If the caliper ends just at the fracture site, it adds a stress on the fracture site) (Figs 38.18 and 38.19).

Case 3

This middle age person presented for symptoms unrelated to the old tibia and fibula injury. I studied his history and the X-ray films, which were well preserved. This case has a historical importance and hence is mentioned:

He had an open fracture of tibia and fibula and was treated with external fixator about 25 years ago. He had local bone loss and in due course, bone grafting was carried out. The defect was made up and the local bone ends were adequately wide, but sclerotic. The fracture remained ununited. *A tibia-pro-fibula procedure* was carried out successfully by a senior surgeon, which was a practice then. The fracture united. As per the X-ray appearance then, if such a situation arose today, one would perhaps consider interlocking nailing, after carefully reaming the tibia (Fig. 38.20).

LESSONS LEARNT FROM THE ABOVE CASES

On day 1, when the first procedure is carried out:

- Copious lavage and thorough wound edge excision needs to be done.
- If the fracture appears unstable, one may consider application of a small plate, to keep the bone ends well aligned, so that bone ends are aligned and remain deep to the skin, reducing tension under the skin. This is preferably done on the day 1.
- One expects the fracture ends to start uniting at the end of three to four weeks. If the fracture ends were comminuted and one expects a possibility of deep lingering infection, the plate may be removed at this stage. This is especially true, if the patient presents late after the initial treatment and the wound was primarily closed then. While the plate is removed, in case some free

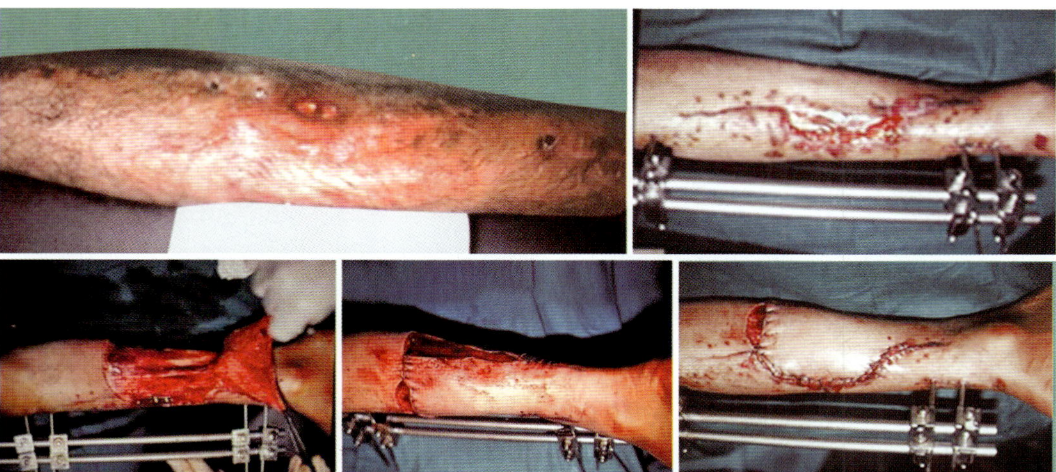

Figure 38.19 External fixator

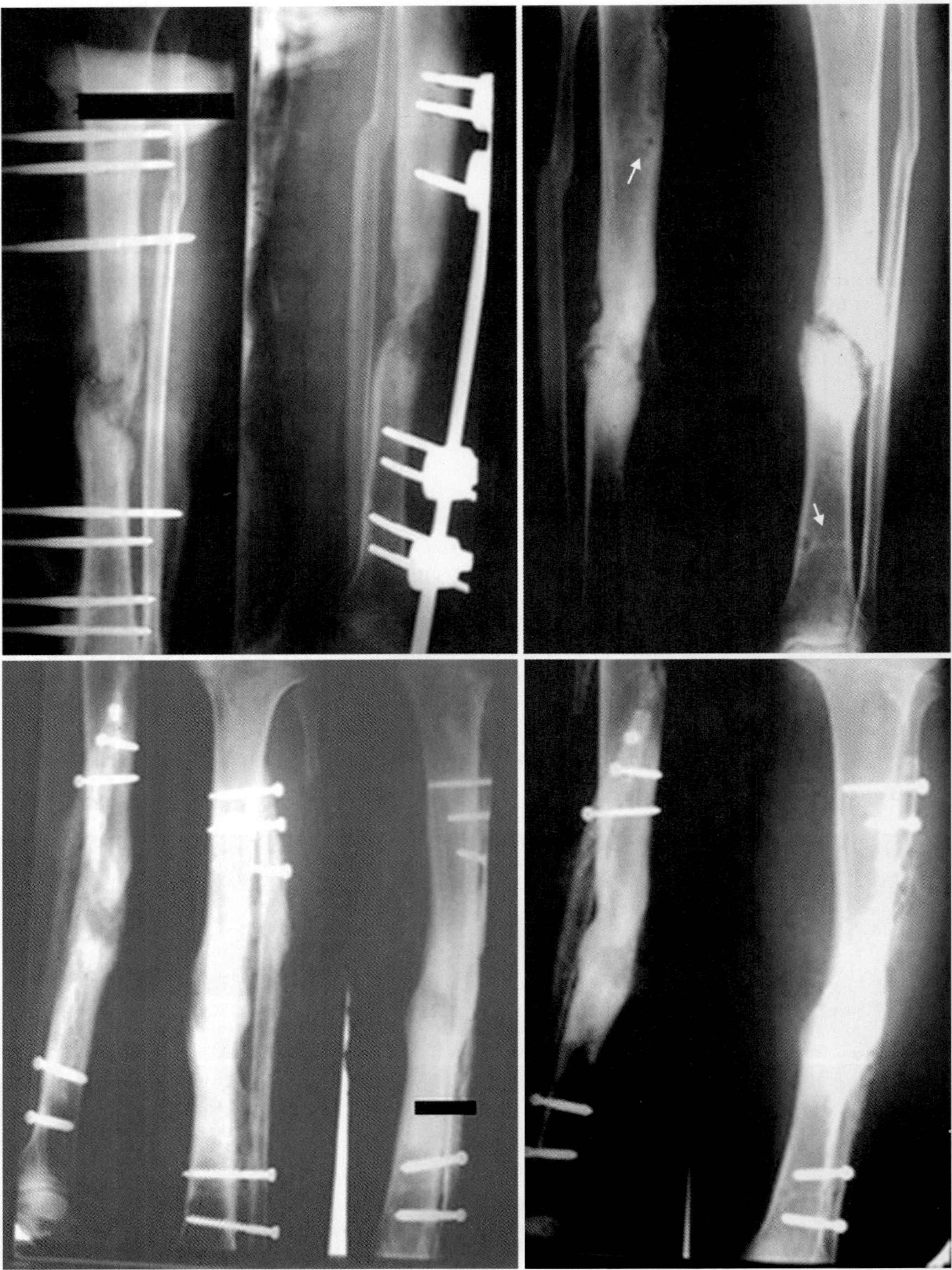

Figure 38.20 Tibia pro-fibula procedure

cortical fragments are visible and appear avascular, they should be removed, to avoid delayed sequestration.

- After this, when one is sure that there is no deep infection and local skin flap is needed, it should be carried out. The flap rotation should not be done, in presence of a possible deep infection or possibility of an avascular fragment underneath. The local flap rotation may be combined with bone grafting, if indicated. If the grafting is delayed, then to make an incision near/through the flap, could devitalize the flap.
- If it a transverse and a stable fracture, one could consider dynamization of the unilateral fixator. The other option is to loosen the fixator and assess the clinical union. If so, the fixator can be removed and a posterior POP slab is given for two weeks, to be changed later to a walking cast. Progressively, more weight bearing is permitted, to help fracture consolidation.
- The patient is alerted that, late sequestration of some small fragments is known to occur and only when the fragment is taken out, the discharge would cease.
- In a tibia, it is preferable to use Schanz pin with short threads. The tip of the pin should just penetrate the far cortex. Fortunately, in this case, the threaded portion did not give way, but is possible. Vide figure 38.20.

CHAPTER

39

External Fixator in Open Fracture of Tibia

Being a subcutaneous bone, open fracture of tibia is common. The aim of treatment is to prevent infection, give a soft tissue cover and achieve optimum stabilization. A rule of thumb cannot be applied to every case. Few typical cases would help to understand various possible methods in the management of a case. In an open fracture with a large wound or a skin loss, a colleague plastic surgeon, who is to carry out a procedure to give a skin cover later, is involved from day 1 procedure of wound excision and application of external fixator. He can guide well, the position of Schanz and Steinmann pin placement, so that at a later date, he can carry out, further procedures with relative ease.

Like other methods of fracture fixation, the external fixation modality needs to be understood well. In a fracture treated non-operatively by either a traction method of a plaster immobilization, unites, in spite of physiological motion around the fracture. The intramedullary nail permits micromotion, which stimulates fracture union, while absolute rigidity conferred by a tension band plating leads to a primary bone union.

External fixator is too rigid, to allow micromotion, while not adequately rigid, to lead to a primary union, without callus formation. An external fixator is a temporary method of treatment, to help obtaining a skin cover and prevent infection. Having achieved this, one should change to a suitable further method of management. Hence, after fracture stabilization with a fixator, following options need to be considered, for fracture union in expected duration.

- Once the soft tissue cover is obtained, remove the fixator and then treat it non-operatively, by plaster method.
- Remove the fixator, curette the tracks and immobilize the fracture till the tracks heal well. Later on internal fixation is carried out at appropriate time.
- If for some reason, either of the above methods cannot be carried out and the fixator has to be continued, then addition of bone grafts is necessary, to achieve fracture union.

FIXATION OF FIBULA

In fractures in lower/3 of tibia and fibula, the fibula is usually fractured at the same level or at a lower level. Being close to the ankle mortise, this lateral column needs to be stabilized well. The fibula fracture, when it is a short oblique or a 3 or 4 part fracture, some shortening by a few mm is likely and is acceptable under the circumstances. The intramedullary nail in fibula , offers the necessary stability to the limb. Often this fixation by IM nailing can be done by a closed method, so there is no additional exposure and the soft tissue cover on the lateral side is not disturbed. (This closed nailing of fibula is important, because, if tibia fracture fixation is to be done by an open method and there is a surgical wound on the fibula as well, the circumferential tissue tension is rather more).

Case 1

This old lady had an open fracture in other country. Fibula plate and a mini external fixator was applied and she arrived here. The assembly was stable. There was some translation.

The plate fixation for the tibia, was not considered, because the medial surfaces of tibia were not aligned well, when she reached India and the medial soft tissue would not have offered a good cover.

Hence bone grafts were added on the tibia and the fixator was continued. After a few weeks, X-ray examination showed, the grafts getting incorporated and fracture area was being bridged. Hence the fixator clamps were made loose and a clinical fracture union and stability was assessed. The fracture was uniting well. Hence, the fixator was removed and an above knee cast immobilization was carried out. The fracture united in expected period. Prior to removal of the cast, weight bearing in the cast was carried out, which helped fracture consolidation (Fig. 39.1).

Case 2

This middle age person had a comminuted fracture of lower/4 of tibia and a fracture of lower fibula. Primary wound excision and fibula IM nailing with a square nail was carried out. The tibia was fixed with a tubular external fixator. At appropriate time, split thickness skin grafting was planned. Bone grafting and split thickness skin grafting was planned, to be done in the same sitting. First, few iliac cancellous bone grafts were laid in the tibia fracture area. Then split thickness skin grafts were laid on the wound and the wound healed well. It is important to know that the stabilization of fibula helped to maintain the leg length and alignment. This is very important contribution of fibula nailing procedure. At the end of six weeks, the fixator clamps were made loose and fracture union was assessed. Since, the fracture was uniting well, the fixator was removed and a plaster slab applied. After a week or so, when the pin tracks healed well, it was changed to a plaster of Paris cast. (This period of delayed cast immobilization, helped to change the dressings at the pin tracks. The blood soaked hard dressing is changed as needed, which adds to the comfort of the patient). This cast was a synthetic one. X-ray examination was carried out at interval of three weeks. When the bone bridge was adequate, gradual weight bearing on the cast with a cast overshoe was encouraged.

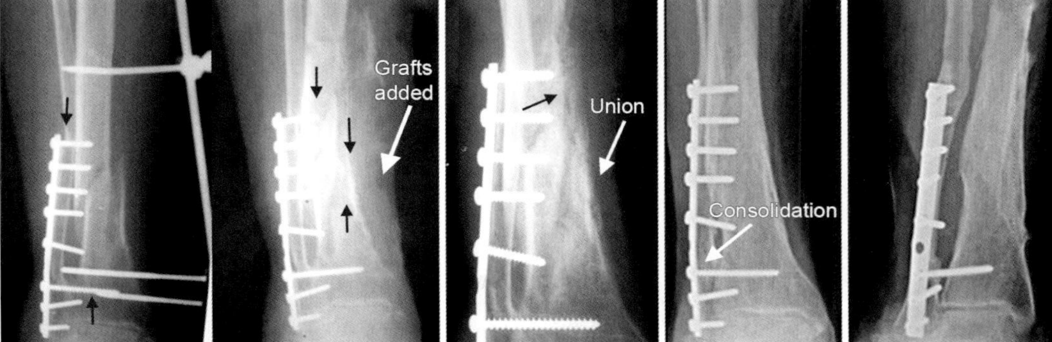

Figure 39.1 External fixator as a definitive method

At the end of approximately four months, full weight bearing was permitted. Follow up X-ray at the end of 15 weeks and at the end of 4 years are shown (Fig. 39.2).

Case 3

This elderly lady has an accident while traveling in a bus and sustained a bilateral open fracture of tibiae. On the right side, there was a rotated 3rd fragment in the mid/3 fracture tibia and the superior tibio-fibular joint was dislocated. There was local degloving of skin on the mid area, due to impact of the shin on the seat in front. On the left side there was a wound on the lower tibia and associated open fracture of the tibia and fibula in the lower/3 area.

On arrival, after assessment, under GA both the legs were cleaned and wound excision was carried out and bilateral above knee plaster slabs applied. After she was stable:

- Closed interlocking nail on the right side was carried out. Due to the local skin condition, the rotated fragment was left as such, to be dealt with later.
- On the left side, fibula was stabilized with a square nail. For tibia, tubular fixator was applied. A transverse Steinmann pin was passed in the proximal tibia. The tibia fracture being very low, another transverse pin was passed through calcaneus. One oblique pin was passed from the anterolateral surface of proximal tibia and another anterolaterally in the mid foot. In such a distal comminuted

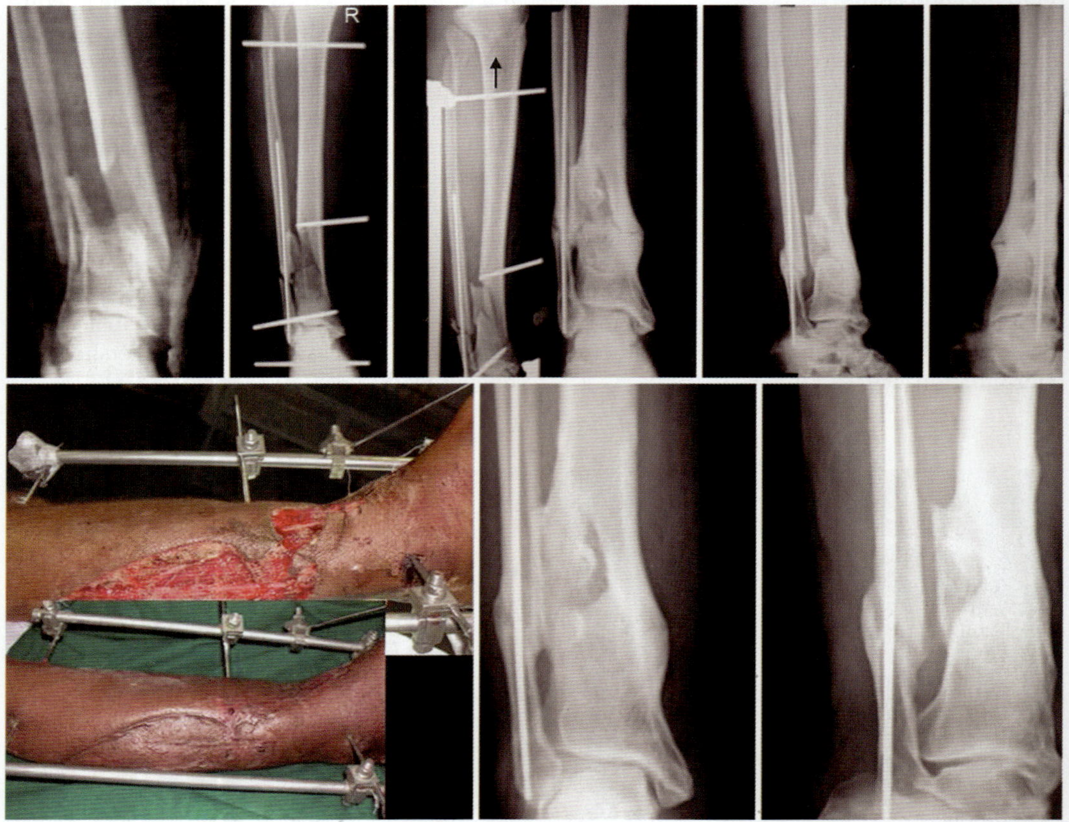

Figure 39.2 Tibia external fixation and skin loss

fracture of tibia. It is necessary to keep the ankle and the foot in neutral position. This was done by passing a 3.5 mm Shanz pin in MT1 and a 2.5 mm pin in MT 5 and linked to the tubes.

- At the end of 7 weeks, the tibia fracture did not show any evidence of union, as was expected to be so. Hence, cancellous grafts were added in the left tibia and fixator continued.
- The degloving on the right tibia in mid/3 area settled. The rotated 3rd fragment was as such and hence grafts were added in the fracture site, to fill the defect created by the rotated fragment. After a month, both the fractures showed some evidence of callus formation. Hence, the right tibia was dynamised. The left tibia external fixator was removed and a left above knee cast was applied. Gradually the patient was made to stand on both the legs and ambulated. The left above knee cast was made a below knee cast and the knee was mobilized. Both the tibiae united and consolidated in due course (Fig. 39.3).

Case 4

This patient of about 50 years, had RTA:

- Ipsilateral segmental femur, open comminuted fracture mid/3 tibia
- Transverse fracture lower/3 fibula
- Fracture of medial malleolus
- Fracture of metatarsals
- Fracture of nasal bone and facial soft tissue injuries
- Fracture head of the right ulna.

He was brought to the hospital with a

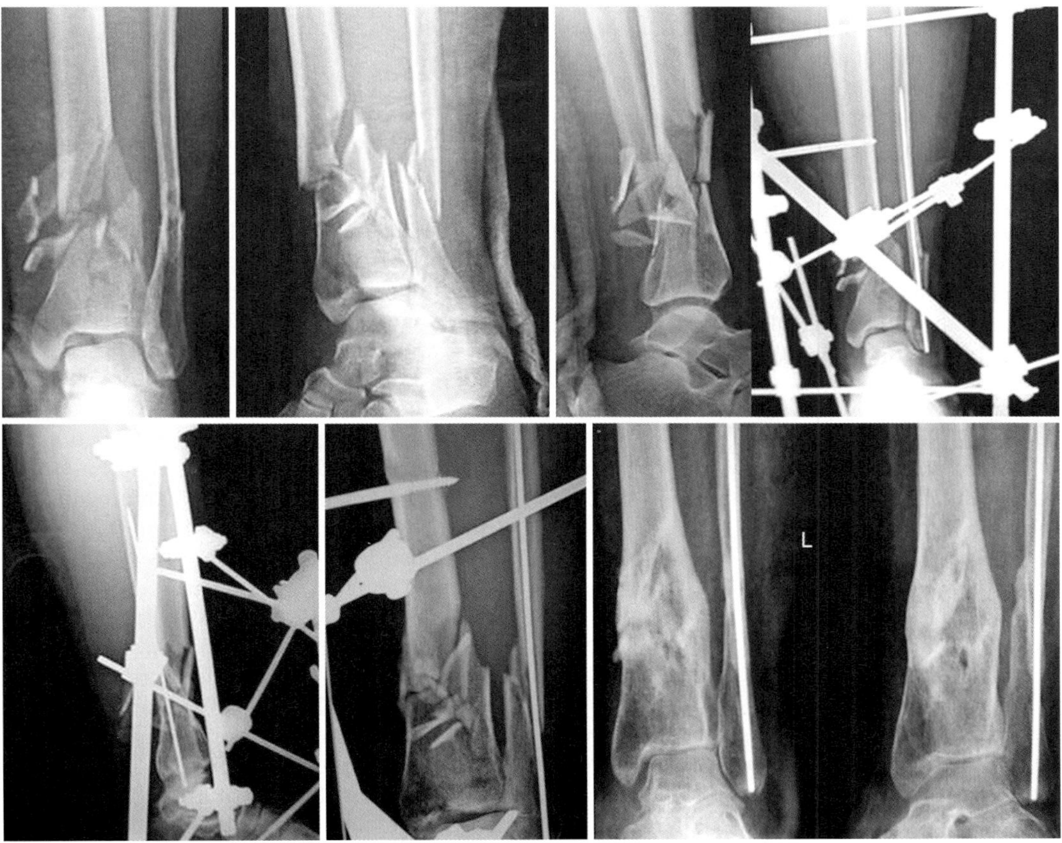

Figure 39.3 Bilateral fracture of tibiae

Thomas' splint on the left leg, which was indeed a good first aid given at the previous hospital. The splint supported both the femur and the tibia as well.

Stages of Treatment

1st Procedure

- Left tibia wound care, wash and wound excision
- Medial malleolus fixation with a 4 mm screw
- Fibula nail with open reduction of fibula. This restored the length of tibia
- Tibia tubular external fixation: Transverse Steinmann pin at the upper end and at lower end, so that it was proximal to the tip of the malleolus screw. Oblique Schanz pins and triangularization done for stability. 3.5 and 2.5 mm Schanz pins were inserted in 1st and 5th metatarsals and linked to the tubes, to keep the ankle in neutral
- The upper most transverse Steinmann pin was also used for attachment of Bohler stirrup, to offer a traction to the femur. Having kept the leg on Bohler frame for traction to the femur, automatically elevated the tibia and the foot, which helped to reduce the edema.
- Right above elbow POP cast in supination for the fracture of head of ulna.

2nd Procedure

- Closed interlocking nail for the left femur and split thickness skin graft for the left tibia wound.
- The interlocking nail had stabilized the femur and hence, the knee was gradually mobilized.

3rd Procedure

After six weeks, bone grafting for the tibia was done. The right upper limb plaster cast was removed and a wrist splint was given. The exercises for that limb were carried out. The forearm and other muscles were especially strengthened, because subsequently, he had used a walker.

4th Peocedure

A month thereafter, the left tibia and foot fixator was removed and an above knee cast was applied and kept for six weeks. Till this time, the knee was mobilized, because the femur was stabilized by a nail. An observation is that, if after an injury proximal to a joint is treated and the joint is well mobilized, one can immobilize it again, without a danger of stiffness developing in that joint.

Gradually he was ambulated, as gained more strength in the right forearm, partial weight bearing was advised, which he carried out.

Both the femur and the tibia united and consolidated in due course (Fig. 39.4).

Case 5

This young man had an open fracture at the mid/3 tibia with a lateral 3rd fragment. Had some facial wounds and head injury as well. On arrival, the facial wounds were taken care off and dermabrasion carried out. The open tibia wound was excised and a POP slab was applied.

After he was neurologically stable, the tibia was stabilized by a tubular external fixator and was triangularized. The fracture tibia was in the mid/3 area and the fibula fracture was still at a higher level. Hence, the fibula was not fixed.

As the open wound granulated, split thickness skin grafting was done and the fixator continued. X-ray revealed that there was medial angulation at the fracture site and it was also corrected by loosening the clamps and adjustment. The other three limbs were uninjured and hence patient was ambulated on a walker.

The facial and tibial wound healed in due course. Locally at the 3-part fracture of the tibia, there was no radiological evidence of union. Hence, bone grafts were added on the tibia and the fixator continued.

At the end of further six weeks, thus at the end of total four months, there was appearance of bridging callus. The fixator was removed

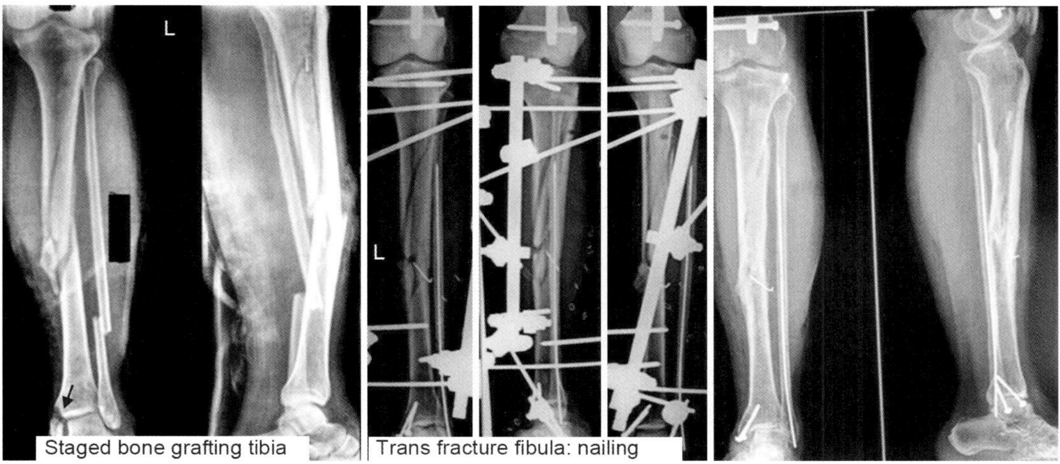

Figure 39.4 Ipsilateral fracture of femur and tibia

and limb immobilized in an above knee cast. Gradually weight bearing was permitted and the callus turned more dense and fracture united well (Fig. 39.5).

Observations

Above cases indicate, in an open fracture of tibia with local bone loss, it takes at least three to four months, for removal of fixator and application of a long leg cast. Gradually partial weight bearing is permitted and takes further six weeks at least, for the fracture to consolidate and to be able to walk without any support.

In cases

- In an ipsilateral fracture of femur and tibia, where femur nailing and tibia fixator is done, the knee was mobile for a few months. Having had a mobile knee, if one has to apply a long leg cast, which includes both the ankle and the knee, the knee does regain good range of motion.

Case 6

A young man had an open fracture of lower/3 tibia with bone loss and a fracture of ipsilateral ulna with bone loss. In a previous hospital, ulna plate fixation and leg plaster was applied. Subsequently for the tibia, an external fixator was applied and then he reported to us for further treatment.

There was anterolateral skin and soft tissue loss in the tibia. The fixator was adjusted. Colleague plastic surgeon rotated a local flap and bone grafting was done for the local defect. The skin cover was restored well and some bone continuity was noted.

Future Plan

The fixator clamps to be loosened and assessment of fracture union to be done. If the stability and union was good, the removal of fixator and cast application was to be done.

While I was away, a colleague carried out as planned and a long leg cast was applied. On table after application of cast, an X-ray examination was not done to confirm the position obtained. On return from my leave, I arranged for an X-ray through the cast, which showed angulation at the fracture site, which needed correction.

I carried out wedging of the cast by open wedge method, under X-ray control. The open wedge was maintained with wooden blocks in the cast wedge and the cast was completed. The restoration of the alignment was maintained

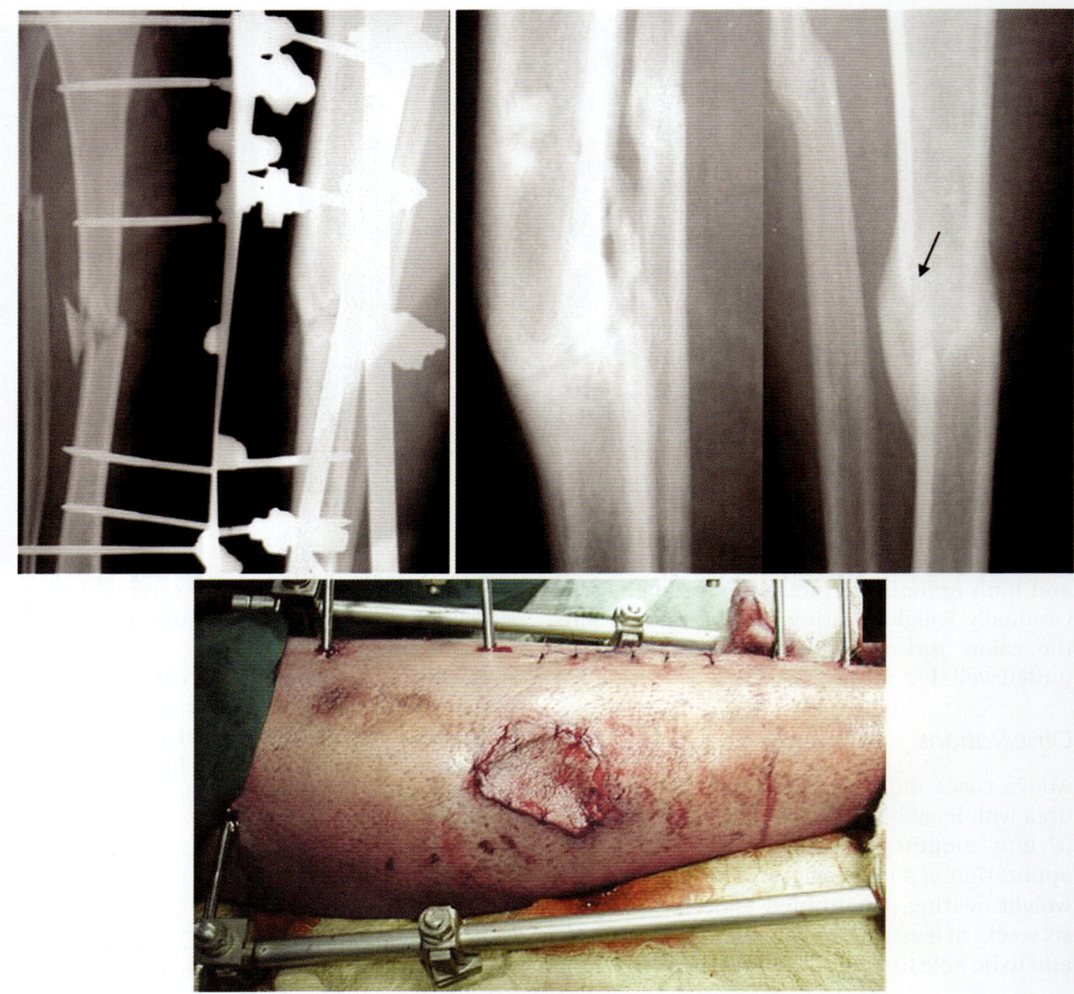

Figure 39.5 Tibia external fixator. Fibula not fixed

well. Since the fracture callus was still soft, one had to wait adequately to permit weight bearing on the cast. It took few weeks more, for bone bridge to appear across the fracture area, and edema to settle. The cast was then bivalved and limb examined. The union was adequate on clinical and X-ray examination. A close fitting long leg cast was applied and gradually weight bearing permitted. The fracture consolidated well, though in the lateral view the tibia looks to be narrow. Gradually it also hypertrophied (Fig. 39.6).

Lessons Learnt

- To assess fracture union, one needs to loosen the fixator. Only if, union is adequate, fixator is to be removed. If not, the alignment is confirmed and the fixator is tightened.
- When the bone has adequately, united, removal of fixator and cast application can be done. The cast is to be well moulded in slight varus and an X-ray to be taken on table through the cast, while the patient is under anesthesia effect.

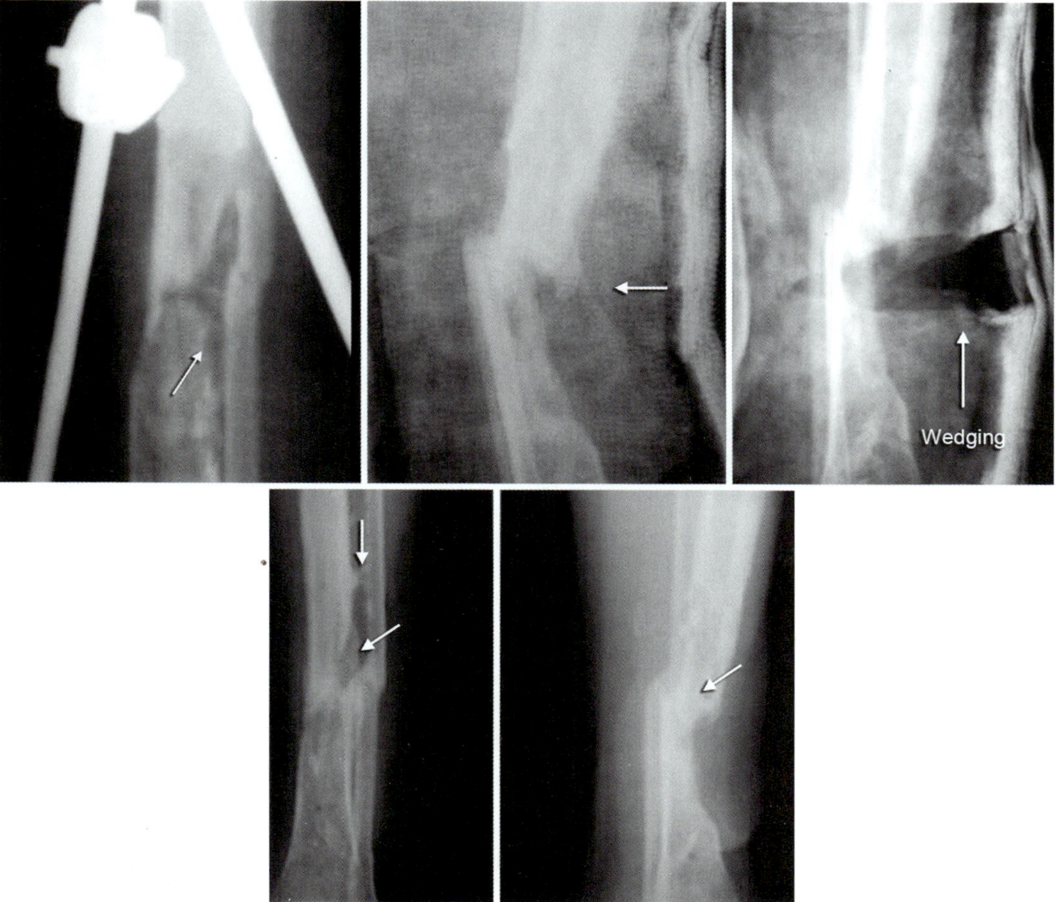

Figure 39.6 Tibia external fixation: Wedging of a cast

REFRACTURE AFTER EXTERNAL FIXATOR REMOVAL

Above cases described, have been subjected to bone grafting, followed by a cast. Later on all the patients were made to bear weight on the cast, till good consolidation had occurred and remodeling started.

Case 7: Tibia External Fixator–Refracture

In this case of a compound fracture of tibia, external fixator was applied in a peripheral place. No bone grafting was carried out. After about 3 months, the fixator was removed and cast immobilization was done. Thereafter, patient continued to walk, though good consolidation and remodeling had not occurred. Perhaps no close follow up and follow up X-ray examination was done. An X-ray taken in between shows partial union and anterior cortex indicates persistence of a fracture line and the fracture still not completely bridged with callus. After a few months, the patient had a refracture at the same area.

The patient reported for further treatment to us. The fibula fracture at the same level had united well.

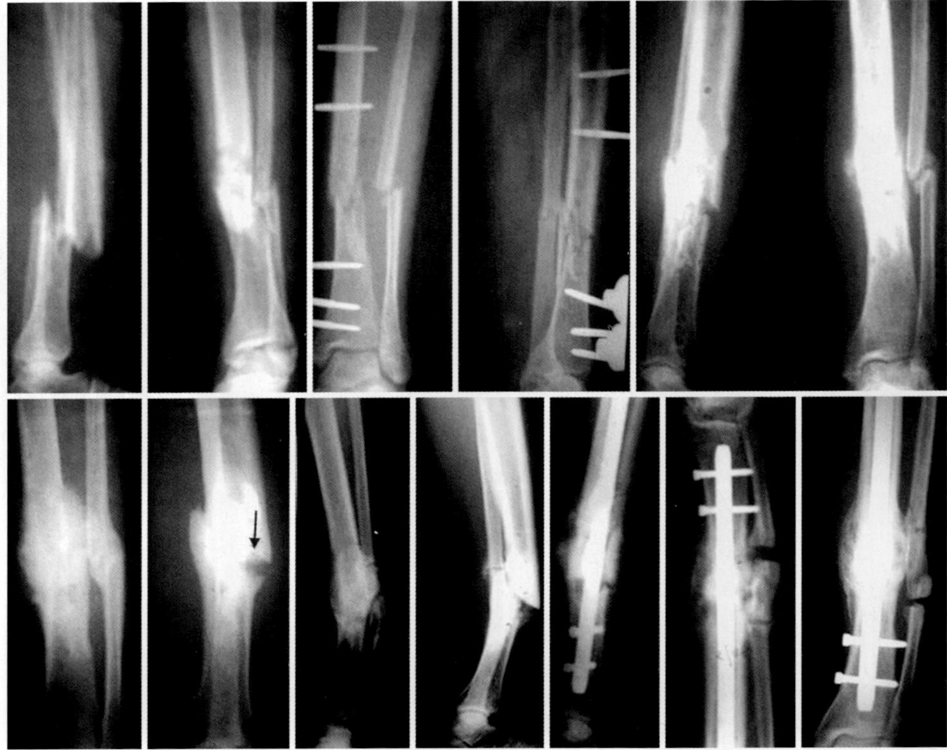

Figure 39.7 Tibia external fixation: Refracture

Treatment Given

Fibula osteotomy followed by interlocking nailing for the tibia was carried out. The fracture consolidated well.

Looking back and review of the X-ray films after removal of fixator:

- It does not show good bone bridging across the tibia fracture. Since the fibula has united, some weight bearing was possible.
- In fact one cannot say, what was advised by the treating surgeon to the patient and if it was followed well.

Message and What One Learns

External fixation stabilizes the open fracture and permits management of the wound on the fracture area. This is a temporary step of management. Once the skin cover is obtained, one of the three options should be followed. The procedure of addition of bone grafts is of lesser magnitude than having a refracture and needs to manage it by another surgery.

A follow up X-ray every 4 to 6 weeks is necessary to monitor the progress of remodeling (Fig. 39.7).

CHAPTER

40

Tibia Interlock Nailing

FEW PREFERENCES

- I prefer to use a wooden quadriceps board, rather than leg hanging on a side technique.
- A padding below the ipsilateral gluteal area, helps to keep the leg in neutral rotation, may be slight internal rotation as well.
- The awl and nail entry whether through splint ligament approach or ligament retraction approach, is individual choice. A slightly curved awl is preferable.
- The awl tip is preferably kept at the junction of plateau and the shaft. Its alignment with the proximal shaft should be checked under a 'C' arm in both the views and then the canal is made.
- Prior to insertion of a beaded guidewire, a 10 ml disposable syringe is taken and its nozzle end cut off. The guidewire is threaded through this cut off syringe barrel, kept above the plateau, so it acts as a tissue protector.
- While the beaded wire reaches the distal end of tibia, it must be in the center of the plafond in both the views, so the nail end will sit exactly in the center. If the wire tip reaches the anterior part of the plafond, it should be withdrawn adequately and reinserted in correct position. If it is accepted as such and reaming done, then the nail would enter this track, resulting in anterior angulation at the fracture site.
- It is adequately preached that the final position of the nail tip be at least 1 cm proximal to the hard distal subchondral bone, so that, when partial weight bearing is started, some distal migration of the nail is possible during weight bearing. If this is not followed, the contact opposition at the fracture site is not adequate and may lead to a delayed union.
- Whenever possible, one should ream adequately, so a nail 1.5 mm smaller can be easily inserted. This difference in diameter to which the canal is reamed and the nail inserted, may help during dynamization as well. If one is able to ream till 10.5 mm or at least 10 mm, then a 9 mm nail can be inserted. The locking holes in this nail accept 4.9 mm bolts. If only an 8 mm nail can be passed, the bolt diameter is smaller and during partial weight bearing, the narrow bolt is known to bend or break.
- During proximal locking with a jig, first the round hole bolt is inserted. After this bolt is inserted, one can check with a guidewire, that the screw is in the nail. Then the oval hole bolt is inserted.
- If one inserts the oval hole bolt first using a jig and then for some reason, removes the jig and then reapply it, following problem is likely. Having done so, attempt to insert the round hole bolt may fail. This is because, the nail may have axially moved proximally, as

the oval hole bolt permits so. Hence the jig should be removed only after both the bolts are inserted.

- During distal free-hand locking, first a full moon appearance of the nail hole is achieved. Then with a 2 mm K-wire mounted on a T handle, the tip should be pierced with some gyration motion, so that a pit is made. Then the K-wire should be further advanced. The slightly tapering hole thus made, helps to stabilize the drill bit and then the bit does not wander about and slide away from the center of the hole.
- A pin with a radiolucent butt end, is a good device. It being strong enough, does not bend, while gentle hammer blows are given (Fig. 40.1).
- After it pierces the near cortex, it is removed. Appropriate diameter drill bit is used to complete the hole in the same direction. After drilling through both the cortices, when a 'C' arm image is taken, the track thus made in the bone, appears more white than the surrounding bone, indicating correct penetration through and through is made in the both the cortices. The drill bit used for the distal locking should be *a short one,* because then the total length of the bit and the drill handpiece is such that, it can be held vertical under the 'C' arm tube well. The usual quick coupling bits are quite long, meant to be used with the proximal jig. If such a long bit is used for distal locking (without a sleeve), there is a chance of its breakage. Besides, the total length of the assembly is such that, the handpiece cannot work under the 'C' arm tube, which needs to be moved away, every now and then.

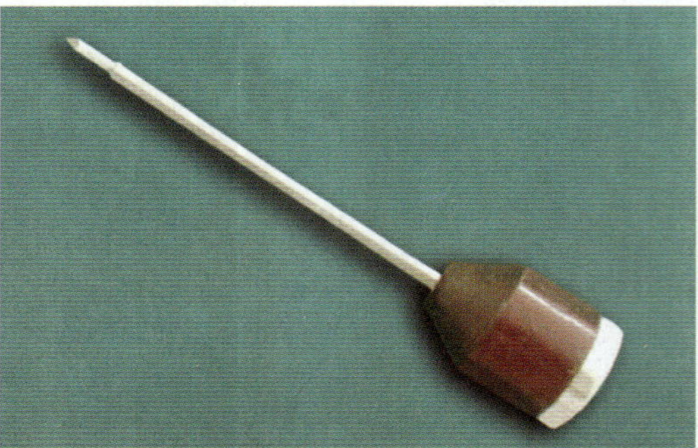

Figure 40.1 Distal hole locking device

- Thus, it is easier to work with a short drill bit with smooth shaft, which is mounted in a Jacob Chuck. Besides, with a short drill bit shaft, the danger of bit breakage is less.
- In case of fracture in lower/3 tibia, with a third or a fourth fracture fragment, with a traction on the foot, one finds that the fragments fall back in place. During distal locking, assistant should maintain the traction on the foot, so that the position of the fragments is maintained and should not leave the foot, till the drilling and screw insertion is complete. This step helps to maintain the length of the tibia.
- The self-tapping bolt has conical tip with tapping flutes. This part of the screw does not contribute to have a hold on the bone. Hence the bolt should be 2 mm longer. Besides, it also helps to remove it from the bone from the other side, should the bolt break.

FEW PRACTICAL OBSERVATIONS IN TIBIA INTERLOCK NAILING

- *Fibula internal fixation:* In a fracture of distal/3rd of both tibia and fibula, the fracture of fibula may be a transverse one and the tibia a transverse or short oblique. In such a fracture morphology, unless the fibula is well reduced, the tibia alignment cannot be achieved. My preference is a square pointed tip nail to stabilize the transverse fracture of fibula. Once a closed reduction of fibula is achieved, the rotational alignment of fibula is confirmed and the nail is advanced further. The nail is adequate enough to hold the reduction well and permits some contact opposition, when weight bearing is started. If the closed reduction of fibula fails, one can do an open reduction of fibula, through a necessary short incision. One can achieve the reduction using a Kuntscher diamond awl, to lever the fragments in place, without the use of bone holding forceps. If fibula fixation is not done first, good tibia reduction cannot be achieved. Hence fixation of the fibula has to be done first (Fig. 40.2).

- In distal/4th tibia fracture, a locking bolt is likely to miss the distal most hole in the nail. This may be due to the obliquity of the tibial surface, along which a drill bit may slide down, missing the mark. In an *oblique fracture at this level,* my preference is to use a plate, rather than a nail, as an implant. Even if both the bolts correctly engage in the appropriate holes, the contact opposition of the fracture surfaces may not be achieved. As against this, a plate achieves a good reduction. The fracture union is more assured, following an open plating than a closed tibia IM nailing, with side to side displacement. However, one should leave the choice to the surgeon (Figs 40.3A and B).

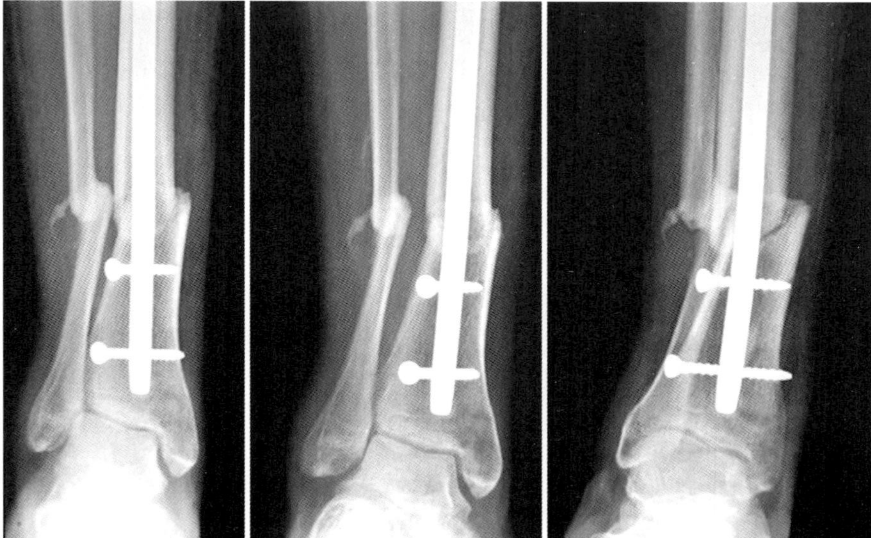

Figure 40.2 Fix fibula first in lower/3 fractures

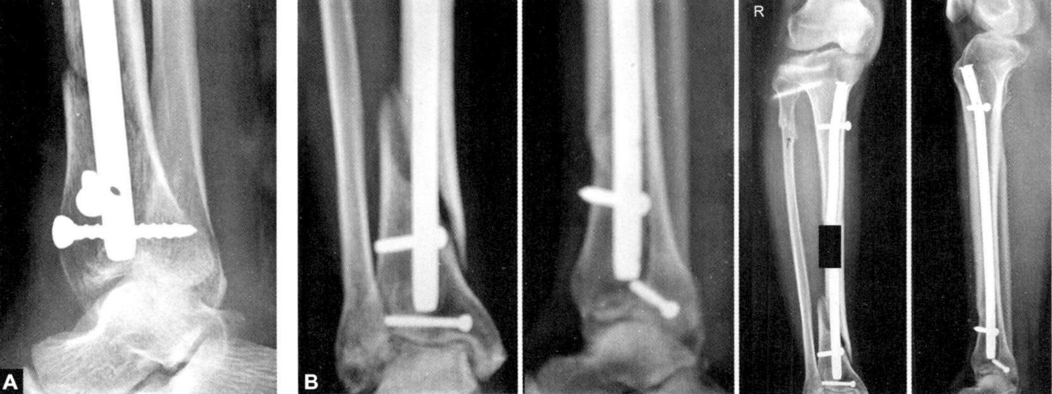

Figures 40.3A and B (A) Missed distal hole; (B) Poor reduction. Missed hole

- In distal tibial fracture, one is tempted to insert all the possible bolts in the distal end of the tibia nail. At times the uppermost bolt may pass through the fracture area and delayed union is observed. Removal of this screw helps fracture union (Fig. 40.4).
- In a spiral fracture in lower/3rd tibia, often the fibula is fractured near the upper end, because it is a torsional injury. Especially, when the fracture is a few days old, closed reduction of the tibia may not succeed. An osteotomy of fibula at the level of fracture helps to attain a successful closed reduction of tibia and the beaded guidewire can be advanced across the fracture well. Having passed the guidewire successfully, the tourniquet, if used, should be released and the fibula wound is closed. This makes the local area a closed envelope, wherein the reaming material is well-accommodated and the fracture healing will be benefited (Fig. 40.5).
- A case presented with a transverse fracture mid/3 tibia and a high fracture of fibula. The injury was a week-old and interlock nail fixation was planned. The fracture was opposed and hitched, with a medial angulation. Exact reduction by doing a translation of fragments was required and was possible only when an osteotomy of fibula was done at the same level. In due course of time, the tibia fracture and both the proximal fractures of fibula and the osteotomy united well (Fig. 40.6).
- Often the fracture line persists at the end of 6 to 8 weeks and no palpable callus is observed in the shin area. In such a situation, it is necessary to carry out dynamization of the fracture by removing the bolt from the round hole at the proximal end. Partial weight

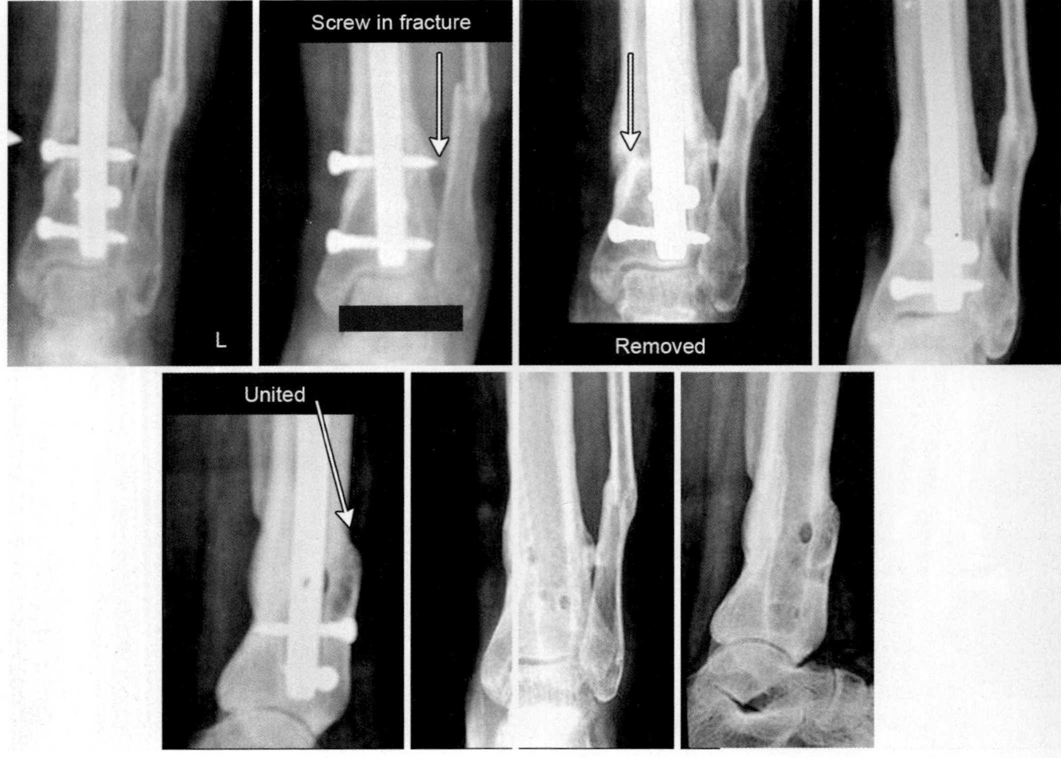

Figure 40.4 Screw in the fracture line

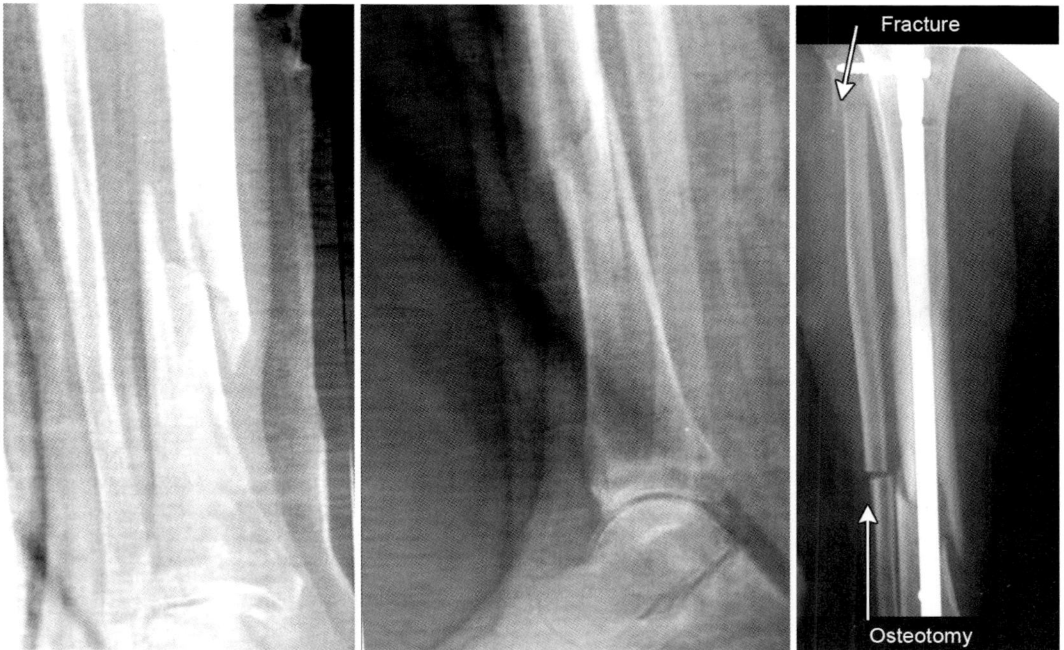

Figure 40.5 Fibula osteotomy in lower tibia fracture

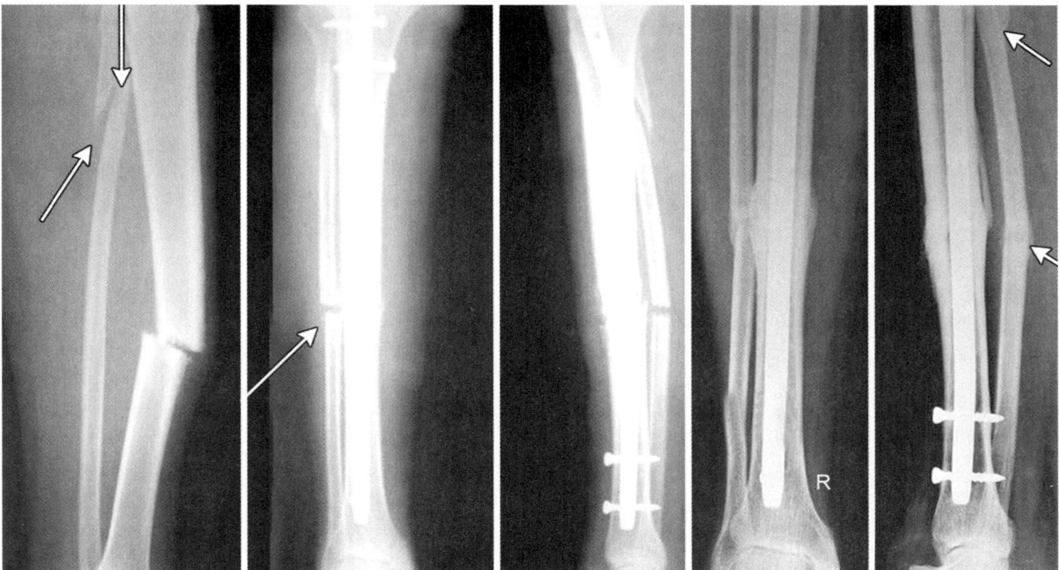

Figure 40.6 Fibula osteotomy in mid-tibia fracture

bearing is advised and executed well. Follow up X-ray every 3 to 4 weeks, does show appearance of callus, bridging the fracture area. In due course, it consolidates well, so the patient can shift from a walker to a stick. At this stage, encouragement to carry out heel raise exercises (Tiptoe) helps to build the calf muscles and improve the contact opposition of the fracture ends (Fig. 40.7).

- This lady had bilateral fracture of tibiae. On the left side external fixator was applied for the open fracture. On the right side, there was internal degloving injury and a successful closed nailing was carried out. There was a fragment medially, which was rotated, so the medullary surface faced, away from the fracture area. It must have lost the soft tissue attachment and was left as such. Some bone bridge was seen on the lateral surface. The hematoma on the mid tibia settled and bone grafting was carried out. The rotated fragment had some soft tissue attachment and was left as such. A month later the nail was dynamised and some weight bearing was encouraged (as per condition on the opposite tibia).

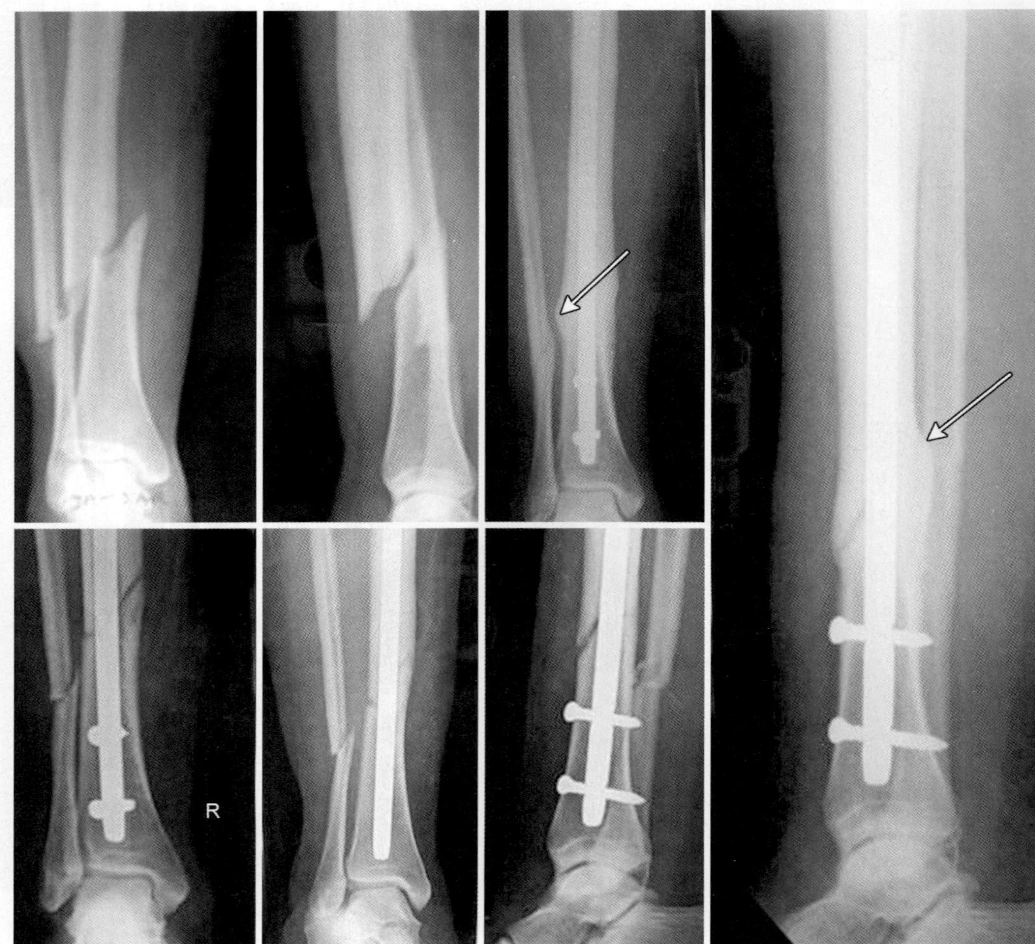

Figure 40.7 Dynamization of tibia

The rotated fragment remained away from the fracture area and looking back, one feels, since the grafting was done, the piece could have been sacrificed (Figs 40.8A and B).

Note: The incision has to be curved, with a wide base medially.

- A few years ago, digital technology for radiography came into vogue and the

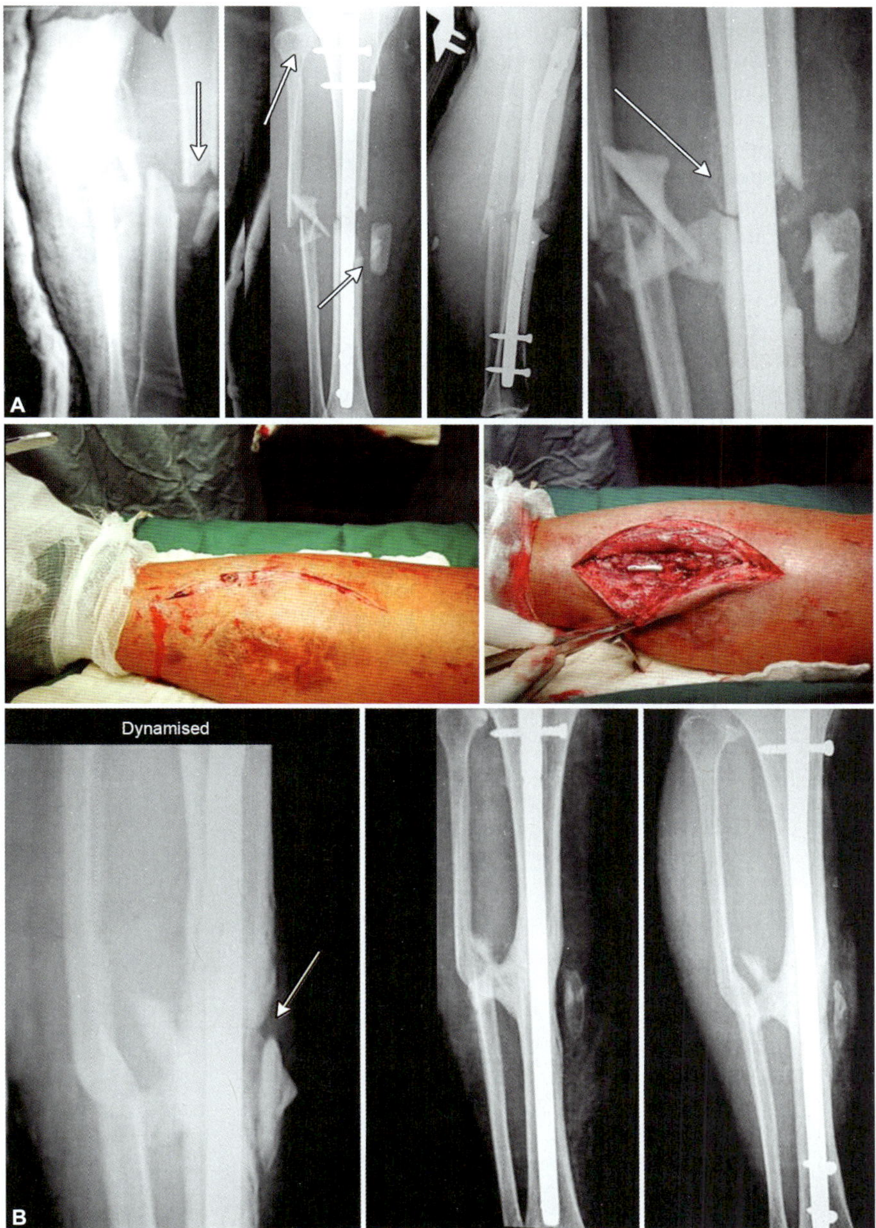

Figures 40.8A and B Rotated fragment and bone grafting

chemical processing gradually became a history. The image processing by the software needs to be carefully done. As seen in the picture, the contrast and brightness needs to be correct. An image of an X-ray film processed by digital technology showed persistence of the fracture line, while another film taken the same week, processed by the chemical method, showed a good bone bridge, so that controlled weight bearing could be safely permitted.

Message: One should keep this possibility in mind and learn to process the image personally. Training of the technical personnel too is equally important (Fig. 40.9).

SEGMENTAL FRACTURE OF TIBIA

- Prior to availability of multidirectional bolts in the proximal end of an interlocking tibia nail, application of plates for both the fractures in a segmental fracture was a common practice. This case had come for *a second opinion,* at the end of three months. The fracture line continued to be visible in the lower fracture area and there was no bridging callus. I recommended bone grafting, which was done by the previous surgeon and the fracture united.

My preferences in the first surgery would be:

- Use of a 12 mm narrow plate for the distal fracture (X-ray indicates presence of a 16 mm plate)
- Being a high-energy injury, addition of cancellous grafts in the medullary cavity and on the lateral side opposite to the plate. This would have assuredly helped union in expected duration. It appears, prebending was not adequate enough, to bring the opposite cortex in good contact opposition.
- Use of a one long plate to span both the fractures is rather difficult to keep the plate exactly on the medial surface.
- The soft tissue care is especially necessary in the distal fracture.
- After the fractures have well-united and remodeled, removal of the plates should be considered. This is important, as the area in between the ends of the

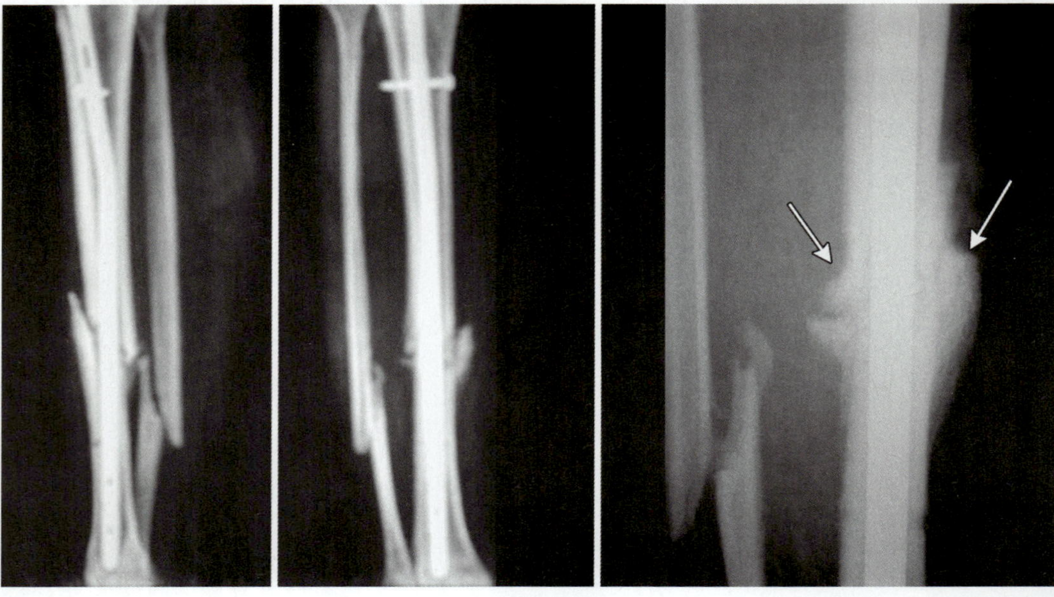

Figure 40.9 Digital processing

two plates, has a different modulus of elasticity and another unfortunate episode may create a fracture in that area. After removal of the plates, one would observe stress shielding of cortex under the plates, especially the distal plate, where the bone is cortical. After removal of both the plates in one procedure, one should apply a back slab and after suture removal, a weight bearing long leg cast for six weeks. This would help to restore the cortical thickness.

- Today a multidirectional bolts nail can be a good option.
- After implant removal and cast removal carefully long-term exercise therapy to restore the muscle strength is very much necessary. A careful long-term follow up is necessary, till the bone remodels well and muscle strength restores to normal (Fig. 40.10).

• Removal of a tibia nail:
Removal of tibia interlock nail with distal broken screw: The X-ray of distal tibia showed a bent screw, which may be perhaps broken also.
One screw was mediolateral, while the other was antero-posterior. 'C' arm was used as required. A wooden quadriceps board was kept under the leg and a good 'C' arm image was confirmed. The board is required for removal of the nail, with the knee flexed.

The Mediolateral screw:
The screw head of the first one was exposed medially. It was removed and being broken, part of the screw came out.
Another incision was taken on the lateral side. The tip of the screw could be seen. Then with a 2 mm K-wire, with the tip cut off, was inserted from the medial side in the screw track and the tip reached the nail cavity. With some pressure, the other part of the screw appeared from the lateral side. The K-wire was kept at the same place and was pressed on the broken shaft of the screw. With the help of a narrow tip nose pliers, the other part of the screw was removed. In place of the K-wire, a distal

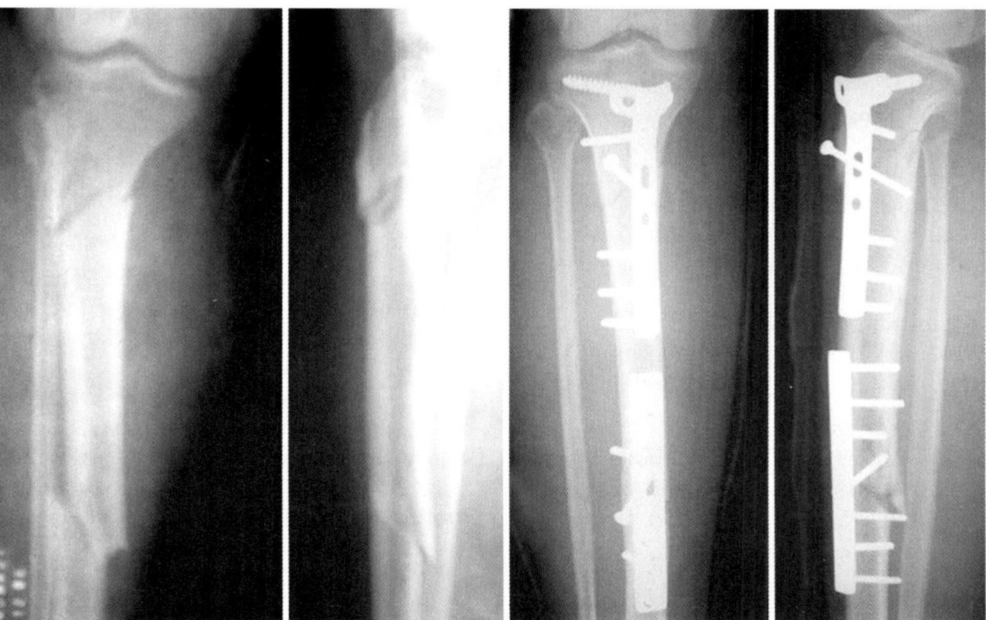

Figure 40.10 Segmental fracture of tibia

aiming device also can be used, as is more broad and rigid.

The AP screw:
The posterior tip of the screw could be palpated lateral to the tendo-calcaneus. The screw head segment was removed anteriorly and a K-wire was inserted through the track and gentle pressure was applied on the other segment. An incision was taken lateral to the tendo-calcaneus and the other segment was removed. Few turns of the segment made it loose and tilted on the posterior tibia surface and it was removed.
The quadriceps board was angulated at the hinge, till the knee was at 60 deg flexion. With a vertical incision on the previous scar, the place of the nail entry was located. If the tip is palpable, it is easy. If it buried under the bone, with a 'C' arm, it is located. With a 5 mm osteotome and a 15 mm gouge, a round track is made, till the nails tip is located. The indigenous available nails do not offer an end cap screw and hence some fibro-osseous in growth is seen at the proximal end of the nail. Having located the nail tip, a groove is dug all around the nail wall, to make it clear from the surrounding bone and extractor bolt is inserted and tightened in it. If the make of the nail, its diameter is not available from the previous record, various types and sizes are fortunately available in the extraction set.

Extraction rod and the ram are attached to the nail. Then the proximal two bolts are removed. If in a case, if any one screw hole was not used to insert the bolt, or if dynamization was done earlier, then some bone growth occurs in the unoccupied screw hole, making nail removal rather difficult.

Why these steps?
If one removes the proximal bolts first and then exposes, locate the nail end, while attaching the extraction bolt to the nail, the nail may move distally or rotate in the cavity. This happens in spite of the Herzog bend and screwing in the extraction bolt in the nail end is time consuming and difficult too.

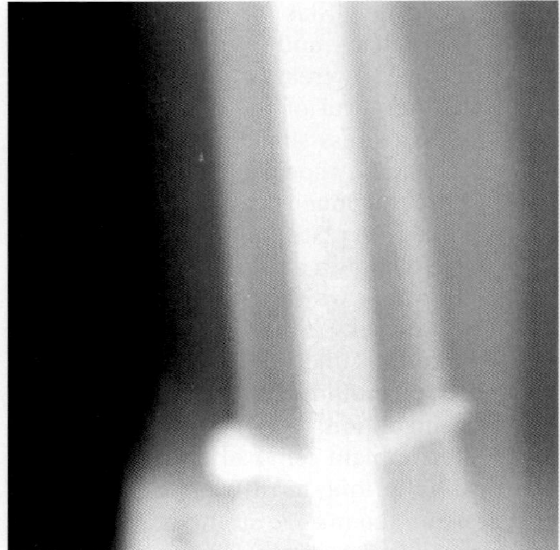

Figure 40.11 Bent distal screw

To remove a broken nail from tibia: A long flexible shaft wire, with a firm hook at the end is inserted through the nail. The hook end should penetrate beyond the nail, which is difficult in the distal tibial subchondral area. The shaft needs to be rotated, maneuvered, to engage the hook on an edge of the nail. When it engages, the long shaft needs to be kept under tension, being pulled proximally, all the while, till extraction blows are given. This is necessary or else, the hook may get disengaged from the nail edge. The extractor shaft is attached to the butt end of the extractor and with a canulated ram, the nail is removed.

In an X-ray film taken prior to nail removal, may not indicate a broken nail. However, during a nail extraction, only a part of the nail comes out. This is usually observed in femur, more often than in the tibia (Fig. 40.11).

CHAPTER

41

Stress Fracture of Tibia

Rheumatoid disease is more common in women. Many factors are responsible for osteoporosis in rheumatoid disease and to name a few:

- Hormonal changes
- DMRD and steroids
- Reduced activity level
- Lack of exercises
- Reduced muscle mass
- Joint deformities, due to muscle spasm, secondary OA, etc.

Often, due to these factors, stress fractures develop in tibiae and often go unnoticed. May be the patient takes it as a part of the disease and/or the primary health providing clinician is unaware of such a possibility. Following few examples would aptly convey the message, so that every clinician would be aware of the pathology and treat the first incidence energetically, to prevent any residual deformity. If a deformity is prevented on the first occasion, incidence of future secondary stress fracture, due to the deformity would reduce.

Case 1

An elderly lady with RA had a fracture of the 3rd metatarsal and dismissed it as some kind of a sprain. She used to walk in an odd way and in due course, the fracture united. (This fracture was noticed only in an X-ray examination done later).

The disease continued to take its toll. She had a minor fall and a bone setter helped her. The pain reduced to some extent and she continued to slowly walk about. After a few months, she noticed some deformity and the clinician noted a united fracture in the distal tibia. It was getting pain free and she continued to slowly move about with support.

Further after a few months, the pain recurred distal to the shin and an X-ray was taken. It revealed another fracture above the previous one. At this stage, she was treated with a ring fixator, followed by a cast application. The story goes ahead. Later had another fracture in the upper/3 tibia, which was then managed (Fig. 41.1).

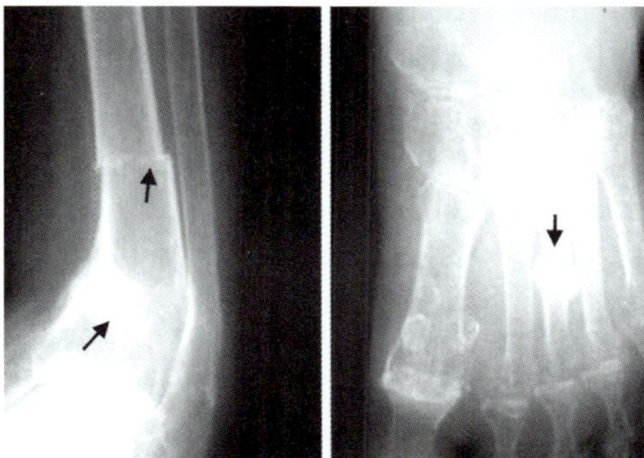

Figure 41.1 Rheumatoid disease—sequential fractures

Case 2

This a story of a brave lady, who faced all the things which came her way, with courage, as a result of rheumatoid disease.

The lady had rheumatoid disease for many years. The fracture history goes back to 1984, when the first episode occurred abroad and a cast immobilization was done: The fracture united with some anterior angulation. After her return back to India, she developed 3 times stress fractures, insidiously, without any specific injury and were treated by a colleague with plaster casts. Gradually, as a result, there was progressive anterior angulation in the mid-tibia, leading to another fracture in lower/3 area. The shin cover was papery thin and any form of surface fixation was not safe. Hence, a surgeon, with prior information, inserted a longer V IM nail (which was in vogue then), so it was purposely passed across the ankle joint in the talus. The aim was to offer good stability to the tibia and keep it well aligned. Stiffness of ankle and subtalar joints was of secondary importance. The fracture was well-stabilized and united.

In between she had a fracture of clavicle and excision of an olecranon bursa as well.

It is a fact that, whenever there is an implant or prosthesis in a bone, delayed insidious infection in that area is observed. This patient too developed so in the operated tibia and since the fracture had united, the nail was removed.

There perhaps appeared another stress fracture in adjacent area and a ring fixator was applied. (The laboratory parameters were within limits). At this stage, not many drugs were available to prevent osteoporosis. The fracture united then.

After 3 years she travelled overseas as well. On returning, she had another fracture in the upper/3 tibia and was managed by a long leg cast.

A few years later, sustained a stress fracture in the mid/3 area and was managed by a ring fixator again.

Later she had some medical problems and passed away. I must admit her courage to face all the events boldly and positively.

A message, therefore, one gets:

- Exercises are important to maintain muscle tone and power well, which in turn, would keep the bone density above the fracture threshold.
- Each clinician must know, what a stress fracture is. Even without one specific episode, one can have a stress fracture and unless this is treated well, progressive deformity would occur. Once the deformity sets in, it is likely to lead another episode of a stress fracture. Deformity in the inferior extremity must be recognized at the earliest opportunity and managed energetically. If it is corrected well, probability of another fracture in the same limb is less.
- Any fracture, including a possible stress fracture in tibia should be diagnosed at the earliest and a nuclear scan is of help, even before MRI can detect the injury. An intramedullary implant is a load sharing device and should be preferred to a plate in managing such an injury.
- Adequate calcium supplements and anti-resorptive agents be given. They should be withheld after use for 3 to 4 years. If the drug is continued for long, the bone tends to be brittle, due to loss of elasticity. A stress fracture at the subtrochanter area of femur is observed after long term uninterrupted use of alendronate, with a trivial injury (Fig. 41.2).

Due to secondary osteoarthrosis in the knees and added osteoporosis, one observes, bow legs. Usually this is seen in untreated primary osteoarthrosis with bow legs or late onset rheumatoid disease.

Case 3

This gentleman over 60, had bow legs and sustained stress fracture in the upper/4 area of the left tibia. The fibula too was fractured and he reported about three weeks after the initial symptom of pain. The fracture had abnormal mobility when he reported.

A multi-directional locking bolt device nail could be passed by a closed method. The fibula fracture being mobile, was automatically well

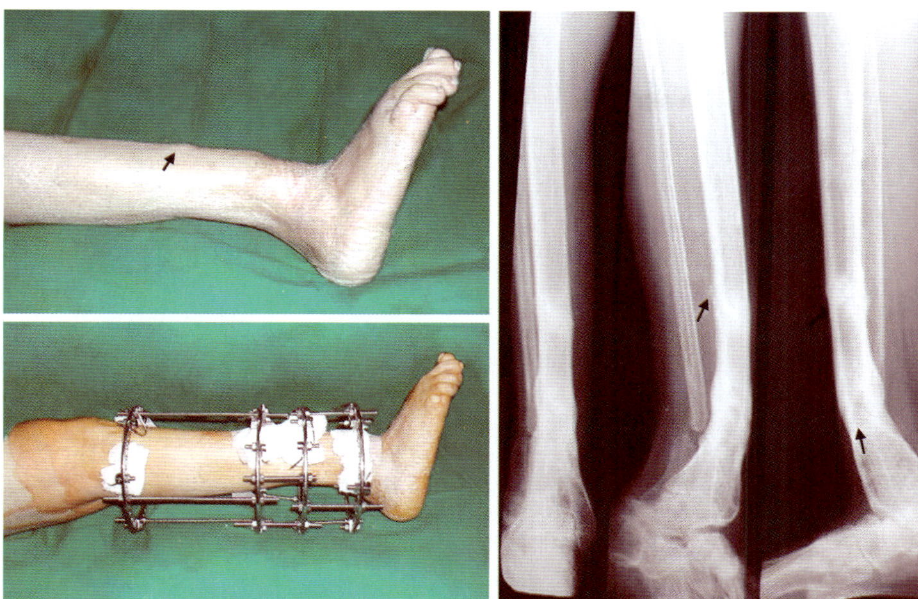

Figure 41.2 Multiple sequential stress fractures in tibia

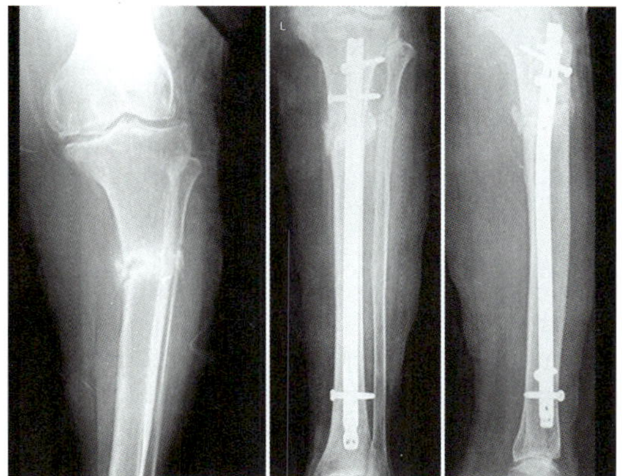

Figure 41.3 Multi-direction bolt nail I

aligned. Both the fractures united in due course (Fig. 41.3).

Case 4

Another fit person over 70 years of age, had bow legs for many years and developed a stress fracture at the upper/4 area on the right side. The fibula was not fractured. It was necessary to correct the deformity, due to the stress fracture. There is a possibility of carrying out a TKR with long stem prosthesis. This could have been useful for both the arthritis and the stress fracture as well. However, he chose to correct the deformity only.

Under anesthesia, the fracture was examined. The intact fibula would not permit correction of the deformity. Hence fibula osteotomy was done at the same level with a narrow blade power saw. The tourniquet was released and the fibula wound was closed over a suction drain.

A multi-directional locking bolt nail successfully fixed the tibia. However, the fracture line persisted longer than expected and he was advised a bone grafting, which he refused (Fig. 41.4).

Comment

In such a high fracture, where the tibia cavity is wide, some translation of the nail is likely on a mediolateral locking bolts. Hence this multi-directional design came in the vogue. However,

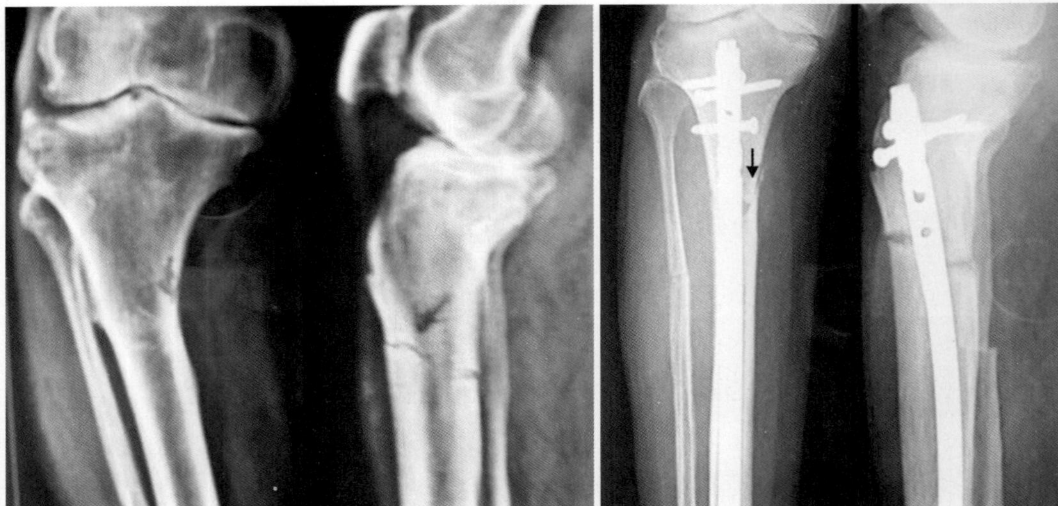

Figure 41.4 Multi-direction bolts nail

as seen in this case, it may not lead to a bony union in each case. If the X-ray appearance continues as such at the end of three months, what are the options?

- Remove few distal most screws and continue to bear weight (dynamization)
- Add only bone grafts on either side of the tibia
- In addition to the grafts, add a derotation plate.

Case 5

In a case of 30-year-old person, having a 3- to 4- part-fracture in the proximal tibia, interlock nailing was done in other city and then he came for follow up in his hometown and reported to us. The fracture was indeed very well managed. At the end of four months, the fracture did not show any evidence of union and the fracture lines continued to be visible. Hence, the proximal bolts were removed, cancellous grafts were added and a 12 mm anti-rotation plate was added. The fracture consolidated well (Fig. 41.5).

Looking at the course of progress in case no.s 4 and 5, I wonder if one has to do only one and final surgery in a given case, whether it would be justified to do a procedure of IM nailing and a complementary plate fixation. This is practised in lower/3 of femur, where the medullary cavity is wide and the nail may not offer absolute rotational stability. A good result is nearly assured and is observed in the distal femur. Hence, I feel, same principle could apply in proximal tibia also.

Case 6

A Nail vs a Plate

One has seen use of a nail in upper tibial fracture. In the given case, a multidirectional bolt nail may be used as an extended indication. However, a plate fixation achieves a better day 1 reduction and a stable fixation and union would be assured more than the use of a nail alone or with a complementary plate (Fig. 41.6).

Case 7

A lady having rheumatoid disease had bilateral bow legs. She started getting pain in the left shin area. The physician was unaware of such a condition. The leg deformity slowly increased and led to a varus deformity. X-ray examination revealed a stress fracture in the upper/4 of

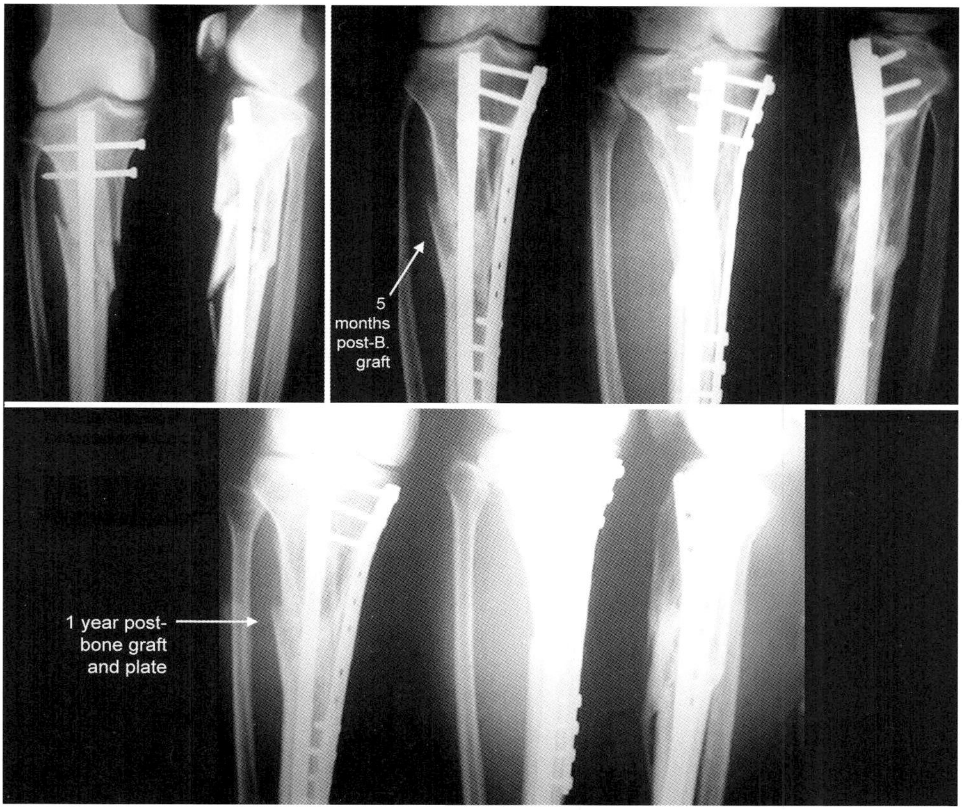

5 months post-B. graft

1 year post-bone graft and plate

Figure 41.5 Derotation plate and bone grafts

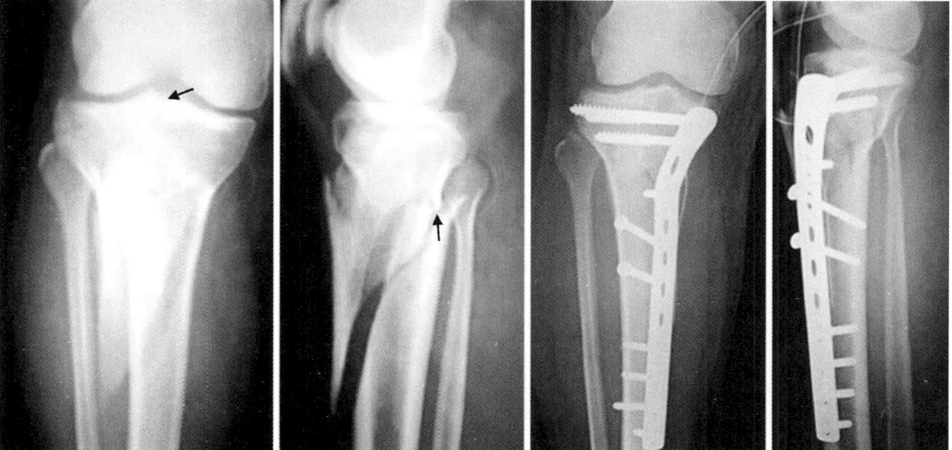

Figure 41.6 Plate better than a nail

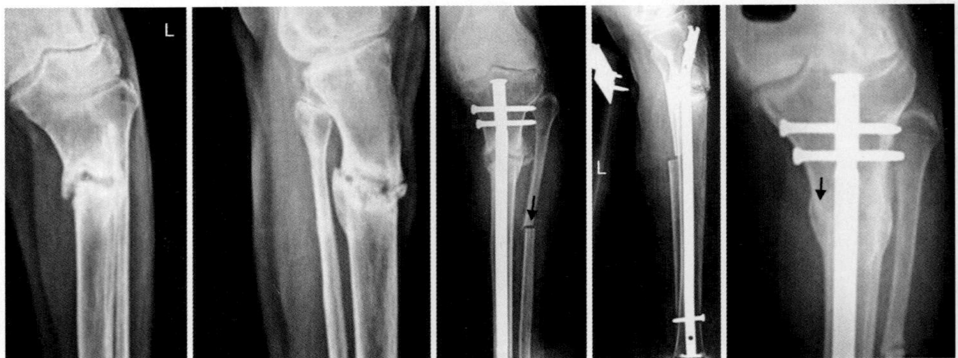

Figure 41.7 Bilateral stress fracture of left tibia (Rheumatoid)

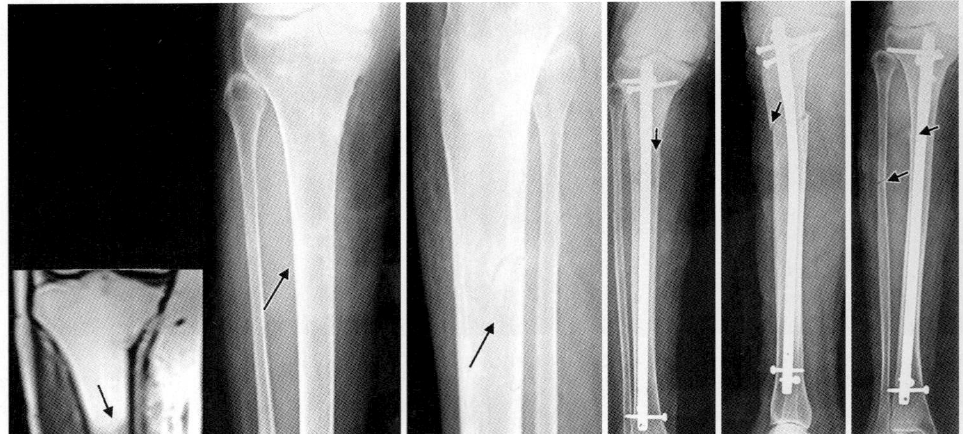

Figure 41.8 Bilateral stress fracture of right tibia (Rheumatoid)

tibia. The fibula was intact. This was prior to availability of a multidirectional bolt design of the nail. She was operated. Osteotomy of fibula and a closed interlocking nail fixation of the tibia led to a good fracture union in expected duration. She could resume her walking again (Fig. 41.7).

Case 8

Having had this experience on the left leg, she was vigilant. The opposite, i.e. the right side tibia alignment was good. After a few days, she had pain in the upper part of the right shin and this was reported by her. X-ray examination revealed a stress fracture in the right tibia. MRI of the right side was done and confirmed the finding of a stress fracture. Osteotomy of fibula and a closed nailing by a multidirectional bolt was done for the right side and the fracture united in due course (Fig. 41.8).

CHAPTER

42

Tibia Plate Fixation

In 80s the trend of rigid fixation of a fracture came into vogue. Soon, the problems and complications of such a procedure emerged and the procedure had quite some complications in early stage.

This was because the technical intricacies were not realized and with time, the surgeon realized them. Thus with experience, a good indication for a plate fixation was understood and practised. Having had experience, one can decide, if a given fracture is suitable for a plate as an implant. If so, which implant? The way it is to be used, whether by an open method or by an MIPO method, etc.

The wound healing was a problem, due to the hardware on a tibia, which has not so adequate a soft tissue cover. Few comments on the use of a plate for fixation of a fracture of tibia:

WIDTH OF A TIBIA PLATE

It was preached that for tibia only a 12 mm narrow round hole or an oval hole plate (with 3.8 mm thickness) should be used. The 16 mm (broad) plate (with 4.8 mm thickness) is meant for proximal segments, i.e. humerus and femur.

Unfortunately, this was not clearly understood or practised and one came across cases, wherein even 16 mm plates put on tibia.

WHICH SURFACE OF TIBIA?

The soft tissue cover on the medial surface is less and hence a plate placed on the medial surface may have some wound healing problem. If one raises a thick skin and soft tissue flap, the wound closure is usually easy.

- In case, there is some difficulty in wound closure, the wound is closed, leaving a few mm of gap in the suture line. A wound closed this way is without tension and chance of flap necrosis is less. If one attempts to close the wound with edge to edge to opposition, there is danger of more width of skin edge loss and related problems.
- The skin incision is preferably a curved one and over a larger area and so the suture line does not fall on the plate directly.
- Can the plate be placed on the lateral surface of tibia?
  Yes. It is covered by lateral muscles and its appearance and presence below the skin is not visible and palpable. However, the screw length has to be exact or else, the tips are palpable under the skin on the antero-medial surface (Fig. 42.1).
- *Prebending a plate:* A plate if fixed by a tension band principle, has to be prebent, as per the width of the bone. This

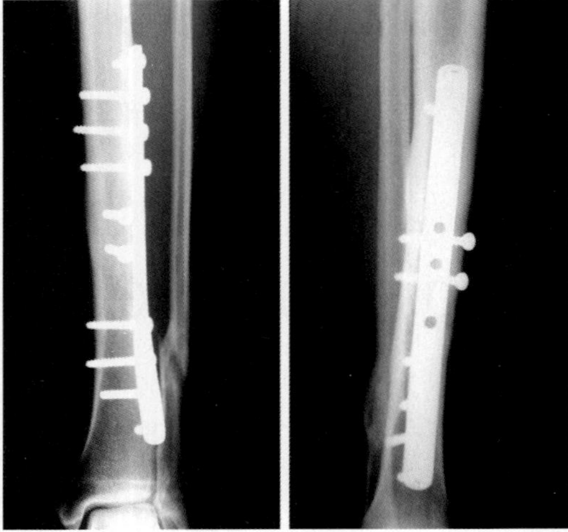

Figure 42.1 Plate on lateral tibial surface

brings the opposite bone surface under compression. Plate bending tools are important and is a necessary investment in the armamentarium, which very few clinicians enjoy. A three-point plate bender, plate bending irons and the most important plate bending press are necessary part of the equipment (Fig. 42.2).

- *Bone grafting:* In fractures with local comminution, bone loss, soft tissue loss, the local perfusion is less. As it is, a fracture of tibia in the distal/3 area is known to unite slowly. Some surgeons believe more in mechanical stability more than biological environment. I would give importance to the later and would not hesitate to add some cancellous grafts, when necessary. In a case where the grafting is likely, it is necessary to drape the donor area accordingly.
- If in preoperative planning, one feels that bone grafting is a must or on exposure of the fracture, one feels so, I find the following technique helpful. A provisional test reduction is done. Then grafts are taken from the iliac crest and *laid down in the medullary* canal and *on the opposite side of the surface*, on which the plate is to be fixed. This is important, because, once a plate is securely applied on the bone, one cannot add grafts in the intraosseous area. I think building up the bone structure this way leads to rapid and assured bone union and further consolidation. Besides, once the fracture is reduced and a plate is applied, adding grafts deep to the opposite soft tissues is rather difficult. Locking plate as an implant merely adds to the stability and not to the biological environment.
- After invention of interlocking nail, internal fixation by a closed method is possible. The soft tissue cover and hence the blood supply to adjacent area is preserved well and hence, the results improved.
- In the last decade locking plate technology and especially availability of precontoured plates, helped the surgeon in many situations. It is up to the surgeon, as to which method of fracture management, one should adopt, from a non-operative method to a locking plate method. Today, the non-operative method is unfortunately going out of vogue and I feel, it should be taken as an important method in management of fracture of tibia, especially, where it is the only injury in the patient.
- In a metaphyseal injury, plate as an implant, still holds good and scores over an intramedullary nail. The description here does not cover each aspect of plate as an implant, but presents certain typical situations, one comes across.

Case 1

One is conversant with a medial approach for fracture fixation in lower half of tibia. At the same time, it is worthwhile considering a lateral approach, where a good soft tissue cover is available. Due to the bone anatomy in this area, one needs to contour the plate over the bone. As per the level of fracture, one can precontour the plate on a bone model, prior to sterilization, so on table, it adds to the ease of procedure. The plate twisting is a difficult part of the procedure, which can be acquired with practice. May be, one may have to sacrifice a few implants. If one chooses to apply a plate on the lateral surface, one has to be careful in selection of a screw of correct length, or else, it may fall short or may become too long and irritate the medial skin (Fig. 42.1).

Case 2

Technique of application and which side to load the plate is governed by the direction of obliquity. In an oblique fracture, if possible an interfragmentary screw adds to the stability.

- In a case where the fracture of fibula is close to the mid/3 area, it may be left as such. When the fibula is fractured in lower/3 area, use of an IM nail for fibula adds to the construct. If one can pass it by a closed method, the skin and soft tissue problems are kept to a minimum.
- In a 3- or a 4- part fracture, the screw holes over the fracture area, often are left as such, as they lie on the fracture lines. In such a situation, this becomes a potentially weak area and usually it is through this area, that a mechanical failure of the plate occurs. I have designed a plate with more span (without holes) in this area, so the plate strength increases and there is more resistance to its failure.
- On the medial surface, there is very less mobile skin with subcutaneous fat tissue, which would offer a good cover for a plate. Hence, rather than a straight incision, a curved incision, with convexity and apex anteriorly is helpful.
- In the presence of local comminution, addition of few cancellous bone grafts assures early and assured fracture union. It is possible to use tibial condyle as a source of cancellous grafts. Drawing about 15 × 15 mm × 15 mm of cancellous bone from this area does not reduce donor site strength. It also reduces morbidity associated with iliac crest as a donor site. Addition of cancellous tissue to lower/3 tibia, which is more of cortical bone, helps the fracture healing (Fig. 42.3).

Case 3

In a fracture, where the fracture line is a long oblique, with additional undisplaced fractures in juxtametaphyseal area, a plate fixation is an absolute indication. It is possible to treat it non-operatively. However, some shortening is likely and there is a possibility of soft tissue interposition. The medial plate has to extend nearly till the medial malleolus and at this area, may cause some wound healing problem. Therefore to achieve a good fracture opposition, a plate of lesser thickness and with its ability to contour well on the bone is useful. A 1.3 tubular plate satisfies the requirement. Besides as per the bone shape, the plate can also be twisted, if need be.

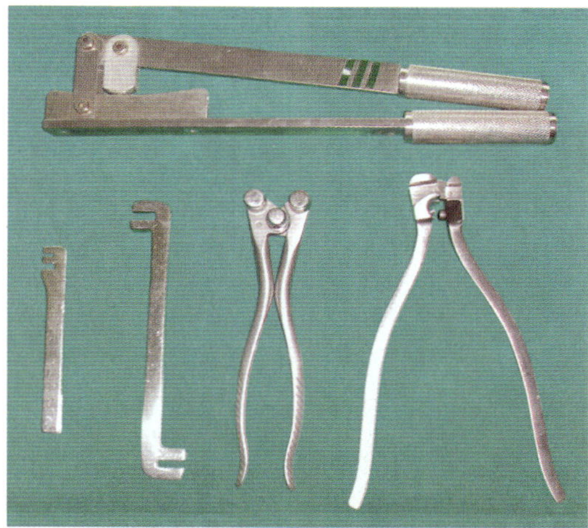

Figure 42.2 Plate bending tools

The advantage of such an implant is:

- Good fracture opposition
- Less need of frequent radiological examination
- Very less wound healing mechanical problems. But one needs to have external immobilization by a plaster cast for the necessary duration. One should look at this method as a non-operative method, with all its advantages. The plate helps to achieve fracture opposition well and prevent its displacement in the cast. It is not, at all, strong enough, to leave the limb without external plaster cast support, till the mid thigh. Needless to say, at the end of

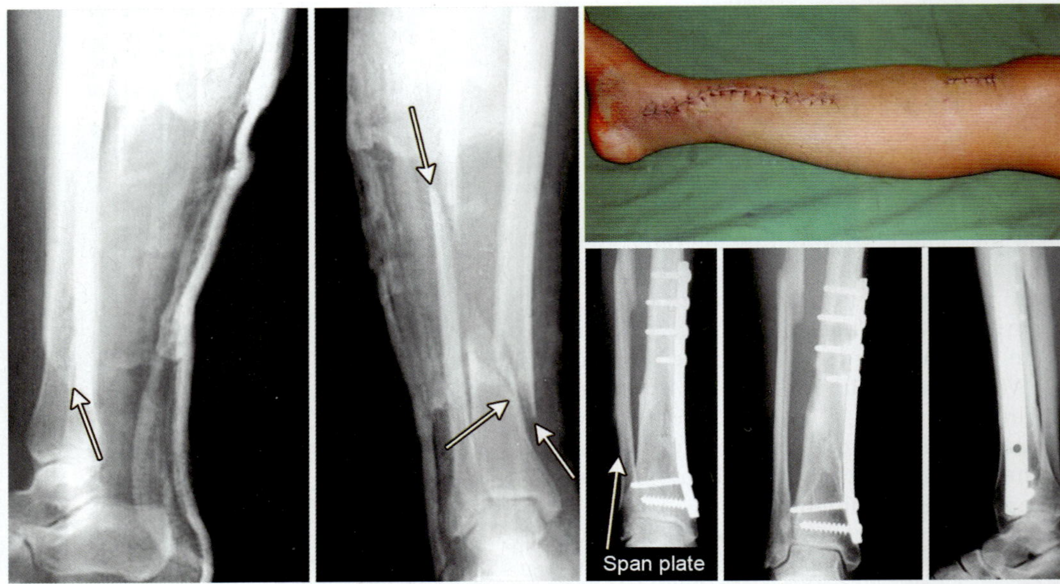

Figure 42.3 Span plate, incision and bone grafts

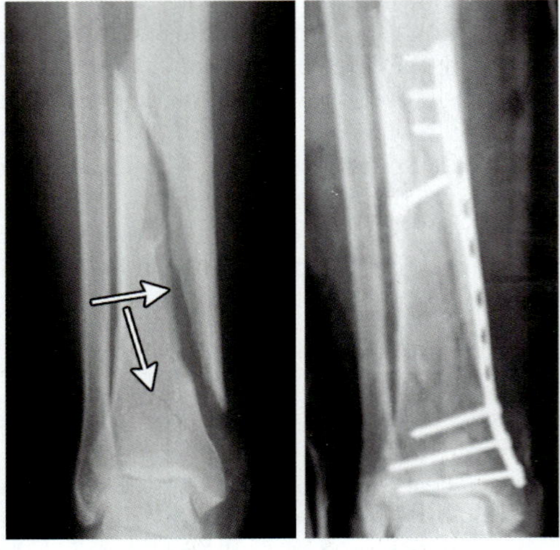

Figure 42.4 Thin plate and a cast

necessary duration, prior to cast removal, weight bearing in the cast must be practised which leads to a better consolidation.

- This method was practiced in mid 90s by a few surgeons and myself, with good result (Fig. 42.4).

Case 4

This patient had a fracture in lower/3 tibia and a fracture of fibula at the same level. A plate was applied on the lateral surface by a colleague. There was some local comminution. After fracture fixation, the X-ray taken revealed some fracture gap, may be exact anatomical reduction was not achieved and adequate interfragmentary compression was not given. The shape of the plate suggests that perhaps adequate prebending was not done, which would have brought the medial surface under compression. In a case with some local comminution, I would prefer to add some bone grafts, which can be taken from ipsilateral tibial condyle area. To achieve stability and contact opposition, I would prefer to use an outboard device: a compression clamp or an articulated tension device. Such a device adds more compression than that offered by an oval hole geometry principle of a DCP (Fig. 42.5).

Case 5

This lady has rheumatoid disease and is under treatment. She sustained a fracture of lower/3

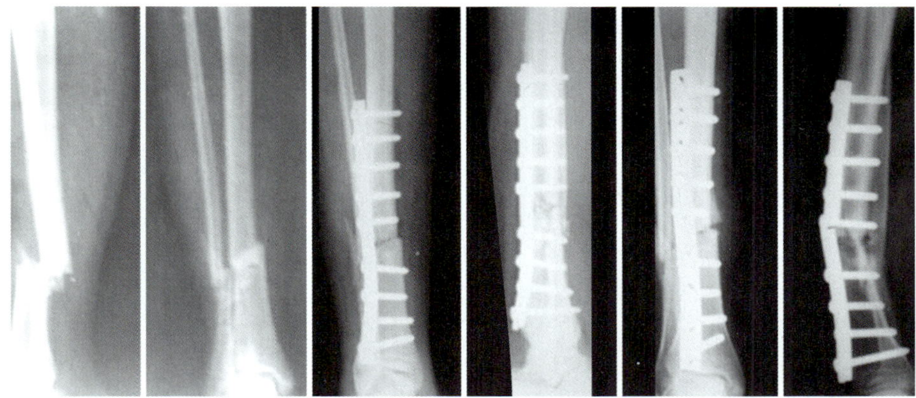

Figure 42.5 Why a plate fails

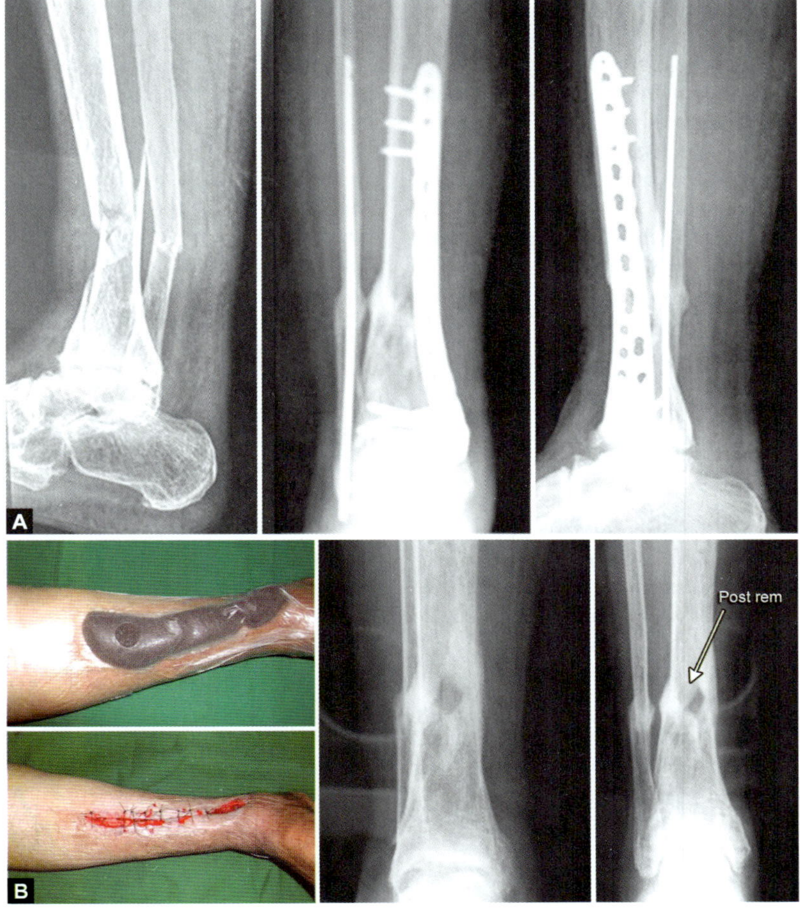

Figures 42.6A and B RA late infection and plate removal

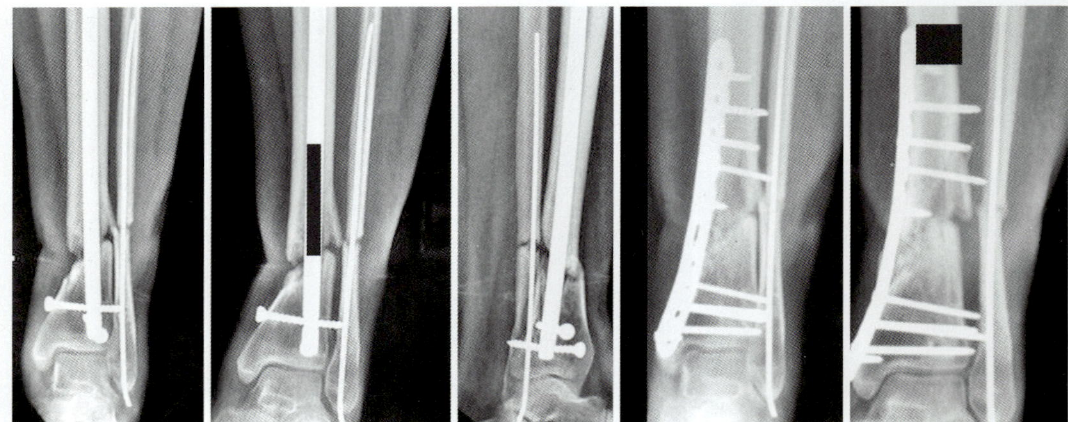

Figure 42.7 Distal tibia plate

tibia and fibula, with few additional local fragments. X-ray revealed osteoporosis. Closed fibula nailing and distal tibia locking plate fixation was done by an MIPO technique. The fracture united in due course and she resumed walking as well.

A year and a half after union, she developed local cellulitis, which was controlled with necessary treatment. A late infection had occurred and the plate and fibula nail was removed at appropriate time. To offer an early and assured wound healing, a VAC suction dressing was applied, which helped for a good wound healing (Figs 42.6A and B).

Case 6

This lady had a grade II open fracture of distal end of tibia, with a bone loss and fracture of fibula in the lower/4th area. There was nearly a 3/4th circumferential wound. Wound excision, lavage, followed by a closed fibula nail and distal tibia interlock nail was done. She was advised to undergo elective bone grafting. The advice was not followed by the patient and the distal bolts started bending. The fracture did not unite. It was revised and a locking plate with bone grafting was done and it united in due course of time.

MESSAGE

In a junctional fracture, with bone loss, it is preferable to carry out an IM nailing, followed by elective bone grafting. However, following a given advice is up to the patient. If the advice is not followed, a revision surgery and change of implant to a stable fixation mode by an LCP would lead to fracture union (Fig. 42.7).

CHAPTER

43

Tibia Lower MIPO Plate

Availability of 'C' arm has made an minimally invasive plate osteosynthesis (MIPO) technique possible and safe. This method to keep the soft tissues intact and undisturbed over the fracture area, has helped to preserve the blood supply to local fragments. Thus while internal stabilization with a plate is done, the exposure is less and often the union is rapid and assured.

The span of the plate over the fracture area is longer, where no screws are inserted. This leads to an elastic module and one observes that when the plate is later removed, the stress shielding is much less, than a case, where nearly all the screw holes are used (Fig. 43.1).

Similar procedure can be done in upper/3 area (Fig. 43.2).

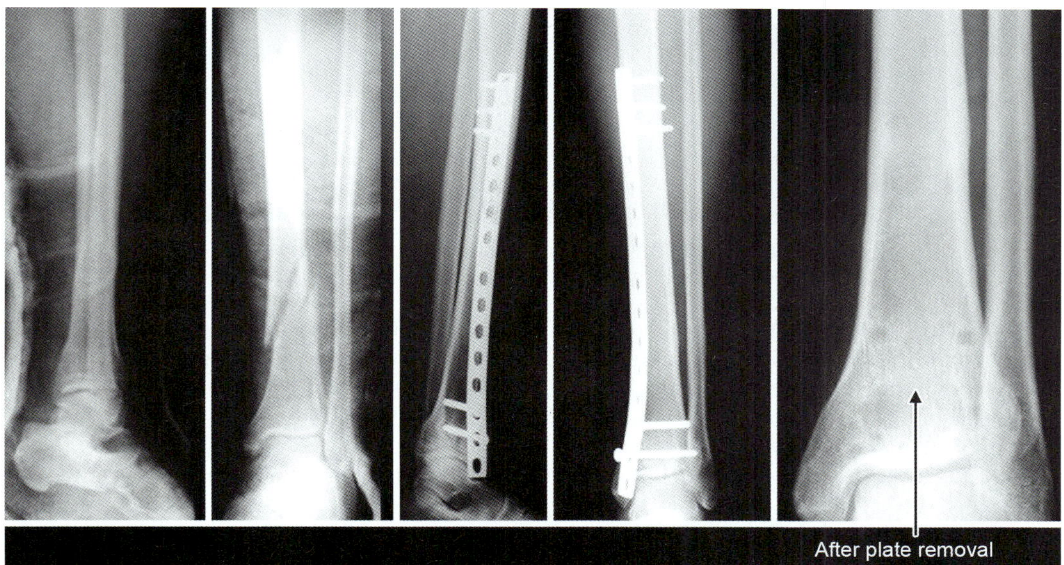

Figure 43.1 MIPO in lower tibia less stress shielding

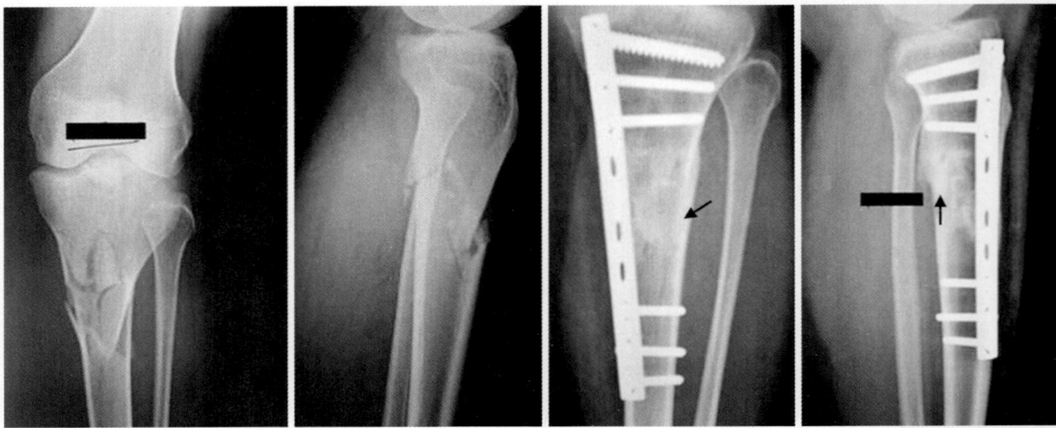

Figure 43.2 MIPO in upper/3 tibia

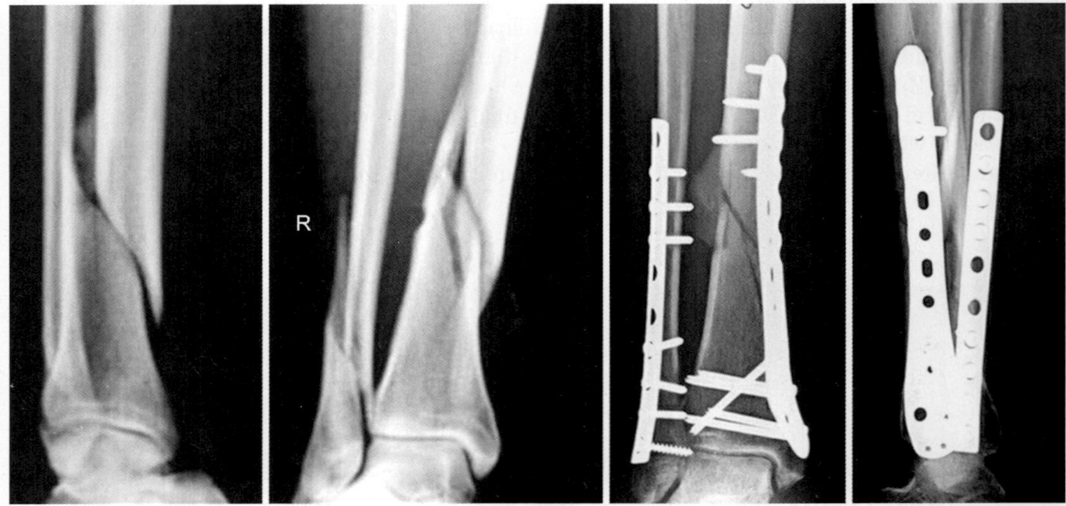

Figure 43.3 MIPO in lower 4 spiral FR tibia and fibula

A spiral fracture in lower/3 level of both tibia and fibula: If the fibula fracture is quite distal, one needs to stabilize it with a plate. Having done so, usually the tibia fracture fragments fall back in place and the reduction is satisfactory, so an MIPO technique is successful (Fig. 43.3).

It is observed that in an oblique fracture, the fracture ends pierce the soft tissue envelope and a good reduction is not obtained. In such a situation, it is necessary to carry out an open reduction, to remove the soft tissue intervention and achieve a good contact opposition. Fracture geometry permitting, an interfragmentary screw enhances the stability also.

Fracture of the lower/4 of the fibula needs stabilization, to restore the mortise and add complementary support to the tibia as well. In a long oblique fracture, an antiglide plate fixation is a better choice. This fixation of the fibula needs to be done first and then tibia is fixed. To carry out plate fixation in both the bones in distal part of the leg needs to be carefully executed. The limb circumference is small and the soft tissues around find it difficult to accommodate the tissue edema, following surgery.

HOW WOULD I PLAN?

- On arrival, keeping the leg hanging from the edge of a bed, aligns the bone well. A padded crepe support and a POP slab is applied. The limb needs to be well elevated and is the important thing to carry out.
- One should wait adequately, till the local reaction is less and wrinkle sign has appeared.
- Under anesthesia, I would reduce the fracture and assess if an MIPO technique would be successful. If so, I would proceed with fibula plate fixation, which in a long oblique fracture confers more stability than an IM nail.
- An important advantage of fibula nail is, often, it is a closed procedure and hence surgical tissue reaction is very less.
- For fibula, both the options: IM nail and a plate be kept ready.
- In exceptional situation, more so as in a diabetic patient, I would not hesitate to carry out the internal fixation of both the bones in two stages, the fibula first and tibia in the second stage, after 4 to 6 days. Though, this increases the hospital stay, means two procedure, added cost, etc. it confers safety to the procedure and prevents repeat procedures, which are presented elsewhere. Unless one has come across a complication, because of not following staged procedure, one may not realize the magnitude of the problem, one has to encounter (Fig. 43.4).

A lady past 65 years having insulin dependent diabetes, sustained a fracture of lower/4 tibia and fibula. The bones were fragile. Fibula was stabilized with a closed nail fixation. The tibia morphology was such that an IFS would enhance the stability. Hence, rather than a MIPO technique, ORIF was carried out. Being elderly, obese, insulin dependent person, one desires assured bone union at the earliest. For her, use of a walker, without putting any load on the injured leg was difficult. Hence, iliac bone grafting was preplanned and explained to her.

Steps

- Closed fibula nailing carried out.
- The tibia fracture was exposed and the fracture morphology and bone quality assessed and a provisional reduction done with traction to the foot.
- Grafts taken from the iliac crest. (It is also possible to take grafts from the ipsilateral tibial condyle, as the quantity required is

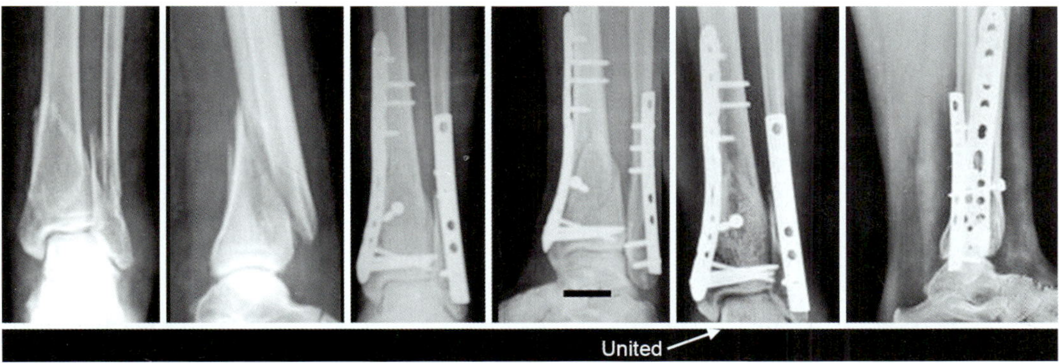

Figure 43.4 ORIF for both tibia and fibula in lower 4

small) and lay in the fracture area. Were laid in the fracture site.

- Locking plate was applied medially. Some local adjustment of plate position was made within permissible limit, so that IFS could be placed across the fracture site.
- Post-operative closed suction drain, padded crepe support and a below knee posterior POP slab was applied, to offer pain relief and to prevent equinus deformity, which is known to occur and is then difficult to correct.
- Depending upon the quality of bone and screw hold, compliance by the patient, physical agility and capacity to carry out non-weight bearing mobilization, either a below or above knee plaster support needs to be given. This is important, because, in almost all the cases, while rising from a chair or sitting down, some weight does pass through the leg. Besides, to confer elasticity to the assembly, often only few screws are inserted on either side of the fracture and this care and protection is needed (Fig. 43.5).

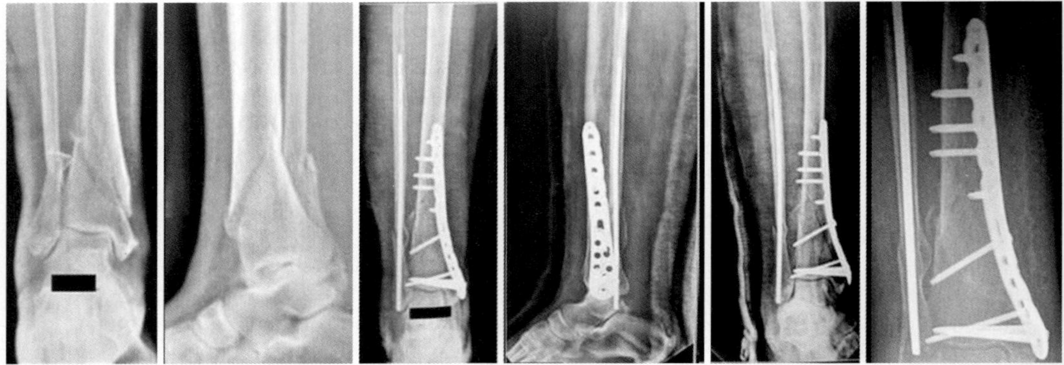

Figure 43.5 Diabetes: Bone grafts and IFS

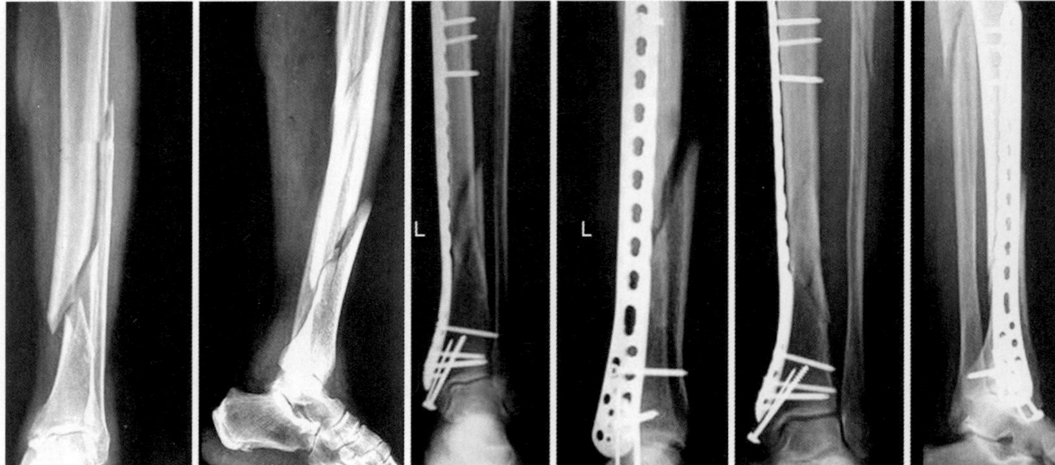

Figure 43.6 MIPO plate

MIPO TECHNIQUE: MUST OBTAIN A GOOD REDUCTION!

Case 1

This lady of 75 yrs. with diabetes, sustained a 3 part fracture of the tibia. An MIPO technique, using a 'C' arm was carried out. Whatever views in 'C' arm, one could take on the table, were taken. However, postoperative X-ray revealed inadequate reduction in only one view. The surgeon thought, being a closed method, blood supply is well maintained and the fracture would unite. Did not so happen. At the end of three months, no bone union was observed and hence decortication and bone grafting was carried out. The fracture united in further three months.

Elasticity conferred to the plate by keeping holes near the fracture ends unoccupied, preservation of blood supply by an MIPO technique is no substitute for a good reduction. It is good reduction and fracture opposition which lead to a sound bone union (Figs 43.6 and 43.7).

Case 2

A young man sustained a three-part fracture of lower/3 of tibia and fibula. A colleague carried out an MIPO plate fixation. At the end of 3 months, the fracture line persisted, as seen in figure 43.8. He reported for further treatment to us. A CT scan was performed for confirmation and documentation, which also revealed persistent fracture gap and ununited fracture. Hence a bone grafting procedure was carried out and in the next three months, the bone consolidated well (Figs 43.8 and 43.9).

Case 3

This person with diabetes sustained a 3- or 4-part fracture of lower/4 of tibia and fibula. (The day 1 X-ray film was not available for me to see). At another hospital, an MIPO technique was used to carry out fixation of tibia. The fibula was also fixed with a plate. As seen in the follow up X-ray film, the plate was not closely in contact with the surface of tibia. The fracture did not unite and he could not bear weight on the limb. There was intermittent discharge from the wound and sinuses developed. As per history, he was advised to take antibiotics a few times, when the discharge would reduce, only to appear after a few weeks.

When first seen approximately six months from the first surgery, for further management, plate was visible through the sinuses. The plate

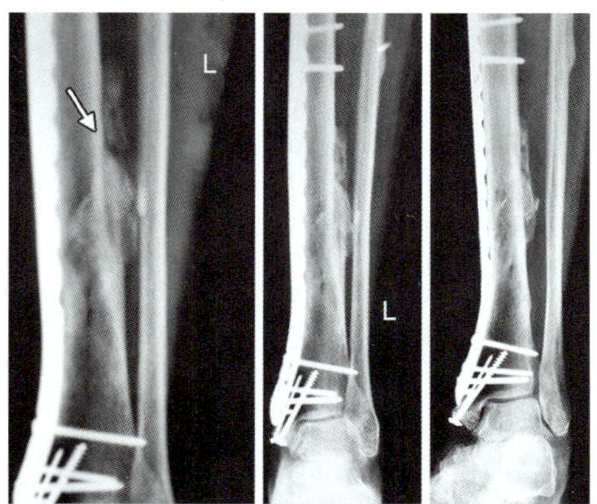

Figure 43.7 MIPO plate

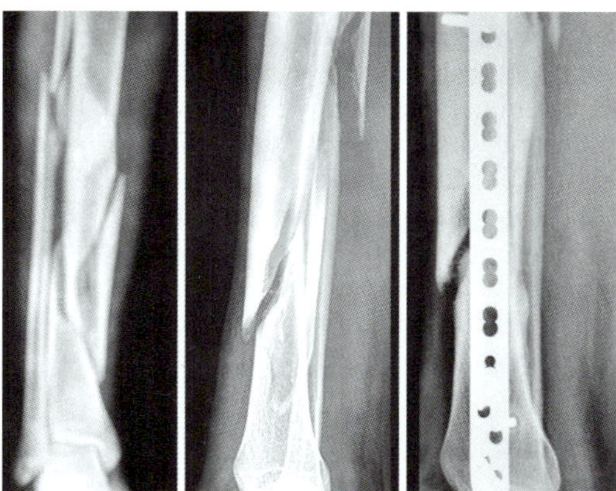

Figure 43.8 MIPO problem

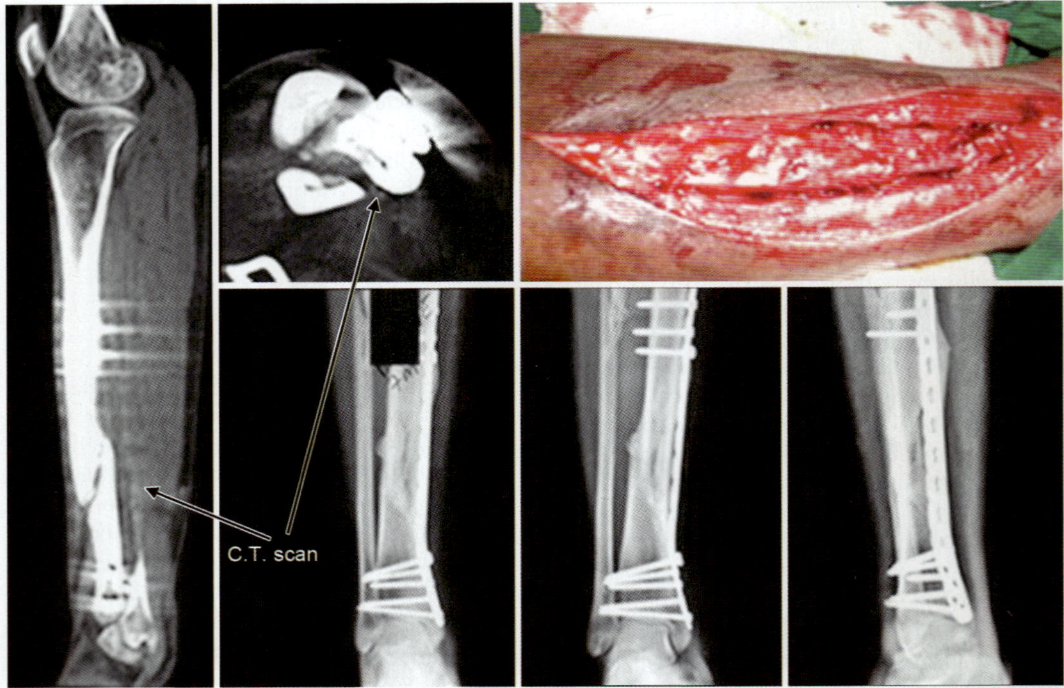

Figure 43.9 MIPO problem

was, therefore, removed and a VAC suction dressing was done. The culture did not reveal any organisms. However, as seen in the picture, presence of local tissue appearance would not permit bone grafting. A long leg cast was applied and window dressing was carried out. Unfortunately, the fracture did not unite. Then a colleague was involved to carry out application of a ring fixator. He removed the fibula plate and bone transport was done. However, the recalcitrant fracture did not unite, though the regenerate healed well.

The fracture continues to be ununited (Figs 43.10 to 43.12).

Message

- In a long oblique fracture line, one needs to be careful, to confirm on table that the fracture is well reduced. If necessary, open reduction needs to be carried out.
- If the local fracture morphology permits, an inter-fragmentary screw fixation should be carried out. The reduction needs to be maintained well with a self-centering forceps, while the IFS is inserted.
- In presence of comminution, the bone voids need to be filled with bone grafts, prior to the reduction and application of the plate.
- A locking plate is described as an internal fixator and that mechanically its close contact opposition and placement close to the bone is not necessary. However, one must remember that biologically, for continued soft tissue cover (at least in a subcutaneous bone like tibia), it is necessary to keep it in close contact with the bone, so that a safe and good soft tissue cover is obtained.

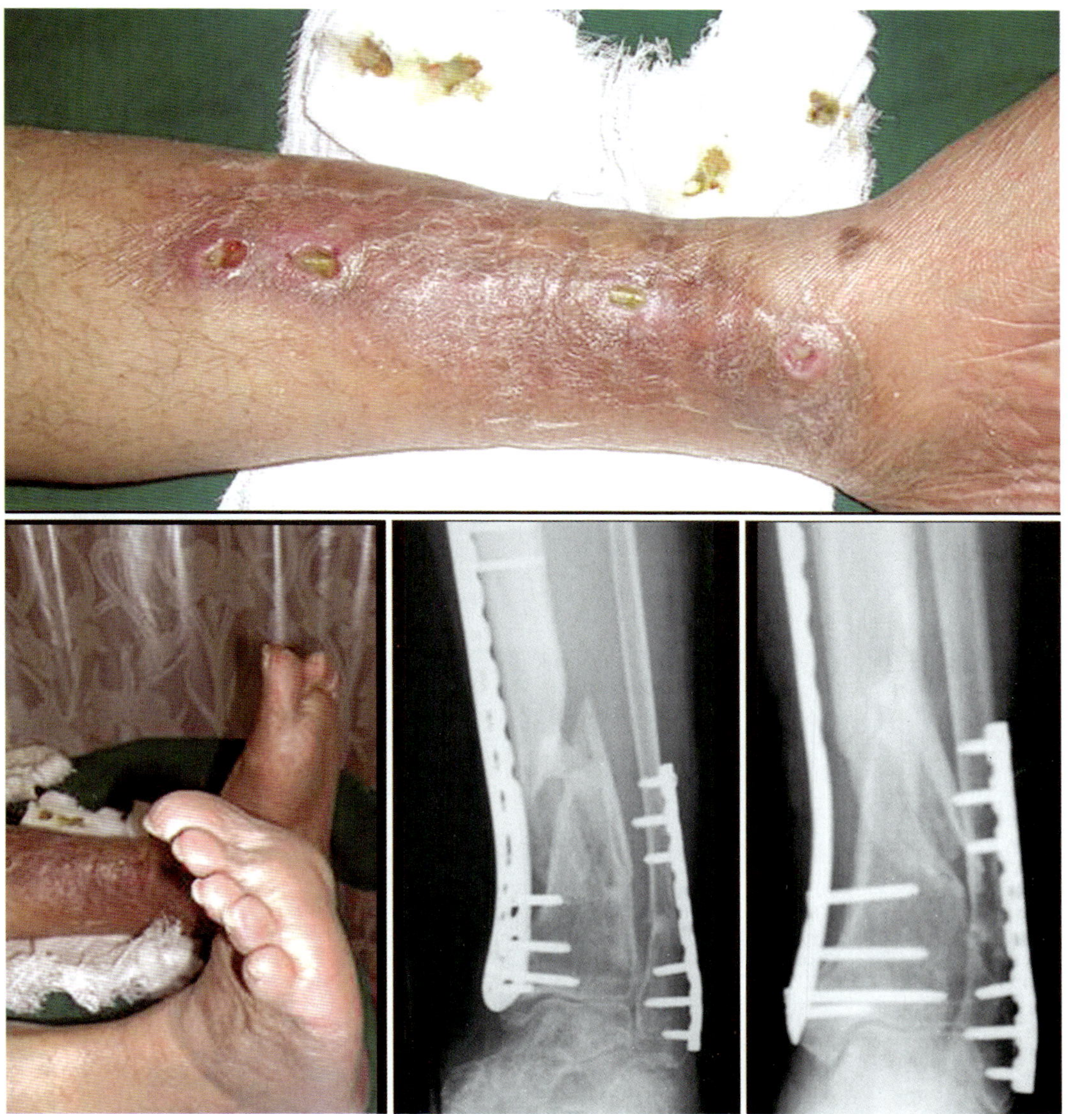

Figure 43.10 MIPO problem

LONG SEGMENT OF TIBIA WITH COMMINUTION

This young man had a comminuted fracture extending from lower/3 area to the middle of the tibia. A successful MIPO locking plate fixation was carried out and a cast immobilization carried out. He was informed that at the end of six to eight weeks, an elective bone grafting would be needed to be carried out, for assured bone union. He moved to his home town and did not come for follow up. He was followed up and called for follow up. Fresh X-ray indicated persistence of fracture

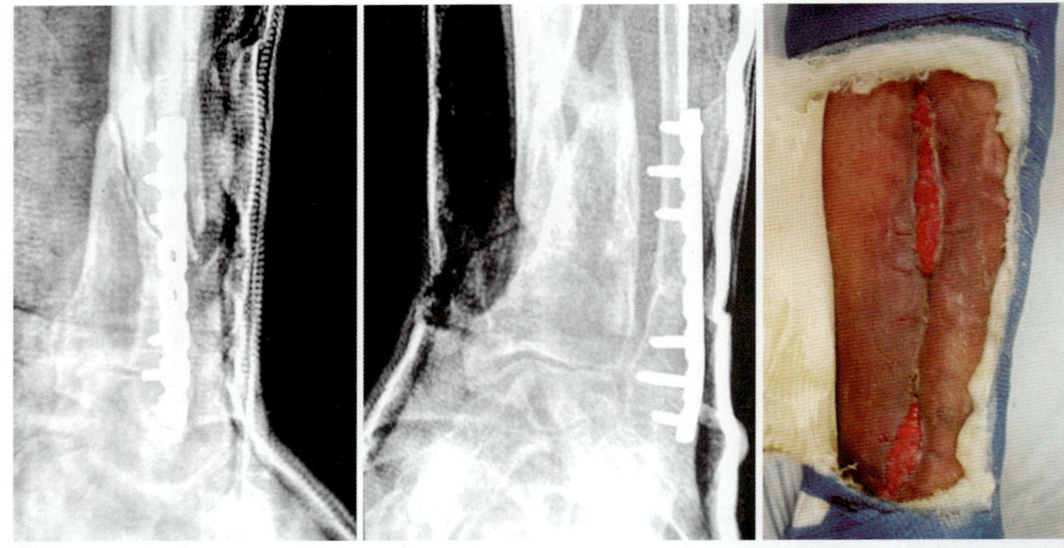

Figure 43.11 MIPO problem

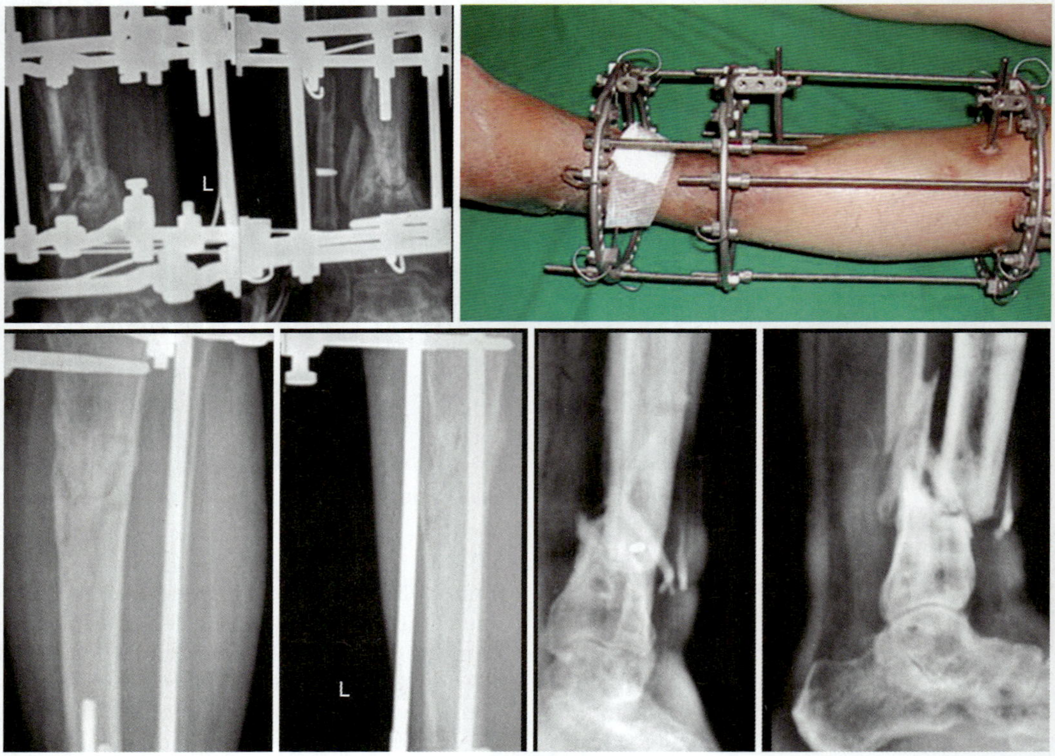

Figure 43.12 MIPO problem

line in one segment and was confirmed by CT scan and for documentation. He was advised bone grafting, but has not made up his mind yet.

In such a situation, unless the bone unites well in expected duration, there is a possibility of implant failure, due to cyclical loading. It is important that the bone unites before this calamity. At the present stage, gentle decortication and bone grafting should result in union of the fracture. If now, should the plate gives way, then the procedure required would be of much more magnitude than only bone grafting. This fact, quite often the patient does not realize, in spite of discussion in detail (Fig. 43.13).

Lessons Learnt

- For tibia, a transverse fracture or a fracture with local comminution, an MIPO technique achieves good alignment, in all views.
- In an oblique, especially a long oblique fracture, good contact opposition by a closed method is difficult. Hence an open reduction with an IFS is necessary.
- Complementary bone grafts are laid down in the marrow cavity, prior to reduction and plate application. The total period of fracture union after such an open reduction is not much longer than an MIPO method, but is more likely to lead to an assured union, without a need of a subsequent surgery.
- In lower/3rd or lower 4th fracture of fibula, in a transverse fracture, a closed fibula nailing is often successful and there is no open surgical wound on it. Hence post-operative tissue edema and tissue reaction is less than when an open fibula fixation is done.
- In an oblique fracture of fibula in lower 4th area, one needs to stabilize it with a 1/3rd tubular plate to restore and stabilize the ankle mortise. This also gives a complementary stability to the tibia. Thus, when both the bones need to be stabilized with a plate, one should wait till the wrinkle sign appears.
- Internal fixation of both the fibula and the tibia, can be considered in two stages, in long-term interest of the wound and the bone healing, as well. Though, it means two procedures in the same stay, in the broad perspective, the entire procedure is of

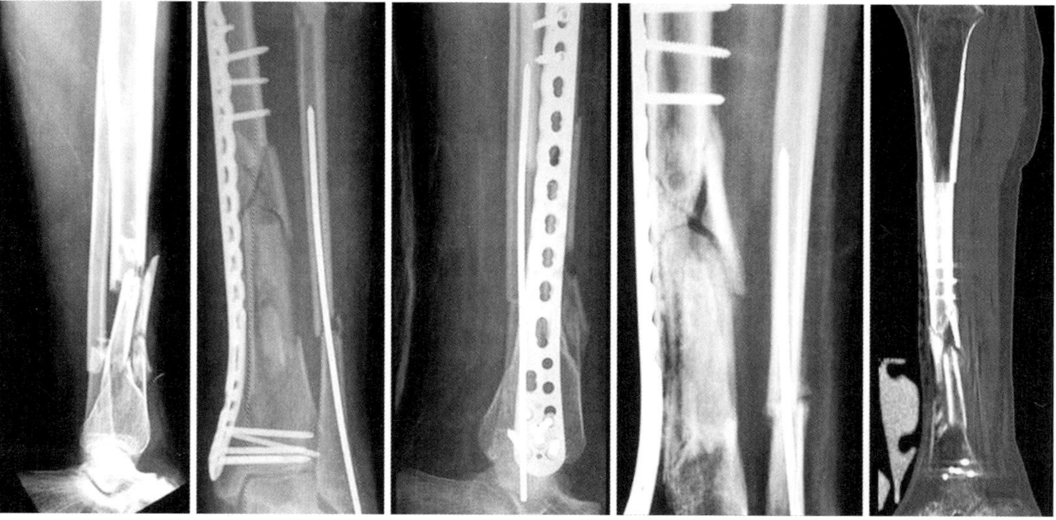

Figure 43.13 MIPO plate may need a staged and planned bone graft

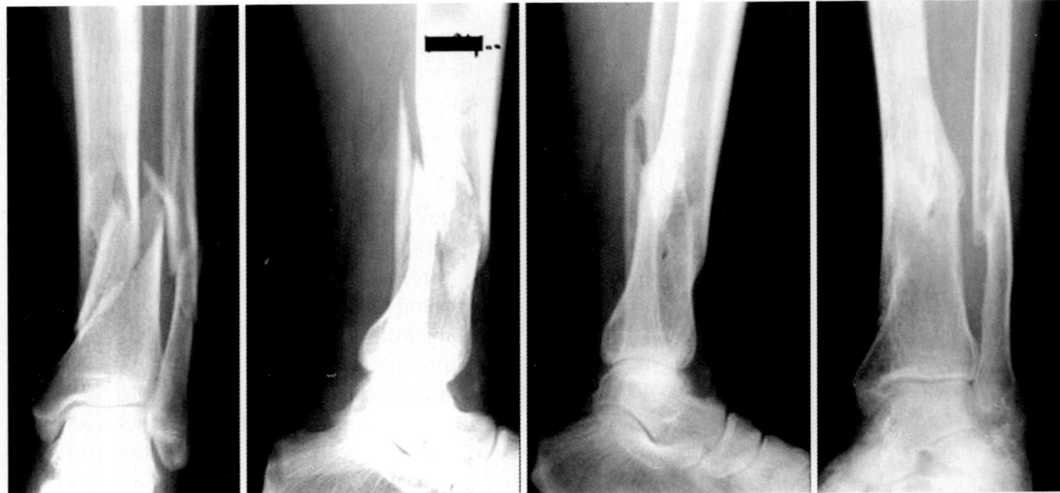

Figure 43.14 Non-operative method

lesser magnitude than having to revise the procedure all over again.

Having seen the problems one may face with the operative method, it is also necessary to look back and understand that a non-operative method also leads to a good outcome. One should be well-versed with this non-operative method as well, which is fast going out of vogue. Even if it leads to a delayed union, decortication and bone grafting is a safe option and the wound healing and fracture union occurs in time (Fig. 43.14).

CHAPTER

44

Ankle Injuries

ANKLE INJURIES: INTRODUCTION

Various classifications are available for ankle injuries. However, here the management is described as per the commonly seen injuries.

In management of any ankle injury, prior to ordering an X-ray or if it is already taken, prior to seeing the film, a clinical examination is necessary (Fig. 44.1)!

Only after a clinical examination, one can judge a case and advise a stress view, if it is not so taken. Having confirmed and documented such a case, one needs to immobilize the ankle for necessary duration, which may be more than that required for a fracture of lateral malleolus alone, without any ligament injury and without subluxation.

A fracture of lateral malleolus can be in the lower end, without injury to the joint as such. A fracture higher up is often associated with lateral dislocation of the ankle and may be associated with a fracture of the posterior malleolus. Hence, such injuries are described together, in respective chapters.

MANAGEMENT IN GENERAL

Whenever, there is an injury with displacement, one should carry out immediate closed reduction and add a padded crepe bandage.

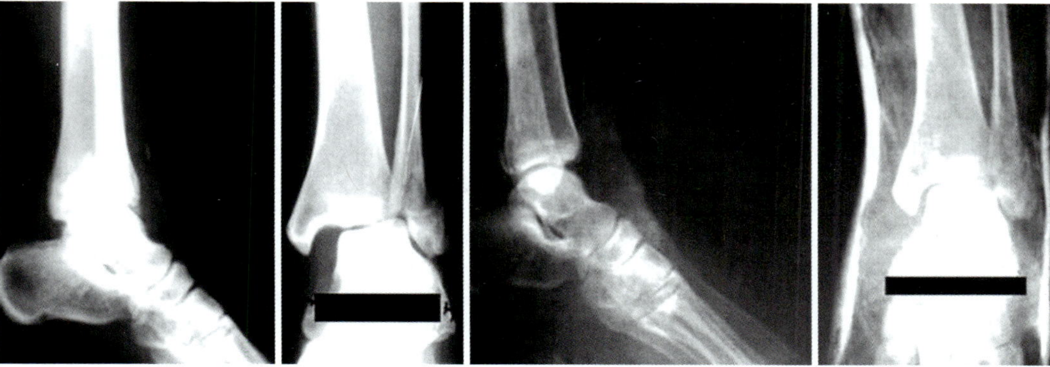

Figure 44.1 Lateral ankle subluxation

On this, a posterior plaster slab is added. Adequate elevation of the injured limb must be carried out, on specially manufactured high Bohler frame. Today, with commonly carried out internal fixation of hip fractures, a non-operative method with skeletal traction is disappearing rapidly. Hence, I have designed flat Bohler frame, without the top pulleys, etc. The frames should be so designed to have different heights and different lengths for the thigh section, so one can choose a frame, as per the length of the femur. Such a well-designed frame is useful during both pre- and post-operative patient care.

If the fracture is painful or is associated with a dislocation of the tibio-talar joint, one should carry out the reduction under anesthesia. It spares the patient of unnecessary pain, achieves a good reduction and restoration of alignment of the tibio-talar joint and permits correct application of the padded crepe bandage and the custom-made POP slab.

Often in a road side ankle injury, the skin is contaminated with dust and dirt. Under anesthesia, one can very neatly clean the skin and the limb in general, so on the day of surgery, the patient enters the theater with a clean limb. Besides, by thorough cleaning, the abrasions are less likely to get infected.

This procedure of closed reduction and addition of padded crepe and a posterior slab, followed by good elevation, keeps the tissue edema and likelihood of any blister formation, to a minimum. This pre-operative period is thus made pain free and is comfortable for the patient. In certain situations, it permits the clinician to think and plan the procedure, as well and if required, a CT scan examination is done. If this step is not carried out, blisters may appear, the definitive procedure is delayed and the result may be compromised.

Thus, after such a first aid, when one operates a few days after the injury, the tissue edema is less and tissue planes are easy to obtain and the reduction too is easy. In spite of this staged procedure, I prefer to open the slab and the crepe on the operation table, prior to the anesthesia, to confirm that the ankle is fit to be operated. On the other hand, if one leaves the ankle as such, without a systematic reduction under anesthesia, the tissue edema and perhaps blisters are observed on table. Exposure of the ankle and reduction, etc. is annoying.

Associated diabetes needs special attention and management. I would prefer to control the blood sugar with insulin, may be a small dose even. This helps to have a better wound and bone healing. In diabetes the pedal pulses may be palpable, but the foot micro-circulation is compromised. This leads to slow tissue healing. In presence of diabetes, I would choose to wait for at least four to five days after the initial closed reduction. If one operates when the initial tissue reaction has subsided, the outcome is far superior and chances of having a complication are much less. This waiting period is safe and of much less duration, should any complication develop.

The thick skin flaps must be raised carefully from the deep fascia which makes the closure neat and without undue tissue tension. In presence of edema, one should suture the skin with some gap left in between the epidermis, which in due course reduces well, leading to a cosmetically good scar. If this is not observed, often the wound gives way and the local tissue loss is quite some, requiring at times, a rotation flap, etc.

- Some groups recommend no external support after an internal fixation and encourage active ankle mobilization. I feel, it is important to add a crepe support and have a plaster immobilization after a surgery. Howsoever, one may advise not to bear weight on the affected ankle, still while rising from a chair, sitting on a chair, in the bathroom, while using a wash basin, certainly some weight does pass through the ankle. The fracture fragments are quite small and the load of the body is quite some and may lead to disruption of the fixation. I, therefore, prefer to have a posterior slab immediately after surgery and change to a cast after suture removal, for necessary duration. Only a crepe bandage in postoperative period, leads to a plantar flexion deformity, which is uncomfortable and later on difficult to correct as well.

Which material? POP or synthetic?

- Quite often in clinical practice, one needs to consider cost and efficacy of any treatment plan. For a first aid, a slab made from POP material is adequate, which, one needs to change after internal fixation. After internal fixation, I prefer to have eight to ten layers of a POP slab and additional roll of synthetic material. After two weeks of this method of immobilization, one removes the sutures and a new cast is given. For such a cast I prefer initial 50% of the cast with POP material and then additional synthetic rolls. The initial part of the cast with POP material permits to have a well-moulded cast and takes the shape of the limb better. The later part of the cast, a synthetic material should be used for additional strength. Such a hybrid cast is quite comfortable and cost effective. After six to eight weeks of such an immobilization, one should change the cast to a similar cast. However, if the cast is well-maintained and strong enough, one can advise to bear weight on the same cast.
- At the end of necessary duration of immobilization, I prefer to start partial weight bearing on the cast with an overshoe. This restores the reflexes of weight bearing. Within two weeks, the patient is able to bear weight on the cast. Now, when one removes the cast, it is interesting to see, how efficiently he can do some weight bearing! If this weight bearing on the cast is not done and if the cast is removed, then for few weeks, the person is unable to bear weight on the unprotected foot. I would, therefore, invest this time in weight bearing or so called walking cast, rather than trying to bear weight on an unsupported foot with only a crepe bandage, which is painful for the patient.
- At appropriate time the cast is removed. Whenever a lower limb cast is removed, any foot or ankle injury does require a crepe bandage support to prevent reactionary tissue edema. In addition, it is necessary to keep the limb elevated to prevent edema for a few days. All these precautions lead to a timely and uneventful recovery and prevent reflex sympathetic dystrophy as well.
- Good skin care and proper ankle mobilization and muscle strengthening exercises, especially tiptoe exercise (heel raising) helps restoration of a good foot and ankle function. One should compare the calf circumference with the unaffected side and convince the patient, the need of exercises, to restore the calf volume.
- It is also important to know, what to do and what to avoid. A young non-diabetic adult sustained an open fracture dislocation of an ankle in a peripheral place. A visiting surgeon cleaned the wound and applied an external fixator to the ankle. Both the medial malleolus and the fibula were left unreduced and were not fixed internally. At a later date fibula was fixed with a plate and medial malleolus with a TBW and plaster immobilization was carried out. There was lingering infection and painful ankle. The next surgeon removed all the implants, which (as expected) did not solve the problem and hence presented for opinion. As can be seen in the photo, the only option now is ankle arthrodesis (Fig. 44.2).

COULD THIS HAVE BEEN AVOIDED?

What Could Be an Alternative for the Day 1?

In a bimalleolar or a trimalleolar open fracture dislocation, the open wound is on the medial side. This needs to be handled on day one only.

- Thorough wound lavage for the medial malleolus wound is given, dirt, foreign material, if any, is removed. If the person was wearing a sock and a shoe, then usually the amount of dirt and dust is less.
- The fibula needs to be reduced. If one can achieve a closed reduction in such a transverse fracture, closed IM nailing

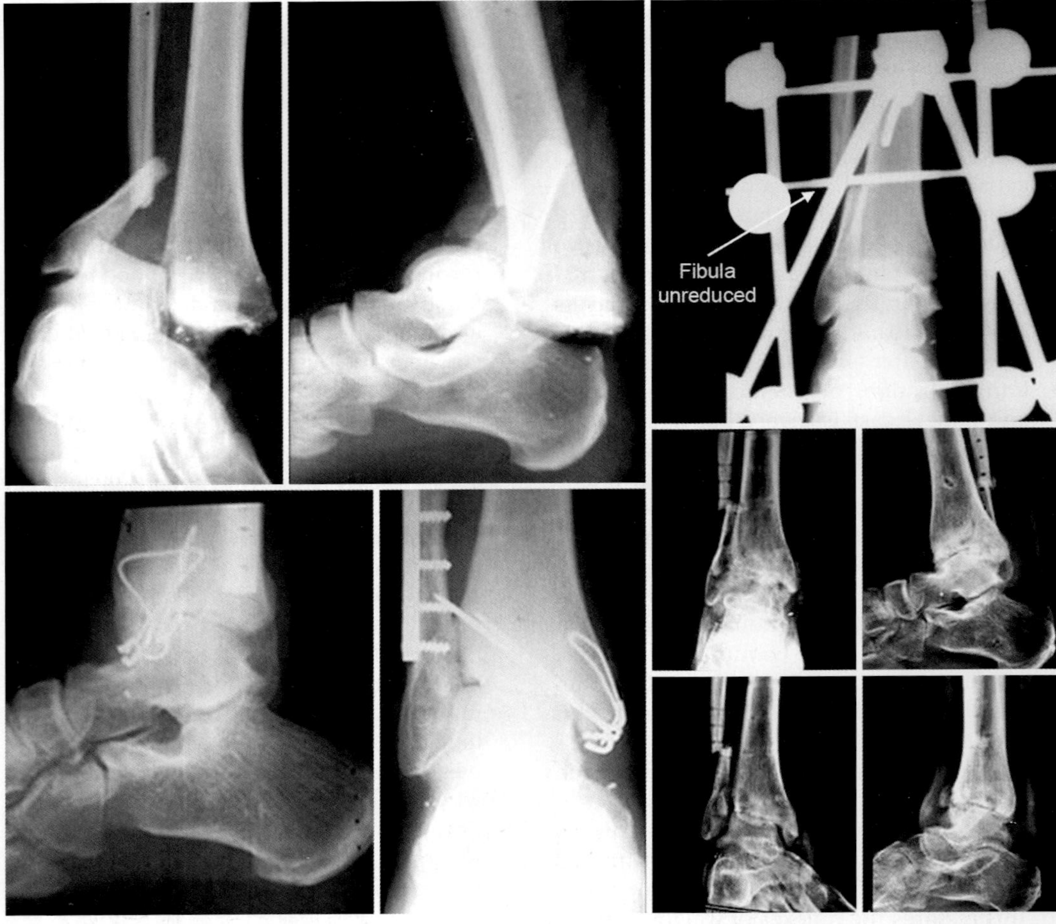

Figure 44.2 External fixation in an open ankle fracture dislocation

is possible. The fracture is above the syndesmosis and an IM nail does offer good stability to the mortise. If closed reduction is not successful, open reduction is done. It is possible to localize the fracture and through a necessary extent of exposure, the fracture ends are visualized. With a narrow awl, the bone ends are levered out and are aligned. This technique does not need use of bone holding/reduction forceps and the soft tissues are well preserved. The deep fascia and the skin are opposed loosely. It is also possible to leave the wound open and close at a later date, when collection, if any, has drained away. This two-stage closure assured reduced chances of infection in such an open injury.

- The medial malleolus may be given another wash. The inverted periosteal ends are everted and fracture surface cleared well. One should carry out minimum dissection, exposure in such an open injury. My preference is to use two 4 mm shaft screws with 7 mm washers, which offer good angular, as well as rotational stability to the fragment. Details are in respective chapter.

The wound is loosely opposed at the ends and the central area may be temporarily left open, as per local condition. Often, there are few abrasions and soft tissue contusion around the medial side of the ankle. The extent of crushing and soft tissue injury may not be clear on day 1.

- Both the wounds are dressed, while padded crepe and a plaster support completes the procedure. In a diabetic patient, one needs to be extra careful in lavage, wound excision and wound opposition, without tension.

THE OUTCOME

Such a primary internal fixation offers restoration of the ankle anatomy and a good soft tissue envelope is offered. Since the wounds are sutured without tension or partly left open, chances of infection are less.

If needed, a secondary skin grafting is possible.

Application of only an external fixator, without internal fixation of the columns, needs a definitive second procedure. During this interval, the soft tissues adhere to nearby osseous tissues and need to be elevated again. This procedure of approaching through the medial open or a sutured wound increases a chance of infection. As against this, when it is done on the day 1, when the tissue planes are supple and mobile, the procedure is easier and the wound heals kindly.

ANKLE FRACTURE MEDIAL MALLEOLUS FIXATION

In a fracture of medial malleolus alone or in a bimalleolar fracture quite often, the fracture is visible, *only in an oblique view*. Hence, this view must be taken in every ankle injury (Fig. 44.3).

REDUCTION TECHNIQUE AND WHICH IMPLANT?

After formal reduction of medial malleolus, one needs to hold the reduction, till the screw fixation is complete. A pointed reduction

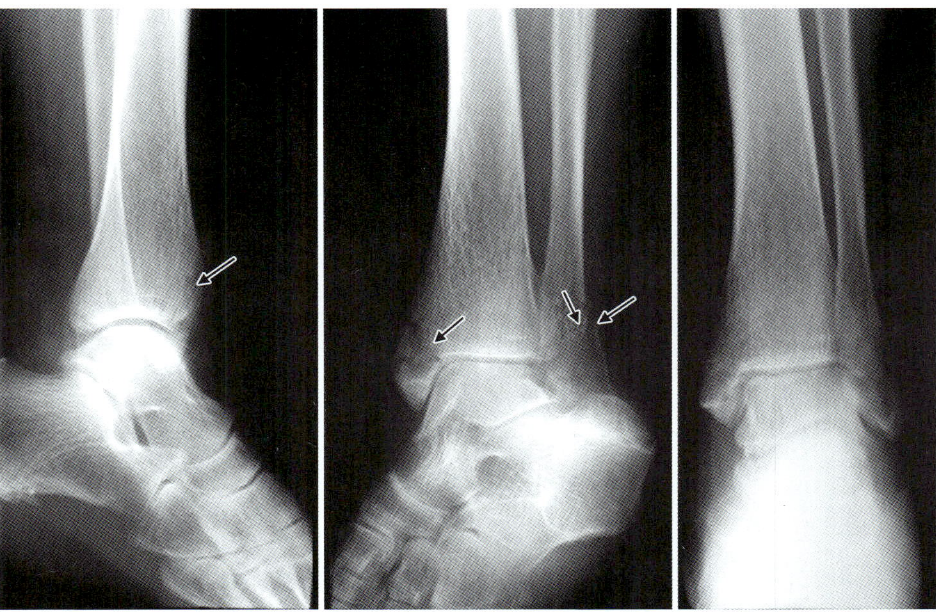

Figure 44.3 Oblique view

forceps or a towel clip is used. One point is anchored at the tip of medial malleolus and the other pointed tip has to have a purchase in the tibia shaft. The tip of the forceps cannot have a purchase on the tibial smooth surface. Hence, prior to reduction, a drill hole is made with a 2.5 mm drill bit, 2 cm proximal to the fracture line in appropriate axis. This hole accepts one pointed tip of the reduction forceps securely, while the other tip catches the tip of the medial malleolus well.

I prefer 2 × 4 mm shaft screws (partially threaded) with a 7 mm washer, to one malleolar screw. These two screws stabilize the fracture better than a single malleolar screw, as rotary stability is more. The height of a 4 mm screw head being smaller than that of malleolar screw, after reconditioning of the soft tissues, the screw head is less palpable under the skin, compared to head of a malleolar screw.

Large Fragment

After reduction of the malleolus, a 1.8 mm K-wire is passed in the center of medial malleolus for provisional stability. Then a 4 mm shaft screw with a small washer is fixed, anterior to the K-wire and another 4 mm screw with a washer is fixed, posterior to the K-wire (Fig. 44.4).

Small Fragment

First a 1.8 mm K-wire is passed at such a place that adequate area is available on the medial malleolus, to insert an additional 4 mm screw with a small washer. In fact, the wire is placed at the final position only, leaving adequate room for a 4 mm screw. After the insertion of the K-wire, a 4 mm shaft screw with a small 7 mm washer is driven in at appropriate level and direction, as per the fracture morphology. Then, the K-wire is first bent acutely and then cut. The K-wire may need some rotation and further bending, so that the wire tip is made to lie in the screw recess.

Alternatively, the wire is bent, cut and gently tapped, so it penetrates the adjacent bone and remains in place.

If a K-wire is first cut, say, 8 mm from the bone surface, then one tries to bend, that short wire segment is difficult to bend. Hence the K-wire should be bent first and then cut (Fig. 44.5).

Still Small Fragment

If the size of the medial malleolus is quite small, only one 4 mm screw with a washer can be inserted (Fig. 44.6).

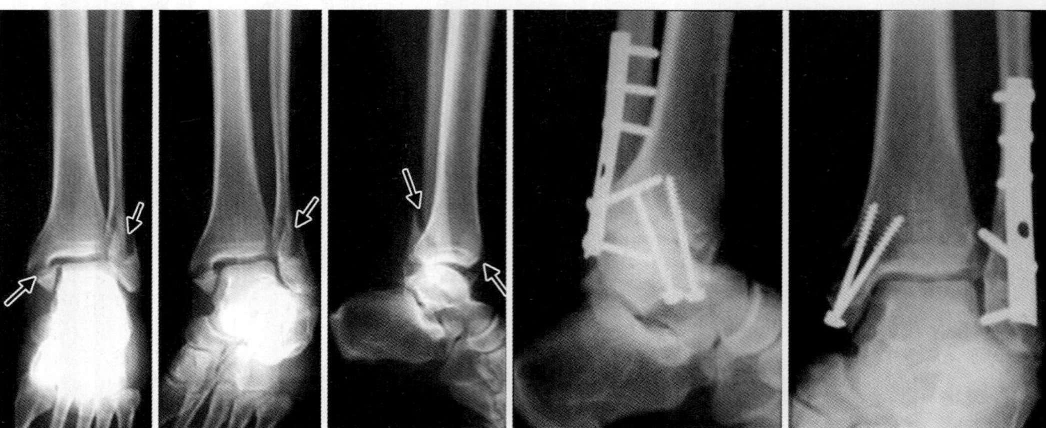

Figure 44.4 2 of 4 mm shaft screws

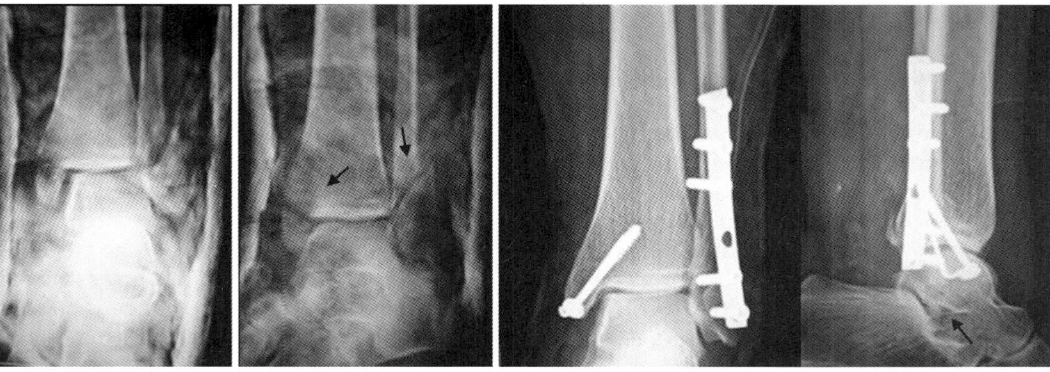

Figure 44.5 4 mm screw and a K-wire

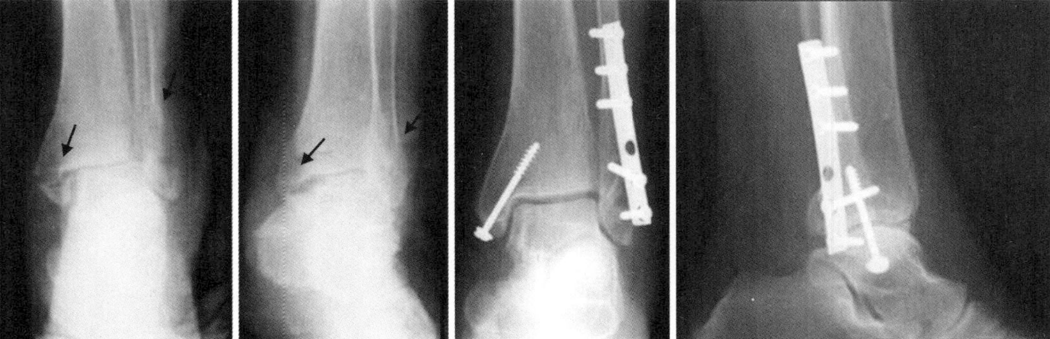

Figure 44.6 Only a 4 mm screw

Other Possible Combinations, As Per Size of the Medial Malleolus Fragment

- A malleolar and a 4 mm shaft screw
- A malleolar screw and a K-wire.

Few Techniques

- *Breakage of a drill bit:* The metaphyseal area in lower tibia is quite dense and offers a good purchase for either a malleolar or a 4 mm shaft screw. Screw inserted in the medial malleolus need not engage the opposite tibial cortex. Besides, when the drill bit hits the opposite cortex, it is at an obliquity and almost always it breaks at the endosteal bone surface. Hence the length of the drill bit outside the chuck is such that it will not hit the opposite cortex, taking into account the length of the drill sleeve also. When a quick coupling device is used, the business length of the bit cannot be adjusted and it is done by the surgeon's judgment only.
- *The length of a malleolar screw:* Usually a 45 mm long screw is the outer limit of length. If one chooses a screw longer than this, since the drill hole is not made in the lateral cortex of the tibia, the screw cannot penetrate the lateral tibial cortex and fracture opposition cannot be achieved. In the given example, the screw needs to be removed. To insert another screw of a shorter length is not a good idea, as it would be in the same track. Hence, perhaps this is a good indication for tension band wire fixation for the medial malleolus. As is discussed elsewhere, the

skin flaps need to be thick and long enough (Figs 44.7A and B).

- *Reduction of the medial malleolus and direction of the screw:* One needs to reduce the fracture under vision. Necessary soft tissue needs to be erased and the tip of medial malleolus should be seen by splitting the deltoid ligament only for the necessary length. As a matter of fact, one should develop a vision to confirm that the fragment is well reduced and then take a 'C' arm image to confirm. (This is how one should develop visual impressions, rather than entirely depending on 'C' arm all the while). To exert an interfragmentary compression, the direction of the screw has to be at right angle to the fracture line. In this example, if the judgment of the screw direction was correct, possibly the fracture line would not be visible. I would always prefer a shaft screw to a full threaded screw, which demands sliding hole and threaded hole technique and may not be rewarding at this site (Fig. 44.8).
- *Only K-wire, perhaps percutaneous, is inadequate:* The case presented with symptoms of osteoarthrosis of the ankle. As seen in the photo, the bimalleolar fracture was stabilized by two percutaneous K-wires in the medial malleolus and a plaster cast by a colleague. Gradually weight bearing was permitted and the patient continued to have pain and lack of confidence to bear weight on the ankle safely.

In the given example it was necessary to stabilize the lateral malleolus with a plate

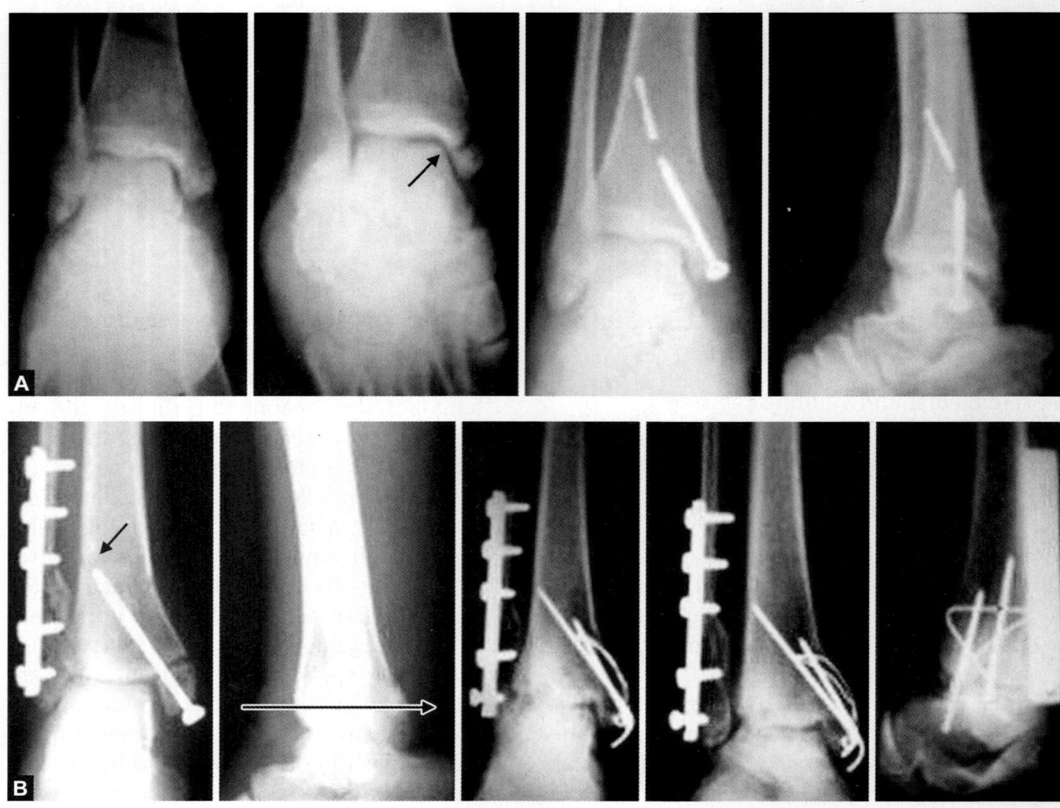

Figures 44.7A and B (A) Drill max 45 mm; (B) Screw max 45 mm

first and then open reduction and a screw fixation for medial malleolus be done. Only 2 K-wires inserted percutaneously in the medial malleolus cannot confer adequate stability to the ankle mortise and lead to lateral subluxation (Fig. 44.9).

- *Large fragments:* As discussed in adduction fracture, if the fragments are adequately large, it is necessary to stabilize them with two 1/3 tubular plates. Voids if any, should be filled with necessary bone grafts, for rapid and complete consolidation (Fig. 44.10).
- *Exceptionally small fragment:* In a case of a bimalleolar fracture, if the medial malleolus is very small, one needs to use one or two 1.6 mm K-wires to stabilize it. The lateral malleolus needs to be stabilized with a plate first and then medial malleolus fixed, as per protocol (Fig. 44.11).
- *MIPO technique:* Almost always the medial malleolus fracture, especially when it is a part of a bimalleolar injury, is rotated and has soft tissue interposition. Trying to reduce and pass K-wires by percutaneous method, is almost always unsuccessful and not justified.

A lady with a bimalleolar fracture presented with such an injury and the attending surgeon did a locking plate for lateral malleolus and percutaneous/minimally invasive K-wire fixation for the medial malleolus. Did not realize the post-operative appearance of X-ray was fallacious. Patient came for a second opinion. X-ray examination in few more views convinced us that the medial

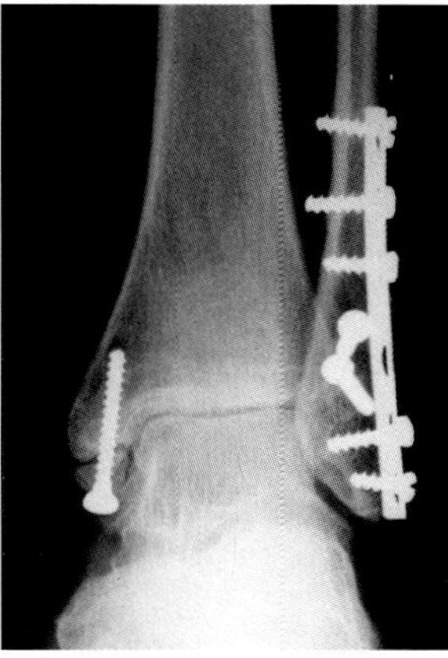

Figure 44.8 Medial malleolus technique

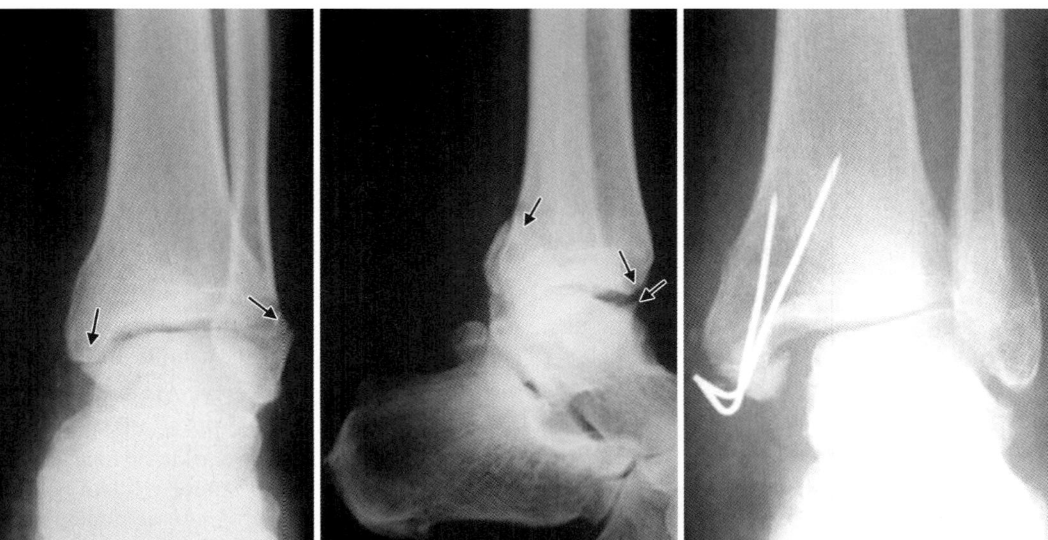

Figure 44.9 Medial malleolus screw and fibula plate needed

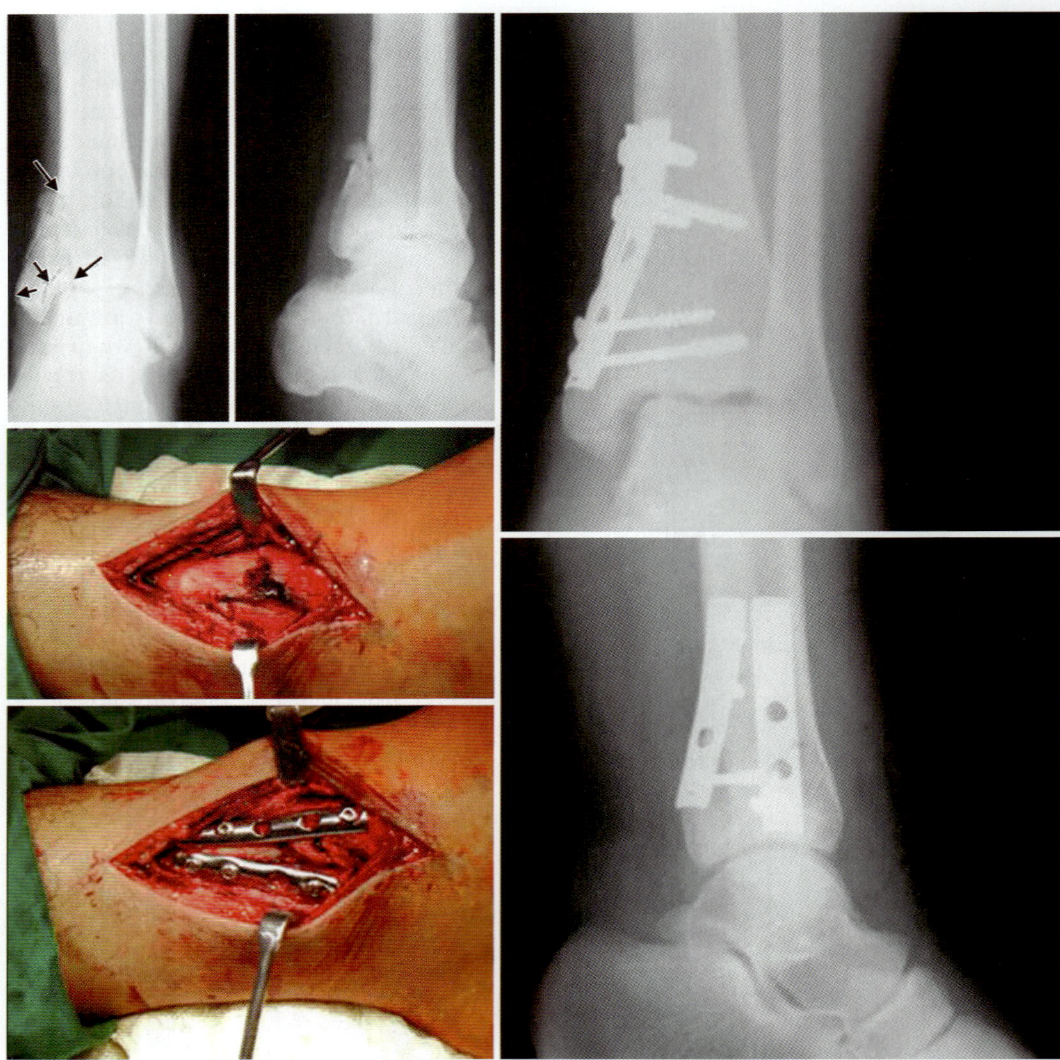

Figure 44.10 Medial malleolus: 2 plates and bone grafting

malleolus required an open revision surgery. It was done (Figs 44.12 and 44.13).

ANKLE LATERAL MALLEOLUS

GENERAL COMMENTS

During dorsiflexion, broad anterior surface of talus shifts fibula laterally and superiorly. Hence, during final reduction and stabilization, the ankle should be held in neutral position.

Talus: Its medial facet for the medial malleolus occupies 1/3 surface and the lateral facet covers 2/3 surface and is for lateral malleolus. This indicates contribution of lateral malleolus is more in keeping the talus and thus the ankle mortise stable.

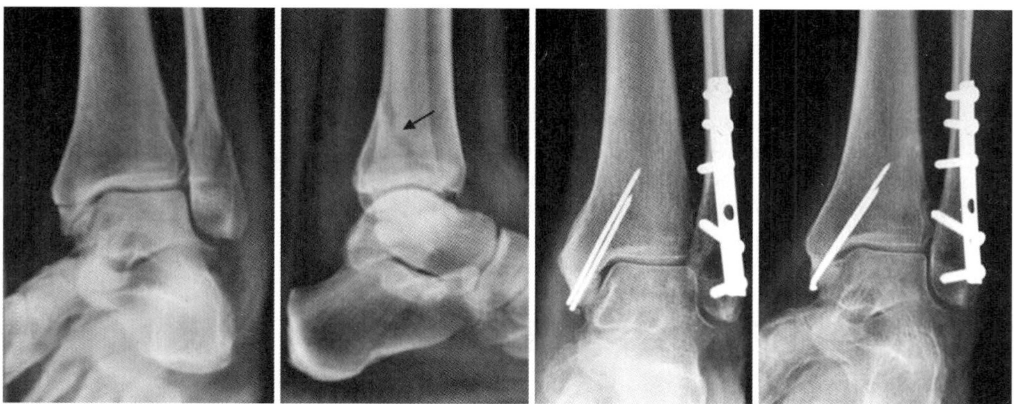

Figure 44.11 Medial malleolus very small fragment

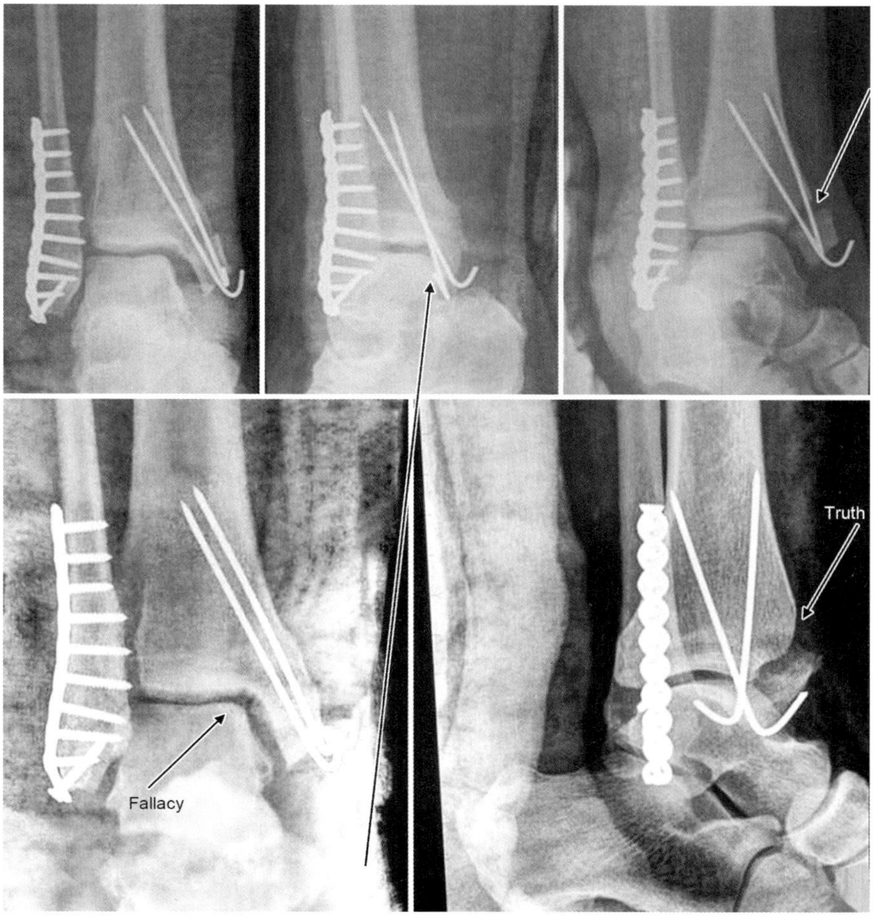

Figure 44.12 Missed in MIPO

The lateral malleolus thus offers more support to the mortise and absorbs static and dynamic forces.

Tibio-talar dislocation occurs only when the lateral malleolus fractures, even without an associated fracture of the medial or a posterior malleolus. This indicates major contribution of the lateral malleolus to the stability of the ankle mortise (Fig. 44.14).

LEVEL OF FRACTURE OF THE FIBULA

The level of fracture of the lateral malleolus indicates the amount of damage to tibio-fibular syndesmotic ligaments.

Higher the fracture, more the damage.

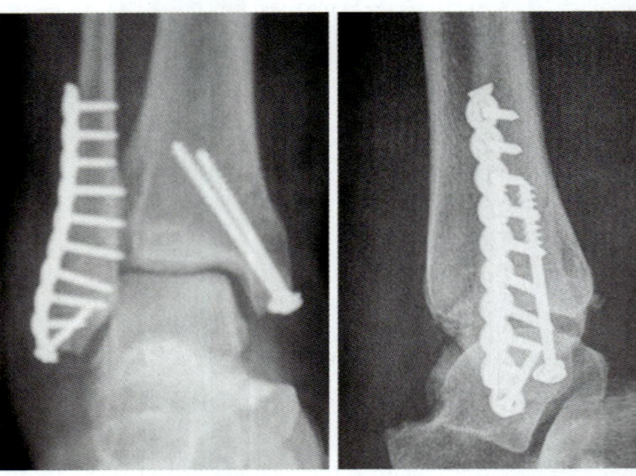

Figure 44.13 Missed in MIPO revised

Lower the fracture, lesser the damage. Hence a high fracture of lateral malleolus needs to be offered more stability, by internal fixation.

X-RAY VIEWS AND POSITIONING

- AP view with internal 30 deg oblique view, for TF syndesmosis.
- Fracture of lateral malleolus may not be visible in AP view, but is usually invariably visible in internal oblique view (Fig. 44.15)
- A lateral view almost always reveals oblique/spiral fracture (Fig. 44.46).
- Stress view of the ankle is necessary to know the ankle stability. In the given example, the fracture was missed on day 1 and consulted after a few weeks. X-ray examination done later for persistent pain, revealed a fracture line. Hence a stress view was taken. It confirmed stability (Fig. 44.17).
- Menert Shenton`s line: If goes above the plafond, indicates shortening in fibula.
- When an injury is suspected either in the foot or the ankle, one needs to give appropriate position for radiological examination for each area. One should not compromise to have a view to include both the foot and the ankle for an AP view. Such a view shows neither the ankle nor the foot, clearly and is unreliable (Fig. 44.18).

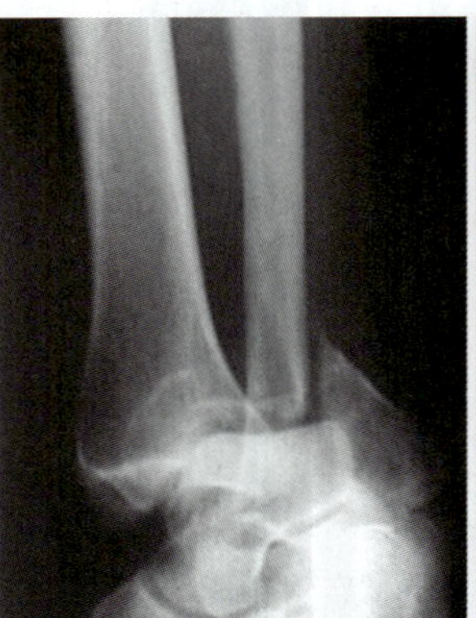
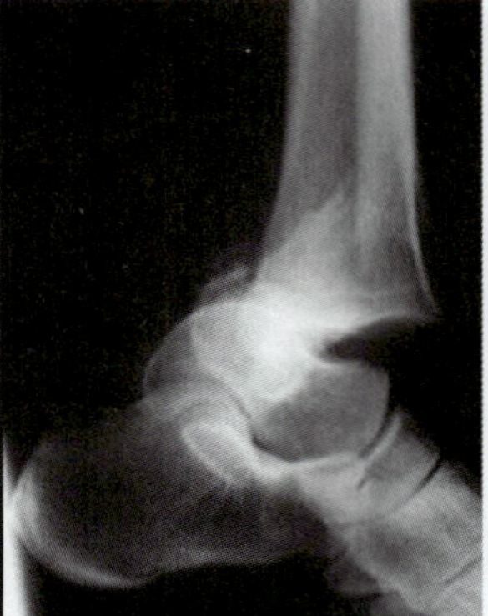
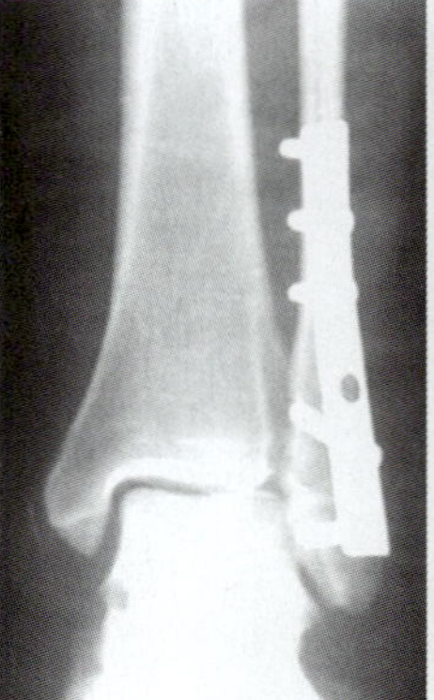
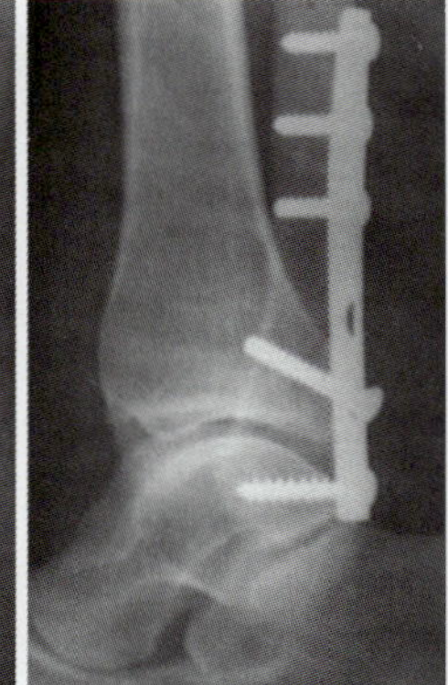

Figure 44.14 Dislocation occurs, only with fracture of lateral malleolus

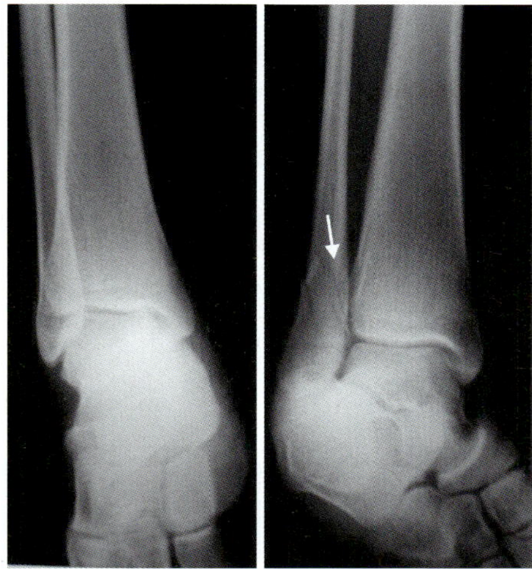

Figure 44.15 Oblique view important in fracture of lateral malleolus

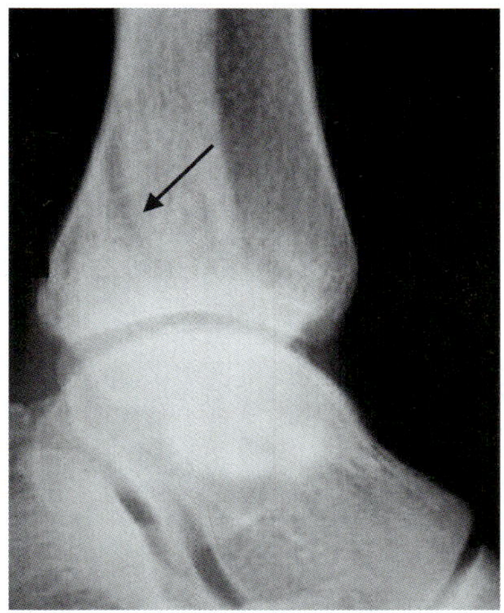

Figure 44.16 Lateral view reveals a fracture lateral malleolus

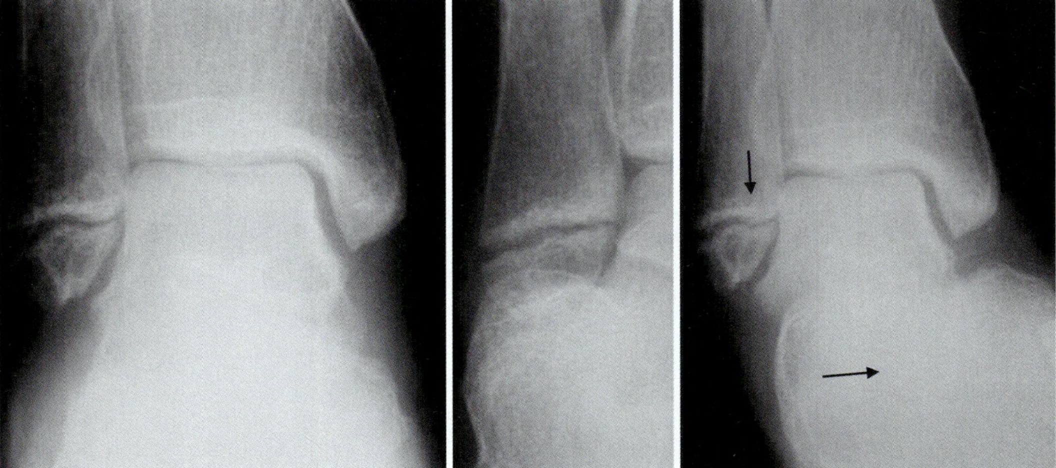

Figure 44.17 Stress view of ankle

- In an old untreated injury, the lateral malleolus fracture ends overlap and tip of the lateral malleolus comes to the same level as that of the medial malleolus (Fig. 44.19).

TIMING OF SURGERY

1. In a fresh injury, surgery is better done within first 4 hours of the injury. However, one wonders, in how many centers, it is possible to have a sound OT condition, availability of the surgeon and willingness of the patient, preparation of the patient, pre-operative tests, etc. possible.
2. If patient presents late, closed reduction under anesthesia should be done and a padded crepe and a posterior plaster slab must be given.

3. In an old untreated bimalleolar or a trimalleolar fracture it should be examined under anesthesia and see if the tip of the lateral malleolus can be brought down. If it cannot be brought down adequately, one should consider calcaneal skeletal traction and is maintained on a Bohler frame. During follow up, for assessment, a portable X-ray must be taken, while the calcaneal skeletal traction is on. Once it comes down adequately, then only a definitive internal fixation should be done (Fig. 44.20).

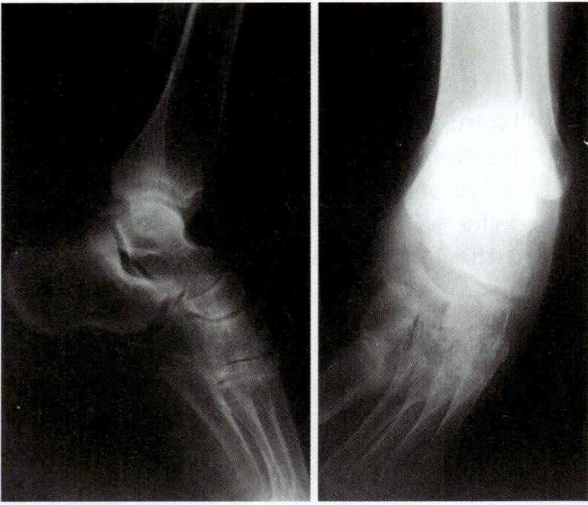

Figure 44.18 Incorrect view for foot and ankle

PATIENT POSITIONING

When both the fibula and the medial malleolus are to be fixed, the lateral malleolus has to be fixed first. When a postero-lateral plate is to be

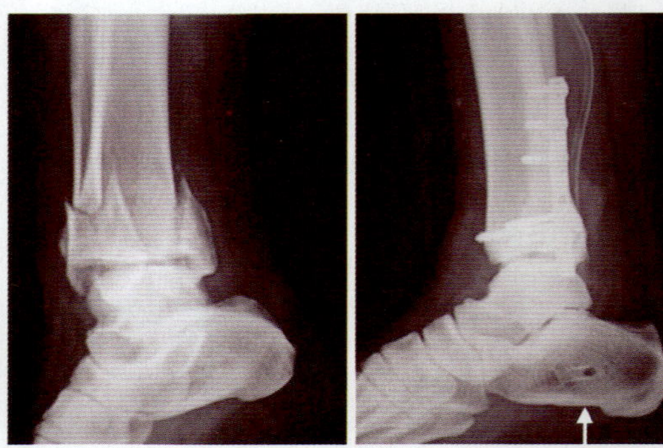

Figure 44.19 Calcaneal traction in fibula proximal migration

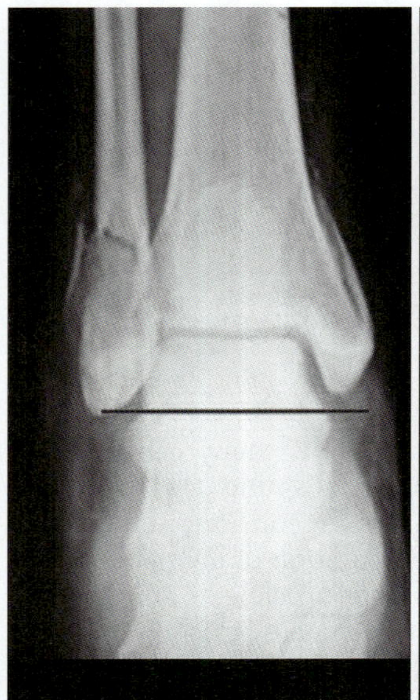

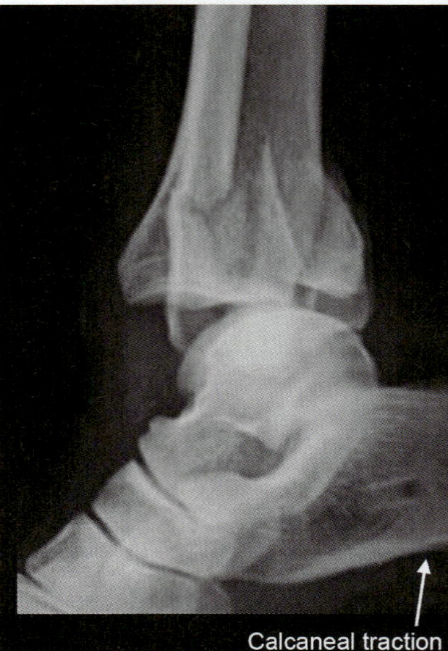

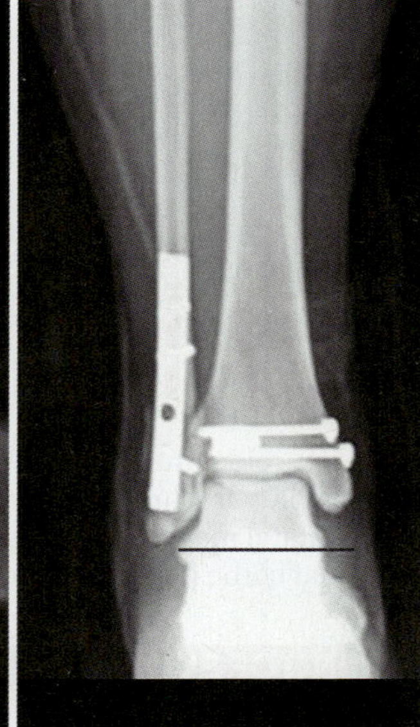

Figure 44.20 Fibula brought down

applied, one must do so with the patient in the lateral position, so a good exposure and access to the posterior surface of fibula is possible.

As is known, an antiglide plate is to be fixed on posterior or postero-lateral surface. In a transverse fracture, the plate on the lateral malleolus is fixed laterally and this can be done in a supine position.

Technique: The patient is given a lateral position, with the leg to be operated towards the ceiling. A towel of 10" width is kept under the gluteal area, with its ends hanging on either side of the table. A bolster is kept on either side, strapped by an adhesive tape. After draping, a pillow draped in a sterile cover is kept in between the calves and the ankles, for support and should not be strapped down to the table, prior to the draping. It has to be taken away, during change of position to a supine position, if the case has a fracture of medial malleolus fracture and needs to be fixed.

The wooden pelvis supports are not to be used, when change of position, with the draping on, as in such a case is to be done (Fig. 44.21).

After fixation of lateral malleolus and closure of the wound, a trained assistant puts hands under the drapes and cuts off the position retaining adhesive strapping, both on the front and the back of the patient. The towel underneath the pelvis is pulled forward, so the patient can be made supine. The free pillow in between the legs is taken away. The scrubbed team takes care of the limb, cautery and suction lines and adjusts the drape. One may have to add additional drape. The leg is slightly externally rotated, to facilitate the exposure of medial malleolus. On the first occasion, the surgeon and the team should try the technique, a day prior to the surgery on a volunteer.

IMPLANTS FOR THE LATERAL MALLEOLUS

- 1/3 tubular plate with 3.5 mm system screws (not to use a 4.5 mm screw with 1/3 tubular plate) is to be used. The 4.5 mm screw is too wide for the morphology of lateral malleolus and the screw head is not well contained within the plate hole. The large screw head may cause skin healing problems and is palpable under the skin, after fracture union and soft tissue reconditioning (Fig. 44.22).
- For the proximal fragment of fibula, 3.5 mm cortical and for the distal fragment (3.5) 4 mm full threaded cancellous screws to be used (Fig. 44.23).
- Antiglide plate fixation for Weber type fracture is rewarding. The plate should be under contoured. The screws are inserted from above downwards towards the lower end, so the distal fragment automatically

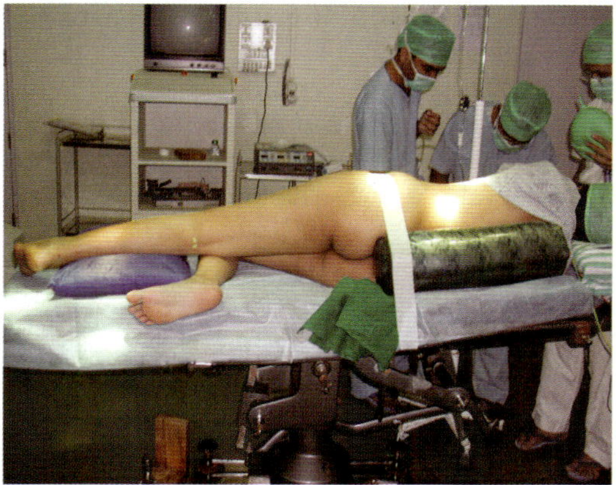

Figure 44.21 Lateral position of the patient

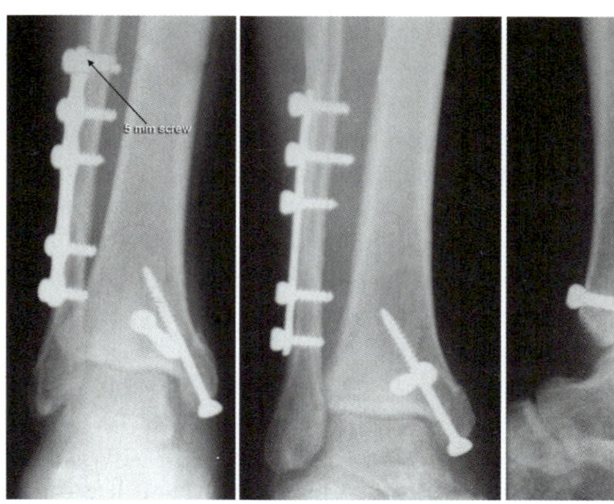

Figure 44.22 No. 4.5 mm screws

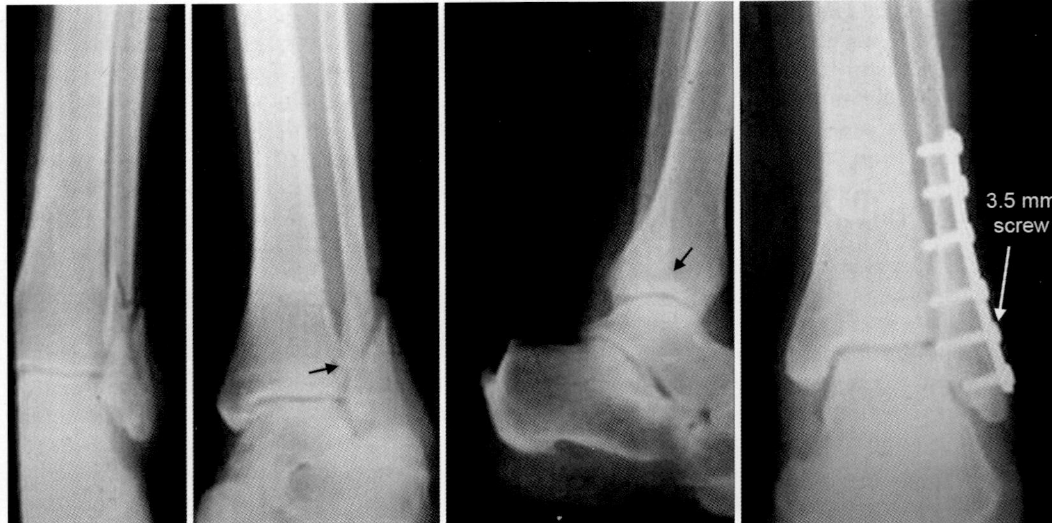

Figure 44.23 3.5 mm screws

moves forward and the reduction becomes stable. The screw just proximal to the fracture line is inserted and finger tightened first, with the traction on, on the foot, to achieve reduction. Some rotational adjustment achieves the reduction and the screw is tightened well. Then one hole is left and screw below it is fixed. Rest of the screws are inserted and in an oblique, especially a long oblique fracture, interfragmentary screw adds to the stability of fixation. If there is a possibility of local comminution the hole over the fracture area, may be left as such. On an X-ray, the fracture line appears adequately long, but the plane of fracture may not be suitable for inserting a screw through the plate hole by IFS technique. I feel, one should use the IFS screw, only if one can insert it through a plate hole and not to use it, outside the plate. The antiglide principle offers adequate stability, even in absence of an IFS (Fig. 44.24).

- If the fracture obliquity is adequate, to accept an IFS, it should be done to confer additional fracture stability. If one finds that the proximal end of the distal fragment is rather too thin, to tolerate gliding hole and threaded hole technique, one can use a 4 mm shaft screw (partially threaded). In exceptional situation, one can insert the oblique screw as a positional screw only, which also would contribute added stability. It is preferable to have such a screw, rather than bone rupture during the gliding hole drilling step with a 3.5 mm bit (Fig. 44.25).
- In an undisplaced transverse fracture of the distal part of the lateral malleolus, an axial screw fixation by a closed technique also offers good stability. A malleolar screw or a 4 mm shaft screw is inserted without a washer (Fig. 44.26).
- If the local skin condition on the lateral malleolus indicates a possibility of delayed skin necrosis, percutaneous two K-wires would also add to stability and safety (Fig. 44.27).

For Undisplaced Fracture of Lateral Malleolus:

Fracture Stability Assessment

If a patient comes walking, especially after 2 to 5 days after an injury and the X-ray reveals a

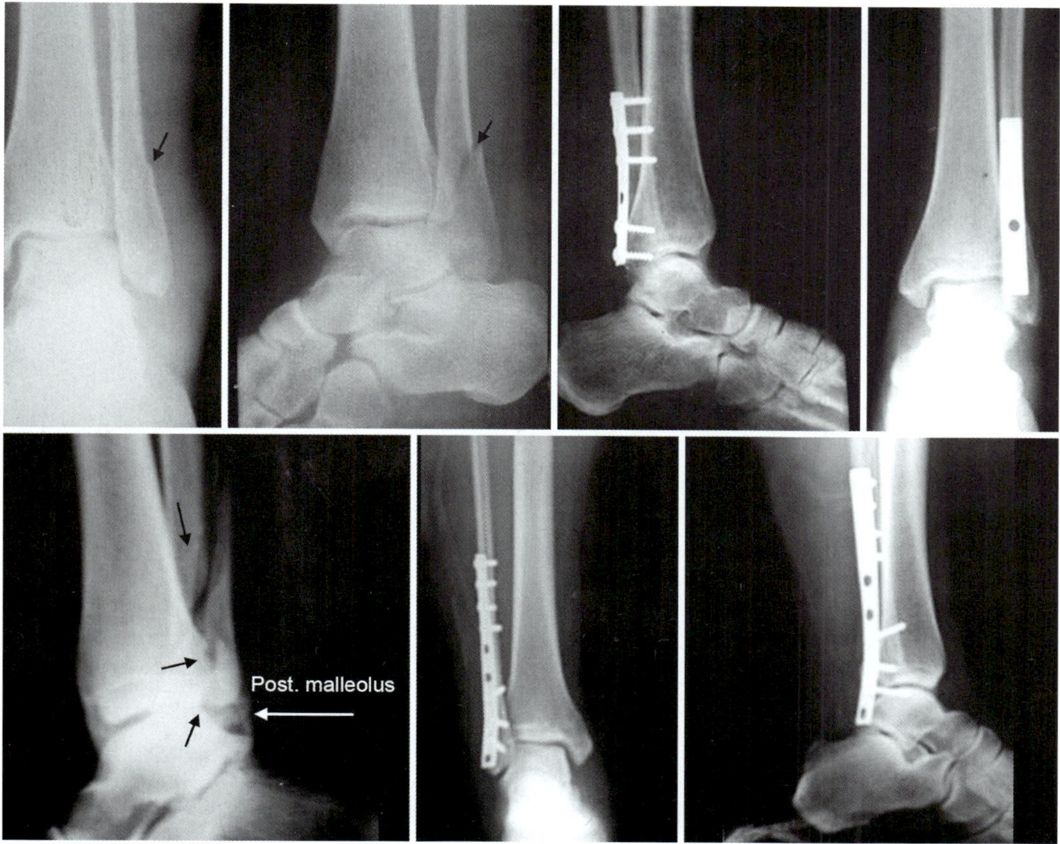

Figure 44.24 Posterior plate and IFS

fracture of lateral malleolus, it usually indicates a stable situation and one may be able to treat it non-operatively. If on the other hand, patient is unable to bear any weight on the leg, it usually means an unstable injury and one may need to consider internal fixation for the lateral malleolus.

In a bimalleolar fracture, if the fracture of the lateral malleolus is at the tip, it is well covered by the ligaments and is stable. Fixation of only medial malleolus is adequate (Fig. 44.28).

NON-OPERATIVE METHOD: PROTOCOL

- A below knee POP cast is adequate. The leg should be off the weight and patient must use a walker or two crutches. Use of a cane is just inadequate to be off the weight.
  - *Follow up*: X-ray every week, for 2 weeks to confirm that the fracture position is well maintained.
- At the end of five to six weeks, as per the fracture geometry, must insist on weight bearing in the cast to facilitate further consolidation and restoration of weight bearing reflexes.

In earlier days, a Bohler walking caliper made from iron, used to be incorporated in plaster cast. However, today with availability of synthetic material, one can permit weight bearing on the synthetic cast itself, with a cast over shoe.

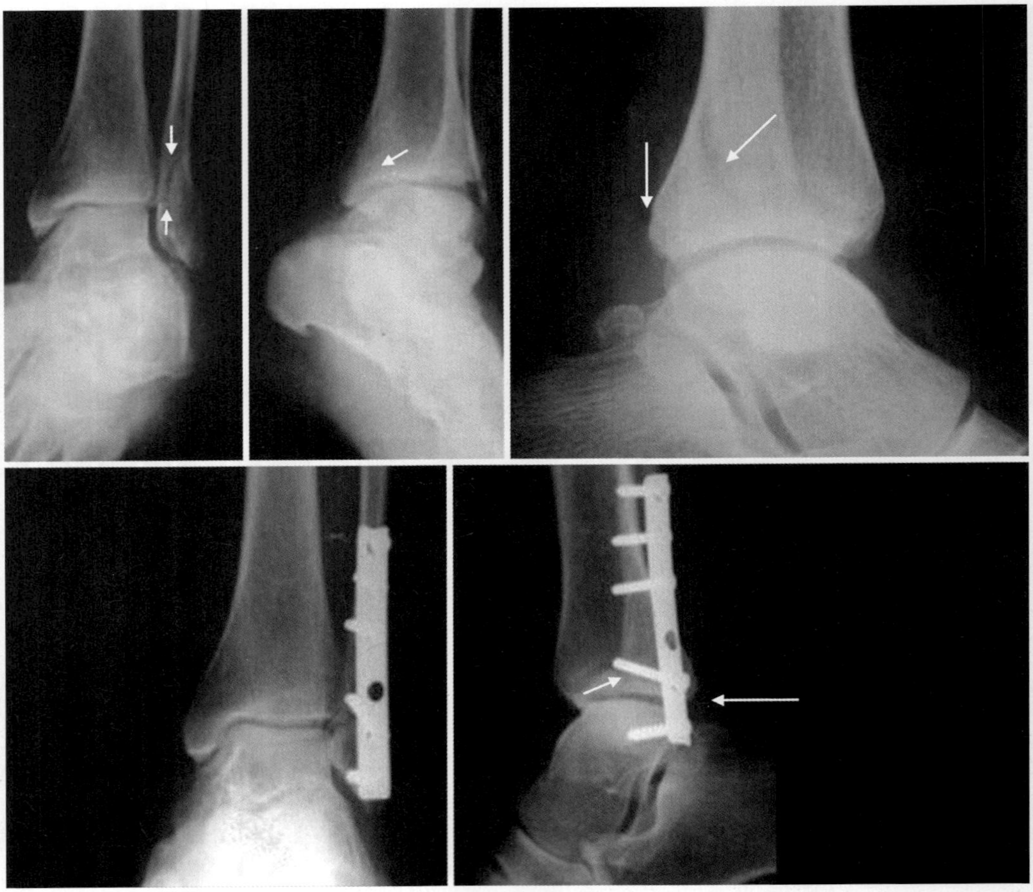

Figure 44.25 Lateral malleolus IFS

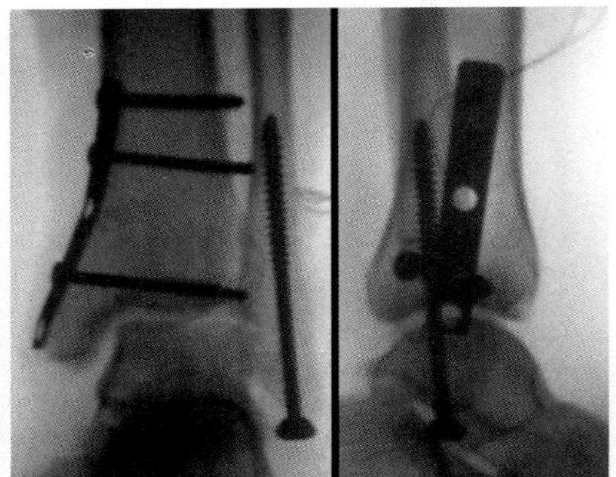

Figure 44.26 Lateral malleolus IM screw

Post-plaster Removal

- Padded crepe support, leg elevation and ankle mobilization is carried out under supervision. The crepe support and elevation is important during the first few days after cast removal. If this is not followed, troublesome edema may come up, which is difficult to control.
  - *In some cases:* The cast is bivalved and the back portion is added on the crepe. This adds to the comfort and confidence of the patient, and is gradually discarded by the patient.
- Progressive weight-bearing is advised and the walker is changed to a walking stick.

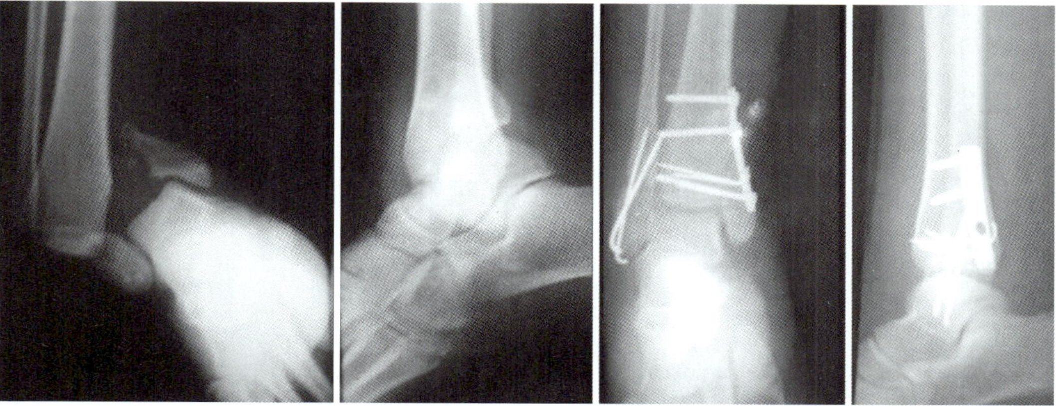

Figure 44.27 Lateral malleolus K-wire

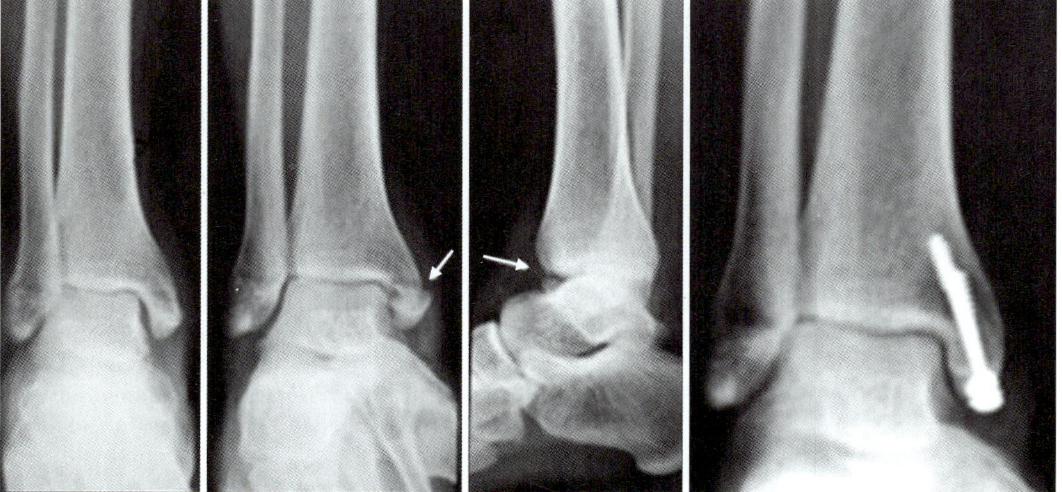

Figure 44.28 Lateral malleolus type A fracture

- Tiptoe (heel raising) exercises are very helpful, till the calf disuse atrophy is corrected.

COMPLICATIONS AFTER A FRACTURE OF LATERAL MALLEOLUS

- More the displacement, more the soft tissue injury and likelihood of stiffness.
- Associated cartilage injury to the tibiotalar joint may lead to osteoarthrosis and is difficult to predict on the day of the injury. Immediate closed reduction of displaced ankle fracture will help to keep the late changes in the joint to a minimum.
- In a fracture of lateral malleolus alone or a bimalleolar fracture, if the lateral malleolus is not well-aligned and stabilized, valgus deformity is observed, leading to osteoarthrosis (Figs 44.29A and B).

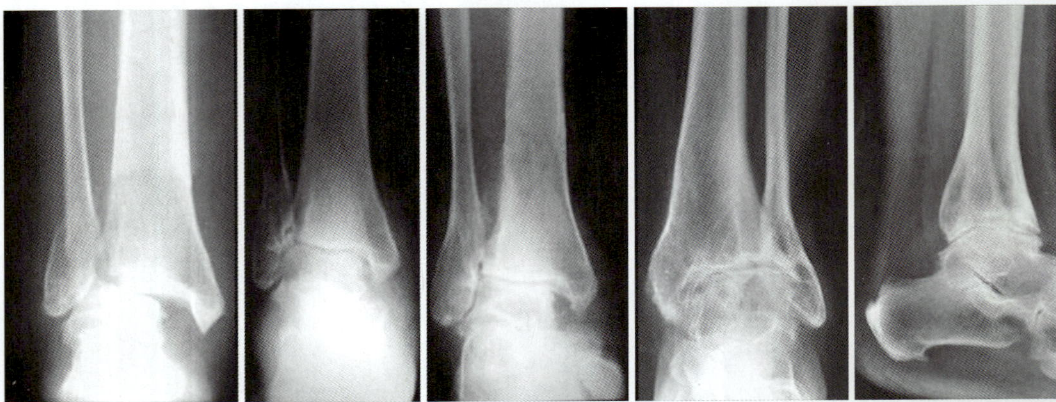

Figure 44.29A Lateral malleolus must be aligned well

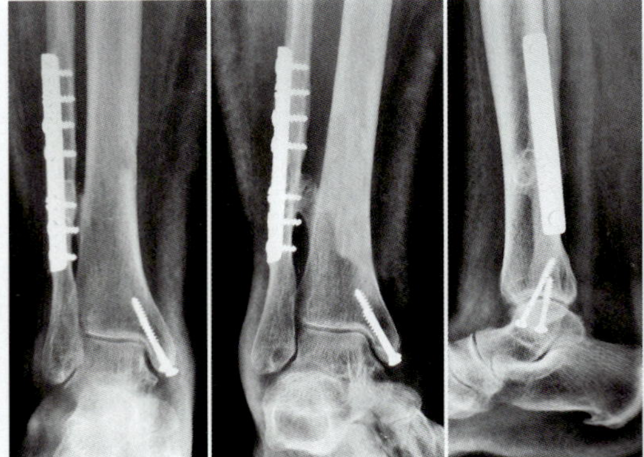

Figure 44.29B Long term result of a well reduced and stabilized injury

LATE PRESENTATION

When a case presents late, primarily or if the fracture was missed on the first clinical and/or radiological examination, bruise appears on the lateral surface.

If a crepe bandage was applied, then the hematoma comes to the skin surface beyond the limit of the crepe bandage, below the tip of lateral malleolus and towards web spaces (Fig. 44.30).

A Spiral Fracture of Lateral Malleolus and Posterior Plate Fixation: Technical Details

In a spiral or an oblique fracture, one needs to practice Weber's method of posterior plate fixation. Such an injury is in the distal end of fibula, above the lateral malleolus and usually is not associated with tibio-fibular diastasis.

Patient position: Lateral, with surgeon standing on the dorsal side of the patient. A draped and free (not strapped to the table) pillow is kept in between the two ankles. A free pillow is especially important, when the patient position has to be changed to a supine position, to fix the medial malleolus, if it is associated with. The instrument trolley be kept next to the surgeon, so he can pick up instruments, as needed and improve the ease in surgery. The assistant stands on the opposite side.

1. The incision should be posterior and should see flexor hallucis longus and peroneus brevis tendons. Take the distal end of the incision distal to the tip of lateral malleolus and curve slightly forward. See flexor hallucis longus medially and peroneus brevis laterally. They are nearly fused and bulge in the wound. Separate them with finger

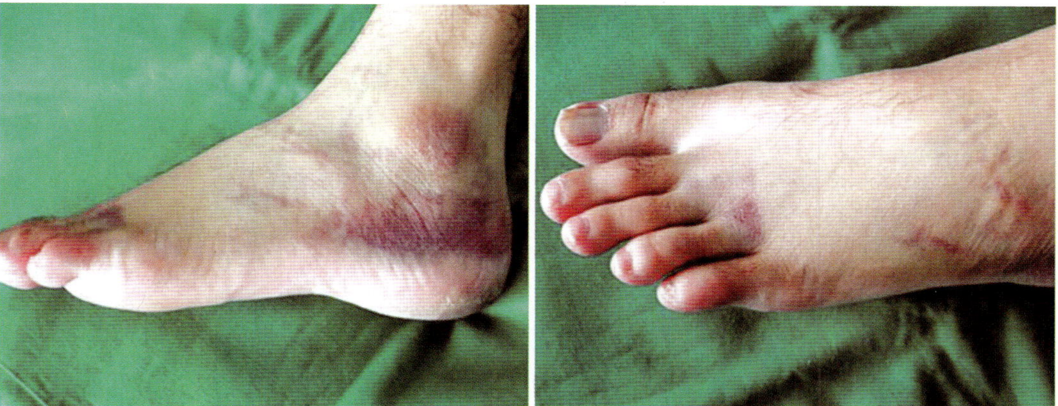

Figure 44.30 Bruise after a lateral malleolus fracture

dissection/scissors from above downwards. Erase FHL above downwards from the fibula and move it medially, while peroneus brevis is shifted laterally. Few veins come in the way, but not the sural nerve.

Which plate: If one thinks, the available 1/3 tubular plate is rather too thin, for a given built of the patient, one can overlap two 1/3 tubular plates, to enhance the strength of the implant. They should be from the same manufacturer, so the metal is the same and the holes overlap precisely.
If the fracture is in coronal plane, a plate is applied exactly on the posterior surface, so the reduction is stable and the antiglide plate stability is more. In some cases, the bone morphology demands, slight lateral position, so the plate sits well on that surface.

Whether to contour the plate?
If a single plate is used, while inserting the screws, it takes the shape of the lateral malleolus. Thus, when a straight plate is bent, as screws are inserted, it creates load, which stabilizes the fracture. While the screws are driven home the plate buttresses the distal fragment well. However, if two plates are overlapped on each other to confer strength, then both together may need to be contoured slightly.

Reduction technique:

1. Traction to the foot and ankle is given with appropriate rotation and is maintained so by the assistant. With a reduction forceps, a provisional reduction is carried out and is confirmed that the reduction is well achieved.
2. A 1/3 tubular plate of appropriate length is laid on the bone and its placement is adjusted with respect to the fracture line, parallel to the shaft. The distal end of the plate is slightly bent, to sit well on the tip of lateral malleolus and would not irritate the tendons crossing the area. A small self-centering forceps is used to hold the plate well co-opted with the bone, while the foot traction is on. The jaws of the forceps are kept *proximal to the fracture site*, so the distal part of the plate shifts the distal fragment anteriorly and reduces the fracture. Fine adjustment may be needed with a sharp 5 mm osteotome to lever the fracture ends in place, while the assistant gives traction to the ankle and slightly rotates the ankle, as advised by the surgeon. The hole immediately distal to the fracture is so placed, that an oblique IF screw can be passed across the fracture and have a good hold on both the fragments.

Order of Screw Fixation

- The first screw is passed through a hole, immediately proximal to the fracture line.
- If a hole comes on the fracture site, it is left void and a hole distal to it is reserved for IFS across the fracture line.
- Then a screw is passed in the next hole on the distal fragment. This is followed by the IFS.
- Thereafter alternate upper and lower screws are inserted.
- In case the bone ends on the oblique fracture are of adequate length and width, then a sliding hole and a threaded hole technique can be used. If not, then, just a positional screw will also confer necessary stability.
- Usually a 6 or 7 hole 1/3 tubular plate is required in most of the fracture morphology. The bone structure is so that in the proximal fragment 3.5 mm cortical and in the distal fragment cancellous screws are inserted.

TIBIO-FIBULAR DIASTASIS

It is an observation, that in a case of a trimalleolar fracture, tibio-fibular diastasis does not occur and almost always, the diastasis is associated with a fracture of fibula alone (Fig. 44.31).

Lower/3 Fibula Fixation: Fracture Fibula in Lower/3 Level, with Associated Diastasis: A Case Report (Courtesy DR Rahul)

After anesthesia, one needs to assess the nature and degree of the tibio-fibular syndesmotic stability. A 'C' arm is used to assess the stability. A valgus stress is given, on lateral strain:

- If the medial joint space increases
- The lateral malleolus with the talus, tilt laterally,
- The distance between the distal tibia and fibula increases, it indicates syndesmotic injury. X-ray in this position should be taken for documentation. This confirms the need of stabilization of the syndesmosis.

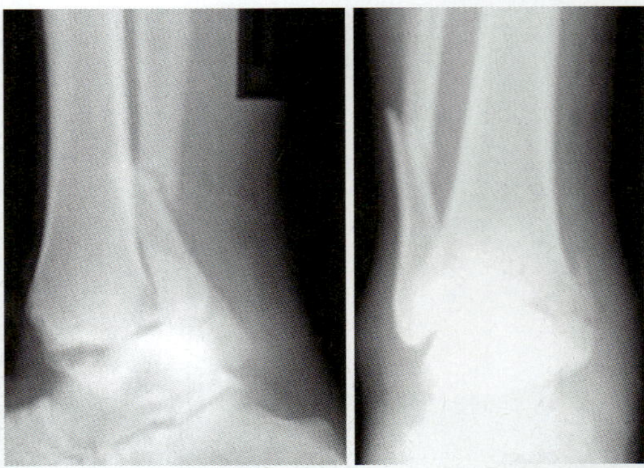

Figure 44.31 Trimalleolar fracture: No diastasis

The Procedure

Patient in a lateral position. Tourniquet. Lateral fibular approach. If there is a long 3rd fragment posteriorly its soft tissue attachment is well preserved in the exposure. Fracture is reduced and a 1/3 tubular plate is selected. It is slightly twisted and contoured to well adapt to both the proximal and distal fragments. Alternate upper and lower 3.5 mm cortical screws are fixed.

Prior to the lowermost screw fixation, the lateral strain test is done under the `C` arm, which may show some lateral shift of the talus. Hence the lowermost hole in the plate is used for a syndesmotic screw fixation.

A malleolar screw is inserted through the plate hole and is directed slightly anteriorly, as the tibia is in an anterior plane. In a patient with small bony frame, one may use a 4 mm shaft screw or a 4 mm fully threaded screw, with a washer.

The screw should cross both the cortices of the fibula and only the lateral cortex of the tibia. It should not hold the medial tibial cortex. This is important. (If the patient does not get this screw removed and starts weight bearing, such a screw anchored in the four cortices, usually breaks, as it cannot tilt within the tibia medullary canal.) If the screw breaks in such a situation, during removal, only the lateral part can be removed, while the medial part fixed in

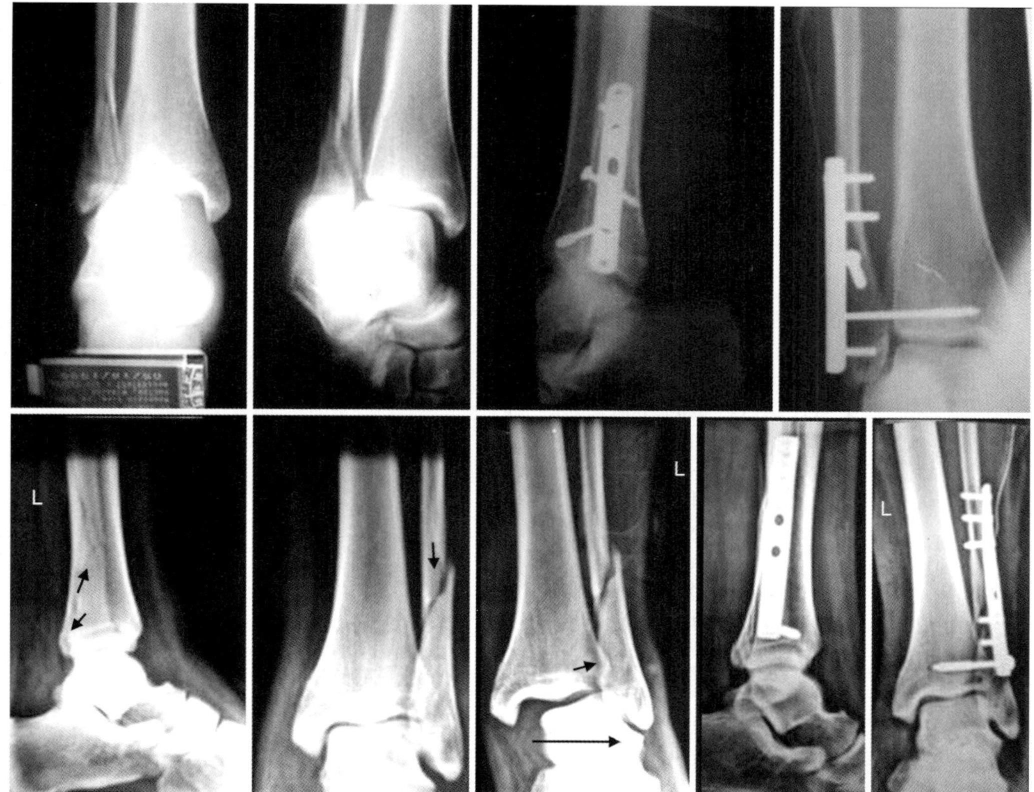

Figure 44.32 Diastasis

the medial tibial cortex remains as such. In such a situation, should the patient have a fracture of the tibia and needs an interlocking nail fixation, mechanical problem would arise.

Stability is checked again under `C` arm, with a valgus strain and is found to be stable, indicating that the decision to stabilize the diastasis was correct (Figs 44.32 and 44.33).

Ankle Lateral Malleolus Fixation, Especially in 4-Part Fracture of Lower/3 Fibula (*Courtesy Dr Rahul*)

The aim is to restore the length of fibula, at the end of the procedure and restore anatomy of the ankle mortice.

In a four-part fracture of lower/3 fibula, aim is to restore the length of the fibula. To achieve this, fix the lower 2 or 3 screws in the distal fragment and give traction to the ankle. This restores the length of fibula and the small fragments fall back in place. With the traction maintained by the assistant, the proximal fragment of the fracture and the plate are held with a self-centering forceps and screws inserted in the proximal fragment. Now, the tip of the lateral malleolus will be lower than that of the medial malleolus and the mortice will be restored well.

ADDUCTION FRACTURE OF ANKLE

This injury is due to inversion strain and the following morphology is observed:

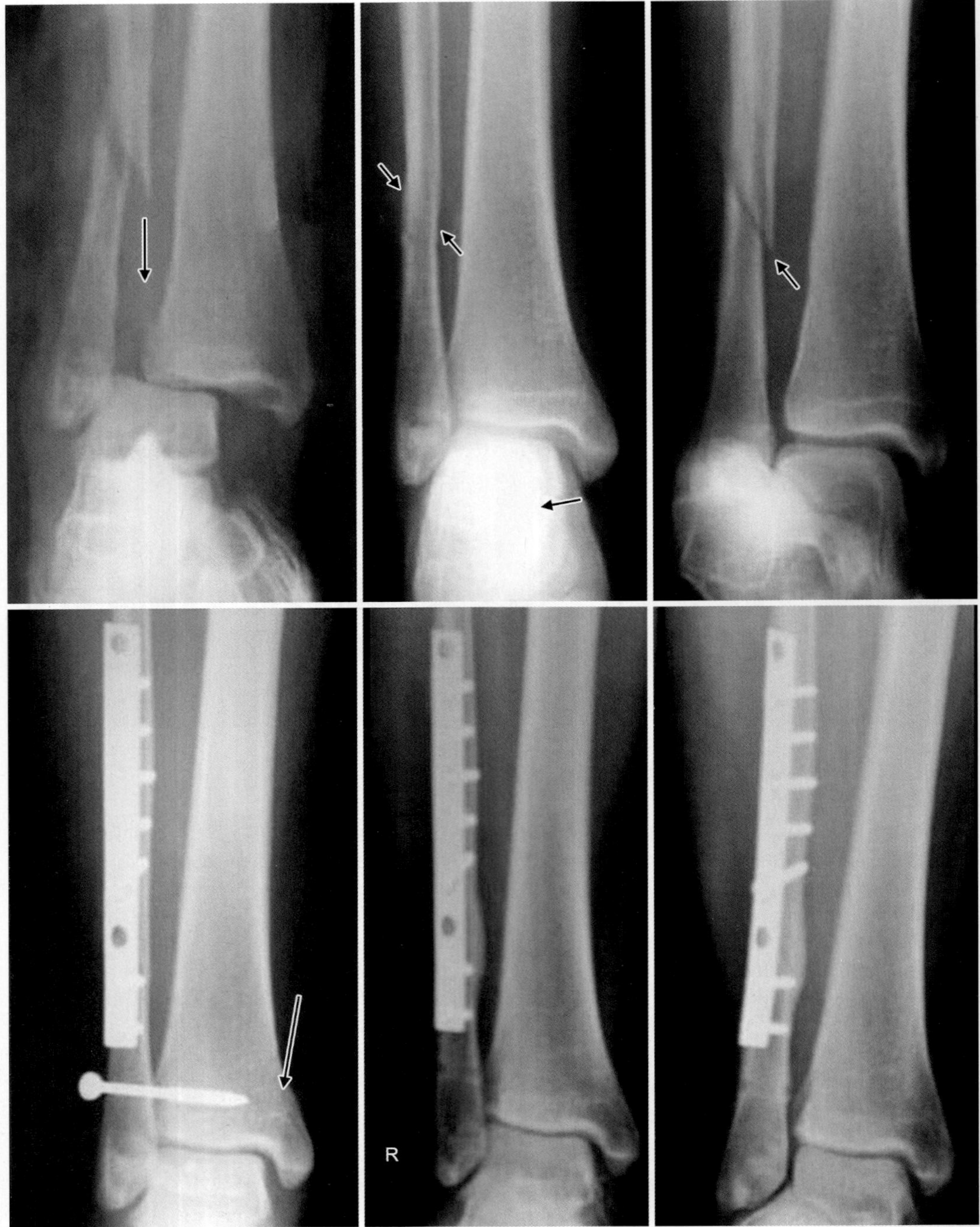

Figure 44.33 Syndesmotic screw removal

- Fibula has a transverse fracture at the syndesmosis
- Medial malleolus has an adduction fracture (with a vertical fracture line) with mild comminution at the plafond angle

First Aid on Arrival

In such an injury, one should immediately reduce the injury under anesthesia, clean the area, add a padded crepe support and immobilize the limb with a posterior plaster slab. I prefer to add an additional anterior slab for more strength of the external support. The limb must be elevated well and should wait for at least 5 days, before ORIF is undertaken. This helps to restore the blood supply to the skin flap and keep a chance of late darkening of the skin to a minimum. This waiting period is much less, compared to what time would be needed, should some skin problem develop. If this protocol is followed, the surgery is far easy and soft tissue problems and wound dehiscence are less likely.

Plan

- The fibula fracture is transverse and hence can be operated in supine and either an IM screw or a lateral plate is applied. (Whenever, there is an oblique fracture with postero-lateral displacement, one needs to apply the plate on the postero-lateral surface and hence a lateral position is necessary).
- This is a serious and major injury to the ankle and hence anatomical reduction and stable fixation is necessary.

In an adduction fracture, often, one finds an impacted area, at the junction of medial malleolus with the plafond. One needs to elevate the impaction and fill the void with cancellous bone grafts. This needs to be discussed with the patient pre-operatively and the ipsilateral tibial condyle needs to be draped accordingly, as a source of donor site. The quantity needed is quite small, it is the same limb and is kept off the weight, because of the ankle fracture and hence the site can be used as a donor site.

Patient Position and the Technique

- As is the usual procedure, the lateral column needs to be stabilized first
- Padding is added below the ischium, to elevate the affected limb and make the exposure of the lateral malleolus easy.
- Fibula is stabilized first and can be done in supine position: Surgeon may choose to do this sitting on a stool or standing on the same side.
- Due to the severe nature of the injury, the lateral subcutaneous tissue is almost always lifted from deeper structures. This needs to be followed up, for fear of skin necrosis.

Lateral Malleolus

Being a transverse fracture, rotary alignment for the fibula needs to be obtained well. This is achieved by the assistant holding the ankle and aligning the distal fragment to the proximal one.

The technique of fixation of the lateral malleolus would depend upon the fracture morphology, skin condition and the soft tissue injury.

- If the distal fragment is undisplaced or minimally displaced, a percutaneous screw fixation is possible.
- If it is rather a large one, a 1/3 tubular plate can be applied which would confer more stability.
- If the skin condition and viability are precarious, one can consider percutaneous 2 K-wire fixation.

On table after exposure, often one finds that the distal fragment is shifted laterally. Hence, with the fracture reduced, place a 1/3 tubular plate on the fracture area, and fix the distal most screw on the proximal fragment. This buttresses the lateral malleolar fragment, which automatically gets aligned with the proximal fragment. Then complete the fixation. Usually a 5- or a 6- hole plate is needed and the middle hole, lying on the fracture area, may have to be left as such. The screws in the distal fragment need to be cancellous, while those on the proximal fragment need to be cortical, due to the type of bone structure.

Warning! The length of the screws in the distal fragment need to be checked under 'C' arm and also by an X-ray film taken on table to confirm, none of the screw tips is touching the talus. It may appear that on 'C' arm the screw length is correct. When an X-ray film is later taken, lit indicates that one of the screws should have been shorter.

It is preferable to release the tourniquet prior to wound closure. A no. 10, closed suction drain is placed and wound closed. The padding under the ischium is removed. This helps to roll the leg laterally and expose the medial malleolus.

Medial Malleolus

The tourniquet is inflated again. The tip of medial malleolus is palpated and a vertical incision is taken. The long saphenous vein is protected, as far as possible. The skin flaps should be thick, because there would be a plate over the medial malleolus and the skin has less subcutaneous fat and wound dehiscence is likely.

Usually the proximal end of the distal fragment is thin, as the fracture is oblique and few flakes/fragments are also observed. The soft tissue attachment is preserved. If the preoperative X-ray film indicated local impaction at the plafond, the fragment is slightly opened and the impaction is confirmed. If so, it is elevated, using a small 5 mm punch, working away from the articular surface and with gentle strokes, it is elevated. Necessary amount of graft is taken from the tibial condyle and laid locally. Too much grafts interfere with a good contact opposition of the fragment with the tibia. Reduce the fracture with traction and gentle pressure on the distal fragment, with a square punch. The assistant should pass a 1.8 mm K-wire through the distal fragment and in the tibia, above the plafond. The position of the K-wire is checked under 'C' arm. This is important, as later on the wire is to be replaced with a screw. Select, usually a 5 hole 1/3 tubular plate: It is slightly contoured and the K-wire is threaded through the second last hole of the plate. The tip of the plate over the medial malleolus should be well contoured, or else, it irritates the skin.

As usual, the reduction is checked at the junction of the medial malleolus and the plafond.

Order of Screw Fixation

The K-wire is through the second hole from below. Through the 3rd hole from below a 3.5 mm cancellous screw is inserted. Then a short screw is inserted in the tip of medial malleolus. (Usually a 10 or 12 mm long screw is required.) The K-wire is replaced with a 4 mm shaft screw, which exerts interfragmentary compression and is the key screw, which confers stability to the assembly. Before insertion of this screw, there is a screw above and below and hence rotation of the plate or the fragment does not occur. The fixation is completed with remaining screw insertion in the proximal part of the plate.

There could be plates on either side of the ankle, in an ankle area where the limb circumference is small and without much soft tissue. Hence, raising thick skin flaps is helpful during the wound closure. The tourniquet is released. The closure needs to be done carefully, without any tension. May be the skin edges may be opposed with few mm space between the skin edges. As the tissue edema reduces, good opposition of wound edges is observed.

Padded dressing and a crepe support keeps the reactionary edema to a minimum. I prefer to apply posterior slab made of plaster of Paris and synthetic rolls. Additional anterior slab contributes to the external support.

Postoperative: Till the effect of spinal and/or epidural anesthesia wares off, elevation on soft pillows is safe. After the effect of the anesthetic has worn off, elevation on a Bohler frame is necessary, to keep the post-operative edema to a minimum. If one keeps the limb on Bohler frame prior to wearing of the anesthesia, there is danger that the leg rolls laterally and the common peroneal nerve is pressed between the limb and the metal bar of the frame.

Case Examples (Figs 44.34 to 44.41)

Next Case

A patient had sustained an ankle injury and was applied a splint in peripheral area. Presented after about 15 days. The fracture was getting sticky and open reduction may have been difficult. Hence, under anesthesia, the ankle was manipulated, to make the fragments mobile and a skeletal traction was applied through the calcaneus for about 10 to 12 days. While

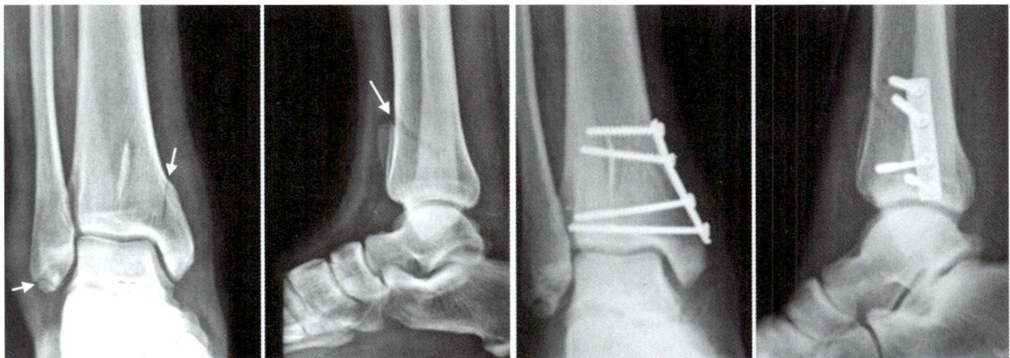

Figure 44.34 The lateral malleolus fragment is just the tip and can be left as such. The ligament over it would maintain the stability

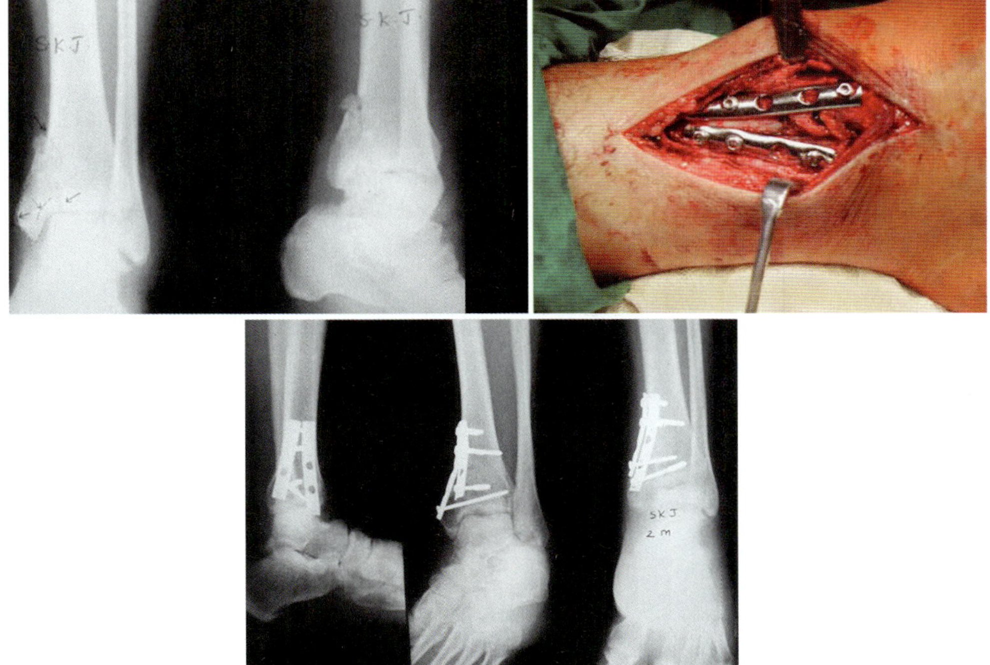

Figure 44.35 Two plates on medial malleolus. The medial malleolus has two fragments. Two plates needed

the traction was on, an X-ray was taken, with the traction on, to know fracture alignment. Then open reduction was carried out. It was a trimalleolar fracture.

- Postero-lateral approach and the posterior malleolus fixed by a posterior to anterior screw. Then fibula plate was applied.

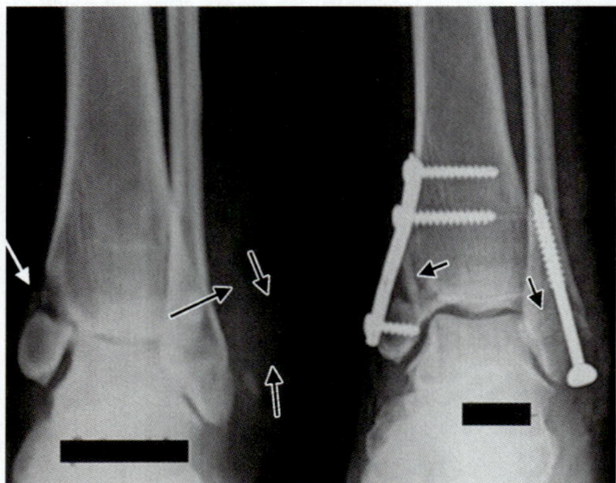

Figure 44.36 Local comminution in medial malleolus. Bone grafts needed. Lateral malleolus undisplaced percutaneous screw is adequate

- Then medially two of 4 mm shaft screws were applied with washers and achieved good stability (Fig. 44.42).

TRIMALLEOLAR FRACTURE OF ANKLE

A trimalleolar fracture injury may be associated with posterior-lateral dislocation of the ankle. Immediate closed reduction and a padded crepe and a posterior POP slab support is necessary.

In appropriate chapters management of medial, lateral and posterior malleoli is described. Here a combination of such injuries is demonstrated.

Case 1

The posterior fragment was nearer to the lateral malleolus. Hence for the lateral malleolus, posterior approach was taken, so that, one was able to access the posterior malleolus and could be stabilized from posterior to anterior side by an IFS (Fig. 44.43).

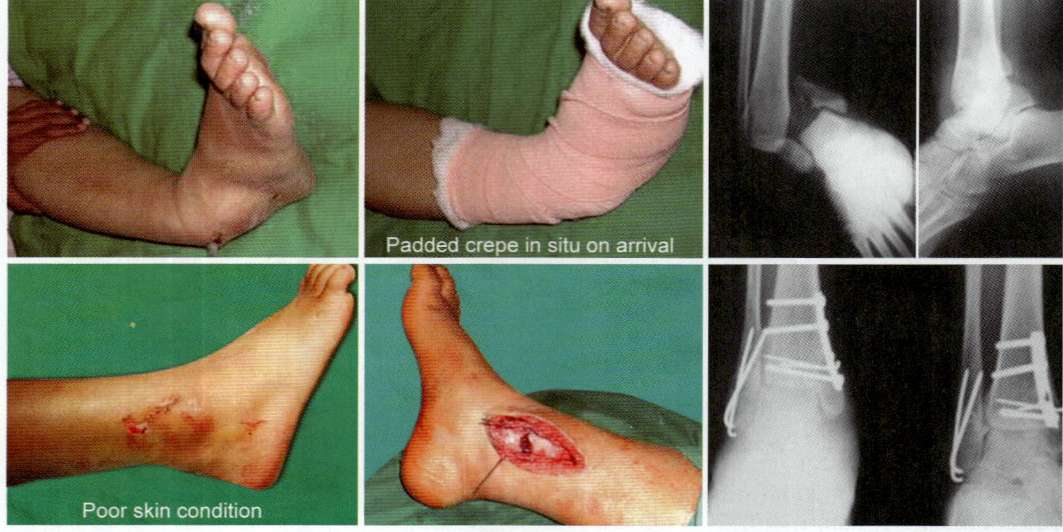

Figure 44.37 Due to local skin condition, immediate closed reduction under anesthesia, padded crepe bandage and plaster support needed. Wait for a few days. Lateral skin condition precarious: only percutaneous K-wires

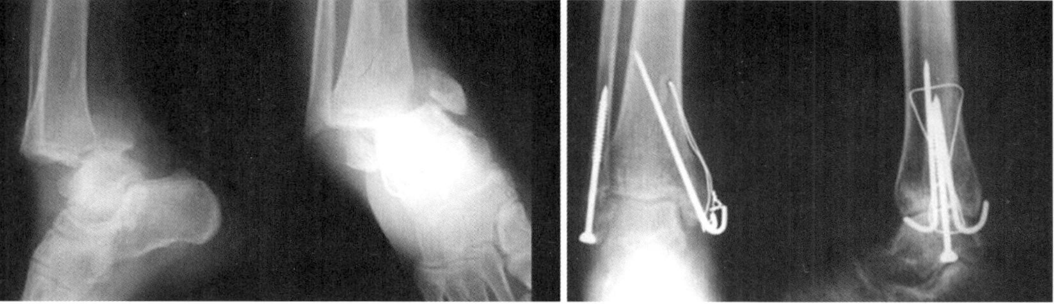

Figure 44.38 For a vertical adduction fracture of medial malleolus, tension band wiring not recommended

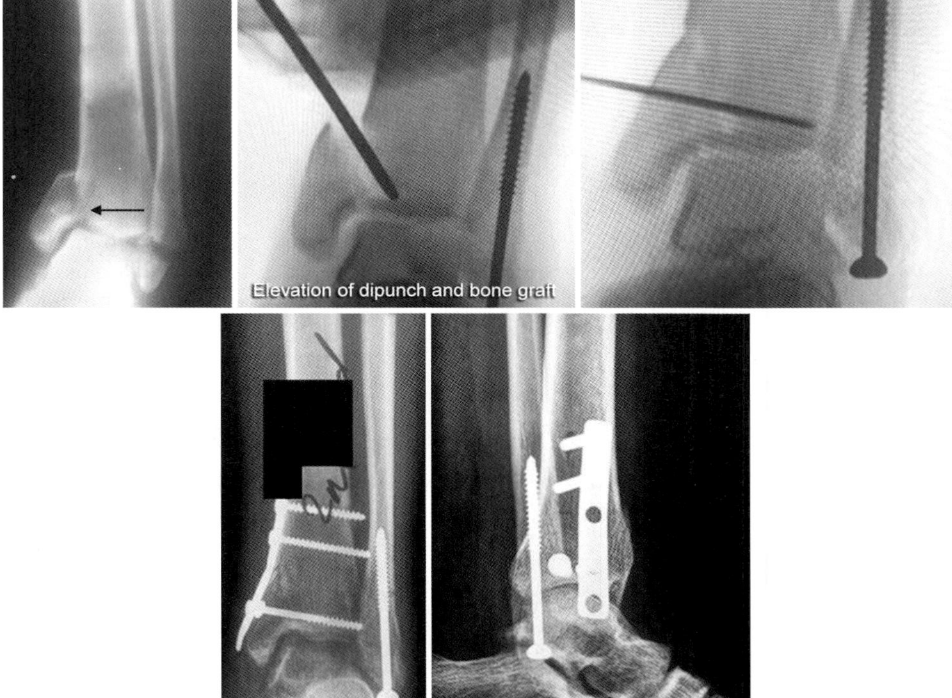

Figure 44.39 Die punch impaction at plafond. Needs elevation and bone grafting

Case 2

This patient had a fracture of the posterior malleolus. The fragment was in the midline and approach from the anterior side was easier. To access it from the posterior approach to the fibula needs extensive retraction and hence this method.

Surgery was started with patient in lateral position, with to-be-operated leg towards the ceiling.

- After exposure of the fibula, the posterior malleolus was exposed, at least its lateral part. Along it, one locates the central portion.
- The anterior part of the plafond was exposed. With pointed reduction forceps, the fracture

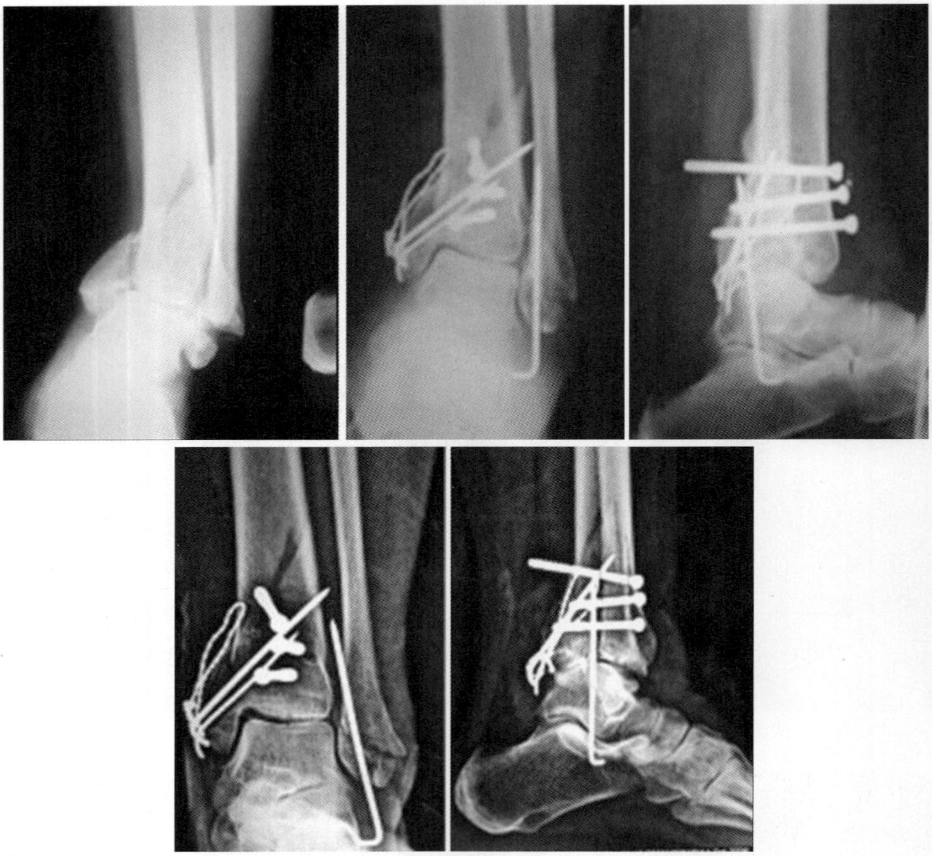

Figure 44.40 No TBW in medial malleolus, as leads to varus

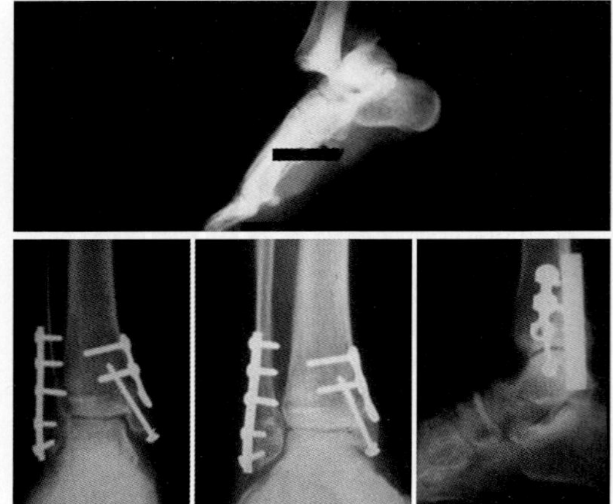

Figure 44.41 Plates on both the columns

was reduced. A place where the K-wire would be inserted was so selected that, by its side, a 4 mm shaft screw can later be inserted. A 1.8 mm K-wire was passed from anterior to the posterior side, for provisional stability and the reduction was confirmed under 'C' arm.

- A drill hole was made with a 2.5 mm drill bit and a 4 mm shaft screw with a 7 mm washer was driven in anterior to posterior side. (The AP width of the posterior fragment was assessed. If it is less than that of the thread length, then a 5 mm longer screw is chosen and part of the thread tip is cut off. This helps to prevent threads staying across the fracture line.)

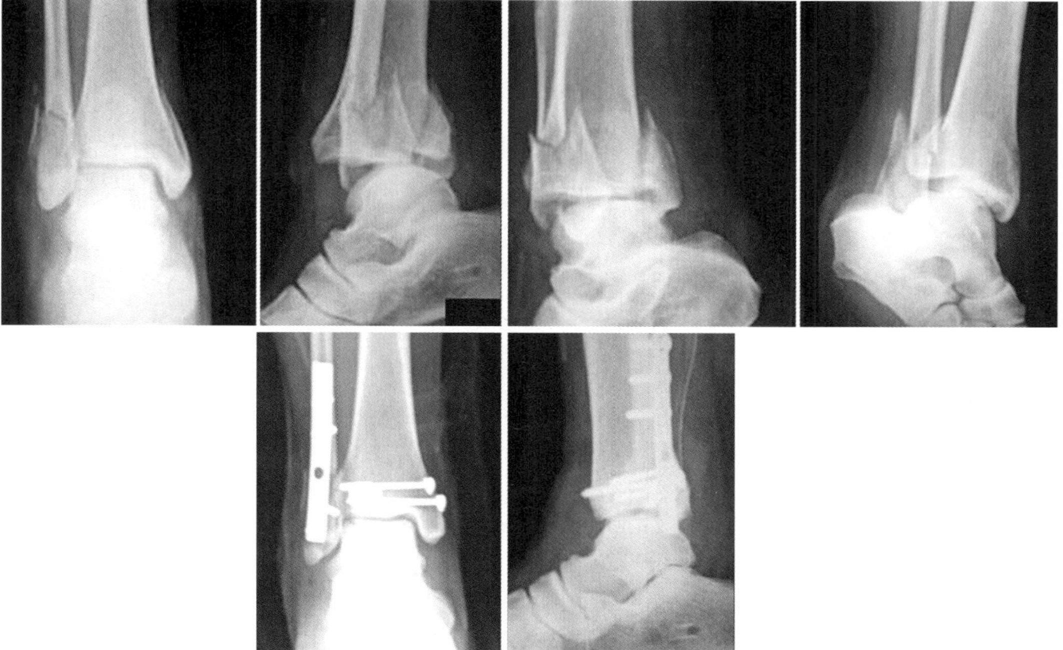

Figure 44.42 Old untreated adduction fracture

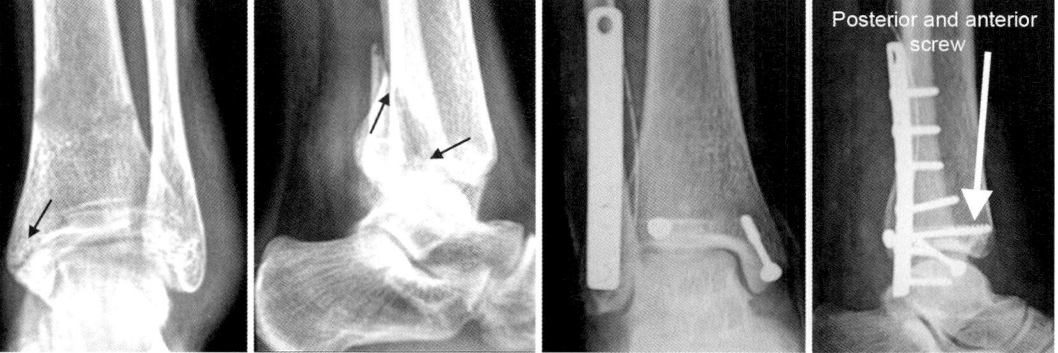

Figure 44.43 Trimalleolar fracture: Posterior to anterior screw

- The fibula was stabilized with a 1/3 tubular plate. The tourniquet was released and a drain no. 10 is inserted and wound closed. Patient was made supine.
- The medial malleolus was stabilized, as per the size of the fragment (Fig. 44.44).

Case 3

Trimalleolar Fracture Dislocation with a Small Posterior Fragment

This lady had a trimalleolar fracture dislocation. The posterior malleolus was a thin small

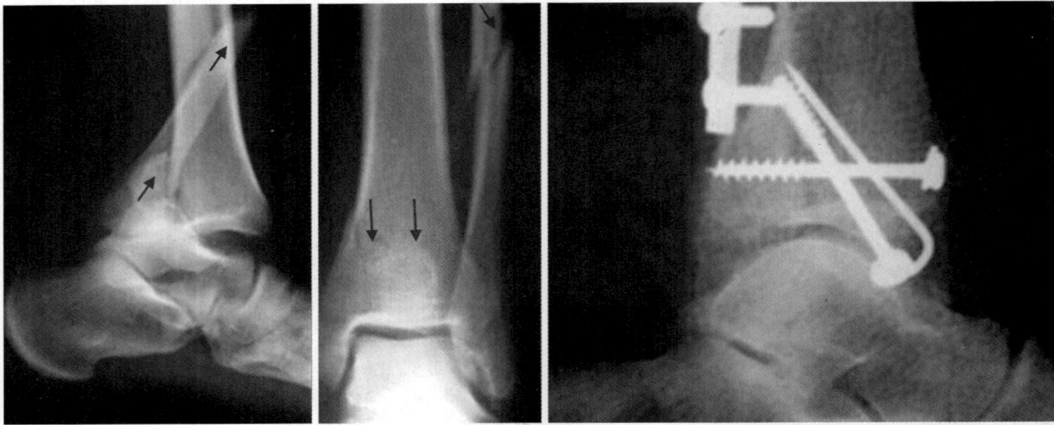

Figure 44.44 Trimalleolar fracture dislocation anterior to posterior screw

fragment. She was operated within four hours of the injury. After closed reduction after anesthesia, the fragment fell back into place. The fibula was fixed with a posterior plate and an IFS through a plate hole. The medial malleolus was fixed with 2 × 4 mm shaft screws with a washer for each. Return of good function obtained (Fig. 44.45).

Case 4

Trimalleolar Fracture Dislocation with a Postero-lateral Fragment

This old lady had a trimalleolar fracture dislocation with osteoporosis. The skin was papery thin. Soon after arrival, a closed reduction and padded crepe was applied. This was in pre 'C' arm era. Study of the arrival X-ray shows the posterior fragment was attached to lateral part of the plafond. The lateral malleolus was exposed by a posterior approach. Medial to it, the postero-lateral fragment was visible. It was reduced and a 4 mm shaft screw was inserted in an oblique direction, so it was at right angle to the fracture area.

The fibula was fixed by a postero-lateral plate. Patient made supine and the medial malleolus was fixed. Good union obtained with good return of function. Has a good function at the end of 12 years now (Fig. 44.46).

Case 5

Large Posterior Fragments

This lady had a trimalleolar fracture in the ankle. CT scan revealed presence of two fragments in the posterior malleolus.

The fibula was exposed by a posterior approach. The incision was placed slightly towards the midline, for better approach to the posterior malleolus. The lateral fragment was larger of the two. It was held reduced and a K-wire inserted at such a place, so that it would be replaced by a screw later on. A 3-hole 1/3 tubular plate was applied over it, so that the K-wire was in the lower-most hole. The plate was fixed with 3.5 mm cancellous screws in the proximal 2 holes. Both the fragments were thus buttressed well under the plate and the screw only through the large one. The K-wire was replaced by a 4 mm shaft screw.

The fibula was fixed with a 1/3 tubular plate. She was turned on the back and the medial malleolus was fixed.

Weight bearing was started only after eight weeks (Fig. 44.47).

ANKLE: WHAT TO AVOID

Time and again, few things are done, which almost always fail and a revision surgery

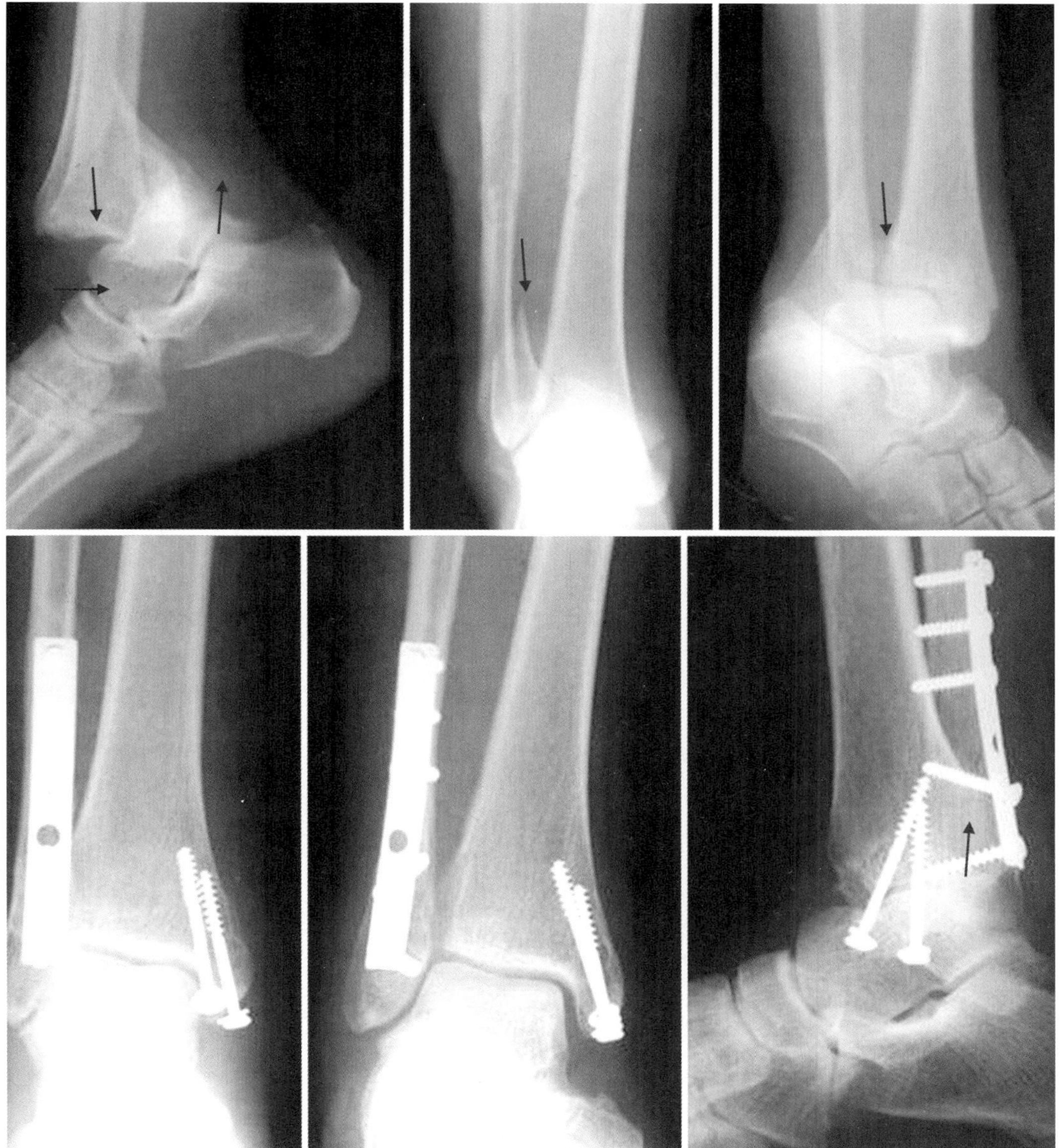

Figure 44.45 Trimalleolar fracture dislocation and a small posterior fragment

is required with delayed recovery, loss of working days and may lead to a stiff and deformed ankle. Such a result is likely to lead to changes of OA which at a later date, may need surgery for that as well. Few examples shown would aptly convince the same.

One should know, how to carry out a procedure. More important is what not to do, to avoid an unfortunate outcome.

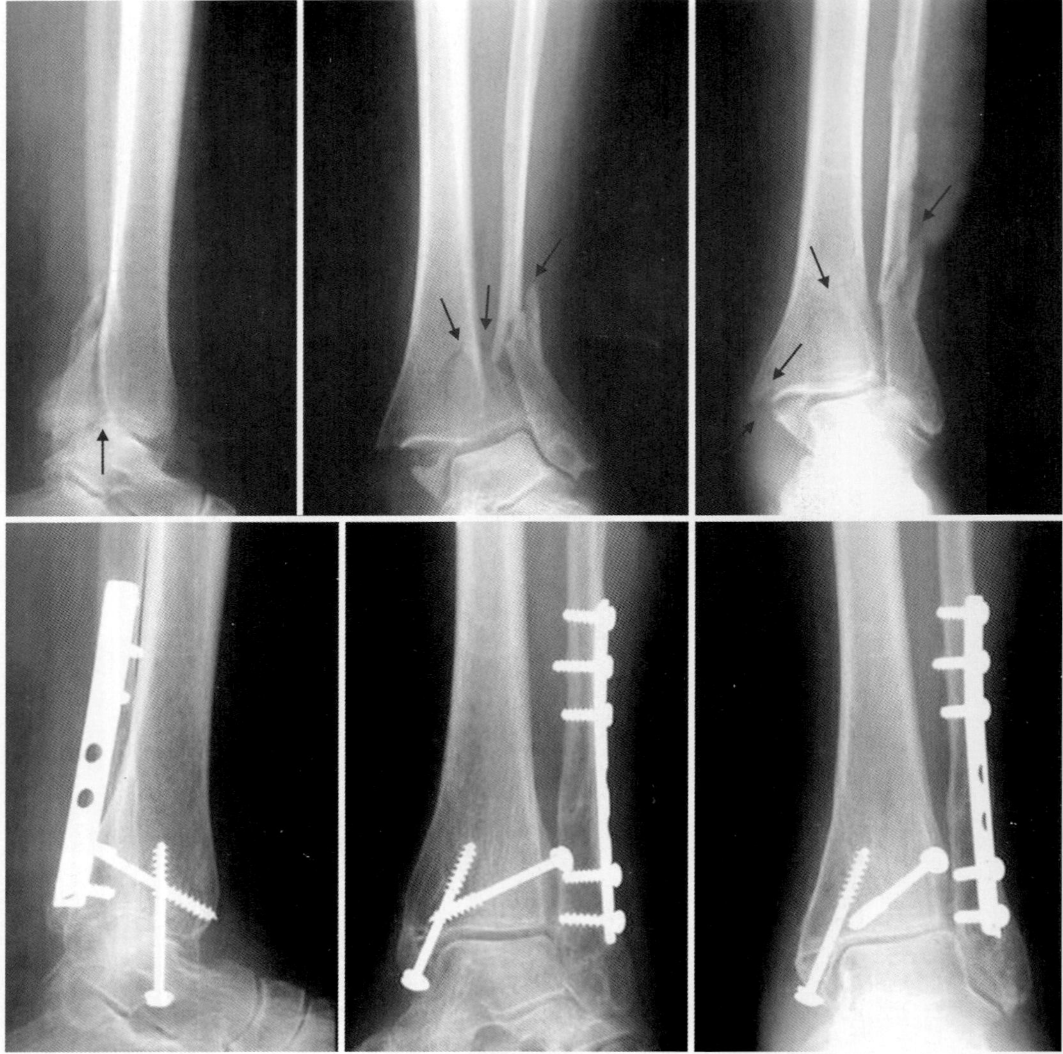

Figure 44.46 Trimalleolar fracture dislocation with postero-lateral fragment

Case 1

Closed Cannulated Screw for Medial Malleolus

An elderly person sustained a trimalleolar fracture of the left ankle. The surgeon carried out:

- Fibula plate fixation by a reconstruction plate.
- Closed percutaneous cannulated screw fixation for the medial malleolus.

At the end of two months, persistent pain in the medial malleolus, local tenderness and instability persisted and hence a second opinion was sought. The X-ray revealed that the cannulated screw was perhaps more than 50 mm and had failed to pass across the fracture line.

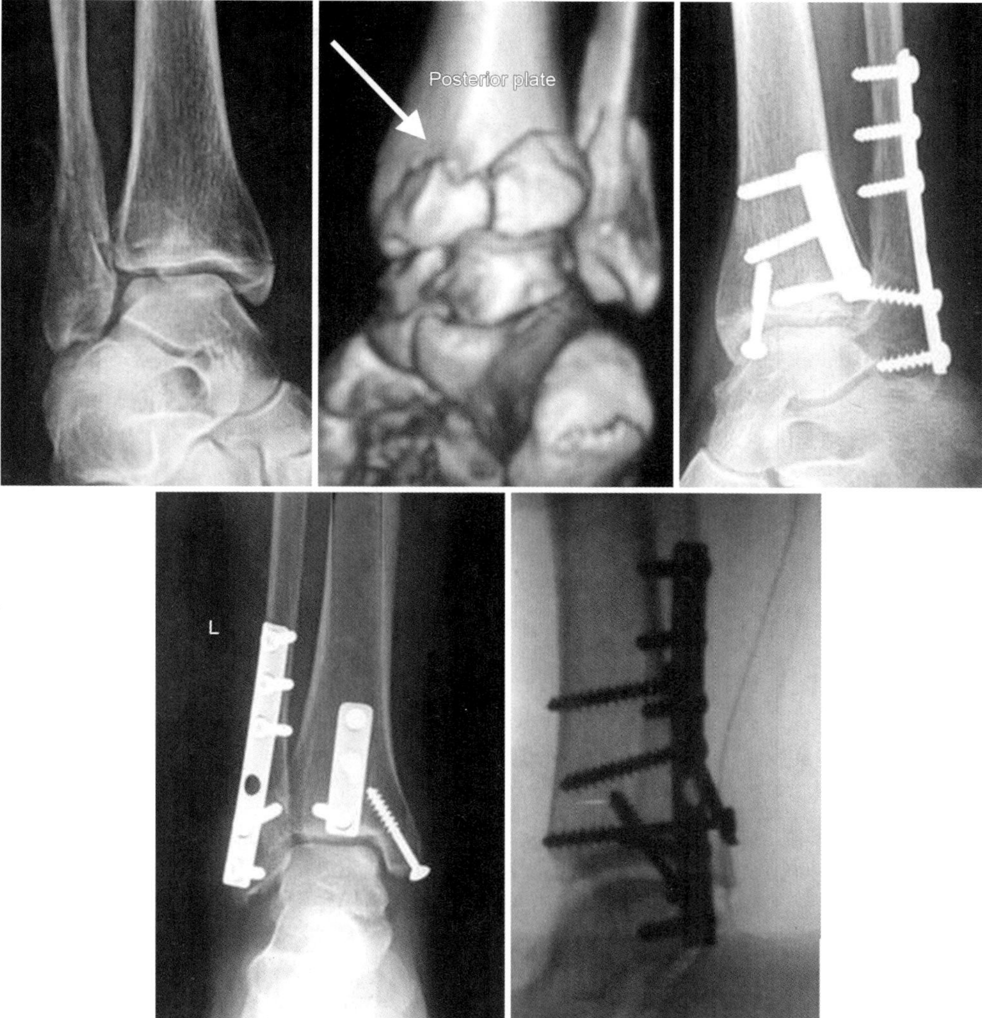

Figure 44.47 Posterior plate

The medial malleolus fixation was revised. The fracture line was mobile, covered with fibrosis. The screw was removed, fracture surfaces were made raw and cancellous graft was laid in 2 of 4 mm shaft screws stabilized the medial malleolus. The fracture union was visible at the end of 10 weeks and gradually weight bearing in a cast was permitted. Good return of motion, stability and walking capacity at the end of 14 months (Fig. 44.48).

Case 2

TBW for Medial Malleolus

The patient had an abduction external rotation injury to the left ankle. As seen in the preoperative film, the medial malleolus has a transverse fracture and the fibula shaft is fractured at a higher level. Posterior malleolus is fractured. Oblique views would indicate,

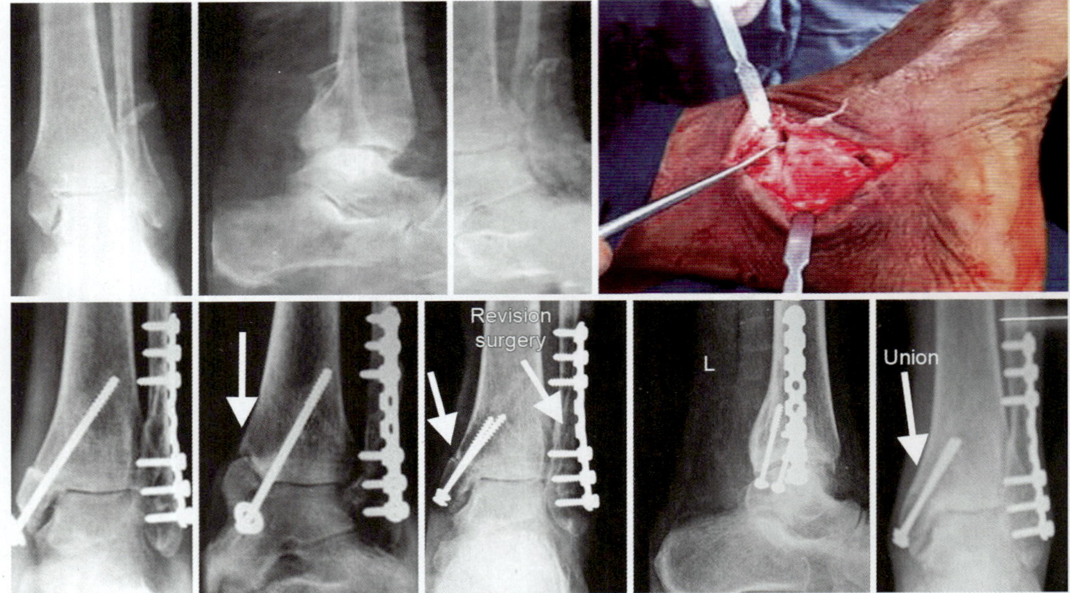

Figure 44.48 Closed medial malleolus screw

whether the posterior malleolus is centrally placed or more on either side. If it is more on the medial side, it is possible to approach it by a postero-medial approach and to fix its posterior to anterior side with a 4 mm shaft screw. Through the same approach medial malleolus can be fixed with 2 of 4 mm shaft screws over a washer. The fibula is stabilized with a plate, as is done here.

What was done prior to second opinion?

TBW fixation was done for the medial malleolus. The adjacent part of the medial malleolus fracture was crushed and the fracture was un-united at the end of seven months and a varus deformity had developed. The circlage and a K-wire have given way.

Revision

- Medial exposure taken and the broken circlage, the medial part of a broken wire and an intact K-wires were removed.
- The fracture surface was cleared off the fibrosis and the cavity was filled with cancellous grafts. A 4 mm shaft screw with a washer and a K-wire stabilized the medial malleolus.
- For additional buttress effect, a contoured 1/3 tubular plate was applied. The gentleman will have to be off the weight for eight weeks at least and then weight bearing on the cast would be permitted (Fig. 44.49).

Case 3

Adduction Fracture of Left Ankle

Fracture morphology on arrival:

- Type A fracture for lateral malleolus
- Adduction fracture for medial malleolus, with a large posterior fragment.

What was done by prior team:

- Medial malleolus fixation with a braided wire
- Anterior to posterior cannulated screws (of incorrect lengths)
- Percutaneous K-wire or lateral malleolus, (which is OK) (Fig. 44.50).

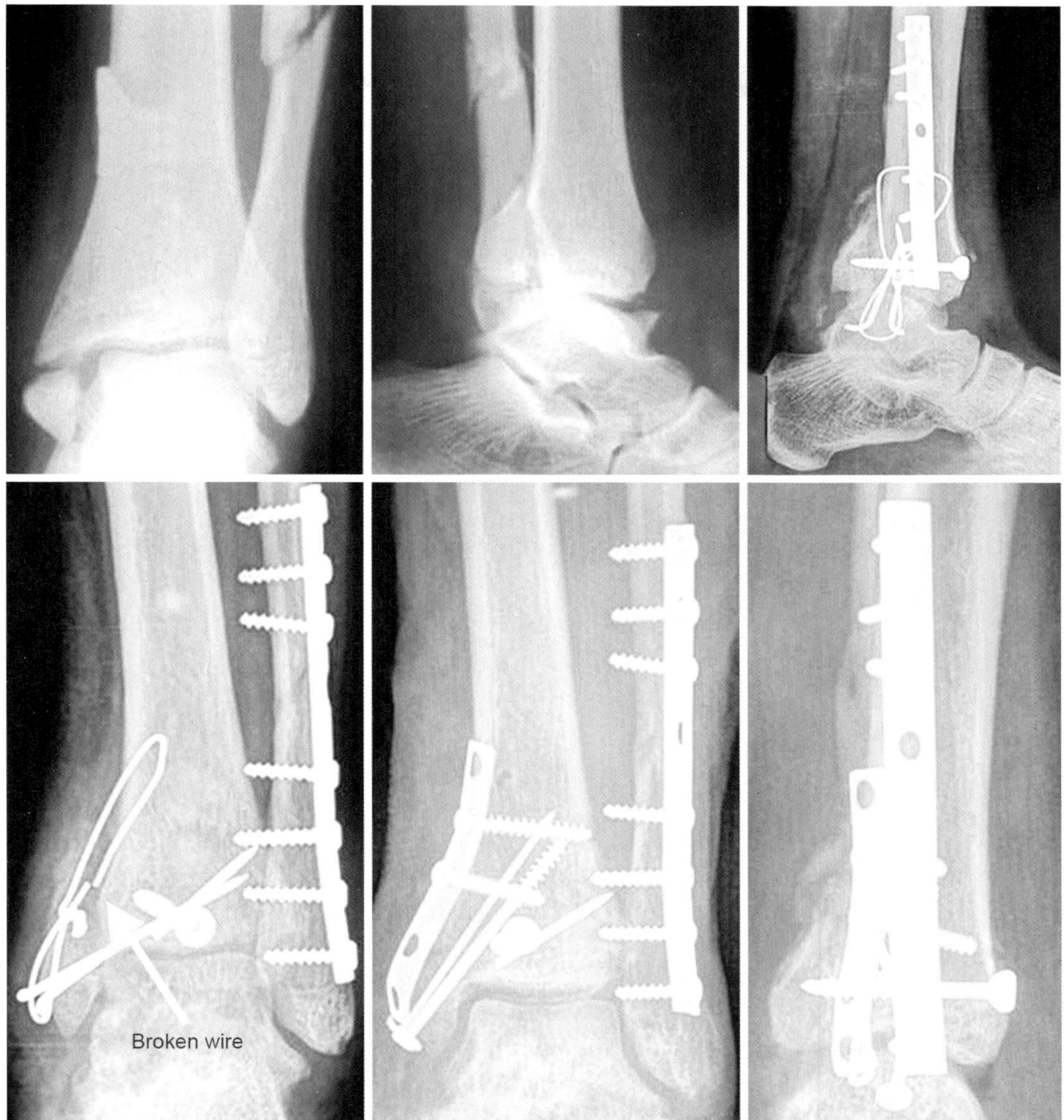

Figure 44.49 TBW broken—for medial malleolus

How I would have thought: Steps

- Generous postero-medial exposure and exposure of the posterior fragments and their provisional fixation with K-wires.
- Medial malleolus reduction and provisional K-wire fixation.
- If voids were seen, cancellous grafts, prior to above reduction.
- Posterior plate application or posterior to anterior 4 mm shaft screws.
- Medial malleolus buttress plate, held with a screw. (TBW in an adduction fracture is mechanically not acceptable).

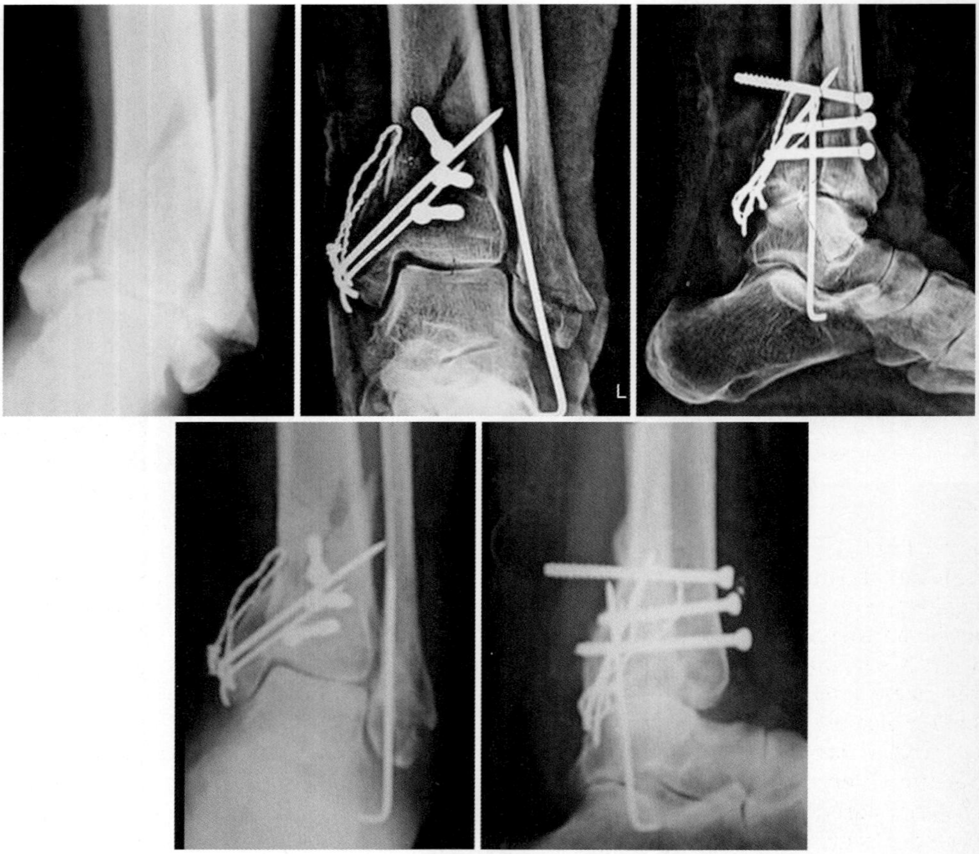

Figure 44.50 Medial buttress plate needed

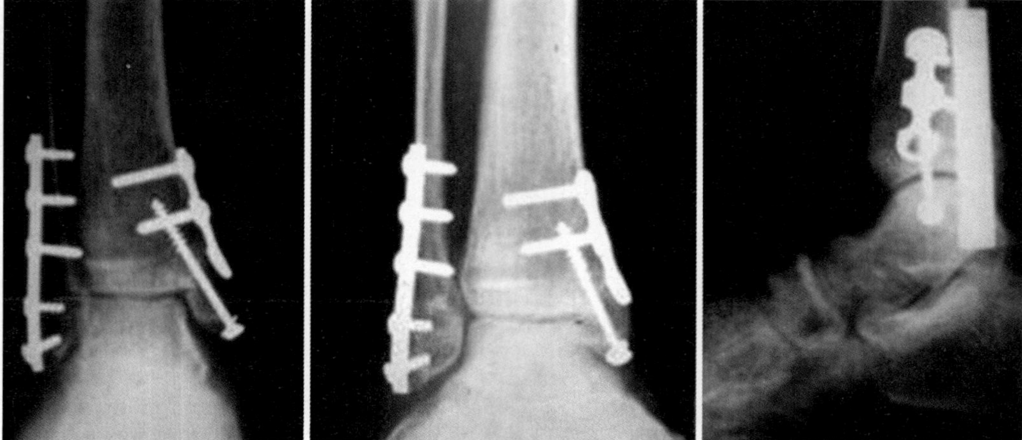

Figure 44.51 Medial buttress plate a must

- Medial malleolus screw fixation. (It is a vertical fracture and as the screw is tightened, the fragment is likely to move superiorly. The presence of the buttress plate would prevent this).
- Complete the buttress plate fixation. The last 3 steps may have to be modified as per local situation (Fig. 44.51).

ANKLE: MEDIAL AND POSTERIOR MALLEOLUS LARGE FRAGMENTS

LATERAL COLUMN SEGMENTAL FRACTURE

A Case

H/o fall from a bike: In fact the case has a trimalleolar fracture. However, the medial malleolus fracture morphology is different and hence is considered separately here.

- 3- to 4-part fracture lateral malleolus. A fairly large 3 rd fragment was - On the lateral surface of lateral malleolus.
- *Fr medial malleolus*: Adduction vertical fracture seen. Was more towards the posterior part of the plafond.
- Posterior fragment was displaced posteriorly and with good contact with the medial malleolus fragment (in CT 3D).
- A die punch fragment of approximately 10 × 12 mm was impaled. In the metaphysis to a depth of 10 mm CT with 3D reconstruction was done to define the injury.

The same day closed reduction under 'C' arm control was done. With axial traction, the impacted fragment could not be brought down and continued to be so. ORIF planned and if need be, bone grafting to be done.

Epidural and spinal anesthesia.

Supine position with a thick pillow below the lower tibia and ankle.

An external fixator was kept ready, in case needed.

A postero-medial approach, curved with convexity posterior, was taken 6 cm proximal to the joint and 5 mm posterior and distal to the tip of the medial malleolus was taken. Tibialis posterior sheath incised and tibialis posterior and flex dig longus were retracted posteriorly. Both the medial and posterior fragments well seen. Few fragments seen with soft tissue attachment. The die punch fragment on the medial plafond, adjacent to the medial malleolus was observed. The fragment had an anterior hinge and cartilage cover was present. Above its proximal limit, a 4 mm elevator was put and with rocking motion, separated from adjacent mataphysis and brought down carefully. With a narrow radius punch the fragment was moved distally and checked in 'C' arm that it was reduced well. A K-wire was inserted from the medial malleolus transversally towards lateral side, 5 mm above the plafond. The reduction was stable. A posteromedial defect was observed.

A 5-hole 1/3 tubular plate was contoured and laid on the medial malleolus. The 2nd hole from below was threaded over the K-wire. Cancellous grafts from iliac crest were taken and laid in this defect.

In the 2nd hole from the upper end, 3.5 cancellous screw was inserted. Due to antiglide pressure the plate buttressed the medial malleolus against the metaphysis and the repositioned (earlier impacted fragment) was thus stabilized.

Then through the uppermost hole 3.5 mm cancellous screw was passed. Then a 14 mm cancellous screw was inserted in the distal most hole over the medial malleolus.

Lastly, the K-wire in the second last hole from below was replaced with 2.5 mm drill and the position checked under 'C' arm (with respect to the plafond) and a 50 mm 4 mm shaft screw was inserted. The entire assembly was found to be stable.

The anterior skin flap was erased little more and the posterior malleolus was reduced with a pointed reduction forceps. The bone being soft, one should exert just necessary pressure to maintain the reduction. Then a 4 mm shaft screw with a washer was inserted from anterior to the posterior, to fix the posterior malleolus.

At this point, the lateral malleolus alignment

was good. It was thought, that if we proceed with fixation of the lateral malleolus, there may be severe edema with possibly skin necrosis. Hence tourniquet was released and wound closed: No drain kept, as no space was available.

Padded crepe + A well-moulded BK slab to prevent posterior ankle subluxation, was applied and the limb elevated.

A week later, the tissue reaction settled down and fixation of the lateral malleolus was carried out, with a lateral plate. The soft tissue attachment to the large lateral fragment was preserved well. The lateral malleolar fragments were well in place, without any defect and did not need bone grafts.

The posterior POP slab was continued, till suture removal was done after two weeks and final cast applied. Non-weight-bearing ambulation was carried on for eight weeks from the second surgery. Then progressive weight bearing was permitted. The patient was very co-operative and accepted the cast willingly for the necessary duration. (In fact, he knew importance of a walking cast and kept it on for two more weeks). The fracture consolidated well, with good function at the end of five years (Fig. 44.52).

ANKLE OPEN FRACTURE

Medial malleolus is subcutaneous bone. A bimalleolar or commonly a trimalleolar fracture dislocation often leads to an open fracture of the medial malleolus and is an inside out wound. The extent of contamination depends

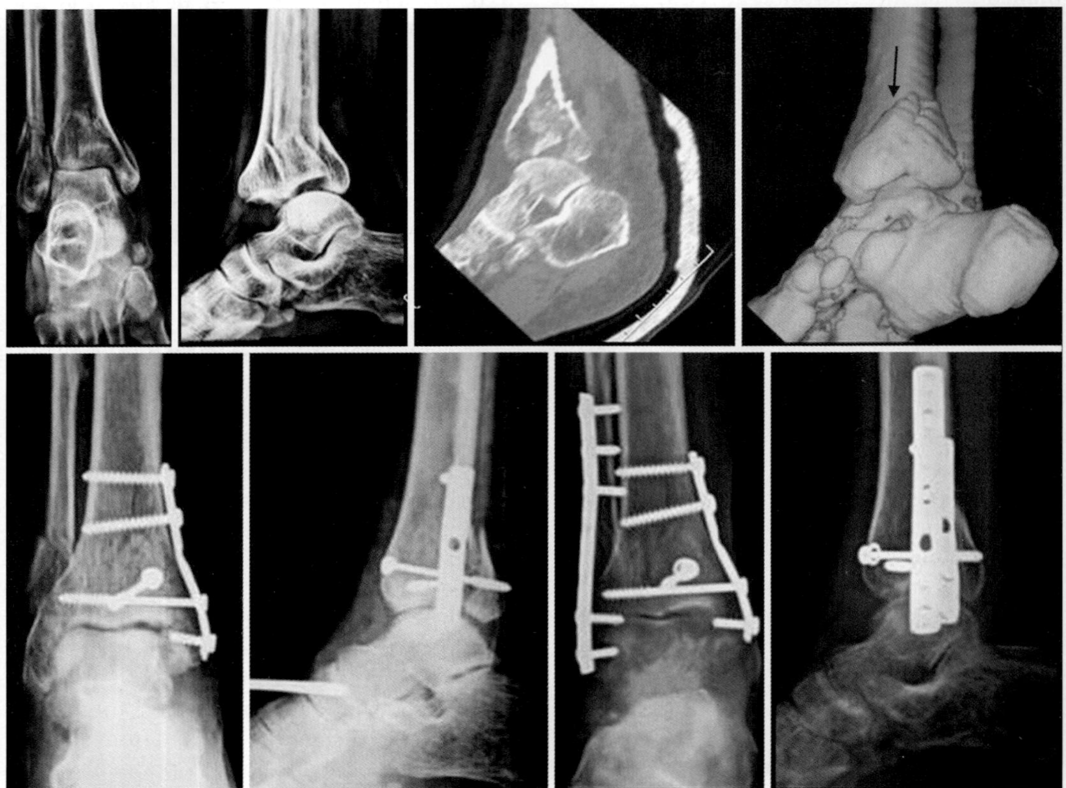

Figure 44.52 Ankle trimalleolar fracture with large fragments

upon whether patient had worn a sock/shoe and the ground, on which he had fallen.

On arrival:
Wound cover with a sterile dressing and a crepe support:

X-ray in 3 views at least.

Padded back slab application. While doing this, at times with some traction, the ankle may get reduced.

Tetanus prophylaxis/antibiotics and a CT scan be arranged.

Preanesthetic tests/ECG/lab, etc. be carried out. In a diabetic BSL control is important and shifting to parenteral insulin considered.

In an open ankle injury, decision regarding control of diabetes, wound condition, duration of injury and fracture morphology need to be considered, prior to emergency internal fixation. The points to be considered:

- The medial malleolus is an inside out injury.
- In a postero-lateral fracture dislocation, there is an associated fracture of lateral and the posterior malleolus.
- After reduction of the dislocation, it is only when the lateral column is stabilized that the posterior malleolus falls back in place and the tension on the small medial malleolus is reduced.

Hence an important decision needs to be taken is that, in the presence of a medial wound, will it be safe to open the lateral malleolar fracture?

SUGGESTED STEPS

Under anesthesia, the ankle is draped and a tourniquet is used. The medial wound is examined and a thorough lavage is given. Wound edges need to be excised and explored for any foreign body. If one finds that the wound is healthy and contamination is minimum and can be taken care off, then one can proceed with fixation of the lateral malleolus.

The medial wound my be sealed with a sterile drape and the entire limb is redraped in a lateral position. The ankle is reduced and examined under a 'C' arm. If the posterior malleolus falls back, well and good, if not, it needs to be fixed, prior to fibula plate application. The fibula is fixed with a posterior plate. Tourniquet is released and wound closed loosely, may be over a drain. It is a safe practice to take deep sutures superficial to the deep fascia and leave them untied, so that any collection may have access to drain it away. After a few days, when the wound permits, the sutures can be tied and wound edges brought closer.

Then the patient is made supine and medial malleolus fixation is carried out. A swab is taken from the wound, at this stage and sent for staining and culture examination. Often, the periosteal flap interposition is observed in the fracture, which needs to be carefully everted out. Again a wash may be given and appropriate internal fixation is carried out. If possible, the periosteum and the deep fascia are sutured back and wound edges opposed, without any tension. It is safe to leave part of a wound open and later obtain a cover with skin grafting.

Padded crepe support and a posterior POP slab, followed by elevation of the limb, help to keep the reactionary edema to a minimum. The wound needs to be dressed in OR after 3 to 4 days and further care taken (Figs 44.53 and 44.54).

If the patient reports late and the local condition is not satisfactory, one has to use judgment. If a closed reduction is obtained well and the medial malleolar fragment is large, one may fix medial malleolus only. The lateral malleolus may be stabilized later on, when the limb swelling, etc. settles.

ANKLE EXTERNAL FIXATION

A diabetic individual working in a factory abroad, sustained an open injury around the ankle. He was dressed and a POP slab support was applied.

Primary internal fixation was carried out. The infection could not be controlled and hence the implants were removed and a back slab was applied. He returned to India. This was about six weeks after the open injury, that he landed in home country.

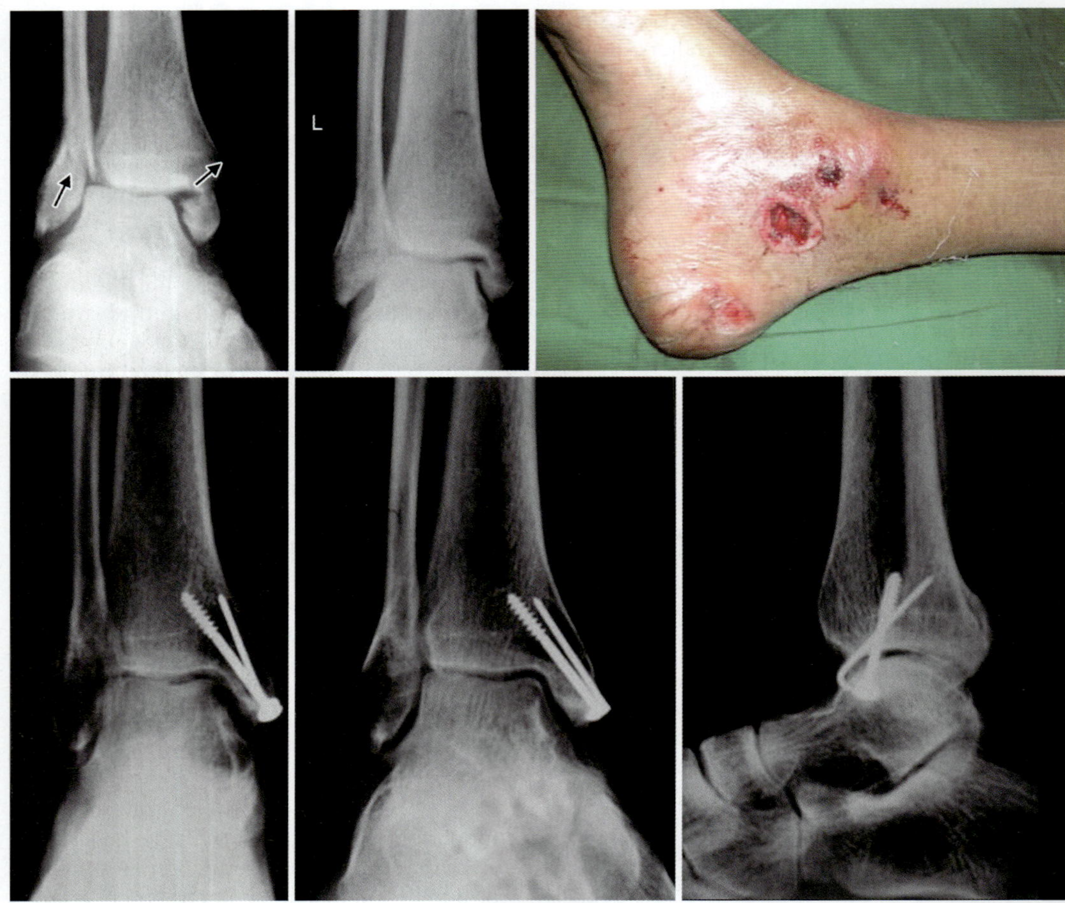

Figure 44.53 Open bimalleolar fracture-primary internal fixation

The right ankle had a few open wounds, local edema. On arrival, the wounds were examined, dressed and a tubular external fixator was applied. Strict elevation was observed. Gradually the local edema reduced and wounds started healing. Split thickness skin grafting helped good wound cover. The fixator was continued for eight weeks. The diabetes was well under control.

The fixator was removed and a back slab given. As the pin tracks healed, a complete cast was given for six weeks. The supramalleolar fracture was in place and uniting well.

At the end of six weeks of the cast, gradual weight bearing on the cast was advised. In due course of time, the cast was removed and he could walk with a crepe support (FIgs 44.55 and 44.56).

Message

In a diabetic person, primary internal fixation if required, is a good procedure. However, the wounds may be left open and closed as a secondary suturing. In case of doubt, one should do only the minimum mandatory internal fixation and apply the external fixator. An open wound is a good wound, as it drains away the discharge.

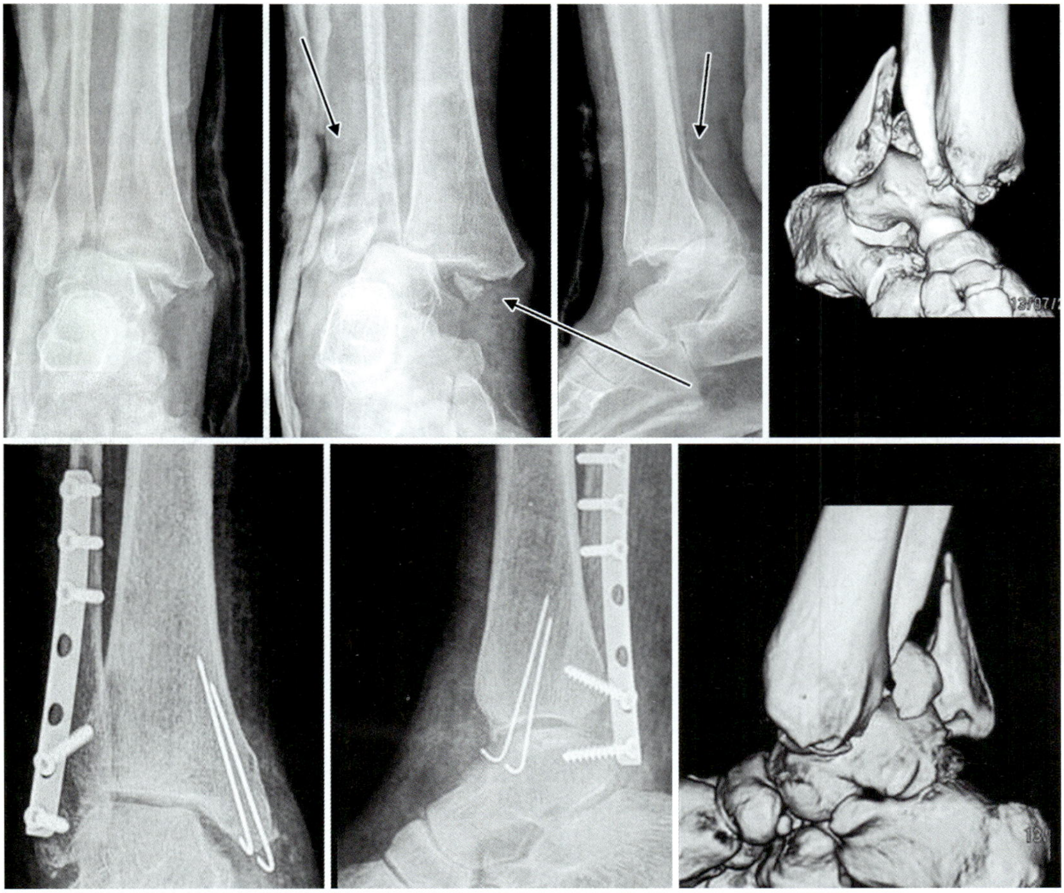

Figure 44.54 Open fracture dislocation of ankle with a small medial malleolus fragment

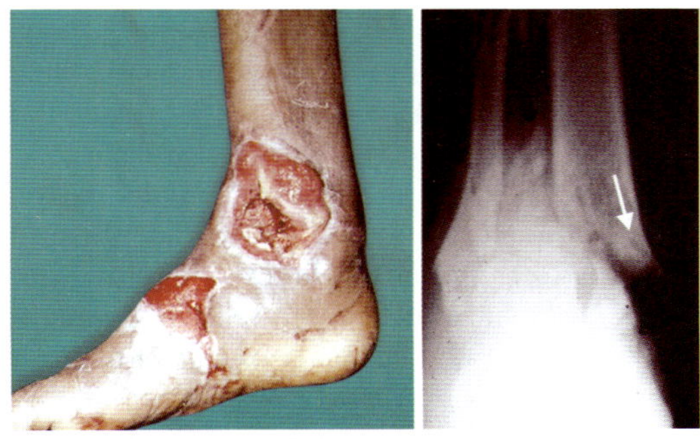

Figure 44.55 Ankle external fixation

ANKLE FRACTURES AND DIABETES

In diabetes, vasculopathy and neuropathy are often seen. Due to reduction in blood supply, often the wound and fracture healing is slow. Here, few cases are presented, which are self-explanatory.

Case 1

The patient had a fracture of the medial malleolus and internal fixation and cast

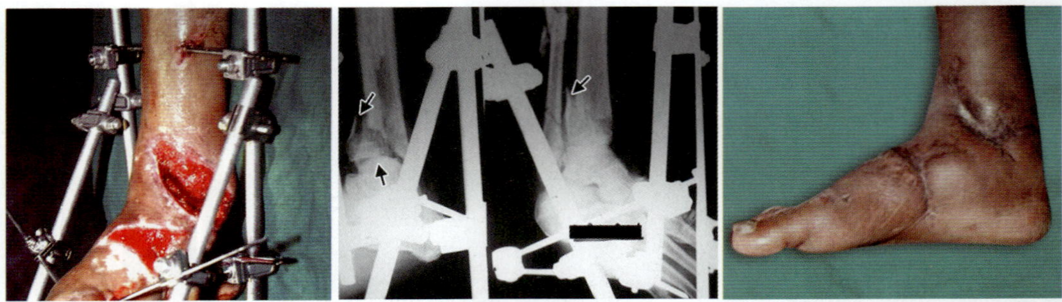

Figures 44.56 Ankle external fixation

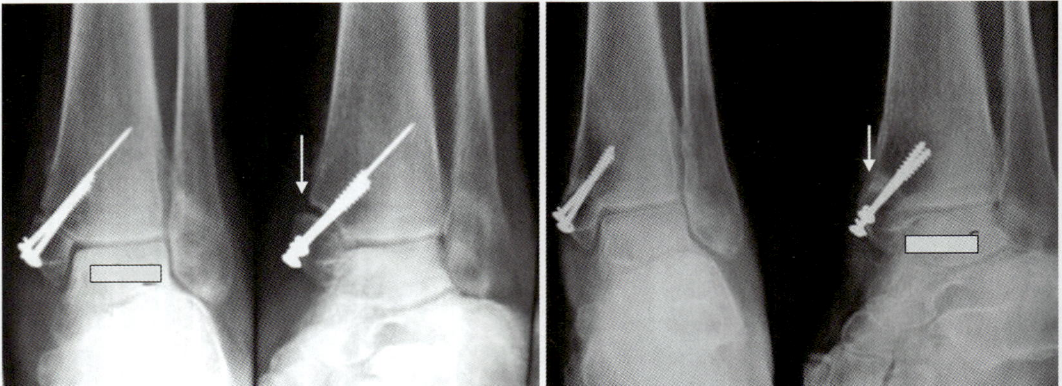

Figure 44.57 Slow fracture union in diabetes

immobilization was carried out. The fracture fragments were well opposed, without any void or a gap in the fracture area. At the end of two months, the fracture line was seen in the superior area and hence bone grafting was considered.

On exposure, one could not localize the fracture area, indicating, fibro-osseous union was taking place. However, since the radiological union had not taken place, we gently cleared the area and the fibro-osseous union was observed. Few cancellous chips were inserted in the area and cast continued. In due course, the fracture united radiologically.

Message

- The fracture union is often slow and if some void is observed during the first surgery, it is safer to insert few grafts, to achieve bone union.
- In a patient with diabetes, even if good contact opposition of medial malleolus is observed on table, the fracture line persists for a longer duration. Especially in such a case of ankle fracture with associated diabetes, after eight weeks from surgery, weight bearing on the cast is necessary. This improves the disuse bone atrophy and helps to remodel the bone well. However, one may have to delay the unaided weight bearing on the limb, compared to other patients.
- Such likely possibilities need to be explained to the patient and the family, during the treatment planning and expectations (Fig. 44.57).

Case 2

In a case of possibly a trimalleolar fracture, the surgeon had done a screw fixation for the lateral malleolus and a tension band fixation for the medial malleolus. The preoperative X-ray film was not available. One does not know, how thick flaps were raised on the medial side. Medially local infection occurred with a discharging sinus. Removal of the implants was suggested, which was done. The wound healed eventually.

Follow up:
- The edema on the foot persisted, with some restriction of motion.
- The foot appeared valgus, the opposite side being normal.

Message

- In a diabetic person, the skin flaps must be thick. If possible, as per the fracture geometry, a screw fixation is better procedure for fixation of either the medial or the lateral malleolus, because the extent of skin flaps to be raised and retracted is less.
- The lateral malleolus is preferably stabilized with a plate, which keeps the ankle mortise well aligned and prevents a valgus alignment of the ankle. A lateral malleolus plate acts as a buttress and chances of a valgus deformity are less.
- In a diabetic person, due to neurological and vascular changes, persistent foot edema is known and hence the crepe support needs to be continued for extended duration (Fig. 44.58).

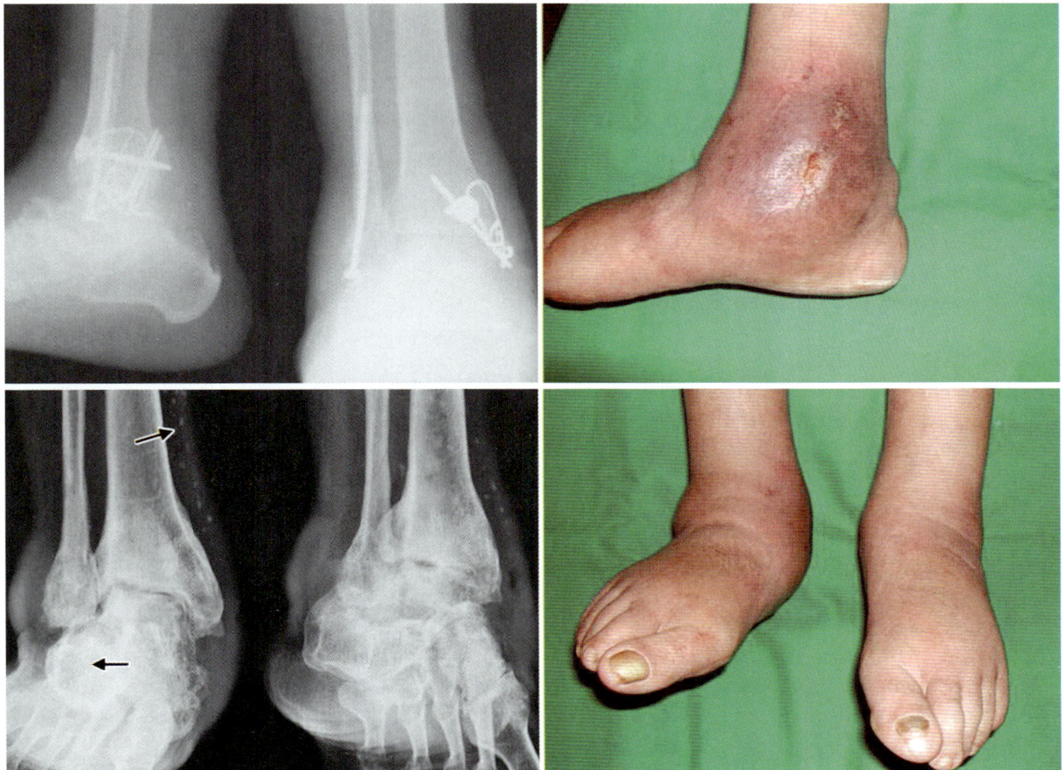

Figure 44.58 Diabetes and infection

Case 3

A patient with diabetes sustained a bimalleolar fracture, with 3-part fracture of the fibula. Plate fixation was necessary for lateral malleolus. On arrival, a padded crepe support and a posterior slab was applied and the limb elevated. Patient was shifted to parental insulin and operated in two stages:

Stage 1: The lateral malleolus was stabilized with a 1/3 tubular plate and a closed suction drain was inserted. As a safety precaution, the medial malleolus fixation was differed to a stage II procedure.

Stage 2: After about 5 to 6 days, medial malleolus was fixed with K-wires and a screw, as per the local fracture geometry. Crepe support and the back slab was continued. After five days, wounds were dressed and a cast was applied. Such a rigid immobilization helps to further reduce the reactionary swelling. An X-ray was taken through the final cast to confirm that the position was well-maintained. If the surgical wounds are dry and without edema, application of a cast, prior to sutures removal is safe. It is preferable to continue parental insulin for better control of the blood sugar, improve the tissue resistance and better healing.

This cast immobilization was continued for five weeks, from the first surgery. At this stage, the cast and the sutures were removed. Another cast was applied, with a synthetic material.

During the post-operative period, exercises for the leg, with the cast on, toe movements, etc. help to prevent disuse atrophy and maintain co-ordination.

As in any ankle fracture, at this stage, X-ray examination through the cast was done. Gradually partial weight bearing was started. Further care and follow up was as in any other ankle fracture.

Message

- It is necessary to shift the patient on parental insulin, may be even a small dose, for better and assured control. Additional oral anti-diabetic drugs may be added, as per the physician.
- Two-stage procedure maintains better tissue perfusion and reduces risks of wound dehiscence/infection, etc. A good end result is important, which a two-stage procedure offers (Fig. 44.59).

Case 4

This elderly lady with diabetes had sustained a Tillaux Chaput fracture with lateral subluxation and was treated elsewhere. May be she had a fracture of the fibula at the upper end (not visible in the X-ray film). Few weeks later on, I was consulted and only X-ray films were brought.

The treatment given till then, as per the reports and X-ray films:

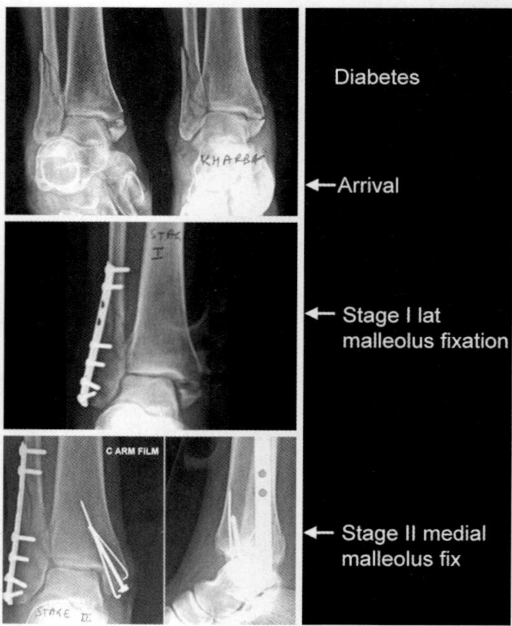

Figure 44.59 Diabetes and 2-stage surgery

Had a Tillaux Chaput fracture with diastasis and perhaps deltoid ligament injury. As seen on the film, deltoid ligament was repaired, using bone anchor and a percutaneous cannulated 4 mm screw was inserted through the lateral malleolus, the Chaput fragment and the tibia. Possibly, wound infection occurred and hence the screw was removed and the ankle stabilized with an external fixator. The fixator was later removed and the X-ray showed changes of continued infection in the ankle. The bones were seen to be resorbed, may be due to the infection and/or neuropathy.

Later on the patient deteriorated and hence was shifted elsewhere and at this stage (when perhaps an amputation was suggested) the films were brought to me. The patient was reported to be very ill and the further course is not known.

Looking back, I wonder if on day 1, a closed reduction, padded crepe and a posterior slab, till the blood sugar was controlled, would have helped. At a later date, may be when the diabetes had stabilized, surgical intervention may have been a good option. This is a conjecture (Fig. 44.60).

Message

- As in every bone and joint injury, blood sugar must be checked.
- If the patient is a known diabetic and on oral for diabetes, should be shifted to parental crystalline insulin.
- On arrival, if there is displacement, immediate closed reduction, padded crepe + a posterior slab must be applied. This may need anesthesia. Un-interrupted elevation of the limb is necessary to keep the tissue edema to a minimum and improve the tissue resistance.
- The blood sugar must be energetically brought under control and then only internal fixation considered.

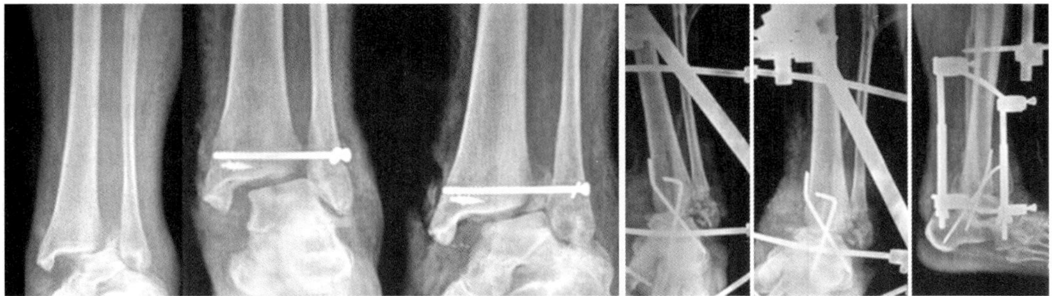

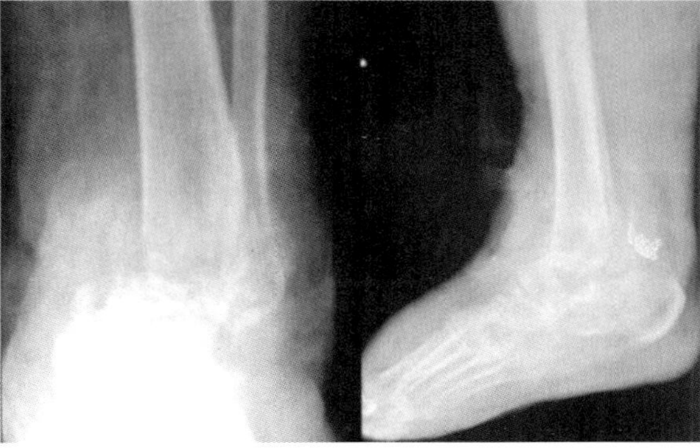

Figure 44.60 Severe diabetes and neuropathy

- Even in presence of palpable pedal pulses, tissue micro-circulation is often compromised and bone and soft tissue healing is slow.
- When both medial and lateral malleoli need fixation, it is worthwhile to do the procedure in two stages.
- The problems, one is likely to come across must be discussed with the patient and relatives, prior to any procedure, including the day 1 closed reduction. In the presence of diabetes after any injury/surgery in and around the ankle, there exists a likelihood of amputation of the limb, as an end result. Unfortunately, in some cases, loss of life is known to occur, in spite of every care taken by the team.

ANKLE FRACTURE IN TREATED CASE OF CLUBFOOT

This a boy, who had a club foot, was treated by the strapping method in the past, with a good outcome. He had sustained an accident and a bimalleolar fracture.

The size and the shape of the medial malleolus is different from the normal ankle. The medial malleolus appears short and shallow. It was stabilized by the usual method, with a good outcome (Fig. 44.61).

ANKLE REFRACTURE

It is an observation that once a diaphyseal fracture treated by a non-operative method has well united, another injury may cause a fracture adjacent to it and not exactly at the same site.

Case 1

Refracture Near Old Adduction Fracture of Medial Malleolus

This elderly lady had sustained a fracture around medial malleolus a few years ago and was treated non-operatively, with a good union. The X-ray films/reports related to that episode were not available.

She had an ankle injury on the same side and inability to bear any weight.

X-ray revealed:

- Old united adduction type fracture of the left medial malleolus.
- A displaced fracture below the united fracture area, of the medial malleolus.
- Fresh fracture of the lateral malleolus, below a united fracture.

Both the fractures were internal fixed, with a good end result. The appearance of AP view indicated a varus deformity in the ankle, which had occurred after the first adduction fracture. Unlike a diaphyseal injury, correction of a deformity, at this level is technically not

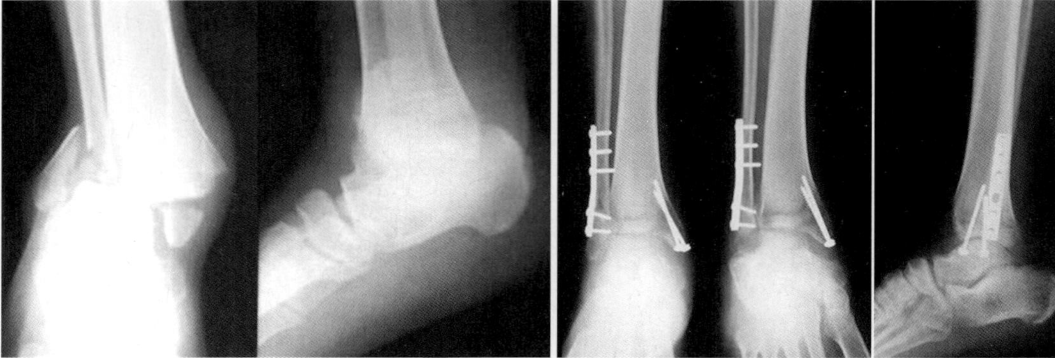

Figure 44.61 Ankle fracture in a treated club foot

possible while stabilizing these injuries. She had returned to her preinjury status.

Message

Any fracture should be so treated that anatomical alignment must be restored back to normal, or else there is a possibility of another injury (Fig. 44.62).

Case 2

Refracture after Internal Fixation

An elderly gentleman of Indian origin had a bimalleolar fracture in another continent and both the malleoli were internally fixed with screws. He was on a holiday and naturally the films were not brought. He had another injury on the same ankle and sustained fracture of both malleoli again. All the screws were bent. (Earlier films would have indicated the status of fracture union).

All the screws were removed and revision plate for fibula and screw fixation for medial malleolus was done (Fig. 44.63).

CHILDRESS PROCEDURE

In a senior citizen, more than 80 years or so, with local foot circulation problems, poor

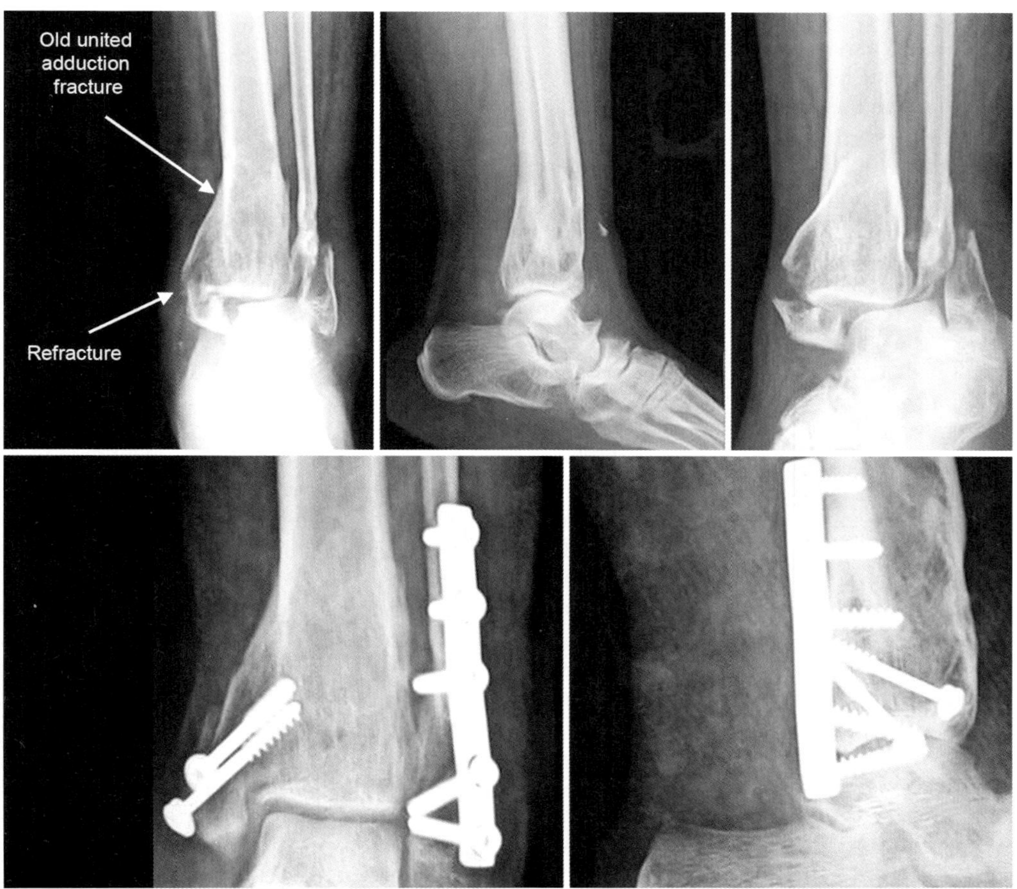

Figure 44.62 Refracture ankle I

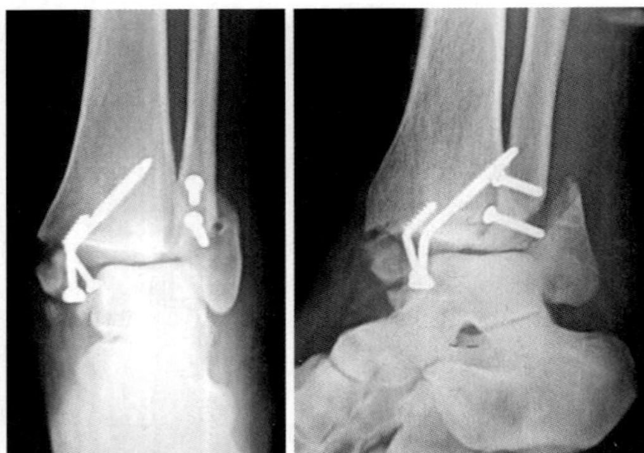

Figure 44.63 Refracture ankle II

skin condition and some associated medical problems, this technique can be used in exceptional situation.

This is a rather semi-invasive method to stabilize the ankle, in a situation, where ankle stabilization is required. Thirty years ago, closed reduction under anesthesia was done and while it was held, axial vertical insertion of a Steinmann pin was done from the plantar surface of calcaneus, across the talus into the tibial medullary cavity. A 4 mm Steinmann pin was used and after insertion, it was necessary to bend it at the plantar aspect, to prevent its axial migration. External immobilization was given with a plaster cast for eight weeks. The 4 mm Steinmann pin can is adequately rigid enough to maintain the stability and also can be bent, compared to a 4.5 mm Steinmann pin.

Initially check X-ray examination was carried out every week and later every 2 weeks or so. At the end of eight weeks, the pin was removed and stability assessed. Then a walking cast was given for 3 to 4 weeks. In this case the fracture united with a fibro-osseous union and the ankle continued to be stable, with good function. He reported after seven years for some other problem and a follow up X-ray is presented. As seen in the X-ray, may be both medial and lateral malleoli may have a fibro-osseous union, but the patient at that age was able to carry out activities of daily living (Fig. 44.64).

ANKLE INJURIES IN CHILDREN

Case 1

Salter Harris Type III Injury

F/6 Fall from a stair: ®ankle injury

1. Lateral malleolus had fracture epiphyseal separation with slight medial displacement. Salter Harris Type I injury
2. *Medial malleolus:* Transepiphyseal injury of epiphyseal plate at medial/3 level. The fragment had tilted medially upwards and Salter Harris Type III injury

   Lateral view: No injury visible.

   Padded crepe + BK slab + elevation given as first aid.

   Operated the next day.

In a child the tip of medial malleolus appears to be small, as its large portion is still cartilaginous.

Hence it is necessary to take an AP X-ray film of the opposite ankle, to know the size and shape of the bone

The Procedure

Under anesthesia, closed reduction was done. The fibular injury was well reduced. However, to achieve an accurate reposition of the tibial epiphysis, open reduction done.

The periosteum in children is always thick and needs to be incised. The incision has to be extended, so the posterior part of the malleolus is also examined for good reduction.

The antero-medial portion was slightly crushed at the time of injury and had a small defect locally. Medial to lateral a 1.2 mm K-wire inserted across the epiphysis. Checked under 'C' arm. Then another K-wire of 1.6 mm diameter was inserted, so that it was also contained in the epiphyseal plate only. Examination in 'C' arm showed good position of the bone fragments and the implant position.

The periosteum was carefully opposed and wound closed. Posterior POP slab was continued. After suture removal, it was changed to a cast. One needs to keep the child off the weight, for total of at least eight weeks. The

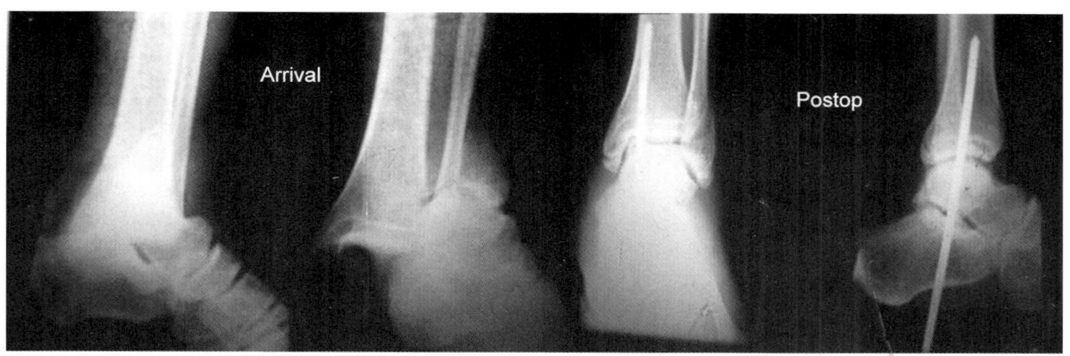

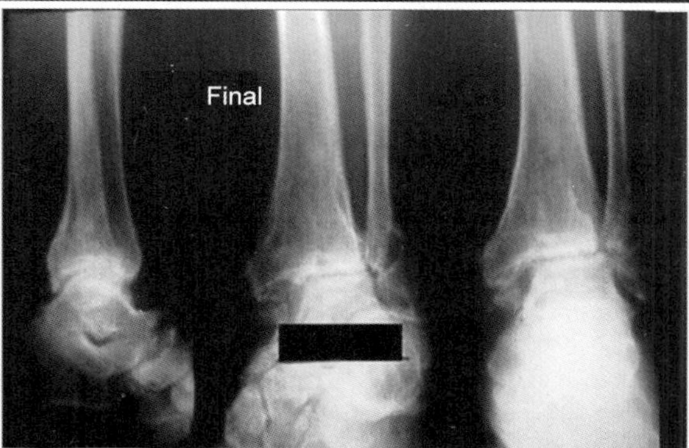

Figure 44.64 Childress procedure

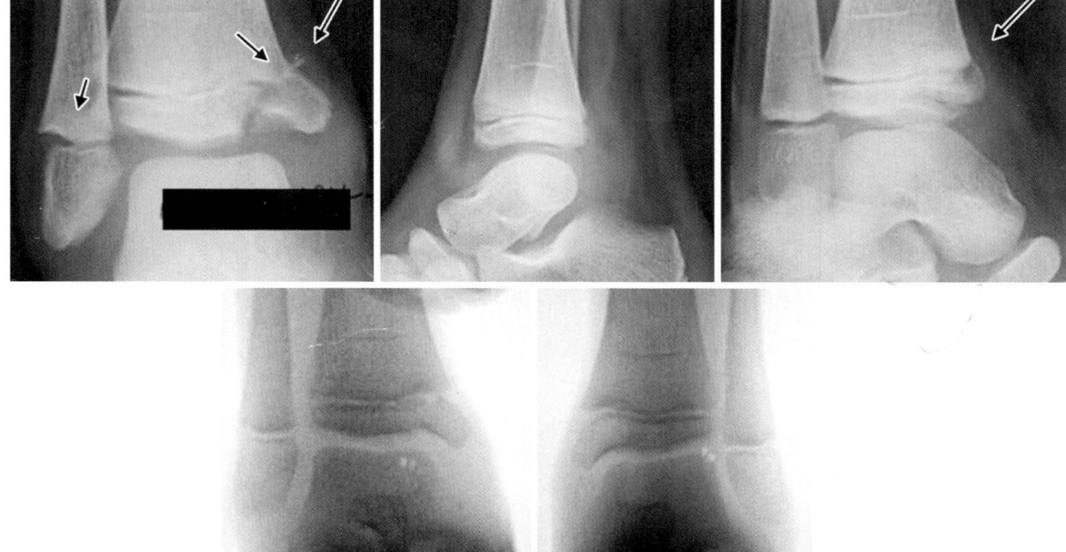

Figure 44.65 Type III injury

injury is in an epiphysis and hence one needs to keep the child non-weight bearing, little longer than a diaphyseal injury. In due course, the K-wires were removed. Follow up at the end of two years showed no growth disturbance (Figs 44.65 and 44.66).

Case 2

Salter Harris Type II Injury

This child had sustained injury to the lower tibial end, with a triangular metaphyseal beak on the lateral side. Closed reduction under anesthesia achieved a good reduction and in due course, the fracture united well (Fig. 44.67).

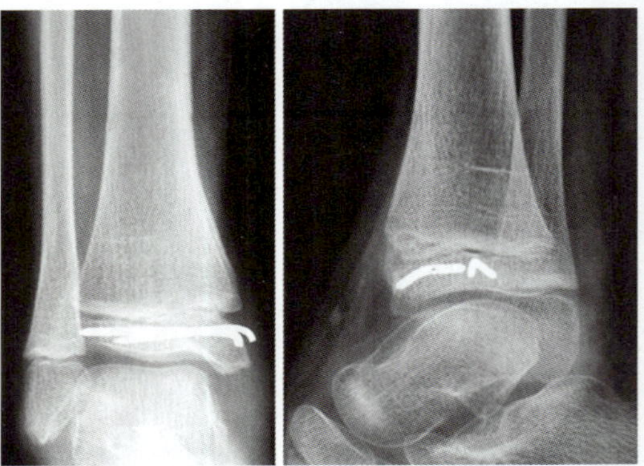

Figure 44.66 Type III injury

TILLAUX INJURY

This child had sustained a fracture of the Tillaux tubercle on the lateral part of the epiphysis. The fragment was large on exposure, which was fixed with a 4 mm shaft screw and a K-wire. Good end result (Fig. 44.68).

ANKLE FUSION AFTER BIMALLEOLAR FRACTURE

Osteoarthrosis is known to occur after an ankle fracture, in untreated cases, treated non-operatively or even after ORIF. The cartilage damage at the time of injury, alignment of the mortise achieved at the end of treatment, govern the long-term outcome.

One needs to explain possibility of some shortening of the limb and loss of ankle movement. The loss of motion is well compensated by the mid-foot motion. However, the pain free and stable ankle makes the patient comfortable.

Prior to advising this procedure, assessment of the limb is important:

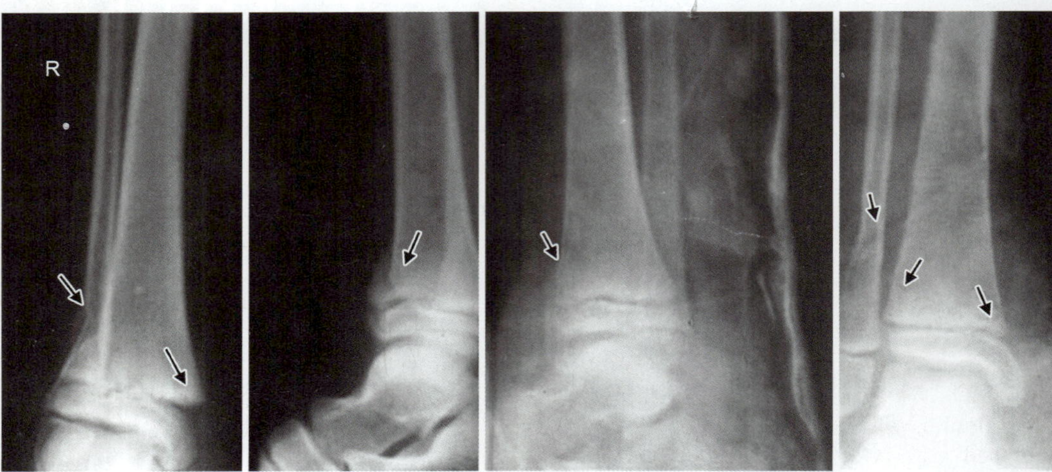

Figure 44.67 Type II injury

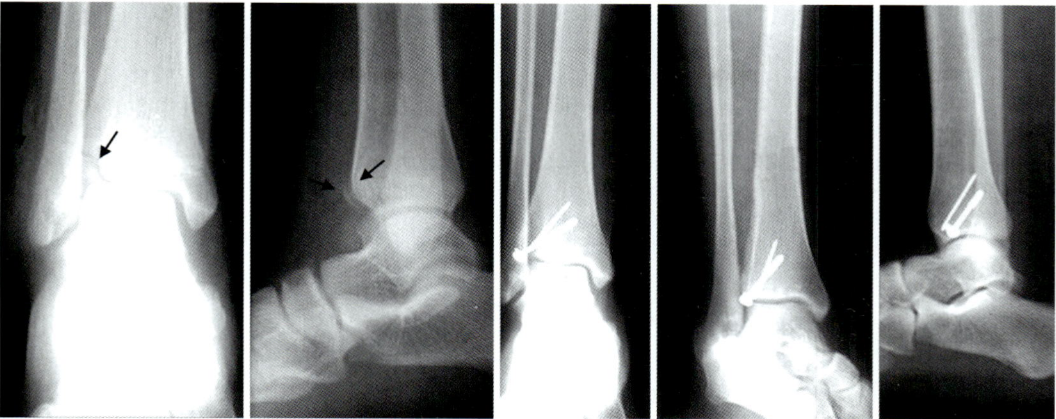

Figure 44.68 Tillaux injury

- Tissue perfusion and palpable pedal pulses
- In presence of diabetes, good glycemic control
- Skin condition and absence of web space infection.
- Absence of neuromuscular disorder.

It is observed in management of an ankle fracture, especially in a diabetic patient, may eventually lead to loss of limb or even life. Hence, adequate time must be devoted in preparation of the skin condition and control of diabetes.

Pneumatic tourniquet is necessary. A pillow below the ankle and the leg.

Surgeon stands on the medial side of the leg, first.

Medial Incision

The upper limit of the incision is preferably so made that the proximal Steinmann pin should be in a different stab incision and not through the same incision.

Any implant, if present in the medial malleolus, is removed. Tibiotalar fibrosis is expected in a case of OA ankle. Insertion of bone levers anterior and posterior to the tibia gives good exposure all around. Tibial plafond is erased anteriorly and posteriorly well, to expose the distal tibial end.

Lateral Exposure

Usually one observes fibrosis all around. Fibular plate or a TBW if any, is removed. Fibular osteotomy done about 5 cm from its tip and levered down, to expose the ankle joint. A lion bone holding forceps is a good instrument to hold the fibula.

With bone levers inserted from the lateral side, anterior and posterior to the tibia, give a good exposure of the plafond all around.

BONE CUTS

Lateral to medial, a transverse 1.8 mm K-wire is drilled approximately 2 cm above the plafond. Distal to it, a saw cut taken to excise the lower end of tibia, protecting the medial structures. This is done at subchondral level, with a power saw, using a blade no: 150. The cut is made till 2/3 of the plafond. Medially the cut completed with an osteotome. If the bone is hard, one may have to use a no. 102 blade. Now the distal tibial fragment with the medial malleolus is removed.

A 1.8 mm K-wire is inserted medial to lateral side, in the talus, distal to the ankle joint: parallel to the expected plane of saw cut. The K-wire comes out, where the talo-fibular ligament is attached to the talus. The trocar tip of the K-wire is cut off, to prevent any injury to the surgeon's hand. The level of insertion of the K-wire be such that usually this is the area, through which a drill hole is made and finally the Steinmann pin is later inserted. Confirm the position under C arm. The talar cut may be planned, so that after final arthrodesis, 5 deg plantar flexion position is achieved in a female patient, to be able to use some heel foot ware. Talar cut is done, just distal to the articular surface, to have good subchondral bone for fusion.

Now, the tibia and talus are co-opted, *shifting the talus slightly posteriorly*. Angular and rotary alignment is checked. Maintaining the alignment, on the medial and lateral side, *vertical marks are made on talus and tibia*, with a cautery point. This is helpful, so that after Steinmann pin insertion, once the marks are matched, the arthrodesis position would be correct in all respects.

Through lower tibia, approximately 5 to 6 cm above the plafond, a 3.5 mm drill hole is made and a 4.5 mm × 9" long Steinmann pin is passed.

Through the neck of the talus a 3.2 mm drill hole is made lateral to medial side and a 4 mm Steinmann pin is passed. As per the size of the dome of talus, a 4 mm Steinmann pin is necessary. (A 4 mm pin needs to be kept ready and is the most important part of preoperative planning).

Sequentially each Steinmann pin is passed in the tibia and fibula. A Steinmann pin mounted in a T handle can be passed by rotary motion because the bone ends are usually soft. It is confirmed that both the pins are parallel to each other and a Charnley clamp is mounted on the Steinmann pins. The cautery marks made previously on the lateral side, are matched. The clamp is so placed that the butterfly nuts are towards the head end. Initially the butterfly nuts are finger tightened and the tourniquet is deflated. Presence of pedal pulses is checked. Check under a 'C' arm image.

Fibula: One is tempted to excise the medial half of the fibula, to make it raw and to fit on the tibia and talus, to serve as a bridge across the fusion area. Thus, though the thickness of fibula is reduced one finds that the skin closure is still difficult and hence one has to excise the distal fibula. The circumference of the ankle is such that this step is necessary. This permits good closure on both the medial and lateral sides.

If satisfactory stability is achieved at the fusion site, one can add a complementary posterior fiber slab. If one is not so sure, additional tubular external fixator needs to be added.

Complementary External Fixator

On the tibial shaft, a 4.5 mm Schanz's pin in inserted antero-medially and another one anterolaterally.

A 3.5 mm Schanz pin is inserted in the distal shaft of MT I and V in appropriate direction, to be parallel with the pins on the tibial shaft. The medial and the lateral pins are linked with 11 mm tubes and prestressed well. Such an additional fixation adds to the stability of the assembly and the posterior slab can be dispensed with. The two 11 mm tubes should be linked to each other, with a connecting bar for additional stability. Such an added fixator helps to keep the entire foot in neutral position with respect to the tibia.

Around the fusion site, bone chips from excised bones are laid down. From the plantar surface, two 2 mm diameter K-wires are passed, parallel to each other across the fusion area in the tibial shaft, for additional stability. The plantar ends are bent and cut off. On table X-ray for documentation is necessary.

Both medial and lateral drains are inserted and wounds closed. A padded crepe is added and if no external fixator is added a padded posterior synthetic slab is added. In absence of a fixator, good pressure bandage application is possible.

Postoperative elevation on soft pillows is a must. After the spinal anesthesia effect has worn off, a high Bohler frame is necessary. In spite of the closed suction drains, one needs to alert the relatives, likel-hood of oozing and soakage of the dressing on both the medial and the lateral side, which needs to be changed, may be on the second day.

FOLLOWUP CARE

The sutures are removed after 12 days or more. Follow up X-ray examination is done every 4 weeks. At the end of *eight to ten weeks*, one expects good union of the arthrodesis. In the OR the clamps are loosened and clinical union assessed. If it is uniting well, the pins and the clamps are removed and a below knee cast applied. Gradually weight bearing is permitted on the cast, usually for four weeks or so. At the end of this period, an X-ray examination is done through the cast. If the position is well maintained, nearly full weight bearing is permitted on the limb. This is necessary and done for further two weeks, which helps to consolidate the fusion area and to restore the reflexes of proprioception.

CAST REMOVAL

The cast is bivalved and clinical and radiological examination is done. The foot and ankle are supported by a padded crepe bandage. My own preference is to add the posterior part of the bivalved cast over the crepe. This offers a sense of security to the patient. The patient is permitted to walk, as much as possible. The back slab and the crepe are removed for bath and skin reconditioning. Prior to application of crepe and the back slab, the forefoot mobilization is done. This helps to restore the range of motion. Usually at the end of two weeks from bivalving the cast, one is able to move about well.

CASE EXAMPLES

Case 1

This elderly person had undergone internal fixation for ankle fracture and had lingering

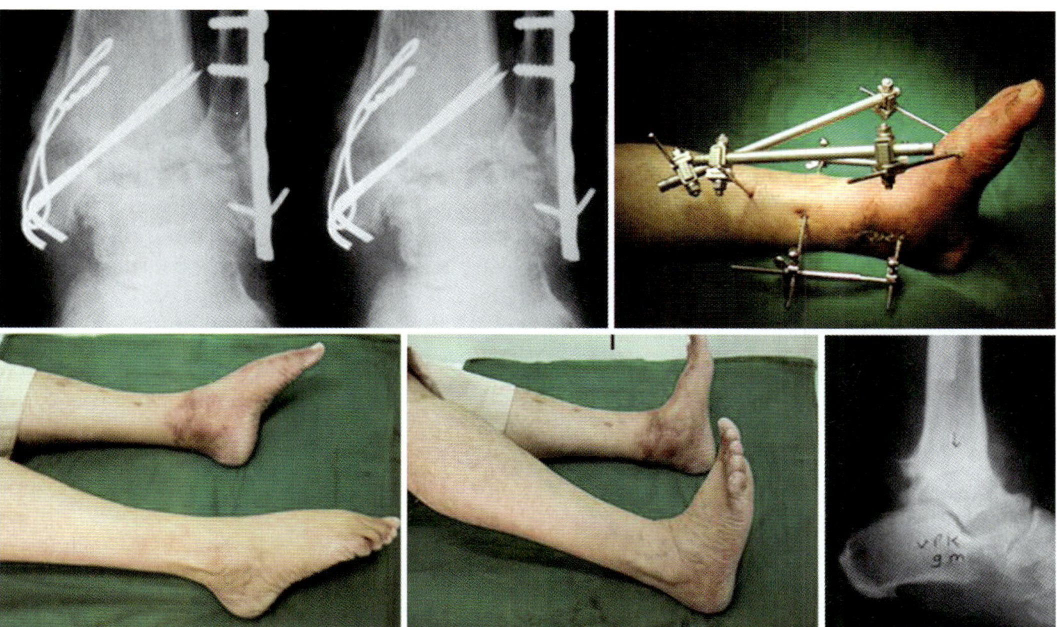

Figure 44.69 Range of motion after ankle fusion

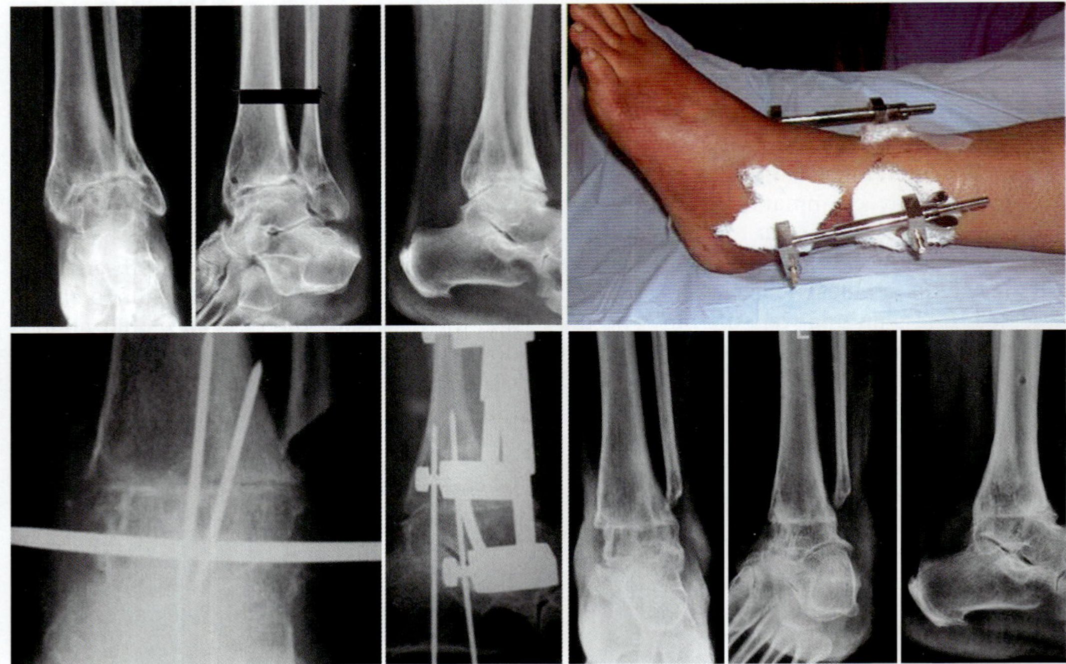

Figure 44.70 X-ray appearance after ankle fusion

infection. The ankle joint was infected and had painful movements. Ankle fusion relived the pain. Due to the infection, one expected muscle spasm and hence the foot was stabilized with external fixator with pins in the first and the fifth metatarsals (Fig. 44.69).

Case 2

This elderly lady had a bimalleolar fracture 30 years ago and was treated with internal fixation of the medial malleolus alone. The medial malleolus screw was later removed. The final alignment achieved showed some valgus. She has been walking on the ankle for many years and started getting pain in the ankle, due to changes of osteoarthrosis. X-ray taken shows valgus alignment and weight bearing, more on the lateral part of the tibio-talar articulation. Ankle fusion achieved good union and offered pain relief (Fig. 44.70).

CHAPTER

45

Foot Injuries

In office room practice, one comes across few common injuries, the common being toe and metatarsal injuries.

STRESS FRACTURE OF METATARSALS

Stress fracture of metatarsal bone is a common thing. Though it is known to occur following some unaccustomed physical activity, it is observed that such a history is not observed in all the cases. The commonly described occurrence is in the 2nd metatarsal.

These two cases reported with insidious pain and fullness in the feet, for few weeks. There was no history of unaccustomed physical exertion. Clinically, mild limp, fullness and diffuse tenderness were observed around the affected area. Having suspected a stress fracture, X-ray examination was done and these two types were observed. In one, diffuse early callus on the 4th MT, while in the other, well formed callus at the neck of the 2nd MT was observed. Since both the patients were able to walk, though slowly, only a padded crepe support was given. Use of a walker or a pair of crutches for two weeks, followed by a stick adds to the relief, because the weight is bypassed. In another month, the pain and swelling reduced remarkably (Fig. 45.1).

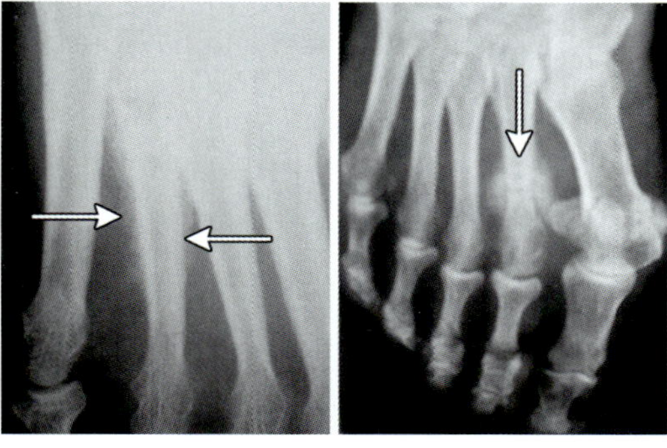

Figure 45.1 Stress fracture detected on day 1

Another elderly person reported with a dull pain of gradual onset, without unaccustomed exertion. Presented with slight limp/fullness on the forefoot and tenderness on the midfoot, near the web spaces. A stress fracture was suspected and explained to him. (If a patient is keen to have a diagnosis beyond doubt, then an MRI or a nuclear scan is useful.)

A crepe support and a posterior synthetic slab was applied and a walker advised. He was followed up every week. X-ray examination was done at interval of every week. With the support and non-weight bearing ambulation, the swelling and pain reduced remarkably and in the 3rd week, callus was palpable and visible on the X-ray film around the neck of the 3rd metatarsal. Having had a diagnosis, patient too was relieved and agreed for a cast three weeks more. Even the existing crepe and the back slab would have been adequate. However, the below knee close fitting cast offered absolute

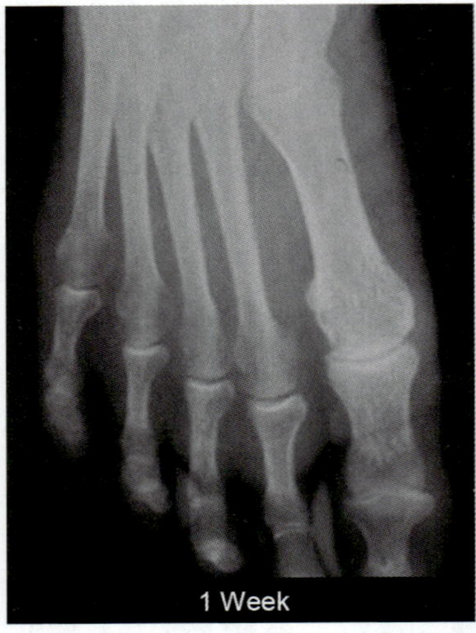

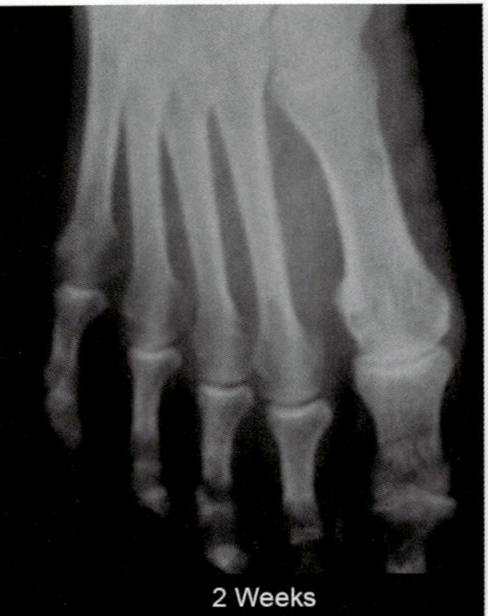

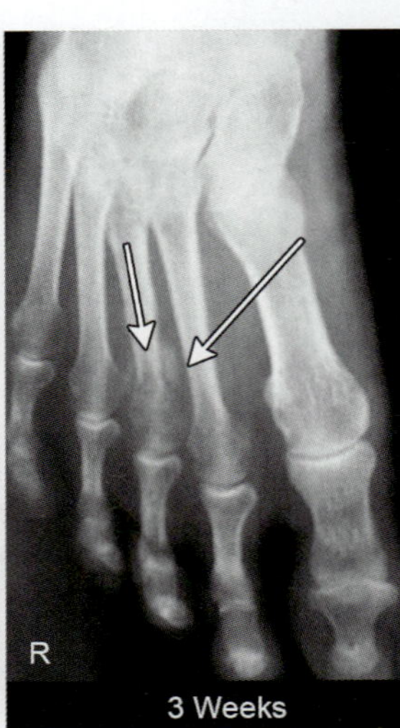

Figure 45.2 Course of stress fracture

immobilization. With a cast overshoe and a stick, he was permitted to walk as was necessary in the home. He being a retired person, willingly accepted this and soon the foot became pain free. Six weeks from day 1, the cast was removed and he could walk well with a crepe support only.

For further assured recovery, crepe support for few weeks and ankle mobilization helps to restore good function. Heel raising (tiptoe) exercises add strain to the injured area and hence is withheld (Fig. 45.2).

NOT TO DO

Twenty years ago, a patient in her thirties came for a second opinion. Clinically, she had a stress fracture, with a palpable early callus, though on X-ray examination it was not visible. I recommended crepe support and that, if the discomfort is too much, a walking cast would help her. She agreed to it. After removal of the cast, palpable callus was observed and on the X-ray film, it was visible beyond doubt.

At this point of time, I was informed the reason why she had taken second opinion. Earlier surgeon had advised her biopsy of the 'Tumor' and that there was a possibility of malignancy! Yes, the appearance of a callus and a neoplasia is said to be similar in histopathological examination, because of the immature cells and great care needs to be exercised in opining on a HPE slide as well.

FRACTURE OF DISTAL PART OF 5TH METATARSAL

A young man had a fall from a bike. He had swelling and abrasions on the lateral border of the foot and difficulty in weight bearing. X-ray examination showed a 3-part oblique fracture in the distal part of the 5th metatarsal. As a first aid, a padded crepe support was given.

The displacement of the fragments was side to side. If the foot is immobilized in a plaster cast, the fracture is expected to unite, though slowly. To reduce the pain and have assured alignment and reduction, percutaneous closed K-wire fixation was done. This restored the length of the metatarsal and fragment contact opposition as well (Fig. 45.3).

Foot Soft Tissue Loss and Fracture of MT

A person had a crush injury on the right foot, with skin loss on part of the dorsum on the dorso-medial part. The wound excision was done. The 1st metatarsal bone had a 3-part

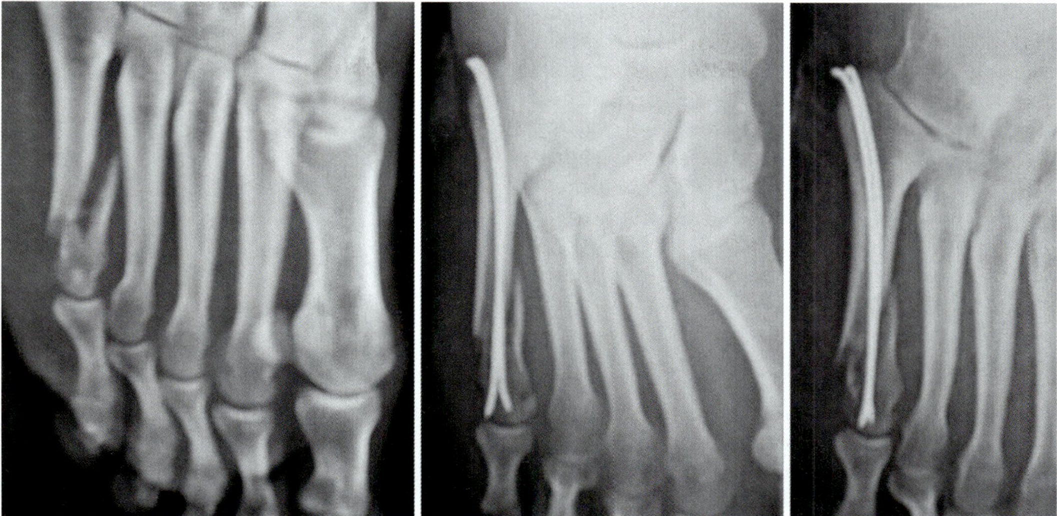

Figure 45.3 Metatarsal shaft K-wire

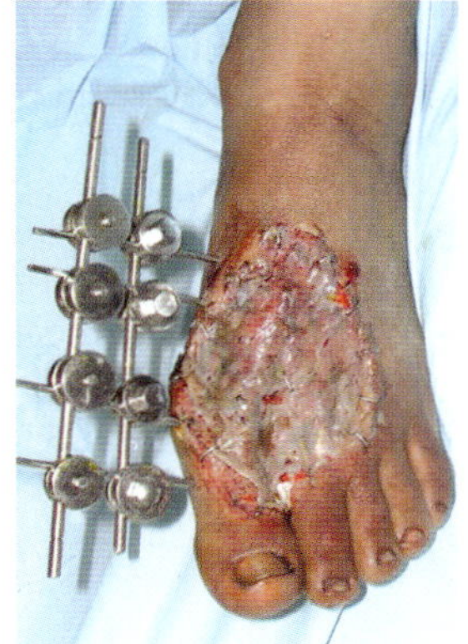

Figure 45.4 Open fracture with skin loss

fracture. It was stabilized by an external fixator. This stabilization helped the bone and the soft tissue healing as well. The skeletal stability is essential for soft tissue healing. Split thickness skin grafting was done, as seen in the photograph.

Midfoot Dislocation

Tarso-metatarsal dislocation is amenable to closed reduction. However, if one can add stability to the reduced foot, redisplacement is avoided. In this injury, the dislocation was soon reduced and few percutaneous K-wires were inserted across the dislocated bones, so that stability was achieved. Such an injury

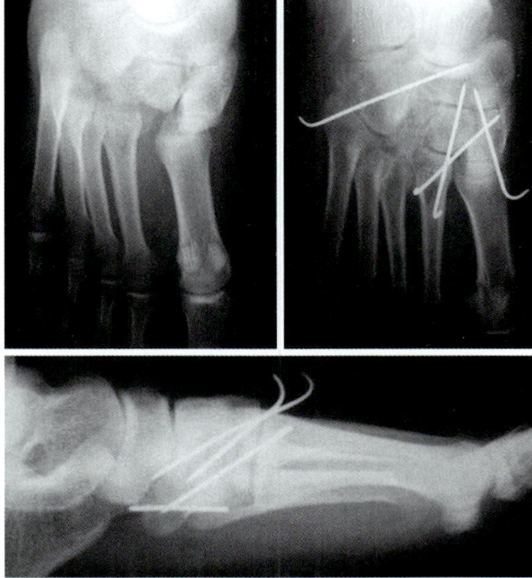

Figure 45.5 Tarso-metatarsal dislocation

needs at least eight weeks of immobilization. My preference would be do radiological examination at the end of seven weeks and confirm that position is well maintained. The cast is removed, so the K wires. The cast is reapplied and gradually progressive weight bearing is permitted. During weight bearing, there is marginal movement in these joints and any chance of breaking of the K wires is less. Still, it is preferable to remove them and then permit weight bearing (Fig. 45.5).

Wounds on Foot (and Other Areas)

This lady had a road traffic accident and the skin flap was avulsed, with a distal base. Fortunately, there was no skeletal injury. After thorough lavage and wound excision, it was studied as to where the flap lies on its own. The flap was anchored to the adjacent skin edges loosely, so there was no tension. Some areas need to be left uncovered. A skin flap thus covering a raw area, gets nourishment from the depth and most of it remains viable. After dressing with a non-adhesive dressing light padded crepe is applied, to avoid tissue edema and help the flap to get its nourishment from the deeper tissues. Pain relief and rest to the area is essential and is given by a posterior slab, keeping the ankle in neutral position.

The photograph is taken 4 days after the accident and surgery. The edges appear viable.

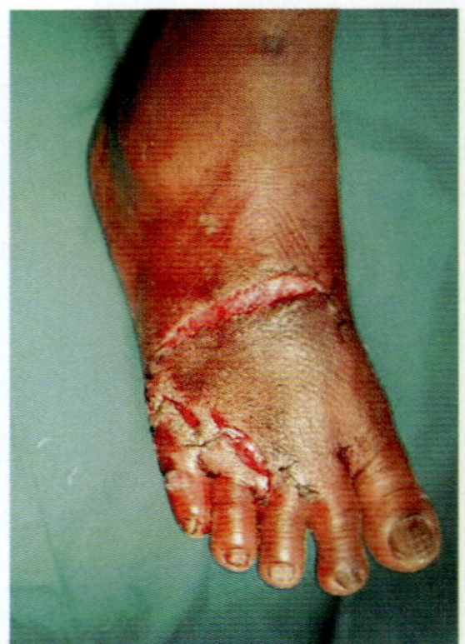

Figure 45.6 Tension free wound

If an attempt was made to oppose the skin edges, then at least few cm wide edge undergo necrosis and the defect appearing is quite wide and unhealthy. With this method of loose opposition and allowing the flap to lie, where it is, the edges are healthy, viable and healing. The edges may epithelialize or may need split thickness grafting, as per the local condition.

Message

In injuries, where such flaps arise after an accident, the suturing needs to be very careful, to preserve its nourishment. A viable flap with some healthy uncovered area is far acceptable than flap necrosis (Fig. 45.6).

CHAPTER

46

Tips for Better Care

In clinical practice, during management

- Knee injury as in MCL/ACL injury/subluxation, etc. needs immediate attention, X-ray examination, etc. Especially a subluxated knee needs immediate reduction. Huge hemarthrosis is expected. I prefer application of immediate padded crepe and an above knee POP slab. In place of the metal clips on the crepe, one should use adhesive strips must be used, so MRI can be done well and safely. Disregard to this step means entire plaster slab needs to be removed prior to the MRI, just to remove the metal clips! Besides, as is known, if the metal clips are on, who is to remove the POP slab carefully and reapply the same when the patient is about to enter the MRI room?
- *My observation*: Another alternative is CMO applies a knee brace. One observes, often as a first aid, without the use of a padded crepe, only the brace is applied, which needs to be removed prior to the MRI. The personnel in MRI may not be trained as how to support the injured knee and remove the brace and reapply it safely with minimum discomfort for the patient. During the duration of the MRI examination, the limb is without any support and is painful for the patient. Besides, there is a possibility of loss of reduction achieved.

Hence, application of a padded crepe, without a metal clip and a POP slab is very necessary, as nothing needs to be removed, when patient has to enter the MRI room.

Message

- If one attends such a case, apply a padded crepe without metal clip
- Preferably a POP slab, which offers more stable support and pain relief, rather than a knee brace. MRI can be done through it with great patient comfort.

Index

Page numbers followed by *f* refer to figure

E

F

N

O

P

T

U

V

W

X